New
Dimensions
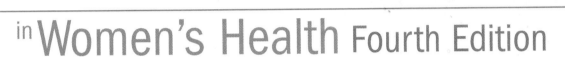
in Women's Health Fourth Edition

New
Dimensions

in Women's Health Fourth Edition

Linda Lewis Alexander, PhD, FAAN

Vice President, Women's Health
Digene Corporation

Judith H. LaRosa, PhD, RN, FAAN

Deputy Director of the Master of Public Health Program
Professor of Preventive Medicine and Community Health
SUNY Downstate Medical Center at Brooklyn

Helaine Bader, MPH

Associate Director, Women's Health
Digene Corporation

Susan Garfield, MSc, SM

Director, Women's Health and Reimbursement
Digene Corporation

Jones and Bartlett Publishers

Sudbury, Massachusetts

BOSTON   TORONTO   LONDON   SINGAPORE

World Headquarters

Jones and Bartlett Publishers
40 Tall Pine Drive
Sudbury, MA 01776
978-443-5000
info@jbpub.com
www.jbpub.com

Jones and Bartlett Publishers Canada
6339 Ormindale Way
Mississauga, Ontario L5V 1J2
CANADA

Jones and Bartlett Publishers International
Barb House, Barb Mews
London W6 7PA
UK

Jones and Bartlett's books and products are available through most bookstores and online booksellers. To contact Jones and Bartlett Publishers directly, call 800-832-0034, fax 978-443-8000, or visit our website, www.jbpub.com.

Substantial discounts on bulk quantities of Jones and Bartlett's publications are available to corporations, professional associations, and other qualified organizations. For details and specific discount information, contact the special sales department at Jones and Bartlett via the above contact information or send an email to specialsales@jbpub.com.

Production Credits
Chief Executive Officer: Clayton Jones
Chief Operating Officer: Don W. Jones, Jr.
President, Higher Education and Professional Publishing: Robert W. Holland, Jr.
V.P., Design and Production: Anne Spencer
V.P., Manufacturing and Inventory Control: Therese Connell
V.P., Sales and Marketing: William J. Kane
Acquisitions Editor: Jacqueline Mark-Geraci
Associate Editor: Patrice K. Andrews
Editorial Assistant: Amy L. Flagg
Senior Production Editor: Julie Champagne Bolduc
Production Assistant: Jennifer M. Ryan
Associate Marketing Manager: Wendy Thayer
Senior Photo Researcher and Photographer: Kimberly Potvin
Associate Photo Researcher and Photographer: Christine McKeen
Text Design: Kristin E. Ohlin
Composition: Publishers' Design and Production Services, Inc.
Cover Design: Kristin E. Ohlin
Cover Image: © Laurence Mouton/PhotoAlto/Jupiterimages
Text and Cover Printing: Courier Kendallville

Library of Congress Cataloging-in-Publication Data
New dimensions in women's health / Linda Lewis Alexander . . . [et al.]. —4th ed.
    p. ; cm.
Includes bibliographical references and index.
ISBN-13: 978-0-7637-4147-1 (alk. paper)
ISBN-10: 0-7637-4147-7
    1. Women—Health and hygiene. 2. Women—Health and hygiene—Social aspects. I. Alexander, Linda Lewis.
[DNLM: 1. Women's Health. WA 309 N5323 2006]
RA778.A438 2006
613'.04244—dc22   2006011490
6048

Printed in the United States of America
10 09 08 07 06   10 9 8 7 6 5 4 3 2 1

This book is dedicated to women everywhere – Witness our complexity and celebrate the strength in our diversity.

This book is also dedicated to a fighter and an inspiration, Julie Garfield Reich.

In memory of three very special women:

Elizabeth A. Bennett, EdD, RN
1926–1998

Diane J. Hunter
1936–1991

Lucille Dorey Lewis
1915–1993

Special Dedication

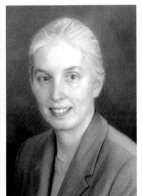

Susan F. Wood, PhD

Dr. Susan F. Wood served as Assistant Commissioner for Women's Health and Director of the Food and Drug Administration (FDA) Office of Women's Health (OWH) from November 2000 through August 2005. The mission of the OWH is to serve as a champion for women's health, both inside and outside the agency, and provide leadership and science-driven policy direction in support of the regulatory, scientific, and public health mission of the FDA.

Dr. Wood's ongoing work with women's organizations results from a commitment to promoting public health and welfare, especially for women. She understands the vital role that federal agencies play in protecting the public health and women's health, and the need for science, not politics, to drive decision-making.

Dr. Wood is currently a Research Professor at the George Washington University School of Public Health and Health Services, where her work focuses on the use of scientific knowledge in public policy. She is also Adjunct Associate Professor at American University in the Department of Government, School of Public Affairs, where she has taught Women's Health Policy at the Women and Politics Institute since 2001. Previously, Dr. Wood has worked in various federal agencies related to Women's Health, and on Capitol Hill for the Congressional Caucus for Women's Issues.

Dr. Wood received her PhD in biology from Boston University Marine Program. She has published a number of research and health policy articles and has received a number of awards in recognition of her work.

We dedicate this book to Dr. Susan F. Wood as an example to all young women of what can be achieved through hard work, scientific rigor, and a commitment to women's health.

Brief Contents

Contents

Preface

New Dimensions in Women's Health, Fourth Edition focuses on women in all their diversity: Women who are physically challenged, women of all racial and ethnic groups, women of different sexual orientations, women of all different ages. The text is intended to be neither traditional nor feminist in tone or scope, but an appreciation of the range of perspectives involved in personal decision-making across the dimensions of women's health. Each chapter includes a global focus that provides an overview of how health issues affect women around the world. This book examines the many factors that affect the health and well-being of women throughout their lifespan. Prevention, health promotion, research, clinical intervention, and public policy form the interlocking basis for considering the different diseases, disorders, and conditions that afflict women. This book is for women, recognizing their outstanding contributions as women, daughters, sisters, mothers, nurses, doctors, scientists, laborers, advocates, and much more.

Organization of the Book

The organization of *New Dimensions in Women's Health* into four areas reflects the various dimensions of women's health.

Part One, Foundations of Women's Health, introduces students to women's health issues through the history of the Women's Health Movement and the political climate around women's health. Chapter 2 is dedicated to the economics around health, including the payer system in the United States, various insurance plans, healthcare reform, and the economics around the aging population. Chapter 3 emphasizes health promotion and disease prevention through the various stages of life.

Part Two, Sexual and Reproductive Dimensions of Women's Health, addresses issues regarding sexual health and sexuality, as well as sexual violence as a public health problem. A discussion regarding various contraceptive methods, abortion, and information for appropriate decision-making is covered in Chapter 5, while the various aspects of pregnancy, childbirth, breastfeeding, and infertility are covered in Chapter 6. Chapter 7 is devoted to the clinical dimensions and treatment issues of sexually transmitted diseases, including HIV/AIDS. Reproductive health throughout the lifespan is explored, with a discussion on menopause and menopause management.

Part Three, Physical and Lifespan Dimensions of Women's Health, offers information regarding nutrition, exercise, and weight issues; cardiovascular disease and cancer; chronic diseases such as osteoporosis, arthritis, diabetes, autoimmune diseases, and Alzheimer's disease; and various perspectives and clinical dimensions of mental health.

The final section, Interpersonal and Social Dimensions of Women's Health, includes discussion of the various dimensions of substance use and abuse, perspectives on violence, abuse, and harassment, as well as current trends and issues for women in the workforce.

Chapter Features

Each chapter of the book comprehensively reviews an important dimension of a woman's general health and examines the contributing epidemiological, historical, psychosocial, cultural/ethnic, legal, political, and economic influences. Special populations of women are recognized in terms of their particular needs or the distinctive factors that influence their well-being. In addition, special features are distributed throughout each chapter, highlighting and summarizing important concepts, and promoting healthy changes:

- **It's Your Health** boxes highlight key facts such as disease symptoms, screening recommendations, and benefits of healthy behaviors.
- **Informed Decision Making** sections provide students with steps for making appropriate decisions regarding their health and well-being.
- **Self-Assessments** provide exercises for students to help them determine their risk of disease and need for modifying behaviors.
- **Quotes** from real women offer students the experiences, opinions, and thoughts from women of all ages, races, and cultures.
- The **Profiles of Remarkable Women** sections highlight women who have made noteworthy contributions to the health and well-being of women. These profiles showcase women as champions of health across all ages and lifespans. The women represented are only a sampling of the remarkable women who have had an impact on women's health.
- **Topics for Discussion** are provided at the end of each chapter to encourage students to consider varying opinions on a topic and to explore the philosophical dimensions surrounding issues of women's health.
- A list of **Web sites** at the end of each chapter enables the student to further explore topics of interest.

New to This Edition

The fourth edition of *New Dimensions in Women's Health* has been updated with the most current health information and statistics, including:

- Updated data on the leading causes of death in women of various ages
- New information on same-sex partnerships
- Updated data on various contraceptive techniques
- Expanded discussion of cesarean sections
- MyPyramid and the *2005 Dietary Guidelines for Americans*
- New information on cardiovascular disease
- New section on cervical cancer screening
- New statistics on epidemiological trends and substance use and abuse issues

- Updated trusted and authoritative resources for students and faculty on each topic

Ancillary Material

New Dimensions in Women's Health, Fourth Edition includes learning tools for students and teaching tools for instructors. The Web site for this book, **http://womenshealth.jbpub.com**, offers self-assessments and Web exercises designed to help students learn to evaluate health information found on the Web. For instructors teaching this course, an instructor's manual, PowerPoint slides, and a computerized TestBank are available on the text's Web site. These resources, along with an Image and Table Bank, are also available on an easy-to-use Instructor's ToolKit CD-ROM (ISBN-13: 978-0-7637-4439-7; ISBN-10: 0-7637-4439-5).

Acknowledgments

This work has benefited greatly from the guidance and understanding of our families and friends. A very special thanks goes to Douglas Skinner, Suzanne and Stewart Bader, Steve Noyes, Frances and Joseph Garfield, and Roslyn Berger. Deep appreciation is extended to William James Alexander, MS, for his editorial support and development of our new Instructor's Manual. Thank you to Jacqueline Mark-Geraci, Acquisitions Editor, Amy Flagg, Editorial Assistant, Julie Bolduc, Senior Production Editor, Jennifer Ryan, Production Assistant, and Wendy Thayer, Associate Marketing Manager.

Reviewers

We also thank the reviewers of this edition for their valuable suggestions:

Dr. Kitty Consolo, Ohio University, Zanesville

Professor Emeritus Maxine Davis, Eastern Washington University

Dr. Lori Dewald, EdD, ATC, CHES, University of Minnesota, Duluth

Peggy LePage, PhD, North Hennepin Community College

Julie A. Lombardi, PED, Millersville University

N. Sue Murphy, MEd, BAEd, Eastern Washington University

About the Authors

Linda Lewis Alexander, PhD, FAAN

Dr. Linda Lewis Alexander has an extensive career in public health and women's health. As Vice President, Women's Health of the Digene Corporation, Dr. Alexander oversees Digene Women's Health initiatives, health education efforts, provider training, and reimbursement and public advocacy programs. Prior to joining Digene, she served for five years as President and CEO of the American Social Health Association. In this capacity, she provided national leadership and worked in close partnership with industry and federal leaders to promote national awareness and resources for all sexually transmitted diseases.

Dr. Alexander is also a retired lieutenant colonel with the U.S. Army Nurse Corps. Her military career included assignments in community health nursing in the United States and Europe, and she was a nurse epidemiologist at the Walter Reed Army Institute of Research. As a health educator, she has held academic positions at the University of Maryland College Park and at the Uniformed Services University of Health Sciences. In her position as Vice President for Women's Health and Science with United Information Systems, she provided leadership with the Department of Defense congressionally appropriated research programs in breast cancer, osteoporosis, and ovarian cancer.

Dr. Alexander is nationally known for her leadership in women's health advocacy and has published extensively on women's health issues. Her many honors include appointments to national advisory panels on infectious diseases and women's health; she is also a fellow in the American Academy of Nursing. Dr. Alexander holds a baccalaureate degree in nursing, master's degrees in education/counseling and community health, and a doctoral degree in health education.

Judith H. LaRosa, PhD, RN, FAAN

Dr. Judith LaRosa's career has spanned education, research, and clinical practice. Her present position is Deputy Director, Master of Public Health Program and Professor of Preventive Medicine and Community Health, College of Medicine, State University of New York Medical Center. Her immediate past positions have been Professor and Chair, Department of Community Health Sciences, Tulane University School of Public Health and Tropical Medicine in New Orleans, Louisiana, and Director, Tulane Xavier National Center of Excellence in Women's Health. From 1991 to 1994, she was the first Deputy Director of the Office of Research on Women's Health, National Institutes of Health. From 1978 to 1991, Dr. LaRosa served at the National Heart, Lung, and Blood Institute (NHLBI) as the first coordinator of the NHLBI Workplace Initiative in cardiovascular disease risk factor reduction. Prior to 1978, Dr. LaRosa was a group therapist in the treatment of heroin addicts and a research assistant in studies of chemical dependency at the George Washington University School of Medicine in Washington, DC. Early in her career, she served as a staff nurse on hospital and clinical research units at the

University of Pittsburgh and the Brigham-Women's Hospital in Boston and as an instructor in psychiatric nursing at Boston University.

Dr. LaRosa has received a number of awards for her work and has been published extensively in the areas of heart disease, women's health, workplace health promotion, and disease prevention. She has appeared on CNN, *Good Morning America*, national and foreign networks, National Public Radio, and in print media such as the *New York Times*, *Los Angeles Times*, *Wall Street Journal*, *Washington Post*, and *San Francisco Examiner*. Dr. LaRosa is a member of the New York Academy of Medicine, is on the editorial board of the *Journal of Community Health*, and has served on numerous committees and advisory councils. She is a fellow in the American Academy of Nursing and the American Heart Association (AHA) and the AHA Council on Cardiovascular Nursing, a member of Sigma Theta Tau International (honorary nursing society), Delta Omega (public health honorary society), and Sigma Chi Scientific Research Society. Dr. LaRosa received her baccalaureate degree in nursing and master's degree in nursing education from the University of Pittsburgh, and her doctoral degree in health education from the University of Maryland.

Helaine Bader, MPH

Helaine Bader has focused her work in the fields of health communications and women's health. In her present position as Associate Director of Women's Health at Digene Corporation, Ms. Bader works to ensure access to cervical cancer screening through developing and implementing advocacy and educational initiatives, with the ultimate goal of eliminating cervical cancer. Ms. Bader came to Digene from GlaxoSmithKline, a leading pharmaceutical company, where she worked in cardiovascular and women's health communications and was responsible for media relations and community outreach within research and development. Ms. Bader has more than 10 years of experience in women's health research, health communications, and health education, including a breast cancer research fellowship with the National Cancer Institute. She has worked on various multimedia and web-based health campaigns in both the public and private sectors and has developed, implemented, and evaluated health education projects for various issues affecting women and children.

Ms. Bader received herbaccalaureate degree in English with a minor in premedical sciences from the University of Pennsylvania and her master's degree in public health from University of Pittsburgh.

Susan Garfield, SM, MSc

Susan Garfield is Director, Women's Health and Reimbursement at Digene Corporation. Ms. Garfield's focus is health policy, reimbursement, and health economics, as well as working with women's health and advocacy organizations to provide patient and provider cervical cancer screening education. Her professional career has focused on innovations in women's healthcare, the economics of practice change, and the role of reimbursement in the adoption of new technologies.

She was a healthcare consultant at Boston Healthcare prior to joining Digene. During her tenure there, Ms. Garfield worked with biotechnology, medical device, pharmaceutical, and diagnostic firms in getting their new technologies to market. Ms. Garfield also worked for the World Game Institute, a nonprofit educational organization, where she marketed and facilitated interactive educational programs that focused on teaching participants about diversity, globalization, gender equity, and the environment.

Ms. Garfield received her baccalaureate degree in English and women's studies from the University of Pennsylvania, a master's degree in population and development from the London School of Economics, and a master's degree in health policy and management from Harvard University School of Public Health. Ms. Garfield is currently pursuing a DrPH at Boston University School of Public Health.

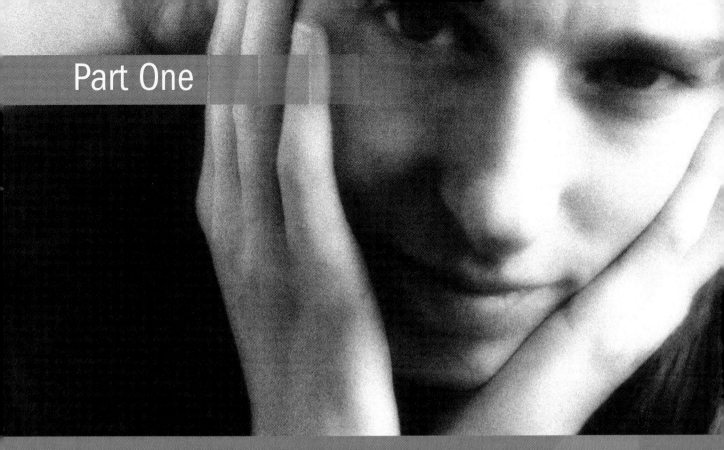

Part One

Foundations of Women's Health

Chapter One

Introduction to Women's Health

Chapter Objectives

On completion of this chapter, the student should be able to discuss:

1. The development of the women's health movement since the early nineteenth century.

2. The contributions to the women's health movement made by individuals, women's health advocacy groups, grassroots organizations, healthcare professionals, and the federal government.

3. Government's role in protecting and promoting the health of the public.

4. Health issues that come into question during a change in the presidential administration.

5. The responsibilities of the Office on Women's Health and the Office of Research on Women's Health.

6. The importance of investing in biomedical research and the inclusion of women and minorities in research studies.

7. The concept of sex/gender-based research.

8. Reproductive rights and the global gag rule.

9. Barriers encountered by women in accessing healthcare providers, services, and information.

10. The need for incorporating women's health and cultural sensitivity training into health professional curricula.

11. The efforts throughout the world supporting women's health and gender equity.

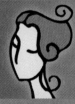

womenshealth.jbpub.com

Women's Health Online is a great source for supplementary women's health information for both students and instructors. Visit

http://womenshealth.jbpub.com to find a variety of useful tools for learning, thinking, and teaching.

Introduction

The increased focus on women's health over the past few decades has brought together a variety of groups that are attempting to improve access to and delivery of health care. Women's health advocates from community groups, government institutions, and healthcare facilities have had significant success at increasing awareness of and creating solutions to key issues that affect women's health. Women have advocated in various organizational forms for issues such as improved healthcare services, respected social status, and control over their own health decisions. Self-help groups, grassroots organizations, political advocacy groups, and healthcare professionals alike have become involved in the women's health movement. As a result, there is now greater recognition of the many factors that contribute to the quality of women's lives and their overall health status. Although significant gains have been made, important challenges remain.

This chapter gives a brief overview of the history of women's health and some of the political issues surrounding the U.S. health system. It provides a framework for understanding key issues related to how priorities are set within the women's health movement and how individuals play a key role in determining the future direction of women's health care. A look at women's health on a global scale is included as well.

Historical Dimensions: The Women's Health Movement

The women's health movement was first noted in the 1830s and 1840s (Figure 1.1). Small groups of women in towns and cities began the wave of women's health advocacy. The movement, focusing on health education and disease prevention, was specifically targeted toward women as the caretakers of families.

1830s and 1840s: The Popular Health Movement

During this time period, women were encouraged to take control of their health as domestic healers and lay practitioners, as opposed to looking to formally trained physicians for treatment.[1] Healthy lifestyles for women encouraged proper diet, exercise, the elimination of the **corset**, and sexual abstinence in marriage to control

■ During the Popular Health Movement, women were encouraged to eliminate the corset. Corsets were worn as an undergarment or outergarment to support and shape the waistline, hips, and breasts.

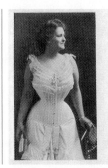
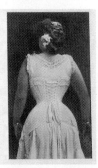

family size. For the first time, a few middle-class women who became interested in their own health sought entry into the medical profession.[1] Elizabeth Blackwell, for example, entered medical school in 1847 and prompted the opening of a series of medical schools for women, including the Female Medical College of Pennsylvania, the New England Medical College, the Homeopathic New York Medical College for Women, and Elizabeth Blackwell's own Women's Medical College of the New York Infirmary. In 1848, the first women's rights convention was held in Seneca Falls, New York; the convention marked the official beginning of the women's rights movement.

1861–1865: The Civil War Period

The Civil War prompted many women to volunteer their services as doctors and nurses to the armies; a number of women even disguised themselves as men to tend to wounded soldiers on the battlefield. Dorothea Dix and Clara Barton were the leaders of a national effort to organize a nursing corps to care for the war's wounded and sick. Dorothea Dix, Superintendent of Nurses for the Union Army, made headway by recruiting numerous women to work with her as nurses, thereby increasing the legitimacy of the role of women as professional healthcare providers. Clara Barton cared for soldiers who were returning to Washington, D.C., and later played an instrumental role in the creation of an American branch of the International Red Cross.

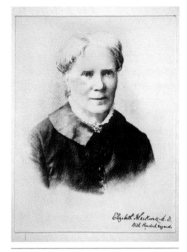

■ Elizabeth Blackwell was responsible for the opening of a series of medical schools for women in the mid-1800s.

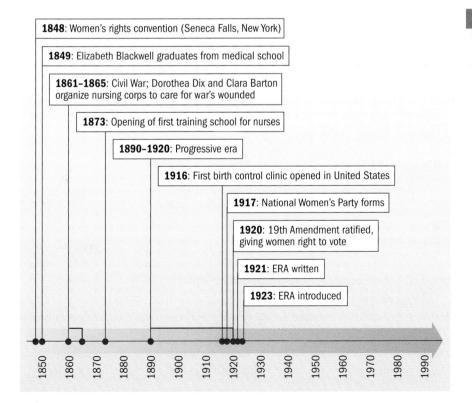

1848: Women's rights convention (Seneca Falls, New York)

1849: Elizabeth Blackwell graduates from medical school

1861–1865: Civil War; Dorothea Dix and Clara Barton organize nursing corps to care for war's wounded

1873: Opening of first training school for nurses

1890–1920: Progressive era

1916: First birth control clinic opened in United States

1917: National Women's Party forms

1920: 19th Amendment ratified, giving women right to vote

1921: ERA written

1923: ERA introduced

1850 1860 1870 1880 1890 1900 1910 1920 1930 1940 1950 1960 1970 1980 1990

Figure 1.1

Timeline of the women's health movement.

My grandmother was a physician at a time when all of her peers were men. I have always admired her but now that I am an adult woman, I have a better understanding of the challenges she must have faced at my age in her time.

24-year-old woman

Women's participation in the war also led to the opening of the first training schools for nurses in 1873, including those at Bellevue Hospital in New York City, Massachusetts General Hospital in Boston, and Connecticut Hospital in New Haven. By 1890, 35 such schools existed. Although this trend represented advancement for women, the relationship between male doctors and female nurses mirrored the domestic sexual division of labor, with males as the authority figures and females as the subordinates.

Mid- to Late 1800s: The Women's Medical Movement

After the Civil War, educational and employment opportunities abounded for women. The Women's Medical Movement was born as a consequence of the rapid growth in the number of women attending medical schools, their struggles to achieve equal status within the profession, and the popularity of challenging historical notions regarding women's fragility.

1890s–1920s: The Progressive Era

The Women's Medical Movement gave way to the intensely active Progressive Era, which advanced not only women's health, but also the roles of women and women's rights in general. In 1920, the 19th Amendment to the U.S. Constitution was ratified, which guaranteed women the right to vote. A few years later, the National Women's Party, formed in 1917, proposed the Equal Rights Amendment (see **It's Your Health**).

During this time, the birth control movement gained force and ultimately led to the legalization and medical acceptance of contraception. The maternal and child health movement also was working to promote healthy motherhood through prenatal care and child health services. Soon after the first birth control clinic in the United States was established in 1916, the Children's Bureau was established, as was the first show of governmental support in the Shepard Towner Act of 1921—legislation that greatly increased the availability of prenatal and child health care.[1]

1930s–1950s: World War II and Postwar Years

World War II opened doors for women's employment opportunities, helping women gain confidence in themselves and bringing their presence in society to the forefront. Advances in anesthetics and delivery techniques made for safer and less painful childbirth; therapies for the treatment of menopause were explored; and a majority of women gave birth in hospitals. As the war drew to a close, many women returned to homemaking from their wartime jobs.

The 1950s were a period of redefining sexuality. Although many women used birth control, the link between sexuality and procreation was constantly reinforced. *The Kinsey Report*, issued in 1953, dispelled this link for some by revealing that marriage was not a prerequisite for sex for many women. During this time, lesbians began to organize groups to change public attitudes and advocate for equal rights.

It's Your Health

Equal Rights Amendment

The Equal Rights Amendment was written in 1921 by **suffragist** Alice Paul. It has been introduced in Congress every session since 1923.

Section 1. Equality of Rights under the law shall not be denied or abridged by the United States or any state on account of sex.

Section 2. The Congress shall have the power to enforce, by appropriate legislation, the provisions of this article.

Section 3. This amendment shall take effect two years after the date of ratification.

1960s–1970s: The Grassroots Movement

During the 1960s and 1970s, grassroots organizations challenged medical authority in the delivery of health care to women and addressed issues ranging from abortion to childbirth reform to unnecessary hysterectomies, cesarean sections, and mastectomies. Women demonstrated on the steps of Congress, and feminist health writers encouraged women to explore their own health. In 1960, the U.S. Food and Drug Administration (FDA) approved the birth control pill, and, for the first time, women were given a real sense of sexual freedom. The Civil Rights Movement also gained force during the 1960s with numerous sit-ins and Martin Luther King's "I have a dream" speech in 1963. In 1964, Congress passed the Civil Rights Act, including Title VII, which protected women against employment discrimination. In 1972, Congress passed the Equal Rights Amendment, although ultimately it was ratified by only 35 states, three states short of the 38 states needed for ratification.

During this time, the self-help manual *Our Bodies, Ourselves* was introduced. In addition, a number of women's health centers and workshops, health advocacy organizations, and disease-specific groups that provided support networks and raised national awareness were formed. By the mid-1970s, more than 250 advocacy, education, and healthcare service groups for women existed, as well as nearly 2,000 self-help groups and other projects focusing on the women's health movement.[1]

Another important development in the 1970s was the establishment of the bipartisan Congresswomen's Caucus by 15 of the 18 women members of Congress. The initial discussions focused on spousal abuse; however, as the women continued to meet, their discussions branched out to cover issues of child care and job training to move women off welfare. In 1981, four years after its inception, the group admitted men and became known as the Congressional Caucus for Women's Issues. Through the years, Caucus members have worked to improve the lives of women and families by opening up opportunities in education and work, promoting women's health, and championing causes such as equitable pay, enforcement of child

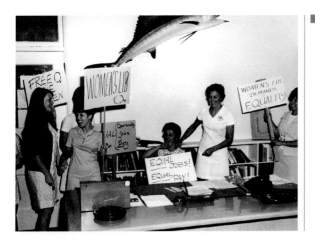

During the 1960s and 1970s, women challenged the authorities on many issues regarding gender equality.

I have an inherited condition that affects most of the women in my family. I don't know what we would have done without the support of an advocacy organization that is focused on our condition.

21-year-old woman

support, and protection for victims of domestic violence and sexual assault. This group was critical in inspiring the formation of two federal offices geared specifically toward women: the Public Health Service on Women's Health in the Department of Health and Human Services (DHHS) and the Office of Research on Women's Health at the National Institutes of Health (NIH). (See the Web sites listed at the end of this chapter for more information.)

As the women's health movement evolved, leadership in the women's groups remained mostly white and middle class. Eventually, organizations specific to certain races or ethnicities evolved and developed agendas that covered general women's health issues, as well as issues focusing on low-income women and diseases and conditions that disproportionately affect women of color. The National Black Women's Health Project (now called the Black Women's Health Imperative) was established by Byllye Avery and is an example of a successful organization dedicated to the promotion of optimal health for black women across the life span. Other nationally recognized groups include the National Latina Women's Health Organization, the National Asian Women's Health Organization, and the Native American Women's Health Education and Resource Center. The women's health movement also was growing globally as health activist groups for women sprouted up throughout the world.

1980s: Changing Public Policy

In the 1980s, the U.S. Public Health Service's Task Force on Women's Health Issues was formed to assess the status of women's health and recommend a course of action to address determined needs. The Task Force issued a series of recommendations, which included increasing gender equity in **biomedical research** and establishing guidelines for the inclusion of women in federally sponsored studies. Although NIH did formulate such guidelines, a 1990 inquiry by the General Accounting Office, requested by the Congressional Caucus for Women's Issues, reported that NIH had failed to implement its policy guidelines across the board. In response, NIH strengthened its guidelines and established the Office of Research on Women's Health (ORWH).[2] The ORWH mandate focuses on ensuring women's participation in clinical trials, strengthening research on diseases affecting women, and promoting the career advancement of women in science. The Women's Health Equity Act also was passed, allocating money to fund health research on particular areas of concern to women, including contraception, infertility, breast cancer, ovarian cancer, HIV/AIDS, and osteoporosis. The Act also included coverage of Pap smear screening and mammography for **Medicaid** recipients, assistance for pregnant women with health care and other services, and increased access for all women to screening and treatment for sexually transmitted diseases.

1990s: Women's Health at the Forefront

The 1990s brought together government, healthcare institutions, academia, and advocacy organizations, which resulted in elevation of women's health and well-being to the forefront of public consciousness. The federal government formed many women's health offices in federal agencies and in regional public health service offices. This trend, in turn, inspired the establishment of a number of women's health centers throughout the country. Existing centers broadened their scope beyond reproductive issues to take a more comprehensive look at health and disease among women.

In the 1993 NIH Revitalization Act, Congress required that women and minorities be included as subjects in all human subject research funded by NIH.[3] This decision was a bold and innovative step. For the first time, women and minorities could not be excluded from studies based on the characteristics of race and sex. The legislation was greeted enthusiastically by many and skeptically by those who predicted a gradual ruin of clinical investigation. Some scientists suggested that recruitment and retention would suffer and costs would overwhelm and ultimately preclude undertaking many studies. These fears have not become reality, however. The inclusion of women in research has instead led to the expansion of the scientific knowledge base necessary for developing sex/gender-specific diagnostic techniques, preventive measures, and effective treatments for diseases and conditions affecting women throughout their life span.

Also in 1993, Congresswoman Patricia Schroeder introduced the Family and Medical Leave Act; the Act, signed by President Bill Clinton, gives employees unpaid medical leave for themselves or for the care of a family member or a newborn or adopted infant. A year later, President Clinton signed into law the Violence Against Women Act, which mandates a unified judicial response to sexual crimes committed against women.

The Future

Recent studies focusing on sex/gender differences have resulted in great promise for the future of research in women's health. The understanding that sex—specifically, being male or female—should be considered when designing and analyzing biomedical and health-related research has helped to validate the scientific study of sex differences. This knowledge has opened the door for scientists to conduct studies that account for sex-based differences and promote the development of new approaches to prevention, diagnosis, and treatment of disease.[4]

The new millennium has continued to bring numerous contributions to improving the health of the public—for example, the identification of the **human genome,** the findings from the Women's Health Initiative, improvements in HIV/AIDS medications, public health programs targeting behavior-related health problems, and the inclusion of children in **clinical trials.** Nevertheless, women still face a number of challenges in the healthcare arena. There has been a rollback of many of the advances made in the 1990s, including curtailment of funding for reproductive health initiatives both domestically and internationally and politicizing of the women's health agenda. Many women struggle to find access to healthcare services; women are living longer but not necessarily with better quality of life; and women across the United States and the world continue to be victims of individual and societal violence and discrimination.

It's Your Health

FEMINISM

Feminism is defined as the policy, practice, or advocacy of political, economic, and social equality for women. It is the principle that women should have economic and social rights equal to those of men.

The first wave of feminism was that of the suffragists and abolitionists who secured basic rights for women, such as the rights to vote, own property, and inherit property.

The second wave of feminism occurred in the 1960s and 1970s. It fought against specific injustices, such as the lack of reproductive freedom, and promoted equal pay for equal work and access to jobs and education. A central tenet of the second wave was making the personal become political by highlighting ways that women were systematically subjugated professionally and legally.

The third wave of feminism continues the work of addressing women's issues, such as domestic violence, access to safe and legal abortions, and sexual harassment, as well as ensuring equal status of women in educational, work, athletic, and social environments. Throughout the 1980s and 1990s, feminists viewed all aspects of society, art, and science through a feminist lens. This perspective provided great insights into where inequality persists and how women often contribute to supporting the status quo instead of actively fighting for change. The third wave has also focused on practical ways to help women achieve equality, such as by promoting flexible work scheduling, demanding the availability of child care, and making time off available for maternity leave and caring for sick family members.

Today, many young women are living out the dreams of the women who started the feminist movement. They pursue careers and family, they demand equality in their relationships, and they support feminist political agendas. However, many young women fail to link their individual achievements back to the feminist movement.

As a result, many groups are trying to "update" their messages to include girls and women who have a strong sense of self and "girl power." These groups are helping to provide a context for the opportunities that girls and women currently enjoy, while also recognizing persistent inequities. At the same time, a rise of conservatism and a return to neo-traditionalism are creating a strong cultural counterpoint to much of the progress that feminism has made in the last 30 years. How this trend plays out and what role women take in defining equality moving forward will shape how feminism continues to develop.

Political Dimensions of Women's Health

By looking at women's health within a political context, many of the advances that have been achieved and the barriers that remain can be better understood. Government at every level plays an important role in protecting and promoting the health of the public. It is involved in six main areas in relation to the health of the population: [5]

1. Policy making

2. Financing

3. Protecting the health of the public

4. Collecting and disseminating information about health and healthcare delivery systems

5. Capacity building for population health

6. Managing of health services

Through policies, regulations, and the law, the government exercises control over many of the areas affecting women's health, both directly and indirectly. Within the context of these six areas, the federal government conducts such activities as ensuring that the food supply is safe, providing federal highway funding for states that adopt a legal drinking age, and regulating businesses that provide medications to the public.

During the 1990s, women's health issues garnered a significant amount of support and attention. Numerous organizations and government agencies devoted to women's health were established. The Department of Health and Human Services' Office on Women's Health (DHHS-OWH) serves as the coordinating agency for all women's health initiatives throughout the agencies and offices of the U.S. DHHS (described earlier), including National Institutes of Health (NIH), Food and Drug Administration (FDA), Centers for Disease Control and Prevention (CDC), and other agencies and departments. OWH works at recognizing and addressing inequities in research, healthcare services, and education that have placed the health of women at risk.[6]

The Office of Research on Women's Health (ORWH) within NIH serves as a focal point for women's biomedical research. ORWH works to ensure that women's health research is present within NIH and the surrounding scientific community:[7]

- ORWH advises the NIH Director and staff on matters relating to research on women's health.
- It strengthens and enhances research related to diseases, disorders, and conditions that affect women.
- It ensures that research conducted and supported by NIH adequately addresses issues regarding women's health.
- It ensures that women are appropriately represented in biomedical and behavioral research studies supported by NIH.
- It develops opportunities for and supports recruitment, retention, reentry, and advancement of women in biomedical careers.
- It supports research on women's health issues.

Since its establishment in 1990, ORWH has been a driving force in these important areas of women's health. It also has been critical in national and international collaborative efforts across government and private organizations to embed women's health research into the scientific and educational infrastructure. Collaborative efforts have ranged from implementing research action on autoimmune diseases and the use and overuse of hysterectomy to returning scientists to active investigations. Working with scientists, practitioners, legislators, and lay advocates, ORWH has identified research priorities and set a comprehensive research agenda for the twenty-first century (outlined in its *Report of the Task Force on the NIH Women's Health Research Agenda for the 21st Century*). In addition, ORWH is an important collaborator in fostering a research agenda that examines the biological differences between the sexes—that is, gender-based biology—in an attempt to more fully understand each and thereby enhance knowledge and practice.

The Healthy Women 2000 initiative was one project that joined DHHS with other federal agencies, nonprofit organizations, and members of various medical industries in a mission to educate women and provide them with the knowledge needed to live long and healthy lives. By identifying diseases that have a significant impact on women, future research direction and goals can be determined.

DHHS also has implemented several programs to provide for family planning, prevent sexually transmitted diseases, and reduce unintended pregnancies. The Title X program provides funding to millions of people for reproductive health and family planning services. Funding has also increased for research and programs aimed at improving the health of older women, demonstrated in part by the development of a resource center launched by the Administration on Aging to educate older women about issues such as income security, housing, and caregiving. In addition, support has been increased for community nutrition services to combat nutrition-related illnesses of the elderly.[6]

The focus on women's health issues is not always a priority in politics, however. Different political parties have different platforms and see healthcare reform in differing lights. Affordable, accessible, quality health care is a central concern for almost every family and is often mentioned as a major priority for both Congress and presidential administrations. Yet each political party envisions a different means of achieving this goal. A change in administration often has implications for health policy; a new president and Congress can bring a different focus and tone to U.S. health policy than that associated with the existing government. Campaign promises, active voters, and special-interest groups all play roles in shaping health policy and influencing the direction of the legislative agenda.

Today, the majority of healthcare reform seeks to address how health care is financed, which services are covered, and who is eligible for public assistance. Women specifically are fighting to ensure that access to vital services is available to all women, regardless of their age, income, or location. Topics high on the current national health agenda include the following:

- Investing in biomedical research for fighting disease
- Maintaining reproductive rights and the freedom of choice
- Ensuring access to healthcare providers and services and to health information

Other issues, such as prescription drug coverage for seniors, genetic testing, malpractice insurance/award reform, the future of Medicare and Medicaid, and federal regulation of health care, may be explored further on the companion Web site for this book (womenshealth.jbpub.com).

Investment in Biomedical Research

The federal government plays a critical role in funding biomedical research. NIH is the main federal agency responsible for distributing money to private and public institutions and organizations for conducting medical and health research. Along with the CDC and other agencies, it helps to advance basic research so as to discover new and better methods of treatment and prevention of numerous health conditions. Funding also comes from the private sector, philanthropic organizations, and voluntary health agencies. Pharmaceutical companies and private corporations invest millions of dollars each year in research and development and continue to introduce hundreds of new drugs, vaccines, and technologies every year. Investment in biomedical research has led to increased **life expectancy,** improved health throughout the life span, and decreased cost of illness. Significant improvements in the understanding of basic science have enabled remarkable discoveries in prevention, treatment, and eradication of disease.

The investment in research also has shown potential in increasing the understanding of biological, psychological, and sociological factors of women's health as well as improving the delivery of healthcare services to women. Research on women's health has seen unprecedented growth in the past three decades, especially with the push for inclusion of women in clinical trials. Policies now ensure that women and minorities are included as subjects in federally sponsored research and in the evaluation of drugs and medical devices. By demanding that women are included in health research, women—not men—become the studied models for the conditions that affect them and the drugs used to treat these conditions. This trend has led to the integration of women-specific data into clinical practice and the formulation of new questions in regard to women and specific diseases. As a consequence, women's health is no longer limited to diseases of the reproductive organs.

Another approach to improving women's health relies on gender-based research—studies that examine the similarities and differences between men and women to learn more about the etiology of disease and responses to medication. Gender-based studies are committed to identifying the biological and physiological differences between men and women. Males and females can manifest different symptoms of a disease, experience the course of a disease differently, or respond differently to pharmaceuticals. By understanding and appreciating the differences between men and women and the way they develop and experience disease, researchers have realized the importance of no longer assuming that males and females are identical. Identifying and studying gender-based differences offers a remarkable potential for understanding disease epidemiology and health outcomes in both men and women. Some examples of areas of women's health research that have benefited from increased funding and attention can be seen in Table 1.1. These topics are discussed in greater detail in later chapters of this book.

Fat and body water content, steroidal sex hormone levels, and **genetic phenotype** all affect drug metabolism through pharmacokinetics (concentration of the drug) and pharmacodynamics (ability to metabolize the drug).[9] Some examples of how women and men metabolize drugs differently are described in the literature for commonly prescribed medications: theophylline, acetaminophen, aspirin, propranolol, and lidocaine.[10] Heterogeneity among women also should be recognized in terms of drug metabolism. Variances to consider include age, hormonal status, race, ethnicity, and socioeconomic factors. The extent to which these differences

The reasons for excluding women from clinical investigations are less obvious than one might expect. In spite of a significant body of opinion to the contrary, the reasons have very little to do with male chauvinism or the gender of the investigating scientist—until the 1990s, female scientists were every bit as likely as men to exclude females from clinical protocols. Even at the most sophisticated academic medical centers, senior investigators taught young scientists that data obtained from male subjects could be extrapolated to women without modification. They assumed that women were essentially small men—identical in all respects except for their reproductive physiology. It is astonishing that in a scientific system that prides itself on its critical sense and accepts no hypothesis as true until it has been rigorously tested, we have tolerated such a leap of faith for so long.[8]

Marianne J. Legato, M.D., F.A.C.P.

(Read about Marianne Legato and her work in the **Profiles of Remarkable Women** section in this chapter.)

Table 1.1	Women and Men: Ten Differences That Make a Difference

When it comes to health, there are many crucial differences between men and women. Yet many women do not know that they react differently to some medications, are more vulnerable to some diseases, and may have different symptoms. The Society for Women's Health Research brought attention to sex differences in initiating the groundbreaking 2001 Institute of Medicine report, *Exploring the Biological Contribution to Human Health: Does Sex Matter?* The report underscored the need to better understand the importance of sex differences and translate that knowledge into improved medical practice and therapies.

Following are some quick but vital facts about sex differences in health care that you probably did not know.

Heart Disease. Heart disease kills 500,000 American women each year—over 50,000 more women than men—and strikes women, on average, 10 years later than men. Women are more likely than men to have a second heart attack within a year of the first one.

Depression. Women are two to three times more likely than men to suffer from depression, in part because women's brains make less of the hormone serotonin.

Osteoporosis. Women account for 80% of the population suffering from osteoporosis, which is attributable to their higher rate of lost bone mass.

Smoking. Smoking has a more negative effect on cardiovascular health in women than men. Women are also less successful in quitting smoking and have more severe withdrawal symptoms.

Sexually Transmitted Diseases. Women are twice as likely as men to contract a sexually transmitted disease.

Anesthesia. Women tend to wake up from anesthesia more quickly than men—an average of 7 minutes for women and 11 minutes for men.

Drug Reactions. Even common drugs like antihistamines and antibiotics drugs can cause different reactions and side effects in women and men.

Autoimmune Diseases. Three out of four people suffering from autoimmune diseases, such as multiple sclerosis, rheumatoid arthritis, and lupus, are women.

Alcohol. Women produce less of the gastric enzyme that breaks down ethanol in the stomach. Therefore, after consuming the same amount of alcohol, women have a higher blood alcohol content than men, even allowing for size differences.

Pain. Some pain medications (known as kappa-opiates) are far more effective in relieving pain in women than in men.

Source: Society for Women's Health Research, 2004. http://www.womenshealthresearch.org/hs/10diff.htm.

prevail among the range of drugs used to prevent and treat disease is still not fully known or understood.

Recent FDA guidelines urge drug investigators to account for pharmacodynamic and pharmacokinetic gender differences throughout the drug development process and to include women of childbearing age in both Phase I and Phase II clinical trials (Table 1.2). In its 1977 guidelines, the FDA excluded women of childbearing potential from clinical trials. Revised guidelines in 1993 called for gender-specific analyses of safety and effectiveness in new drugs and removed

It's Your Health

Research Studies

1. **Descriptive Studies** examine general characteristics of distribution of a disease in relation to person, place, and time using indices such as basic demographic factors (i.e., age, sex, race), geography, and seasonal or yearly patterns.

   - Population or Correlational Studies: use data from entire populations to compare diseases between and among groups during the same time period or the same groups during different time periods.

   - Individual Studies: case report studies detail a profile of a single patient; case series describe a number of patients with a given disease; cross-sectional surveys involve questionnaires that inquire about presence or absence of disease and exposure or specific risk factors in groups of people.

2. **Analytic Studies** involve groups of individuals who are investigated to compare risk of disease in people exposed to a specific factor with those people not exposed.

   - Observational Studies: researcher observes course of events in either a case-control study or cohort study. A case-control study involves observing patients without a disease and comparing them with a control group of people with a disease. Cohort studies group people based on the presence or absence of a specific factor of interest and then follow the group to determine development of a disease.

     —Retrospective Observational Study—both disease and exposure have occurred and investigator is determining whether the exposure caused the disease.

     —Prospective Observational Study—the exposure has occurred but the disease has not; therefore, population is observed in comparison with unexposed subjects.

   - Intervention Studies: viewed as a type of prospective cohort study; however, the exposure status of the population is assigned by the researcher.

     —Clinical Trial—a research study designed to answer specific questions about vaccines or new therapies or new ways of using known treatments. Clinical trials are used to determine whether new drugs or treatments are both safe and effective.

the FDA's policy of excluding women of childbearing potential from early drug studies. These measures have helped the FDA acquire better information on drug effects in women.[11]

A serious issue in gender-based research has been the concern of pharmaceutical manufacturers that by identifying drugs as effective in only one gender, the

Table 1.2 Phases of a Clinical Trial

- **Phase I:** new drug tested in a small group of healthy volunteers (20–80) to evaluate its safety, determine a safe dosage range, and identify side effects.

- **Phase II:** study drug is given to a larger group of people (100–300) to further evaluate its safety and effectiveness.

- **Phase III:** study drug is given to large groups in clinics and hospitals (1,000–3,000) to confirm its effectiveness, monitor side effects, and compare it with other treatments.

- **Phase IV:** study done after drug is marketed to continue collecting information regarding the drug's effects in various populations.

potential market for their drugs could be limited, thereby decreasing their expected profits. Recently, however, the pharmaceutical industry has been instrumental in meeting the special needs of women by increasing research devoted to medicines for treating diseases that disproportionately affect women. Pharmaceutical companies are currently developing over 350 new medicines targeting more than 30 diseases that disproportionately affect women. The potential medicines, all either in clinical trials or awaiting final approval by the FDA, target breast cancer, ovarian cancer, arthritis, diabetes, depression, osteoporosis, and multiple sclerosis. In addition, companies have medicines in their pipelines for heart disease, stroke, and lung cancer, three leading causes of death in women.[12]

Even with all of the advances toward inclusion of women and minority groups in research studies, one barrier to women's participation in biomedical research still exists. Many women are unable to take part in clinical trials because of a lack of insurance coverage. A growing number of states have passed legislation or instituted special agreements requiring health plans to pay the cost of routine medical care that a woman may receive as a participant in a clinical trial. In 2000, **Medicare** began covering **beneficiaries'** patient care costs in clinical trials.[13] Clinical trials still are considered experimental by some insurance companies, however, and therefore are not covered under all standard health policies.[14]

Including women in clinical studies may pose challenges, but leaving them out courts disaster through ignorance. Using women, particularly women of childbearing age, presents challenges to the investigation as the researchers must consider the effect of hormonal cycling on the hypothesis being tested. Furthermore, the potential for pregnancy and possible **teratogenic** effects in the fetus must be considered. These factors weigh heavily in designing and conducting any study.

Although information continues to emerge from ongoing women's health research, additional studies are needed to discover optimal preventive measures and interventions to reduce risk factors and improve health outcomes for women. This is particularly so in the case of sex differences in disease presentation, progression, and response to therapies. Standards of medical care and public health policies that recognize biological and psychosocial differences must be developed. Action on examining sex/gender differences in health has been promulgated by many of the federal agencies and organizations that initially brought about equity in women's health research. Several of these agencies and other private organizations commissioned a study by the National Academies of Science's Institute of Medicine to examine these differences. That study, *Exploring the Biological Considerations of Health: Does Sex Matter?*, was published in 2001 and has provoked a more intense focus on sex/gender differences in research and practice.[4] The current challenge in women's health research is to establish a scientific knowledge base that permits reliable diagnoses and effective prevention and treatment strategies for all women.

Reproductive Rights

The history and politics of abortion are long and complex. (See Chapter 5 for a detailed history.) For nearly a century, abortion was illegal in the United States. On January 22, 1973, it was legalized in the United States through the landmark

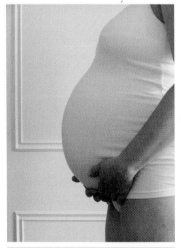

■ The potential for pregnancy and possible teratogenic effects in the fetus must be considered in clinical trials.

Supreme Court decision *Roe v. Wade.* On January 22, 2001—President George W. Bush's second day in office and the twenty-eighth anniversary of the *Roe v. Wade* decision that legalized abortion—the "global gag rule" on international family planning assistance was reinstated. Previously known as the "Mexico City Policy" when the Reagan Administration imposed it in 1984, the rule had been eliminated by the Clinton Administration in 1993. Under the global gag rule, foreign family planning agencies may not receive U.S. assistance if they provide the following services, even if the funds used for these services are from another source:

- Perform abortion in cases of pregnancy that are not life-threatening to the woman or the result of rape or incest
- Provide counseling and referral for abortions
- Lobby to legalize abortion or increase its availability in the country in which the NGO is operating[15]

Restrictions on funding can lead to an increase in unplanned pregnancies, abortions, maternal and infant deaths, and transmission of HIV in countries around the world. The global gag rule represents a step toward limiting reproductive freedom, just like the recent push to overturn the *Roe v. Wade* decision. Although the Supreme Court's decision on abortion still stands, state restrictions have been imposed that limit a woman's access to reproductive health services.

Access to Healthcare Providers, Services, and Health Information

Advances in public health and medicine have created significant improvements in the prevention, diagnosis, and treatment of disease. Many people are living longer and healthier lives as a result. Over the years, women have learned to seek out medical information on their own, thereby becoming informed consumers of medicine. As new findings lead to improved methods of prevention, public health officials and healthcare practitioners focus on encouraging healthcare consumers to practice health promotion and disease prevention.

Unfortunately, healthcare promotion and disease prevention are not simple. Many women encounter barriers to adequate health care, such as the following:

- Low socioeconomic status
- Lack of health insurance
- Lack of access to healthcare facilities
- Inability to understand medical personnel because of language barriers or illiteracy
- Unfair treatment by medical personnel because of race, ethnicity, or sexual orientation
- Inability to pay for the costs of medications needed for treatment
- Declined coverage for healthcare costs that are deemed unnecessary or experimental
- Fear of doctors and avoidance of seeking health care altogether

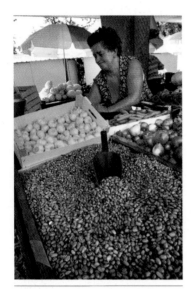

■ Millions of Americans work, but do not have access to health care.

Lack of adequate access to healthcare services and information is a serious issue in the United States, with a lack of health insurance being one of the most formidable barriers. In 2001, 41.2 million Americans were uninsured[16] and millions more were underinsured, meaning their health insurance coverage had limitations that restricted access to necessary services. Such restrictions could mean lack of coverage in the event of a serious illness, exclusion for preexisting conditions, increased co-payments and deductibles, increased patient responsibility for payment of prescription medications, gaps in Medicare service, and lack of coverage for long-term care. Often, as unemployment rates rise, the number of people covered by insurance steadily declines. **Premiums** for private health insurance are extremely expensive and, therefore, many people opt to take a chance and remain uninsured when an employer does not sponsor them. (For more information on this issue, see Chapter 2.)

Lack of cultural and gender sensitivity and failure to fully understand women's health needs also create barriers for women. To bring women's health into the mainstream of medical education, ORWH developed a model curriculum in women's health for medical schools. Research findings and guidelines for the health care of women are being incorporated into education and training curricula for **osteopathic** and **allopathic** schools; dental, nursing, and pharmacy programs; and medical schools. Incorporating women's health as part of the curriculum for medical students, nursing students, and other healthcare practitioners has reiterated the uniqueness of being female, along with emphasizing the heterogeneity of women as a population. Medical school graduates are now being trained in cultural and gender sensitivity and the use of medical interventions appropriate to different cultures and women. This minimization—and ideally elimination—of physicians treating all patients as a homogenous group should improve access to health care by removing the cultural and gender barriers for minorities and women. Other strategies for ensuring the inclusion of women's health in educational curricula include sponsorship of residency training and fellowship programs in women's health and demands for state licensing boards to evaluate a physician's competency in women's health.[17,18]

Global Perspective on Women's Health

Throughout the world, inequities remain in women's health care and research. Furthermore, there is a great difference in the leading causes of morbidity and mortality between developing countries and developed countries. Global threats to women's health include poverty, underweight and malnutrition, HIV/AIDS, violence, and **maternal morbidity and mortality.** Women are burdened not only by disease, but also by violations of their human rights that directly affect their health. These problems include domestic and societal violence, **female genital mutilation, honor killings, trafficking,** and barriers to reproductive health services. The social, political, and economic determinants of health greatly affect women and children throughout the world. Access to clean water, nutritious food, and medical care, as well as protection from violence and poor working conditions, are basic rights that should be afforded to all for the improvement of health on a global scale. So-cial inequalities, such as lack of education, money, and decision-making freedom, pose a greater threat to women than to men, as women consequently end up with a disproportionately higher burden of disease, poverty, and maternal morbidity and mortality. Women also have the double burden of work and family drawing on them. Alignment among women across the world has become a powerful force for change.

Since 1975, five world conferences on women convened by the United Nations (UN) have worked for the advancement of women to achieve gender equality. The first world conference on the status of women met in Mexico City and developed a World Plan of Action, which offered guidelines for governments and communi-ties throughout the world to follow. The focus of these guidelines was to secure equal access for women to resources such as education, employment opportunities, political representation, health services, housing, nutrition, and family planning.

In 1980, the second world conference on women met to review and appraise the 1975 World Plan of Action. Significant progress had been made, including the adoption of the "Convention on the Elimination of All Forms of Discrimination Against Women," also referred to as "the bill of rights for women." It legally binds 165 member states of the UN to report on steps they have taken toward achieving women's equality. Despite the progress, members at the conference recognized that a discrepancy existed between secured legal rights and women's ability to exercise those rights. A variety of factors were noted as causing the discrepancies, includ-ing a lack of men involved in improving women's role in society; a lack of women in decision-making positions; insufficient supportive services for women and fami-lies, such as childcare facilities; and a lack of awareness among women about opportunities available to them.[18]

By the third world conference, held in 1985 in Nairobi, the women's movement toward gender equality had achieved international recognition. This conference became known as the "birth of global feminism." While successes were being cele-brated, evidence pointed to only a minority of women benefiting from the ad-vances. A new approach toward the women's movement was identified—all issues

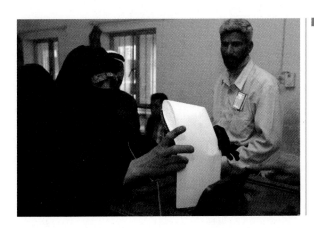

In many developing areas of the world, voting is new or not yet available for women.

were now declared to be women's issues. Women's active involvement in all issues, from education and employment to health and science to industry and the environment, was necessary if women were to attain equality.

In 1995, the fourth world conference on women was held in Beijing and was considered a great success. The conference led to the recognition that "the entire structure of society, and all relations between men and women within it, had to be re-evaluated."[19] Twelve critical areas of concern were highlighted as the greatest obstacles to women's advancement (Table 1.3).

In the five years since Beijing, culminating with the New York conference "Women 2000: Gender Equality, Development and Peace for the 21st Century," also known as "Beijing + 5," the achievements of governments have been evaluated and new action plans have been prepared. Additionally, the UN's Millenium Development Goals specifically look at how the UN and other groups can measure countries' progress toward promoting gender equity and empowering women. Indicators used to measure progress include the ratio of girls to boys in primary, secondary, and tertiary schools; the ratio of literate women to men; the percentage of women in waged employment; the proportion of seats held by women in parliament; the maternal mortality rate; and the percentage of births attended by a skilled health professional.

Advances have been recorded, although women still face discrimination and marginalization, and they continue to account for the majority of the world's poor.[19] Much work remains to be done; yet the accomplishments that have arisen from the five world conferences deserve to be celebrated. By uniting the international community, women and men throughout the world have created a set of common objectives with the one final goal of equality for everyone.

Table 1.3	**Beijing Conference's Platform of Action—Twelve Critical Areas of Concern**

- Women and poverty
- Education and training of women
- Women and health
- Violence against women
- Women and armed conflict
- Women and the economy
- Women in power and decision making
- Institutional mechanisms for the advancement of women
- Human rights of women
- Women and the media
- Women and the environment
- The girl child

Source: United Nations WomenWatch. (2000). The 4 global women's conferences, 1975–1995: Historical perspective. United Nations Department of Public Information: DPI/2035/M.

Profiles of Remarkable Women

Marianne J. Legato, M.D., F.A.C.P. (1935–)

Marianne J. Legato, M.D., F.A.C.P., is an internationally known academic physician, author, lecturer, and specialist in women's health. She is a Professor of Clinical Medicine at Columbia University College of Physicians and Surgeons and the Founder and Director of the Partnership for Women's Health at Columbia, which is the first collaboration between academic medicine and the private sector focused solely on gender-specific medicine. She also is a practicing internist in New York City. Over the years, Dr. Legato has helped to make significant progress in the area of research on women's health and gender-specific medicine.

Dr. Legato has spent her research career doing cardiovascular research on the structure and function of the cardiac cell. Her work was supported by the American Heart Association and the National Institutes of Health. She has won numerous awards and has been listed as one of New York's best doctors.

Dr. Legato was a member of the National Heart, Lung and Blood Institute's study section on cardiovascular disease and has served as a charter member of the Advisory Board of the Office of Research on Women's Health of the National Institutes of Health. She was co-chair of a task force that authored a report from ORWH, *An Agenda for Research on Women's Health for the 21st Century.* In 1992, Dr. Legato won the American Heart Association's Blakeslee Award for the best book written for the lay public on cardiovascular disease with her publication of *The Female Heart: The Truth About Women and Heart Disease.* Her film, *Shattering the Myths: Women and Heart Disease,* won first prize in the category of Women's Health at the 1995 International Health and Medical Film Festival. In 1997, she published another book: *What Women Need to Know: From Headaches to Heart Disease and Everything in Between.* In 2003, her book titled *Eve's Rib: The New Science of Gender-Specific Medicine and How It Can Save Your Life* was published. Dr. Legato is the editor of *The Journal of Gender-Specific Medicine,* published for the scientific community, and *Gender and Health,* published for the lay public. She is on the editorial board of *Cardiovascular Risk Factors and Prevention* magazine. Dr. Legato writes continuously for both the scientific and lay communities and is a consultant in health for *Ladies Home Journal* and *MORE* magazines. She is a consultant to several multinational corporations, to which she provides expertise in the area of women's health. Dr. Legato is truly one of the nation's leading advocates of women's health.

Informed Decision Making: Take Action

There are a number of ways to become involved in women's health advocacy. Many women's health organizations encourage becoming members by donating, getting involved by sending letters to legislators and helping to organize events, and educating oneself on women's health issues. Visiting the Internet can be a good first step in learning about various organizations and deciding where to focus personal interest and commitment. A number of organizations that offer ways for individuals to start becoming involved are listed in the Web sites section.

Summary

Women's health has become part of mainstream medicine, brought to the forefront of national attention and out of the auspices of solely feminist advocacy groups.

Profiles of Remarkable Women

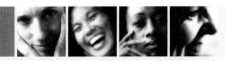

Gloria Steinem (1934–)

Gloria Steinem, well-known feminist leader, activist, and journalist, is the daughter of a newspaperwoman and the granddaughter of the noted suffragette, Pauline Steinem. Steinem's interest in activism and writing was sparked following her graduation from Smith College in 1956. She won a fellowship to study in India for two years, an experience that made her aware of the extent of human suffering in the world. Steinem returned from India strongly motivated to fight social injustice and thus began her career as a journalist.

Although her initial search for work as a professional journalist was not successful, Steinem eventually landed a job as an editorial assistant. In 1960, she moved to New York and began working as a freelance writer for popular magazines. One of her first major assignments in investigative journalism was a two-part series for *Show* magazine on the working conditions of Playboy bunnies. To do research for the article, Steinem worked as a Playboy bunny for three weeks. The articles that she wrote exposed the poor working conditions and meager wages of the Playboy bunnies and the discrimination and sexual harassment that occurred at New York's Playboy Club.

In 1968, after finally landing an important political assignment covering Senator George McGovern's presidential campaign, Steinem joined the staff of *New York* magazine as a contributing editor and political columnist. She established a column, "The City Politic," and wrote in support of causes on the American left. During these years Steinem moved into politics more directly, covering everything from the assassination of Martin Luther King, Jr., to demonstrations of United Farm Workers led by Cesar Chavez. She also worked for various Democratic candidates. Steinem's shift to the current women's liberation movement and feminism were sparked while attending abortion hearings. She found herself deeply moved by the stories, realizing that women were oppressed as a class by society.

By the late 1960s, Steinem had positioned herself as a leader of the women's liberation movement through her research, writing, and activism. In 1971, she joined Bella Abzug, Shirley Chisholm, and Betty Friedan to form the National Women's Political Caucus, encouraging women's participation in the 1972 election.

Steinem had become friendly with Dorothy Pitman Hughes, an African American childcare pioneer. Steinem and Hughes spoke together publicly throughout the United States to promote women's rights, civil rights, and children's rights, and in 1971 they formed the Women's Action Alliance to develop women's educational programs. Although the alliance folded in 1997, its offshoot WISE (Women Initiating Self-Empowerment) continues.

In 1972, Steinem gained funding for the first mass-circulation feminist magazine, *Ms.* The preview issue sold out, and within five years *Ms.* had a circulation of 500,000. As editor of the magazine, Steinem became an influential spokesperson for women's rights issues, while continuing in her active political life. In 1975, she helped plan the women's agenda for the Democratic National Convention, and she continued to exert pressure on liberal politicians on behalf of women's concerns. In 1977, Steinem participated in the National Conference of Women in Houston, Texas. The conference—the first of its kind—served to publicize the number of feminist issues and draw attention to women's rights leaders.

Steinem has published a number of books, including *Outrageous Acts and Everyday Rebellions* (1983), *Marilyn: Norma Jean* (1986), *Revolution from Within: A Book of Self-Esteem* (1992), and *Moving Beyond Words* (1994). As a writer and an activist, Gloria Steinem continues to be a leader in the women's rights movement.

Although tremendous progress has been achieved in expanding the scope and depth of women's health research, major challenges remain. Continued success in the women's health movement is predicated on a series of factors: legislative mandates; sufficient funds; educated and interested scientific and lay communities; advocacy by professionals, patients, and the public; and involvement of women, men, and communities in working for equality. These factors have been catalysts driving the explosion in women's health research and are responsible for both the present state of success in developed countries and the advancements being made throughout the world. Biological, behavioral, and social sciences have provided critical insights and important data that have enhanced women's health and well-being. The research success from developed countries is slowly kindling international awareness such that women's health and gender equity are improving across the world, albeit at a slower pace than many might desire.

Topics for Discussion

1. The women's health movement has played a critical role in bringing women's health issues to the forefront. Has the success of the movement made it obsolete for the future? Why did the women's health movement advance so rapidly during the 1990s?

2. Numerous women's advocacy organizations exist today. What challenges do they face in representing their constituents? How can they maximize their impact while also competing for scarce funding resources?

3. How has the modern information age influenced women's advocacy in both positive and negative ways?

4. What areas of health could benefit from gender-based research?

5. What are some gender inequities that are present throughout the world?

6. Discuss the ways the government is involved in the following areas in relation to health:

   - Policy making
   - Financing
   - Protecting the health of the public
   - Collecting and disseminating information about health and healthcare delivery systems
   - Capacity building for population health
   - Managing of health services

Web Sites

Black Women's Health Imperative: http://www.blackwomenshealth.org

Centers for Disease Control and Prevention: http://www.cdc.gov/health/womens menu.htm

The Children's Bureau: http://www.acf.dhhs.gov/programs/cb/

Equal Rights Amendment: http://www.equalrightsamendment.org

Feminist Women's Health Center: http://www.fwhc.org

Global Health Council: http://www.globalhealth.org

National Organization for Women (NOW): http://www.now.org

The National Women's Health Information Center: http://www.4woman.gov

The Office on Women's Health: http://www.4woman.gov/owh/index.htm

Office of Research on Women's Health: http://orwh.od.nih.gov

Planned Parenthood Federation of America: http://www.plannedparenthood.org

Society for Women's Health Research: http://www.womenshealthresearch.org

U.S. Food and Drug Administration (FDA): http://www.fda.gov

Women's Issues in Congress: http://www.womenspolicy.org

■■■■

References

1. *The History and Future of Women's Health: Seminar Highlights.* (1998). Sponsored by the Office on Women's Health and Public Health Service Coordinating Committee on Women's Health.

2. U.S. Department of Health and Human Services, Public Health Service, National Institutes of Health. (1999). *Agenda for Research on Women's Health for the 21st Century: A Report of the Task Force on the NIH Women's Health Research Agenda for the 21st Century,* vol. 1, Executive Summary. Bethesda, MD. NIH Pub. No. 99-4385.

3. Legato, M. J. (1998). Report of the task force on research on women's health for the 21st century: a personal overview. *Journal of Gender-Specific Medicine* 1(1).

4. *Exploring the Biological Contributions to Human Health: Does Sex Matter?* (2001). National Academy of Sciences.

5. Hamburg, Margaret A. (2001). National perspective: United States. *Women's Health Issues* 11(4): 282–292.

6. *About the Office on Women's Health.* (2002). Office on Women's Health.

7. Office of Research on Women's Health, National Institutes of Health. *Overview.* Available online: http://orwh.od.nih.gov/about.html.

8. Legato, M. J. (1998). Belling the cat: clinical investigation in vulnerable populations (a good idea, but who's going to volunteer?). *Journal of Gender-Specific Medicine* 1(2).

9. Owens, N. J., and Hume, A. L. (1994). Pharmacotherapy in women: do clinically important gender-related issues exist? *Rhode Island Medicine* 77: 412–416.

10. Merkatz, R. B., Temple, R., Sobel, S., et al. (1993). Women in clinical trials of new drugs: a change in the FDA. *New England Journal of Medicine* 329: 292–296.

11. FDA Backgrounder. (1994). *Food and Drug Administration's Role in Women's Health Issues.*

12. Holmer, A. F. (2001). *New Medicines in Development for Women.* Presented by America's Pharmaceutical Companies.

13. National Cancer Institute. (2002). *Clinical Trials and Insurance Coverage—A Resource Guide: Summary.*

14. Howe, J., and Bass, M. (1999). Including women in clinical trials: the need for insurance coverage. *Journal of Gender-Specific Medicine* 2(4).

15. Center for Reproductive Rights. (2003). *The Bush Global Gag Rule: Endangering Women's Health, Free Speech and Democracy.* Item: F033.

16. U.S. Census Bureau, Population Division, Population Projections Branch. (2002).

17. Rios, E. V., and Simpson, C. E. (1998). Curriculum enhancement in medical education: teaching cultural competence and women's health for a changing society. *Journal of American Medical Women's Association* 53(3).

18. Pardes, H. (1998). Changing medical education for the 21st century. *Proceedings of the National Conference on Cultural Competence and Women's Health Curriculum in Medical Education.* Washington, DC: U.S. Department of Health and Human Services, II-4.

19. United Nations Women Watch. (2000). *The 4 Global Women's Conferences, 1975–1995: Historical Perspective.* United Nations Department of Public Information: DPI/2035/M.

Chapter Two

The Economics of Women's Health

Chapter Objectives

On completion of this chapter, the student should be able to discuss:

1. The third-party payer system.

2. The fee-for-service model versus managed care.

3. Factors to consider when choosing an insurance plan.

4. Types of public health insurance, including Medicare and Medicaid.

5. The significant risks associated with being uninsured.

6. Ways that women as healthcare consumers affect demand within the healthcare system.

7. Healthcare reform and the arguments for and against a universal health system.

8. The financial burden of aging and how it disproportionately affects women.

9. Long-term care and its associated costs.

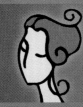

womenshealth.jbpub.com

Women's Health Online is a great source for supplementary women's health information for both students and instructors. Visit

http://womenshealth.jbpub.com to find a variety of useful tools for learning, thinking, and teaching.

Introduction

In the United States, the economics of health care—how it is financed, what the individual's responsibility for payment is, which services should be paid for, and which social factors influence the availability of care—are the key issues behind most healthcare-related decision making and policy. Participants in the healthcare system, including physicians, patients, hospitals, health insurers, health education firms, and pharmaceutical, medical device, and diagnostic companies, all work to shape the direction of health care. Although most individuals believe that all people have a right to health care, significant debate has arisen regarding the best pathway to achieving that goal.

Increasingly, health care is becoming a consumer- or patient-oriented industry. As in other markets, goods and services are being developed to court consumers and drive demand for specific services. At the center of the healthcare paradigm, the patient is becoming a vital healthcare decision maker and is increasingly being targeted by information on diseases and available treatments. Patients are showing a growing willingness to shop around for different providers, an increasing demand for wide access to services, and a growing eagerness to pursue litigation in cases of perceived substandard care.

Understanding the effects of women's growing economic power on women's health and the persistent limitations that marginalized women face in accessing quality women's health care is critical. A discussion of the way in which the healthcare system is funded identifies how the system functions and leads to an examination of the factors that create inequities in women's health care. Other important issues include the economics of aging and the effects of an aging population on women's health, public policy that influences the economics of health care, and the roles that women as caregivers have in the delivery of health care.

Paying for Health Care

Health care functions within the parameters of a market setting, offering goods and services that carry costs to healthcare consumers and patients. Unlike in other markets, like real estate or retail, all individuals are healthcare consumers at one stage or another of their lives. People do not have control over the degree to which they need to interact with the healthcare system in the same way that they do when deciding whether to purchase a TV. If a woman has heart disease and needs to go to a cardiologist, she has very little choice except to purchase the services needed or go without care. In addition, a patient must trust her physician to tell her which goods and services she needs instead of making that decision on her own. The necessity of health care, and an individual's inability to have full information to make purchasing choices, make health care a unique market from an economic perspective.

In the United States, the healthcare system is based on a **third-party payer system** in which most individuals do not pay directly for the delivery of care (Figure 2.1). Instead, many have health insurance, which, in return for a monthly or yearly payment called a premium, provides coverage for health-related goods and

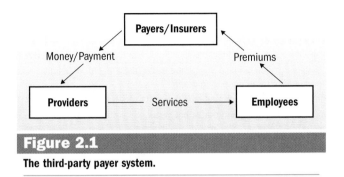

Figure 2.1
The third-party payer system.

services. Before third-party payers became a mainstay of the U.S. system, patients would pay out-of-pocket for health care, either to their doctor or to hospitals. Medical care was purchased and delivered much like most other commodities. Private health insurance was introduced in the early 1930s as a method to minimize the risk associated with hospital care costs. At that time, if an individual became sick or was injured on the job, the financial repercussions of paying for medical care could be significant. In response, health insurance was developed and based on an **indemnity** or **fee-for-service** system. Through this system, hospitals were reimbursed by health insurers based on a list of charges for services rendered. As the third-party payer system matured, it grew to include fee-for-service payments to physicians and other outpatient providers of health care (Table 2.1).

Today, most people (71%) are covered by private health insurance either provided by their employer or purchased individually. Much of private health insurance is now structured within a managed care plan. **Managed care** was introduced

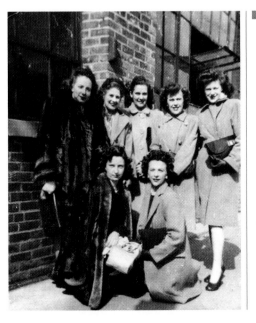

Before World War II, few Americans had health insurance.

Employment-based health benefit programs have existed in the United States for more than 100 years. In the 1870s, for example, railroad, mining, and other industries began to provide the services of company doctors to workers. In 1910, Montgomery Ward entered into one of the earliest group insurance contracts. Prior to World War II, few Americans had health insurance, and most policies covered only hospital room, board, and ancillary services. During World War II, the number of persons with employment-based health insurance coverage started to increase for several reasons. When wages were frozen by the National War Labor Board and a shortage of workers occurred, employers sought ways to get around the wage controls in order to attract scarce workers, and offering health insurance was one option. Health insurance was an attractive means to recruit and retain workers during a labor shortage for two reasons: unions supported employment-based health insurance, and workers' health benefits were not subject to income tax or Social Security payroll taxes, as were cash wages. Under the current tax code, health insurance premiums paid by employers are deductible for employers as a business expense, and are excluded, without limit, from workers' taxable income.[1]

Table 2.1   Paying for Health Care Timeline

1900s:
- American Medical Association (AMA) becomes a powerful national force.
- In 1901, AMA reorganizes as the national organization of state and local associations. Membership increases from about 8,000 physicians in 1900 to 70,000 in 1910—half the physicians in the country. This period is the beginning of "organized medicine."
- Doctors are no longer expected to provide free services to all hospital patients.
- America lags behind European countries in finding value in insuring against the costs of sickness.
- Railroads are the leading industry to develop extensive employee medical programs.

1910s
- American hospitals are now modern scientific institutions, valuing antiseptics and cleanliness, and using medications for the relief of pain.
- American Association for Labor Legislation (AALL) organizes first national conference on "social insurance."
- Progressive reformers argue for health insurance and seem to be gaining support.
- Opposition from physicians and other interest groups, plus the entry of the United States into the war in 1917, undermine the reform effort.

1920s
- Consistent with the general mood of political complacency, there is no strong effort to change health insurance.
- Reformers now emphasize the cost of medical care instead of wages lost to sickness. The relatively higher cost of medical care is a new and dramatic development, especially for the middle class.
- The cultural influence of the medical profession grows—physicians' incomes are higher and prestige is established.
- General Motors signs a contract with Metropolitan Life to insure 180,000 workers.
- Penicillin is discovered. It will be 20 years before this antibiotic is used to combat infection and disease.

1930s
- The Depression changes priorities, with greater emphasis being placed on unemployment insurance and "old age" benefits.
- The Social Security Act is passed, omitting health insurance.
- There is a push for health insurance within the Roosevelt Administration, but politics begins to be influenced by internal government conflicts over priorities.
- Against the advice of insurance professionals, Blue Cross begins offering private coverage for hospital care in dozens of states.

1940s
- Prepaid group health care begins; it is seen as radical.
- During World War II, wage and price controls are placed on American employers. To compete for workers, companies begin to offer health benefits, giving rise to the employer-based system in place today.
- President Roosevelt asks Congress for an "economic bill of rights," including the right to adequate medical care.
- President Truman offers a national health program plan, proposing a single system that would include all of American society.
- Truman's plan is denounced by the American Medical Association (AMA), and is called a Communist plot by a House subcommittee.

1950s
- At the start of the decade, national healthcare expenditures are 4.5% of the gross national product.
- Attention turns to the Korean War and away from health reform; America will have a system of private insurance for those who can afford it and welfare services for the poor.
- Federal responsibility for the sick poor is firmly established.
- Many legislative proposals are made for different approaches to hospital insurance, but none succeeds.
- Many more medications are available now to treat a range of diseases, including infections, glaucoma, and arthritis, and new vaccines become available that prevent dreaded childhood diseases, including polio. The first successful organ transplant is performed.

Source: Adapted from *Healthcare Crisis: Who's at Risk?* Healthcare Timeline, PBS. Produced by Issues TV, 2000. Reprinted with permission.

(continued)

1960s
- In the 1950s, the price of hospital care doubled. In the early 1960s, those outside the workplace, and especially the elderly, have difficulty affording insurance.
- More than 700 insurance companies sell health insurance.
- Concern about a "doctor shortage" and the need for more "health manpower" leads to federal measures to expand education in the health professions.
- Major medical insurance endorses high-cost medicine.
- President Lyndon Johnson signs Medicare and Medicaid into law.
- "Compulsory Health Insurance" advocates are no longer optimistic.
- The number of doctors reporting themselves to be full-time specialists grows from 55% in 1960 to 69% by 1969.

1970s
- President Richard Nixon renames prepaid group healthcare plans as health maintenance organizations (HMOs), with legislation that provides federal endorsement, certification, and assistance to them.
- Healthcare costs are escalating rapidly, partly due to unexpectedly high Medicare expenditures, rapid inflation in the economy, expansion of hospital expenses and profits, and changes in medical care, including greater use of technology, medications, and conservative approaches to treatment. American medicine is now seen as in crisis.
- President Nixon's plan for national health insurance is rejected by liberals and labor unions, but his "War on Cancer" centralizes research at NIH.
- The number of women entering the medical profession rises dramatically. In 1970, 9% of medical students are women; by the end of the decade, the proportion exceeds 25%.

1980s
- Corporations begin to integrate the hospital system (previously a decentralized structure), enter many other healthcare-related businesses, and consolidate control. Overall, there is a shift toward privatization and corporatization of health care.
- Under President Reagan, Medicare shifts to payment by diagnosis (DRG) instead of by treatment. Private plans quickly follow suit.
- Growing complaints are voiced by insurance companies that the traditional fee-for-service method of payment to doctors is being exploited.
- "Capitation" payments to doctors become more common.

1990s
- Healthcare costs rise at double the rate of inflation.
- Expansion of managed care helps to moderate increases in healthcare costs.
- Federal healthcare reform legislation fails again to pass in the U.S. Congress.
- By the end of the decade 44 million Americans, 16% of the nation, have no health insurance at all.
- The Human Genome Project to identify all of the more than 100,000 genes in human DNA gets under way.
- By June 1990, 139,765 people in the United States have HIV/AIDS, with a 60% mortality rate.

2000s
- Healthcare costs are on the rise again.
- Medicare is viewed by some as unsustainable under the present structure and must be "rescued."
- Changing demographics of the workplace lead many to believe the employer-based system of insurance cannot last.
- The Human Genome Project was expected to be completed a full two years ahead of schedule, in 2003.
- Direct-to-consumer advertising for pharmaceuticals and medical devices is on the rise.
- Medicare expands to include a prescription drug benefit as of January 2006.
- Employers continue to cut down on health insurance benefits in an attempt to address persistent increases in costs.
- Medical savings accounts become common.

It's Your Health

Drive-Through Deliveries

In the 1990s, HMOs and other managed care plans shortened average maternity stays for normal births. Such programs were dubbed "drive-through deliveries." Because women were being discharged from hospitals only 24 to 48 hours after giving birth, many lawmakers, alarmed that the practice would endanger newborns, adopted laws to require insurance coverage for at least 48 hours of care after delivery.

In a study conducted at Harvard Medical School, researchers found that newborns needed the same number of later emergency room visits and hospital readmissions, regardless of whether they had longer initial stays or shorter ones. In essence, the shorter stays were not adding risk to the newborns, even though the "common sense" of many women and legislators suggested that it would. The study looked at 20,366 normal deliveries in the 1990s. During the period studied, newborn visits to emergency rooms kept steady at an average of about 1% every three months. Hospital readmissions hovered around 1.5%. The same pattern held for a more vulnerable group of young, lower-income mothers with less education.

In an article on this subject published by the Associated Press (December 18, 2002), Larry Akey, a spokesman for the Health Insurance Association of America, said that short-stay programs were designed "not entirely as cost-saving measures, but an opportunity for the mother to get home" faster. The debate continues among women's advocacy groups, health insurers, and hospitals.

as a method to control costs by changing how the delivery of care is coordinated and how health care is reimbursed. In contrast to a fee-for-service model, managed care requires patients to go to specific providers, have access to care only when certain criteria are met, and, in some cases, the payer pays physicians a lump sum for all care delivered as opposed to a fee for each service rendered. Managed care has been perceived both as a driver of positive change by keeping costs down and providing broad access to services and as a villain by placing limits on care. It is blamed for decreased access to care, shorter physician office visits, higher co-payments, and more restrictions on which doctors patients can see. Managed care is not a static concept; in fact, the types of products that are offered are continually evolving to meet the changing needs and demands of patients, employers, and providers.

The limitations on access that lead patients and physicians to vilify managed care ended up slowing the rate at which health-related expenditures grew in the United States in the 1990s (see Figure 2.2). This goal was accomplished by managed care organizations asking for more stringent proof of medical necessity before services are paid for—for example, by requiring physicians to get prior authorizations from the payer before certain care is rendered. Another method for controlling costs has been to allow members to get care only from a specific network of physicians who have contracted with the payers to offer low-cost care, or to make

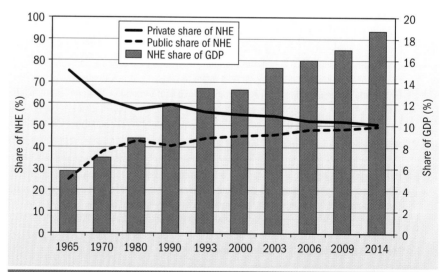

Figure 2.2

National Health Expenditures (NHE) Share of Gross Domestic Product (GDP) and Private and Public Shares of NHE, 1965–2014.

Note: The left axis (public and private spending's share of NHE) relates to the two line graphs. The rights axis (NHE's share of GDP) relates to the gray-shaded bars. Data for 2006, 2009, and 2014 are projections.

Source: Centers for Medicare & Medicaid Services, Office of the Actuary, National Health Statistics Group.

patients pay higher co-payments if they see doctors who are not members of the network. By controlling the supply of healthcare resources, however, managed care organizations have been able to provide patients with access to a wider range of services at a relatively reasonable cost, such as pharmaceuticals and rehabilitation services, than fee-for-service models are now able to offer. More recently, health care as a share of the gross domestic product (GDP) has begun to rise fairly rapidly.

Managed care plans differ based on the level to which they control what services are provided to patients. Types of managed care plans include preferred provider organizations (PPOs), health maintenance organizations (HMOs), and point-of-service (POS) plans. Table 2.2 describes the various types of managed care plans. Almost all health insurers today offer some form of managed care products or include elements of managed care products such as physician networks or tiered co-payments into their existing product lines.

In paying for health care, insurers decide which types of services they will cover (see Figure 2.3). Hospital care, outpatient care, physician office visits, diagnostic tests, preventive services, prescription drugs, mental health services, durable medical equipment like wheelchairs, and home health care are all elements of health care that most people would consider important; however, all of these are separate services that may or may not be covered under a given insurance plan. As patient demand evolves, many alternative therapies and preventive care services, such as massage, acupuncture, and chiropractic care, are beginning to be covered by health insurance.

Table 2.2 Types of Managed Care Plans

Health Maintenance Organization (HMO): An HMO is a managed care plan that offers a full range of services for a fixed prepaid fee, rather than charging patients for each service provided. Patients normally pay only a small co-payment for care. With some plans and for some services, patients also have to satisfy a deductible. Usually, patients don't have to file claims.

HMO plans typically fall into one of two categories:

- **Staff Model:** A staff model HMO has salaried physicians who provide services only to plan members. They offer care at a hospital, clinic, or health center in the community.

- **Independent Practice Association (IPA):** An IPA maintains contracts with a number of physicians and/or physician group practices. These physicians see patients in their own offices.

Point-of-Service (POS) Plan: POS plans function much like IPAs. Patients select a primary care physician who coordinates all care within the participating provider network, including specialist referrals.

Preferred Provider Organization (PPO): A PPO plan functions much like a POS plan, but it eliminates the primary care physician. As with the POS plan, patients can use a healthcare provider outside of the preferred provider network for an additional cost. Patients can usually see any participating provider—whether a primary care physician or a specialist—without a referral, at no additional cost.

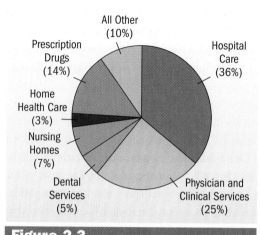

Figure 2.3

National health expenditures, 2006.

Source: Centers for Medicare & Medicaid Services;
National Health Expenditure Data Projections, 2004–2014.

Choosing an Insurance Plan

When people choose between different insurance options, their choices are often influenced by which services are covered or what percentage of the total cost the insurer will pay. If a woman thinks that she is unlikely to use many services, as a 26-year-old woman without any existing medical conditions might, she may opt for a less expensive insurance program like an HMO that has more restricted coverage. Regardless of the insurance program selected, an individual is at significant financial risk if her insurance does not cover or only partially covers the services that she uses. This issue commonly arises with individuals who have mental health problems that require ongoing outpatient psychotherapy. Many health insurers do not cover psychotherapy, or cover only a limited number of visits per year, leaving the individual responsible for paying for the care out-of-pocket. The inability to pay for health care, beyond insurance premiums, leads many people to avoid going to the doctor when necessary or to cut short therapy if it becomes too expensive.

As a method to manage rising costs, patients are increasingly being required to pay out-of-pocket for a portion of their health care. A **co-payment** (or **co-pay**) is the amount of money that a patient is responsible for paying to receive healthcare services. Co-pays can be either a fixed amount of money, like a $5 or $10 co-pay for a routine office visit, or a percentage of the overall charge for a given service (referred to as a co-insurance), like the popular 80% covered/20% patient responsibility payment schemes.

With prescription drugs, many payers have introduced a tiered co-pay system, in which different levels of payment are required for different types of medications. Most tiered co-pays try to reward patients for purchasing lower-cost generic drugs, as opposed to more expensive brand-name drugs. **Generic drugs** are the chemical equivalents of brand-name drugs, but are far less expensive. Within a tiered co-pay

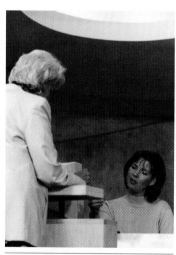

■ A co-pay is the amount of money that a patient is responsible for paying to receive healthcare services; co-pays are either a fixed amount of money or a percentage of the overall charge for a given service.

system, for example, a patient may pay $5 for a generic antibiotic, $15 for a preferred brand-name drug, and $25 for the premium-cost brand-name drug. Women often are forced to expend significant co-pays for birth control pills, with many prescriptions falling into the highest co-pay tier. As a result, a woman may have to pay $20 to $40 per month to control her fertility. Health insurers have lists of drugs for which they provide reimbursement called **formularies,** which describe to patients and doctors which drugs are covered, into which tier each drug falls, and how much each drug will cost the patient.

Out-of-pocket costs to women continue to be a significant barrier to appropriate care and compliance with taking medication. A report by the Kaiser Family Foundation found that one in five (21%) non-elderly women did not fill a prescription because of the cost, compared with 13% of men.[1] This issue was also a problem for 40% of uninsured women, 27% of women with Medicaid, and 15% of privately insured women.

Types of Health Insurance

Employer-sponsored health insurance, as well as health insurance purchased by individuals, is considered **private health insurance.** Most private health insurance in the United States is purchased and subsidized by employers. When an individual has a full-time job, health insurance is often a central benefit. Employer-sponsored health insurance can often be extended to cover the family of the insured individual.

Public health insurance is insurance provided by the government. The federal government is the largest health insurer in the United States through its Medicare, Medicaid, Veterans Administration, Department of Defense, and Bureau of Indian Affairs insurance programs (see Figure 2.4). Medicare is the result

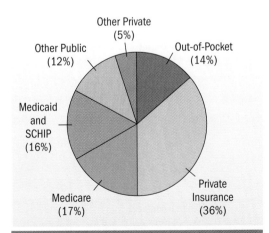

Figure 2.4

The U.S. health dollar, 2003: where it came from.

Source: Stephen Heffler, Sheila Smith, Sean Keehan, Christine Borger, M. Kent Clemens, and Christopher Truffer, *Health Affairs Trends: U.S. Health Spending Projections for 2004-2014,* February 23, 2005.

■ Due to the aging population and the fact that women live longer than men, an increasing majority of Medicare beneficiaries are women.

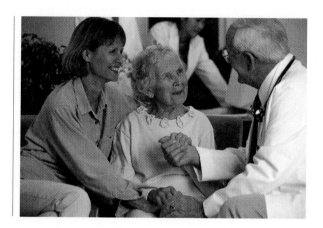

of a bill enacted by Congress in 1965 to provide health insurance at a reasonable cost to Americans aged 65 and older. Medicare is provided in several parts:

- Part A is provided to all enrollees and covers inpatient hospitalization.
- Part B is optional and covers outpatient services.
- Part D is optional and covers a portion of prescription drug costs.

Since 1965, the program has grown to cover disabled individuals and patients with end-stage renal disease. Most recently, it has grown to include a portion of prescription drug coverage. Medicare's prescription drug coverage is expected to have a significant impact on who pays for prescription drugs in the United Staates (see Figure 2.5). Today, Medicare is the largest single insurer in the United States,

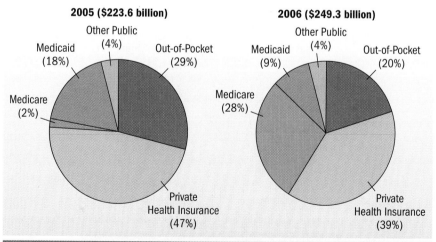

Figure 2.5

Projected prescription drug spending, by payer, 2005 and 2006.

Source: Centers for Medicare & Medicaid Services, Office of the Actuary, National Health Statistics Group.

covering more than 40 million people. Due to the aging of the population and the fact that women live longer than men, an increasing majority of Medicare beneficiaries are women (see Figure 2.6).

Medicaid is a program jointly administered by federal and state governments that provides health insurance for low-income Americans. Whereas Medicare is a federally controlled health system, Medicaid is largely run at the state level. In some states, such as California and Tennessee, Medicaid has a state-specific name (MediCal, TennCare). The vast majority of Medicaid recipients are low-income women and their children; the children are covered through State Children's Health Insurance Programs (SCHIPs). Medicaid and the benefits it provides are fundamental to the provision of health care to economically disadvantaged women and children in the United States.

Currently, Medicaid covers nearly 40 million people. Individuals qualify based on income status, level of disability or need for long-term care, or by being a dependent of a Medicaid recipient. Medicaid is accepted as a payment method by all hospitals and most physicians, although some private physicians refuse Medicaid patients due to the lower reimbursement rates the system provides as compared to private insurance. All states cover the following basic services for Medicaid recipients:

- Inpatient and outpatient medical care
- Laboratory and X-ray services
- Chronic care facilities for persons older than 21 years

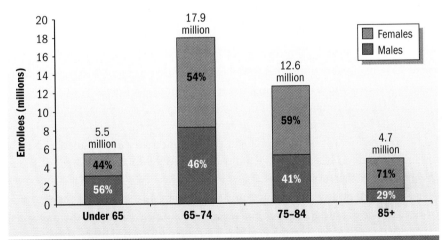

Figure 2.6

Age and gender of the Medicare population, 2000. The proportion of women increases as the population grows older.

Note: Fifty-six percent (23 million) of all Medicare beneficiaries are female, 44% (18 million) are males. Data reflect Medicare beneficiaries ever enrolled in the program during the year.

Source: Centers for Medicare and Medicaid Services Office of the Actuary. National Health Statistics Group, January 2005.

- Home health care for those eligible for nursing facility services
- Services provided by a physician or nurse practitioner
- Necessary transportation

States may provide optional services to eligible patients, including prescription drugs, case management, dental care, prosthetic devices, medical transportation, intermediate care facilities, optometry, and tuberculosis-related services. Federal law requires the delivery of services that are "medically necessary," but states exercise substantial independence in determining the amount and duration of services covered by establishing criteria for medical necessity and utilization control.

In addition to Medicare and Medicaid, the federal government provides health insurance to veterans through the Veterans Administration (VA), active-service military personnel through the Department of Defense (DOD), government workers through the government's own health insurance program, and Native Americans through the Indian Health Services. These programs are all separately administered and have differing organizational structures. For example, the VA is not only a payer for health care, but also a network of providers. Veterans covered within this system are eligible for care at VA hospitals and clinics. This approach is similar to how the DOD provides health insurance and healthcare services to active-duty military personnel.

Uninsured Americans

In addition to those people with private insurance and those with public insurance, 45.8 million Americans were uninsured for all of 2004[2]—more than the populations of Texas, Florida, and Connecticut combined (Figure 2.7). According to a report by the Robert Wood Johnson Foundation, 74.7 million people were uninsured at one point during 2001–2002. That means that close to one in three Americans were uninsured for all or part of that period. Of those 74.7 million people, two-thirds were uninsured for six months or longer. [3]

Like Medicaid recipients, the uninsured are largely (58%) women and children. These individuals are more likely to have poorer health, have significantly less access to care, and die prematurely than their counterparts with insurance. Nearly one in five families has at least one uninsured member. Most uninsured individuals are younger than age 30.

People without health insurance are at significant financial risk if they get sick or have an accident that requires emergency medical care. Because the uninsured must pay out-of-pocket for medical services, such as doctors' office visits or prescription drugs, they often avoid preventive care or proper follow-up care due to cost concerns. In addition, the uninsured end up paying more for medical care because they are not eligible for the discounted pricing structures that health insurance companies negotiate with hospitals and doctors. As a result, the cost of care often strains family finances, jeopardizing families' physical, emotional, and economic health.[4] Long-term implications from being uninsured may include worsening of health status due to lack of appropriate care and not being accurately monitored by a physician, leading to suboptimal care.

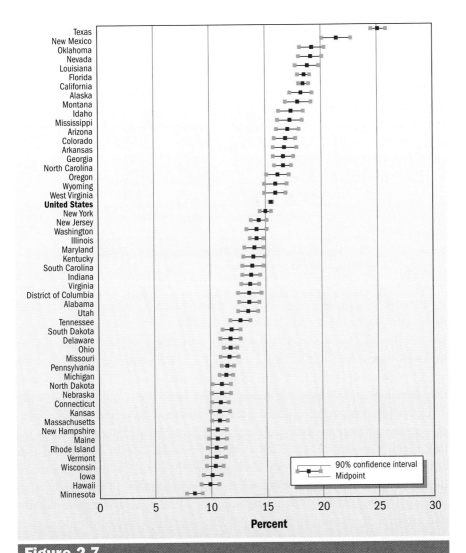

Figure 2.7

Percentage of people without health insurance coverage, by state, 2002–2004.

Source: U.S. Census Bureau, Current Population Survey, 2003 to 2005 Annual Social and Economic Supplements.

Minorities, including African Americans and Hispanic Americans, have higher rates of uninsurance than white or Asian Americans (see Figure 2.8). Although lower-income people have the highest rates of being uninsured, the profile of who lacks health insurance is changing. The largest increases in 2001 were seen in the $75,000-plus income bracket, making lack of insurance an increasingly middle-class issue. In this same time period, unemployment increased significantly due to a weakening U.S. economy and rising healthcare costs for employers; as a result, many individuals who were formerly covered by their employers suddenly lost their

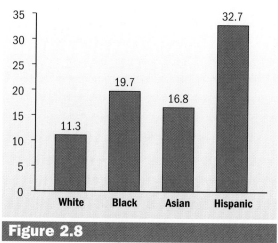

Figure 2.8

Rates of uninsurance by race.

Source: National Center for Health Statistics, *Health, United States 2004*.

health insurance. A decline in coverage through employer-based health plans, rising out-of-pocket costs associated with these plans, and skyrocketing costs for insurance premiums are seen as major drivers of this trend.

Lack of health insurance affects access to health services and contributes to poorer health, higher hospitalization rates, and more advanced disease states by the time health services are finally received. While more than 1 in 10 children still lack health coverage, the expansion of Medicaid and the State Children's Health Insurance Program is helping to keep the number of uninsured children steady at 8.5 million.[3] Overall, the scope of the uninsured problem is vast and requires significant attention by the American public if the goals related to equity in delivery of and access to health care are to be achieved.

Preventive Care and a Focus on Women's Health

Managed care plans have been successful at using evidence-based medicine and economic analysis to determine the value of new medical technologies, procedures, and drugs to the plan and its members. A positive outcome of this trend has been widespread support for many preventive services, such as mammograms, cervical cancer screening, and smoking cessation programs. The old saying that "an ounce of prevention is worth a pound of cure" has been proven true in most studies. (See Chapter 3 for more on primary, secondary, and tertiary prevention.) Payers have been shown that investing in preventive services and education leads both to members with fewer major medical problems, such as heart disease, and to the ability to diagnose diseases, such as breast cancer, at an earlier stage. Through their positive effects on healthcare outcomes, many preventive and educational services have shown their ability to decrease overall healthcare costs.

Preventive services and health education are the cornerstones of women's health. As awareness and support of these and other women-specific health issues increase, many payers have established whole departments dedicated to women's health. These departments help to ensure that patients and physicians are educated about best practices and newly available treatments specifically for women; they also analyze the benefits of new technologies. Women's health departments within payer organizations have enjoyed success in prioritizing women's health issues—for example, by supporting prenatal check-ups and strict monitoring regimens for pregnant women, promoting women's cardiac health, and ensuring universal coverage of gynecological exams.

Women as Healthcare Consumers

Women have been recognized as the primary decision makers relating to health care and as a growing economic force to be courted. In one large survey, women were reported to make 90% of health-related decisions for their families.[5] As a group, women have seen their economic power and ability to affect the overall demand within the healthcare system increase significantly. They have increased their participation in the workforce, in government, and in decision-making positions over the last 40 years. In the United States, women earn more than $1 trillion annually, and according to a study by the Commonwealth Institute, more than 68% of women say they manage the bills in their household, compared to 55% of men. Women's growing economic power has made them increasingly important in the eyes of pharmaceutical, medical device, and diagnostics manufacturers. More and more, research and development dollars are being poured into discovering both necessary and voluntary treatments for women. In addition, women are taking a more active role in their own health care, by learning more about their health status, by taking part in preventive health care, and by articulating their needs to providers, payers, manufacturers, and legislatures. Together, these factors work to raise awareness of women's health issues and force the healthcare industry to make women's health a priority.

Although women's overall economic position has been improving, many women still find themselves in economically disadvantaged circumstances. Whether due to being unemployed or underemployed, not having adequate childcare support, lacking education, being in poor health, lacking access to resources, or just not having adequate support, they do not have the decision-making freedom that other women with greater access to resources enjoy. Today, lower-income women are disproportionately affected by poor health. Those women with the least resources thus carry the largest burden of healthcare costs, disability, and responsibility in caring for others. Women with health problems often have the most difficult time obtaining care because of coverage restrictions, high costs, and logistical barriers, such as transportation. For many women, coverage and access to care are unstable. Health coverage, involvement with health plans, and relationships with doctors are often short lived, resulting in spotty and fragmented care. A survey by the Kaiser Family Foundation found that one quarter (24%) of non-elderly women delayed or went without care in the past year because they could not afford it, compared with 16% of men.[6]

Healthcare Reform

In many countries, such as Canada and the United Kingdom, the government provides health insurance to all citizens through a system of **universal health insurance.** Universal healthcare systems are aimed at allowing all citizens access to a minimum level of care that is deemed acceptable. Individuals are then allowed to purchase supplementary insurance to pay for items not covered under the national health systems. Proponents of these types of systems argue that health care is a right, not a privilege, and should therefore be available to all citizens. Their opponents counter that universal health care is an overly costly approach and prefer that the private sector manage and fund health care through a free-market approach. In the early 1990s, President Bill Clinton led a major drive for establishing universal health insurance in the United States. Although those efforts ultimately failed, healthcare reform has remained a major political topic. (See **It's Your Health** for more information.)

In the future, health care is likely to be significantly affected by the research and development of new technologies. Major advances in women's health issues are likely to arise from research into genetic engineering, stem cell research, microscopic surgical techniques, and molecular diagnostics. How the system will pay for these advancements and make them accessible to the majority of people remains a challenge.

■ Healthcare reform is a major political topic in the United States.

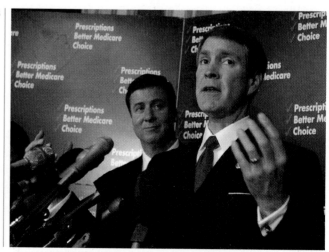

It's Your Health

Universal Health Care

The lack of healthcare coverage is detrimental to individuals, their families, and the community at large. Due to the high costs of health care, uninsured individuals and their families have difficulties getting quality health care when they are sick. They tend to delay treatments until their illnesses become serious, and they are less likely to seek routine preventive health services that can avert or detect major illnesses early on. As a result, they tend to die sooner than people with health insurance.

The lack of health insurance aggravates the financial burden placed on the community as a whole. Because the uninsured tend to delay necessary treatment, they are often sicker and therefore more expensive to treat when they finally seek care. Also, they frequently turn to the nearest hospital emergency room, which is an expensive and inefficient way to get care. Furthermore, the primary providers of care to the uninsured—such as public hospitals, teaching hospitals, academic health centers, and nonprofit community hospitals—incur heavy losses from high rates of uncompensated care. In turn, these providers are forced to cut back on their services to all patients or even close their facilities.

The American Public Health Association has advocated the following:

- Universal coverage for everyone in the United States, to include comprehensive benefits, affordable prices, and quality services

- Organization and administration of health care through publicly accountable mechanisms to assure maximum responsiveness to public needs, with a major role for federal, state, and local government health agencies

- Attention in the organization, staffing, delivery, and payment of care to the needs of all populations, including those confronting geographic, physical, cultural, language, and other nonfinancial barriers to service.

Source: American Public Health Association; www.apha.org. Related APHA Policy: Support for a New Campaign for Universal Health Care. 20007, 9502. Accessed Jan. 1, 2000.

To ensure the ongoing improvement of our healthcare system in general, and in women's health issues in particular, healthcare reform must take into account the disparities in care and outcomes related to the socioeconomic positions of patients. The American public must identify their priorities as they relate to health care, whether that entails equity, access to new technology, or improved outcomes. Reform should attempt to manage rising costs while recognizing and addressing the diverse needs of women within the system.

Economics and Aging

The population of the United States is getting older as disease prevention, health promotion, and innovative treatments prevent or delay disease and prolong life. In 2004, the average life expectancy for all Americans was 77.3 years of age: 74.5 years for men and 79.9 years for women.[7] On average, women now live six years longer than men. In 2000, there were only 70 men per 100 women over age 65; there were only 41 men per 100 women aged 85 or older (see Figure 2.9). Note, however, that these figures are an aggregate of all American women.

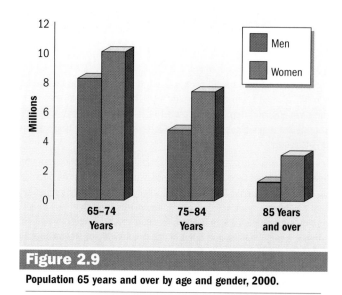

Figure 2.9

Population 65 years and over by age and gender, 2000.

Source: U.S. Census Bureau, U.S. Census 2000 Summary File.

When examined by race and ethnicity, life expectancy varies among both women and men.

As a result, the majority of the burden of aging rests on women, and increasingly women are aging into their oldest years without the support or help of spouses.[8] The aging trends have enormous economic ramifications. As women age, they become increasingly more likely to suffer from chronic disease such as heart disease, cancer, and arthritis. These illnesses create significant morbidity as well as costs to affected individuals.[9] Currently, Medicare provides health insurance for all Americans over the age of 65, ensuring that all older Americans have at least some access to health care. Because Medicare covers only 80% of costs, however, a significant financial burden is often imposed on older patients when seeking care.[10]

The economic realities faced by elderly women can have a significant impact on women's health. As women age, they are likely to need increased access to prescription drugs, perhaps specialty medical assistance, durable medical equipment (such as walkers and orthopedic beds), and other expensive goods and services. A survey of 2,380 elderly California residents by the Kaiser Family Foundation and Tufts Medical School found that nearly one in five California seniors (18%) was without drug coverage in 2001. Roughly the same number said they did not fill a prescription or skipped doses of a prescribed medication to make their medications last longer. Higher rates of such behavior were reported among seniors in poor health and those without drug coverage. In an effort to decrease their out-of-pocket drug costs, nearly 20% of those studied were putting themselves at increased health risks by not taking their medication correctly. This behavior leads to increased illness and disability among seniors, and increases costs to the healthcare system as

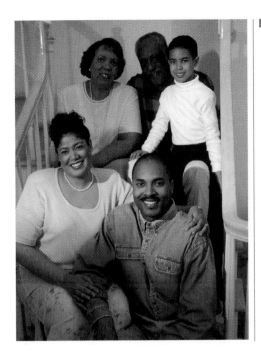

■ Many women are "sandwiched" with requirements for elder care and child care.

a whole. It remains to be seen whether the new Medicare Part D prescription drug benefit will mitigate this problem.

Taking Care of the Population: Long-Term Care and Women as Caregivers

Once an individual or her family becomes unable to take care of an elderly or disabled person any longer, long-term care or assisted living communities are available. In direct correlation to the percentage of women and men in the oldest age categories, the vast majority of residents in these facilities are women.

Long-term care provides ongoing care for people who need lengthy or even lifelong assistance with daily living due to an illness, injury, or severe cognitive impairment (such as Alzheimer's disease). It can be provided either in a nursing home, assisted living facility, or at the patient's home. According to the Federal Long-Term Care Insurance Program, sponsored by the U.S. Office of Personnel Management, the average annual cost for home care substantially exceeds $20,000. The national average annual cost for care in a nursing home exceeds $74,000 for a private and $64,000 for a semi-private room, according to a recent survey by MetLife's LifePlans in 2005. This was an increase of 6% from the year before. Costs are expected to continue to increase dramatically.[11] Two insurance options are available to cover these expenses:

- Private long-term care insurance programs are very expensive, and are predominantly purchased by wealthier Americans.

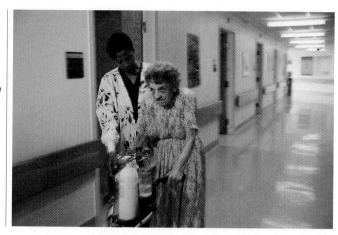

■ Most older women in nursing homes spend down their life savings to pay for services until Medicaid begins to cover the remaining costs of care.

- Medicaid covers Americans in long-term care facilities once they have spent out all other resources. Most older women in nursing homes spend down their life savings to pay for services until Medicaid begins to cover the remaining costs of care.

As the U.S. population ages and life spans increase, informal caregiving by family members has become a vital component of the healthcare delivery system in general and elder care in particular. One national study estimates the value of unpaid caregiving at approximately $257 billion per year. That is twice as much as is spent on home care and nursing home servcies.[12] Women continue to provide the majority of this informal caregiving today, even though most working-age women now participate in the labor force. As a result of shouldering the stress and burden for caregiving, women caregivers tend to suffer more adverse health events than non-caregivers. According to the Commonwealth Fund, one-fourth (25%) of women caring for a sick or disabled family member rate their own health as fair or poor, compared with one-sixth (17%) of other women. More than half (54%) of women caregivers have one or more chronic health conditions, compared with two-fifths (41%) of other women. In addition, half (51%) of all caregivers exhibit high depressive symptoms and sleeplessness, while 38% of other women do so.

Informed Decision Making

Choosing health insurance is often a baffling undertaking, with many options meaning little to the individual other than being associated with different monthly premiums. As most people receive their health insurance through their employers, they usually have a small menu of plans from which to pick.

When choosing a health insurance plan, it is important to consider the following:

- **Deductibles.** Often different plans have a certain amount that the individual must pay out-of-pocket before the benefit kicks in. For example, if a woman has a $500 deductible on her insurance plan, she must pay for the first $500 worth of healthcare services she receives before the insurance plan will begin to pick up the cost. Usually, the less expensive the plan, the higher the deductible. Deductibles are common in all types of insurance programs.

- **Benefits.** Look closely at the list of covered services. For example, does the insurance plan cover prescription drugs? Does it cover open access to relevant specialists or provide medical equipment needed for specific health problems?

- **Network.** Consider the implications of a restrictive network to the costs of care and access to care. Does the insurance plan restrict access to a specific network of physicians? Is the preferred doctor a member of that network? If not, what are the costs for going to a doctor that is out of the network? Are the major local hospitals part of the health plan's network?

- **Co-insurance.** Many plans today require patients to pay a set percentage of charges, often 10–20%. While this can keep premiums affordable, patient costs can be very high if hospitalization or long-term care is required. Consumer should inquire whether their insurance plan has a maximum amount that a patient required to pay if a hospitalization or other high-cost event occurs.

- **Emergency Services.** Often health insurance programs have very restrictive criteria for use of emergency services. What is the process for receiving emergency services? Is prior authorization needed before going to the emergency room?

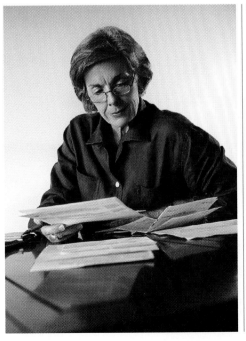

Choice of health insurance plans is often a baffling undertaking; there are many important factors to consider other than simply the monthly premium.

- **Co-payments.** Co-payments are fixed amounts of money a patient is required to pay to receive health-related goods or services. Co-pays usually have to be paid out-of-pocket, either at the doctor's office, at the pharmacy, or at the hospital.

- **Benefit Cap.** Is there a maximum amount of money for which the insurer is liable, after which the patient has to pay for services? This is usually only a concern for very ill people, or people who have very serious accidents.

By considering these factors when choosing health insurance, a woman is more likely to get a package that is right for her and her family.

Summary

The delivery of and access to health care in the United States is significantly affected by the way that it is funded. The U.S. system includes both public and private health insurance that helps individuals to afford high-quality health care. The way that health insurance is structured affects the amount that individuals have to pay out-of-pocket for healthcare goods, such as prescription drugs, and services, such as physician office visits. There are still significant inequity issues within the healthcare system, as demonstrated by the fact that more than 45 million Americans do not have health insurance. Among the elderly population, issues of access to and payment for healthcare goods and services continue to be a major problem. Although most are covered by Medicare and Medicaid, the elderly, who are predominantly women, face a unique set of economic challenges in managing their health.

Topics for Discussion

1. How can a person's health insurance status affect his or her health status?

2. Should everyone have access to health insurance, even if she can't afford it?

3. Is access to health care a right or a privilege?

4. What are some common health-related items that often are not covered by health insurance?

5. What role do employers have in the delivery of health care?

6. What are potential implications of Medicare becoming more like a managed care program and less of a fee-for-service program?

7. How can health insurance status be affected by women's different stages of life?

Profiles of Remarkable Women

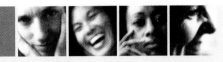

Katherine Swartz (1950–)

Katherine Swartz is a Professor of Health Policy and Economics at the Harvard School of Public Health. She is a demonstrated leader in health policy research, with a focus on the issue of the uninsured. She has been involved in research concerning health insurance issues since she graduated from college and went to work at what was then the U.S. Department of Health, Education, and Welfare (now the Department of Health and Human Services). Particularly for the last 20 years, Prof. Swartz's research interests have focused on the population without health insurance and efforts to increase access to healthcare coverage. Her research contributed to policy makers' understanding that people without health insurance are not all alike—many different types of people lack insurance. Prof. Swartz also was the first researcher to show that people differ in terms of the length of time they may go without health insurance. In fact, many spells without health insurance last less than six months but a significant percentage of uninsured spells last more than two years. The dynamic nature of health insurance coverage means that over the course of a year, many more people are at risk for the financial costs of medical care than the number estimated to be uninsured when a survey is conducted.

Prof. Swartz's interest in how health insurance might be made more affordable and more accessible to the uninsured has led her to analyze the markets for health insurance, particularly for individuals who may not be covered through work in a group insurance plan. This research has focused on insurance companies' fear of being left with the sickest and therefore most expensive people in these markets. Findings from her research have emphasized the need for government policy to reduce such fears so as to allow the nongroup insurance markets to expand health insurance coverage. One such policy that Prof. Swartz has proposed is that government act as the reinsurer and take responsibility for the extremely high-cost people each year in the nongroup markets. Her most recent book, *Reinsuring Health: Why More Middle-Class People Are Uninsured and What Government Can Do*, was published in 2006.

Prof. Swartz has been a member of the faculty in the Department of Health Policy and Management at the Harvard School of Public Health since 1992. Prior to joining the faculty at Harvard, she was with the Urban Institute in Washington, D.C. She also has been on the faculty in the Economics Department of the University of Maryland and was a visiting professor at the Center for Public Policy at Brown University. In November 1995, Swartz became the editor of *Inquiry*, a journal that focuses on healthcare organization and financing. She has a Ph.D. in economics from the University of Wisconsin and a B.S. in economics from the Massachusetts Institute of Technology. Katherine Swartz is married to an economist, and the couple has two grown children.

8. What are some central issues related to the elderly population's healthcare needs?

Web Sites

Academy Health: http://www.academyhealth.org

America's Health Insurance Plans: http://www.ahip.org

Center for Medicare and Medicaid Services: http://www.cms.hhs.gov

Kaiser Family Foundation: http://www.kaisernetwork.org

National Center for Quality Assurance: http://www.ncqa.org

■■■■

References

1. *EBRI Health Benefits Databook,* 1st ed. (1999); *EBRI Databook on Employee Benefits,* 4th ed. (1997); and Field, M. J., and Shapiro, H. T., eds. (1993). *Employment and Health Benefits: A Connection at Risk.* Washington, DC: National Academies Press.

2. U.S. Census Bureau, Population Division, Population Projections Branch. (2005).

3. *Going Without Health Insurance, A Report Prepared by Families USA for the Robert Wood Johnson Foundation.* (March 2003). Publication 03-103.

4. Harris Interactive. (April 11, 2002). *Many Patients Willing to Pay for Online Communication with Physicians.*

5. Pew Foundation. (May 22, 2002). *Vital Decisions: How Internet Users Decide What Information to Trust When They or Their Loved Ones Are Sick.*

6. Salganicoff, A., Beckerman, J. Z., Wyn, R., and Ojeda, V. D. (2002). *Women's Health in the United States: Health Coverage and Access to Care. Kaiser Women's Health Survey May 2002.*

7. National Center for Health Statistics. (2004). *Health, U.S., 2004 with Chartbook on Trends in the Health of Americans.* Hyatville, MD.

8. Schulz, R., and Beach, S.R. (1999). Caregiving as a risk factor for mortality: the Caregiver Health Effects Study. *Journal of the American Medical Association* 282: 2215–2219.

9. *Women and Retirement Security.* (October 27, 1998). Prepared by the National Economic Council Interagency Working Group on Social Security.

10. Collins, K. S. (May 2001). *Midlife Women: Insurance Coverage and Access.* Women's Research and Education Institute.

11. Trevor, T. (October 3, 2005). Average annual nursing home costs hits $74,000, survey finds. National Underwriter Company. *National Underwriter, Life and Health/Financial Services Edition* 10.

12. Arno, P. S. *Economic Value of Informal Caregiving.* Presented at the American Association of Geriatric Psychiatry, February 24, 2002.

Chapter Three

Health Promotion and Disease Prevention

Chapter Objectives

On completion of this chapter, the student should be able to discuss:

1. Concepts of health promotion and disease prevention.

2. Definitions of epidemiology, incidence, prevalence, morbidity, and mortality.

3. Primary, secondary, and tertiary levels of prevention.

4. Diversity of women based on such factors as race, ethnicity, age, and sexual orientation.

5. Diversity as a barrier to healthcare access.

6. Global health issues and the difference in the burden of disease in less economically developed versus more economically developed countries.

7. Differences in life expectancy according to gender and race.

8. Healthcare concerns and preventive measures for adolescents.

9. Healthcare concerns and preventive measures for young adults.

10. Healthcare concerns and preventive measures for women in midlife.

11. Healthcare concerns and preventive measures for senior women.

12. Taking responsibility for one's own health.

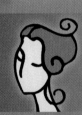

womenshealth.jbpub.com

Women's Health Online is a great source for supplementary women's health information for both students and instructors. Visit

http://womenshealth.jbpub.com to find a variety of useful tools for learning, thinking, and teaching.

Introduction

Being a woman is not a homogenous state. Just as major biological and social differences exist between men and women, so women as a group are made up of many disparate and often overlapping subgroups. These subgroups can be described in any number of ways: racial, ethnic, social, economic, physical, and psychological. In considering women's issues and health-related needs, one should consider these factors:

- The cyclic variability of women of reproductive age
- The changes in women throughout their life span as adolescents, pregnant women, premenopausal women, postmenopausal women, and older women
- The special needs of women of varying racial, ethnic, cultural, socioeconomic, and demographic backgrounds

Mindfulness of women's diversity ensures thorough and equitable analysis of the issues that affect women's lives.

Recognizing the heterogeneity of women is important for understanding the factors that may influence causes, diagnoses, progression, and treatment of disease. These differences create a need for tailored approaches to the delivery of health education and healthcare services. Some women are systematically mistreated or have their needs ignored; examples include women with disabilities or rare diseases, women in prison, and lesbians. This marginalization often prevents their different perspectives from being considered. Certain subgroups of women, such as elderly women, black women, and Hispanic women, are having significant success at getting their voices heard. These women have organized to create a collective voice that is having influence in health-related decision making. The recognition of heterogeneity among women requires an approach to women's health care that addresses a diverse population.

■ Women are not a homogenous population.

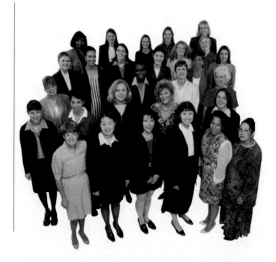

Political Dimensions

There are a number of players in the health system, including government agencies, international agencies, national health education associations, hospitals, and volunteer groups. The federal health infrastructure starts with the Secretary of Health. The Assistant Secretary for Health, who is the principal advisor to the Secretary on public health and scientific issues, is supported by the Surgeon General. The Surgeon General has numerous responsibilities, including protecting and advancing the health of the nation through educating the public; advocating for effective disease prevention and health promotion programs and activities; and providing a highly recognized symbol of national commitment to protecting and improving the public's health. Reports, workshops, conferences, and calls to action from the Surgeon General on various issues, including the adverse health consequences of smoking, nutrition and health, mental health, violence, overweight and obesity, suicide, and sexual health, have heightened awareness of important public health issues and generated major public health initiatives. One of these initiatives, Healthy People 2010, grew out of the 1979 Surgeon General's Report, *Healthy People—The Surgeon General's Report on Health Promotion and Disease Prevention.* Healthy People 2010 is a set of national disease prevention and health promotion objectives for the United States to achieve over the first decade of the new century. States, communities, and professional organizations can use Healthy People 2010 as a basis on which to develop programs to improve health.

The Department of Health and Human Services (HHS) is the U.S. government's principal health agency and includes more than 300 programs. HHS works with state, local, and tribal governments and provides funding for a number of services offered at the local level. The department's programs are administered by 11 HHS operation divisions, including eight agencies in the U.S. Public Health Service and three human service agencies (Figure 3.1).

The eight agencies of the U.S. Public Health Service have differing mandates:

- *National Institutes of Health (NIH).* NIH is the world's premier medical research organization, supporting some 35,000 research projects nationwide in diseases such as cancer, Alzheimer's disease, diabetes, arthritis, cardiovascular disease, and AIDS.

- *Food and Drug Administration (FDA).* FDA assures the safety of foods and cosmetics, and the safety and efficacy of pharmaceuticals, biological products, and medical devices.

- *Centers for Disease Control and Prevention (CDC).* Working with states and other partners, CDC provides a system of health surveillance to monitor and prevent disease outbreaks, implement disease prevention strategies, and maintain national health statistics.

- *Agency for Toxic Substances and Disease Registry (ATSDR).* ATSDR helps prevent exposure to hazardous substances from waste sites on the U.S. Environmental Protection Agency's National Priorities List, and it develops toxicological profiles of chemicals found at these sites.

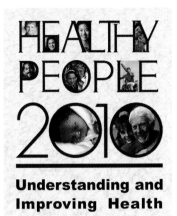

Understanding and Improving Health

Healthy People 2010 is a set of national disease prevention and health promotion objectives for the United States to achieve in the first decade of the century.

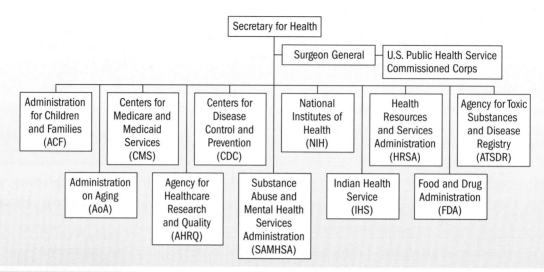

Figure 3.1

The U.S. Department of Health and Human Services (DHHS).

- *Indian Health Service (IHS).* The IHS provides health services to nearly 1.5 million American Indians and Alaska Natives of 557 federally recognized tribes in 35 states.

- *Health Resources and Service Administration (HRSA).* HRSA provides access to essential health services for people who are poor, who are uninsured, or who live in rural and urban neighborhoods where health care is scarce. Working in partnership with many state and community organizations, HRSA also supports programs that ensure healthy mothers and children, increase the number and diversity of healthcare professionals in underserved communities, and provide supportive services for people fighting human immunodeficiency virus (HIV) infection and acquired immunodeficiency syndrome (AIDS) through the Ryan White Care Act.

- *Substance Abuse and Mental Health Services Administration (SAMHSA).* SAMHSA works to improve the quality and availability of substance abuse prevention, addiction treatment, and mental health services. This agency provides funding to the states to support and maintain substance abuse and mental health services through federal block grants.

- *Agency for Healthcare Research and Quality (AHRQ).* AHRQ supports research designed to improve the quality of health care, reduce its cost, improve patient safety, address medical errors, and broaden access to essential services. It provides evidence-based information on healthcare outcomes; quality; and cost, use, and access.

The Assistant Secretary for Health oversees these eight health agency divisions of HHS as well as the Commissioned Corps, a uniformed service of more than 6,000 health professionals who serve at HHS and other federal agencies. The Surgeon General is head of the Commissioned Corps.

The HHS also includes three human service agencies:

- *Center for Medicare and Medicaid Services (CMS).* CMS administers the Medicare and Medicaid programs, which provide health care to approximately one in every four Americans. Medicare provides health insurance for more than 41 million elderly and disabled Americans. Medicaid, a joint federal–state program, provides health coverage for more than 44 million low-income individuals, as well as nursing home coverage for low-income elderly people. The Children's Health Insurance Program covers more than 4.2 million children.

- *Administration for Children and Families (ACF).* ACF is responsible for some 60 programs that promote the economic and social well-being of families, children, individuals, and communities. This agency administers the state–federal welfare program, the national child support enforcement system, and the Head Start program.

- *Administration on Aging (AoA).* AoA supports a nationwide aging network, providing services to the elderly, such as home meal delivery and transportation services, that enable them to remain independent.

Economic Dimensions

Individual behaviors and environmental factors are responsible for approximately 70% of all premature deaths in the United States. Developing and implementing policies and preventive interventions that effectively address these determinants of health can reduce the burden of illness, enhance quality of life, and increase longevity. Also, preventive care is often significantly less expensive than medical intervention. By changing individual behavior, such as modifying diet and increasing exercise, individuals can have a huge impact on defraying healthcare costs down the road. For example, according to the National Institute of Diabetes and Digestive and Kidney Diseases (NIDDK), obesity costs America $123 billion in direct and indirect costs.[1] Much of these costs could be averted by making health behavior choices that would lead to weight loss (Figure 3.2).

Total costs associated with diseases are often significantly less for people who take part in preventive care measures, as disease is often detected at earlier stages. For example, according to the American Cancer Society, the five-year survival rate for cervical cancer detected at the earliest invasive stage is 92%. The costs and associated morbidity of treating women with early cellular changes, or minor cervical cancers, is significantly lower than that associated with treating women for invasive disease. Total costs should be considered in terms of both true financial costs and human costs counted in pain, suffering, and anxiety.

Health insurers have grown to understand the economic value of health promotion and preventive care, and they recognize their importance by increasingly covering these services. Many insurers now offer some benefit for joining a health club, or provide some payment for alternative therapy services such as massage or chiropractic adjustments.

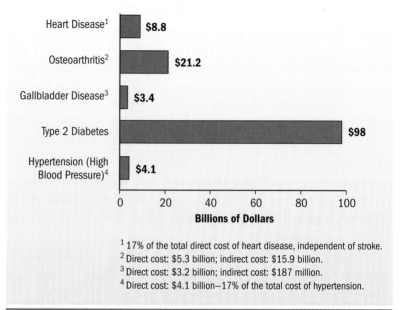

1 17% of the total direct cost of heart disease, independent of stroke.
2 Direct cost: $5.3 billion; indirect cost: $15.9 billion.
3 Direct cost: $3.2 billion; indirect cost: $187 million.
4 Direct cost: $4.1 billion—17% of the total cost of hypertension.

Figure 3.2

Cost burden of obesity-related conditions to society and the health industry.

Source: The Endocrine Society and The Hormone Foundation. (2004). *The Endocrine Society Weighs In: A Handbook of Obesity in America* 43. Available at http://www.obesityinamerica.org. Reprinted with permission.

Important Terms

Epidemiology is the study of patterns of disease in the population. It is concerned with the frequency and types of disease in groups of people and the factors that influence the distribution of disease. The following list defines some of the terms used to describe the epidemiology of a given disease within a population:

- **Incidence:** new cases of a condition that occur during a specified period of time.
- **Prevalence:** the total number of people affected by a given condition at a point in time or during a period of time.
- **Mortality rate:** the incidence of death in a given population during a particular time period. It is calculated by dividing the number of deaths in a population by the total population.
- **Morbidity rate:** the incidence of illness in a given population during a particular time period. Morbidity rate is calculated in a similar manner to mortality rate.

Rates of incidence and prevalence are used to determine changes in the impact that a condition or disease is having on the population and to understand the relative effects of one condition versus another. Morbidity and mortality rates can be cal-

It's Your Health

Important Epidemiological Terms

Measures of Morbidity (illness)

$$\text{Incidence} = \frac{\text{number of new cases of a disease during a given period of time}}{\text{total population at risk}}$$

$$\text{Prevalence} = \frac{\text{number of existing cases of a disease at a given point in time}}{\text{total population at risk}}$$

Measures of Mortality (death)

$$\text{Mortality rate} = \frac{\text{number of deaths in a population in a given period of time}}{\text{total population}}$$

culated across the entire population or within a specific subpopulation, such as age, gender, or race, to show relevant variations across those groups.

Health education is defined as "any combination of learning experiences designed to facilitate voluntary adaptation of behavior conducive to health."[2] One of the principal facets of health education is its voluntary nature. Health education can cover any issue of health, including prenatal care, screening for cancer, or recognizing signs of a stroke. By contrast, health promotion is defined as "the combination of educational and environmental supports for actions and conditions of living conducive to health."[2] While health education deals with the voluntary actions of people in terms of decision making, values, and perceptions, health promotion deals with enabling factors on a societal level. The objective of health promotion is to enable people to make informed decisions regarding behaviors and actions related to health with societal, political, and environmental support. For health promotion to be effective, it must include the component of health education. Health promotion deals primarily with lifestyle and chronic disease factors, such as smoking, drinking, use of primary care medical facilities, and sexual activity.

Many diseases and conditions are a result of lifestyle factors, such as poor nutrition or smoking, and are therefore preventable. Through health promotion efforts, people are increasingly learning to make more informed decisions regarding lifestyle behaviors and disease prevention practices. Prevention is practiced at three different levels—primary, secondary, and tertiary.

- **Primary prevention** is prevention of disease by reducing exposure to a risk factor that may lead to the disease. Primary preventive measures include healthy nutrition, regular physical activity, cessation of smoking, and safe sexual practices.

- **Secondary prevention** refers to early detection and prompt treatment of disease. Screening tools such as mammography and cervical cancer screening are considered examples of secondary prevention because they may detect disease before it spreads, thereby preventing further complications or disease progression. The use of medications and lifestyle behaviors to control chronic diseases that cannot be prevented, such as diabetes or asthma, are also examples of secondary prevention.

- **Tertiary prevention**, which takes place once a disease has advanced, involves alleviating pain, providing comfort, halting progression of an illness, and limiting disability that may result from disease. It consists of rehabilitation in situations where a person can work on restoring certain functions, such as those lost after suffering a stroke.

Primary prevention is largely the responsibility of the healthcare consumer. Secondary prevention requires both the guidance of the healthcare provider and the compliance of the consumer. Tertiary prevention remains a goal of both healthcare providers and caregivers.

The Diversity of Women

Throughout the United States, the diversity of the population, in terms of race and ethnicity, continues to evolve. This changing diversity is seen particularly with the growth of the Hispanic and Asian American sectors of the population, as well as increased numbers of people of mixed racial backgrounds. By 2030, 1 in 5 American women will be of Hispanic heritage, and 1 in 14 will be Asian (Figure 3.3). Significant diversity exists among women based on age as well. By 2030, 1 in 4 American women will be over the age of 65.[3] With the majority of the elderly population in the United States being women, the needs of the elderly represent a significant women's health issue.

Figure 3.3

Projected U.S. population by race and Hispanic origin, 1995–2030.

Source: U.S. Census Bureau. (2004). U.S. interim projections by age, sex, race, and Hispanic origin. Available at http://www.census.gov/ipc/www/usinterimproj/.

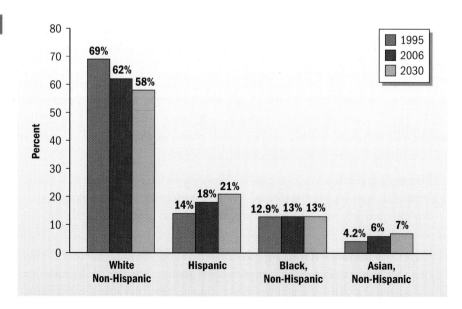

Women's increased educational attainment adds to the diversity of the population. Educated women tend to be more educated healthcare consumers. Differing education levels create heterogeneity among women, as women with little or no education and women with advanced education may have differing health and health education needs. The increased number of women in the workforce also presents new opportunities in women's health, providing another venue for disseminating health education information to women. Women work in a variety of settings, creating differences in their healthcare needs. For example, women working at home, in factories, in offices, in agriculture, and in retail will encounter different work-related health issues.

Another area of diversity relates to the many ways and stages of life in which women choose to become mothers. Many women are delaying marriage and family to focus on careers, and thus are having children in their later years. This trend creates new issues surrounding childbirth, fertility, and parenting that target women in their thirties, forties, and fifties as opposed to solely focusing on women in their twenties. Other women are having children at younger ages, becoming teenage mothers. These women are either working to raise children alone or having their parents take a leadership role in childrearing responsibilities by raising their grandchildren. Some women choose not to have children, instead pursuing careers and other opportunities.

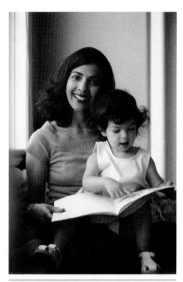

■ By 2030, one in five American women will be of Hispanic heritage.

Diversity also is reflected in women of different sexual orientation. Health concerns specific to lesbian women are often overlooked, leaving many women without proper guidance and medical attention. Lesbians share many health concerns and risks with heterosexual women, but misconceptions about the health needs of lesbians by healthcare providers and lesbians themselves often create barriers to receiving adequate care. Both lesbians and healthcare providers often believe that women who have sex with women do not need cervical cancer screening, routine gynecological care, or contraception to protect them from sexually transmitted diseases (STDs), including HIV/AIDS. Other barriers to health care may include homophobia among providers and lack of health insurance coverage, as many lesbians are unable to share their partner's benefits or are eligible for less complete benefit coverage than a heterosexual spouse would be.[4]

Incarcerated women face special health-related challenges. Many have unmet medical needs that relate to drug addictions, mental health, and reproductive health.[5] Women in prison complain of "lack of regular gynecological and breast exams and argue that their medical concerns are often dismissed or overlooked." Many women in prison are survivors of physical and sexual abuse, putting them at increased risk for high-risk pregnancies, HIV/AIDS, hepatitis C, and cervical cancer. Pregnant incarcerated women face significant hurdles.[6]

Women with disabilities also contribute to the landscape of diversity and stand out as having been the focus of less research and clinical attention than is warranted. Physical barriers, such as inaccessible facilities or examination equipment, present major problems for these women in obtaining adequate health care. Communication barriers may pose a problem if a patient has visual, hearing, or verbal disabilities.

Women with disabilities, as well as uninformed healthcare professionals, may have the misconception that they are less likely to acquire diseases or infections. Many times, healthcare providers focus on the woman's disability and associated issues, rather than on basic routine healthcare needs.[7] Whether a woman's disability is a mobility, vision, hearing, speech, or cognitive challenge, greater levels of research, support, and compassion are needed to adequately address her health concerns.

The heterogeneity of women as reflected in differences of race, ethnicity, socioeconomic status, geographic location, sexual orientation, country of origin, and employment status contributes to the diversity of women's needs. As the medical community has begun to embrace the diversity of women, significant emphasis has been placed on health promotion and disease prevention efforts targeted toward specific populations of women.

Global Health Issues for Women

Women from countries outside the United States have health needs specific to their cultures and socioeconomic status. In developing countries, the health needs of women are extensive and often differ from the needs of American women. According to *The World Health Report 2004,* a report from the World Health Organization (WHO), 10 factors globally account for more than 40% of the disease burden worldwide[8] (Table 3.1). Behavioral and environmental risk factors that are major contributors to death and disease worldwide include the following:

- Underweight
- Unsafe sex
- High blood pressure
- Tobacco consumption
- Alcohol consumption
- Unsafe water, sanitation, and hygiene
- Iron deficiency
- Indoor smoke from solid fuels
- High cholesterol
- Obesity

All ages are at risk for **underweight,** but this condition is most prevalent among children younger than five years of age.

Unsafe sex closely follows underweight as a risk factor and is the major factor in the spread of HIV/AIDS. HIV/AIDS is now the world's fourth leading cause of death. More than 19 million women are living with the disease, the majority of whom reside in Africa. In 2002, 2 million women were infected with HIV worldwide and 1.2 million died from AIDS.[9] AIDS is a devastating disease that is affecting both adults and children and wreaking havoc on already fragile health systems in many of the countries most dramatically affected.

Table 3.1 Leading Causes of Disease Burden for Males and Females Aged 15 Years and Older, 2002

Males	% DALYs	Females	% DALYs
1 HIV/AIDS	7.4	1 Unipolar depressive disorders	8.4
2 Ischemic heart disease	6.8	2 HIV/AIDS	7.2
3 Cerebrovascular disease	5.0	3 Ischemic heart disease	5.3
4 Unipolar depressive disorders	4.8	4 Cerebrovascular disease	5.2
5 Road traffic injuries	4.3	5 Cataracts	3.1
6 Tuberculosis	4.2	6 Hearing loss, adult onset	2.8
7 Alcohol use disorders	3.4	7 Chronic obstructive pulmonary disease	2.7
8 Violence	3.3	8 Tuberculosis	2.6
9 Chronic obstructive pulmonary disease	3.1	9 Osteoarthritis	2.0
10 Hearing loss, adult onset	2.7	10 Diabetes mellitus	1.9

Note: DALYs are disability-adjusted life years, a measure used to calculate the total amount of healthy life lost to a given cause.

Source: *The World Health Report 2004.*

Many of the pharmaceutical treatments for the disease are very expensive and are produced in the United States and other developed countries. Significant debate is currently focusing on how to provide those people in most need with access to these life-saving medicines at reduced costs. Private companies are working with both non-governmental organizations (NGOs) and governments to address the issue. The World Bank defines NGOs as "private organizations that pursue activities to relieve suffering, promote the interests of the poor, protect the environment, provide basic social services, or undertake community development." In wider usage, the label NGO can be applied to any nonprofit organization that is independent from government, including a large charity, community-based self-help group, research institute, church, professional association, or lobbying group.

Risk factors caused by exposure to harmful substances, such as tobacco, or risk factors influenced by unhealthy eating, such as high blood pressure, high cholesterol, and obesity, affect people throughout the world. The conditions they produce are often considered diseases of excess, though they affect people in low-resource settings as well as their counterparts in wealthy communities. Environmentally caused diseases, such as cholera and tuberculosis, are often caused by people not having access to clean water or regular trash removal, and lack of regulations providing bacteria-free meat and food sources. People in developed countries often take for granted the infrastructures that make these systems available and reliable in their countries. In contrast, many developing countries have no system in place for sanitation and often use the same polluted water sources for bathing, drinking, and washing clothes. Parasitic infections from contaminated water and food sources are major causes of morbidity and mortality in countries throughout the world. Increasing access to preventive care, vaccinations, safe drinking water, and proper sanitation has been a primary focus of global health initiatives. The World Health Organization and various NGOs have played leadership roles in trying to effect change in countries that do not have adequate resources.

In almost every country in the world, women are the primary caregivers for children and elderly family members. Although family composition varies from culture to culture, women consistently shoulder the burden of reproduction and feeding, clothing, and caring for children and elderly across the world. The health risks associated with motherhood in developing countries are astronomically higher than those experienced by women in more developed countries. Iron deficiency, one of the most prevalent nutrient deficiencies in the world, most severely affects young children and their mothers because of the high iron demands of infant growth and pregnancy. Regular sources of iron, such as meat, fish, and beans, are not often available to families living in developing countries. Indoor smoke from solid fuels also directly affects women in developing countries because they are inside cooking for their families and working in the home far more often than men. In developing countries, about 700 million people—mainly women and children in poor rural areas—inhale harmful smoke from burning wood and other fuels. They are increasingly at risk from acute respiratory infections, especially pneumonia.[10] According to the World Health Organization:

> In some communities, inequality of girl children and women is the transcending risk factor that explains the prevalence not only of maternal mortality and morbidity, but also of higher vulnerability of girls to childhood mortality. Risk factors like malnutrition of girl children resulting in anemia, and early marriage resulting in premature pregnancy, can be traced to the fact that women do not enjoy the status and significance in their communities that men enjoy … Barriers to improving women's health are often rooted in social, economic, cultural, legal and related conditions that transcend health considerations. Social factors, such as lack of literacy and of educational or employment opportunities, deny young women alternatives to early marriage and early childbearing, and economic and other means of access to contraception. Women's vulnerability to sexual and other abuses, in and out of marriage, increases risks of unsafe pregnancy and motherhood.[11]

By creating guidelines for prevention and developing health promotion programs, practitioners, policy makers, and healthcare activists are encouraging women both in the United States and abroad to become empowered and knowledgeable healthcare consumers.

Stages of Life

Health risks and concerns change as a woman ages during her life span. Certain factors remain constant at any age: good nutrition, regular physical activity, and adequate sleep are essential for health at all stages of life. Healthy living also encom-

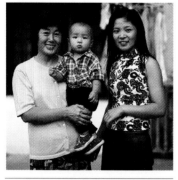

■ Health risks and concerns change as a woman develops from a child to an adolescent, from a young adult to an older adult.

passes avoidance of harmful substances, such as tobacco, drugs, and excessive alcohol. Mental health is equally as important as physical health. Maximizing mental health requires recognizing signs and symptoms of mental health threats, such as depression, drug or alcohol abuse, and physical or mental abuse. In addition, healthy sexuality and responsible sexual behavior are important for a woman's overall health. Healthy sexuality is expressed throughout life by exploring one's sexuality in adolescence, establishing long-term intimate relations in adulthood, and maintaining sexual pleasure in the senior years.

Health risks and concerns change as a woman develops from a child to an adolescent, and then from a young adult to an older adult. Aspects of health promotion must be accompanied by methods of disease prevention. The risk of disease often varies throughout life, and, therefore, the methods of prevention differ depending on one's age as well as multiple other factors. Table 3.2 highlights the major primary preventive measures that should be taken throughout one's life span. Nevertheless, the need for one practice remains constant for all women: Women should learn, understand, and listen to their bodies and empower themselves by becoming informed healthcare consumers.

Adolescence

The transition from childhood to adolescence is a time of major change. Adolescence begins with the onset of puberty and continues until the approximate age of 17, when adult physical development is generally realized. During adolescence, a girl is transformed into a woman and begins to form her identity and sense of independence. As girls set off on this journey, they face a host of issues that threaten their physical and mental well-being. It is important for parents to provide guidance and

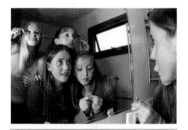

Adolescence is a time when friends become an important influence in a girl's life.

Table 3.2	Primary Preventive Measures Throughout the Life Span

Avoid alcohol, drugs, and tobacco.

Consume a healthy diet.

Participate in regular physical activity.

Learn appropriate and effective weight-management techniques.

Practice safe behaviors, such as using seat belts, wearing motorcycle and bicycle helmets, not driving under the influence of alcohol, and not riding with someone under the influence of alcohol.

Learn nonviolent measures to achieve conflict resolution.

If engaging in sexual activity, use condoms to reduce the risk of STDs, HIV/AIDS, and pregnancy.

Maintain an overall sense of well-being through stress reduction techniques, relaxation methods, socializing with friends and family, and seeking counseling if needed.

Strive to balance work, school, family, friends, and time for oneself.

It's Your Health

Challenges of Adolescence

Increased independence from parents

Adjustment to sexual maturation

Establishment of new and changing relationships with peers

Decisions regarding educational and career goals

Developing a sense of self-identity

Threats During Adolescence

Smoking and substance abuse

Sexually transmitted diseases, including HIV/AIDS

Pregnancy and decisions regarding keeping the baby or having an abortion

Unhealthy eating behaviors and poor body image leading to eating disorders

Unhealthy quest for thinness

Source: Benderly, B. L., for the Institute of Medicine. (1977). *In her own right: The Institute of Medicine's guide to women's health issues.* Washington, DC: National Academy Press.

support during this time and to help their children make appropriate decisions. Adolescents should be encouraged to learn on their own and begin to understand how to take responsibility for oneself and one's actions.

Puberty is a process that encompasses changes in nearly every aspect of development, from physical to intellectual maturation. During this period in life, girls begin to differ in appearance from boys. Secondary sexual characteristics appear, such as widening hips, breast development, height and weight gain, and bodily hair growth. Perspiration and body odor increase, and vaginal discharge creates a new awareness of sexuality for girls. Menstruation, the onset of a woman's reproductive capability, also begins. As these changes occur, adolescents begin to separate from their parents and assume greater independence. Their friends emerge as important factors in their lives, and teens may display rebelliousness. Peer pressure often becomes a strong influence in decisions that teenagers make and may be a factor in their self-esteem and self-perception. Adolescent girls often focus on and define themselves through their relationships with both friends and romantic interests. Their concerns often revolve around popularity, attractiveness, and body weight. They face many challenges as they adjust to their sexual maturation and their increased independence.[12]

Specific Health Concerns for Adolescents

In the United States, the top four causes of death for female adolescents age 15 to 19 are accidents (unintentional injuries), malignant neoplasms, assault (homicide), and intentional self-harm (suicide) (see Table 3.3). Mortality rates for boys in the same age group are more than twice as high as for girls.[13] Behaviors such as not using seat belts, not wearing motorcycle helmets and bicycle helmets, riding with a driver who has been drinking alcohol, and driving after drinking

---

Table 3.3   Leading Causes of Death for Females, 2002*

10–14 Years	Rate	15–19 Years	Rate	20–24 Years	Rate
Accidents	5.3	Accidents	21.8	Accidents	18.4
Malignant neoplasms (cancer)	2.2	Malignant neoplasms (cancer)	3.0	Assault	4.6
Congenital and chromosomal abnormalities	1.0	Assault	2.9	Malignant neoplasms (cancer)	4.2
		Suicide	2.4	Suicide	3.5
Assault	0.8	Heart disease	1.3	Heart disease	2.1
Suicide	0.6	Congenital and chromosomal abnormalities	1.0	Congenital and chromosomal abnormalities	1.1
Heart diseae	0.6				
Chronic respiratory disease	0.4	Flu and pneumonia	0.3	HIV	0.6
Flu and pneumonia	0.3	Pregnancy and childbirth	0.3	Pregnancy and childbirth	0.6
Septicemia	0.3	Septicemia	0.3	Cerebrovascular disease	0.5
Cerebrovascular disease	0.3	Diabetes	0.3	Diabetes	0.5

Source: Anderson, R. N., and Smith, B. L. (2004). Deaths: leading causes for 2002. *National Vital Statistics Reports,* vol. 53, no. 17. Hyattsville, MD: National Center for Health Statistics.

*Rates are per 100,000 population in selected group.

alcohol are responsible for many of the injuries that result in death. Homicide is the second leading cause of death for adolescents age 15 to 19 years and the third leading cause of death for adolescents age 10 to 14 years.[14] Current statistics show that guns kill 10 to 12 children (ages 0–19) in the United States every day on average. Two or three of these children take their own lives, and the other deaths are homicides or unintentional injuries. In contrast, in the developing world, major health issues for young people currently focus on infections, diarrheal diseases, and other communicable diseases like tuberculosis.

Although many adolescents display moody behavior and signs of rebelliousness (normal behaviors during the teenage years), this should not be confused with depression, a significant concern during adolescence. As girls reach adolescence, there is a noted increase in the rate of depression and the rate of suicide attempts. At any given time, between 10% and 15% of children and adolescents have some symptoms of depression. After age 15, depression is two times as common in girls and women as in boys and men.[15] Suicide is the third leading cause of death for adolescents aged 15–19 years and the fourth leading cause of death for younger adolescents.[16] In the Youth Risk Behavior Surveillance survey, 19% of students had seriously considered attempting suicide and 8.8% of students had attempted suicide. Of the students surveyed, girls were more likely than boys to have considered attempting suicide (23.6% versus 14.2%) and more likely to actually attempt suicide (11.5% versus 5.4%).[16]

Trying new behaviors is a key aspect of the period of adolescence and is essential for healthy development; however, risky behaviors may lead to negative health consequences. Sexual experimentation is one example of a behavior that has potentially life-altering consequences. Sexual relations often occur before adolescents have gained experience and skills in self-protection, before they have acquired adequate information about STDs, and before they have access to health services and supplies (such as condoms). This problem is often amplified in developing countries, where girls typically have even less access to health care and information. Each year, approximately 1 million teenagers become pregnant, though teen pregnancy rates have been steadily dropping for much of the 1990s and into the 2000s.[17] According to the National Center for Health Statistics, increased condom use, the adoption of the effective injectable and implantable contraceptives, and the leveling off of teen sexual activity are some of the factors believed to be driving this downturn in teen pregnancies.

Despite these positive trends, only 57.9% of students who were currently sexually active reported that they had used a condom during their last act of sexual intercourse,[16] putting themselves at risk for various STDs, including HIV infection. Approximately 3 million cases of STDs occur annually among teenagers.[18] HIV infection is the seventh leading cause of death among persons age 15 to 24 years in the United States, but its incidence varies greatly among races. Chlamydia infection during adolescence is more likely to result in pelvic inflammatory disease and, as a consequence, lead to infertility.

Globally, more than half of all new HIV infections affect members of the 15–24 age group. According to UNAIDS, "7,000 girls and women become infected with

It's Your Health

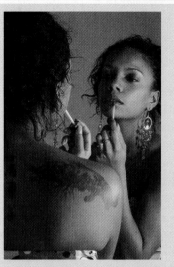

Tattoos

The following advice has been prepared by professional tattooists working with local, state, and national health authorities.

1. Always insist that *you see* your tattooist remove a new needle and tube set-up from a sealed envelope immediately prior to your tattoo.

2. Be certain that *you see* your tattooist pour a new ink supply into a new disposable container.

3. Make sure your artist puts on a new pair of disposable gloves before setting up tubes, needles, and ink supplies.

4. Satisfy yourself that the shop furnishings and tattooist are clean and orderly in appearance—much like a *medical facility.*

5. Feel free to question the tattooist about any of his or her sterile procedures and isolation techniques. Take time to observe the tattooist at work and do not hesitate to inquire about his or her *experience and qualifications* in the tattoo field.

6. If the tattooist is a qualified professional, he or she will have no problem complying with standards above and beyond these simple guidelines.

7. If the artist or studio does not appear up to these standards or if the person becomes evasive when questioned, seek out a different professional tattooist.

Source: Alliance of Professional Tattooists, www.safe-tattoos.com. Reprinted with permission.

HIV every day. In South Africa, Zambia, and Zimbabwe, young women (aged 15–24) are 5 to 6 times more likely to be infected than young men of the same age."[19] In one study in Zambia, more than 12% of the 15- and 16-year-olds seen at antenatal clinics were already infected with HIV. Girls appear to be especially vulnerable to infection. Although statistics from Uganda show that, in some areas, infection rates among teenage girls have dropped 50% since 1990, incidence rates are still six times higher in these girls than in boys of the same age.[20]

Substance use is another risky behavior with which some adolescents begin to experiment. Alcohol and drug use are detrimental activities on their own (see Chapter 13), but they also lead to other situations that may compromise one's health. According to the Youth Risk Behavior Surveillance Survey (YRBS), more than 13% of high school students reported having driven a vehicle after drinking alcohol, and more than 30% have ridden with a driver who had been drinking.[16] Alcohol and drug use also can lead to unsafe sex. Another harmful behavior that can cause illness later in life is smoking. Most adults who smoke regularly began the habit as adolescents and consequently are at greatest risk of diseases attributed to smoking. According to the YRBS, 40% of students in grades 9–12 reported having tried cigarettes and 35% were engaging in current cigarette use. [16]

Recently there has been a dramatic increase in overweight and obesity among adolescents (Figure 3.4). Obese children are at risk for type 2 diabetes, low self-esteem, and many other adverse health outcomes. According to the Youth Risk Behavioral Survey 2003, 43.8% of students in the United States are trying to lose weight.

Other behaviors that have become popular with adolescents are tattooing and piercing. These activities hold inherent risks of infection and have been associated with more serious complications. Increasingly, people are choosing to have body parts such as the lips, eyebrows, septums, or genitalia pierced, in addition to the more standard ear piercing. These piercings increase risks of infections, scarring, and nerve damage. Individuals can minimize the risks associated with these behaviors by choosing experienced professionals who uphold high safety and cleanliness standards. For more information, individuals can contact organizations like the Association of Professional Piercers and the Alliance of Professional Tattooists, which have created tattoo, piercing, and jewelry guidelines. In many cases, primary care physicians have ear-piercing kits and can perform the service in the safety of a clinical setting. To further ensure safety, anyone getting either a piercing or a tattoo should be fully sober.

Preventive Behaviors

Many of the common health risks and challenges facing adolescents are linked to the health-related behaviors that adolescents choose to adopt. These damaging behaviors include smoking, alcohol and drug use, unhealthy dietary behaviors,

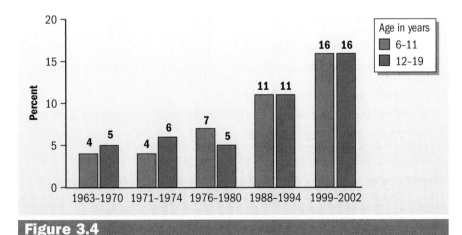

Figure 3.4

Prevalence of overweight among children and adolescents ages 6–19 years.

Results from 1999-2002 National Health and Nutrition Examination Survey (NHANES), using measured heights and weights, indicate that 16% of children and adolescents ages 6-19 years are overweight. This represents a 45% increase from the overweight estimates of 11% obtained from NHANES III (1988-1994).

Note: Excludes pregnant women starting with 1971-1974. Pregnancy status not available for 1963-1965 and 1966-1970. Data for 1963-1965 are for children 6-11 years of age; data for 1966-1970 are for adolescents 12-17 years of age, not 12-19 years.

Source: CDC/NCHS, NHES, and NHANES.

It's Your Health

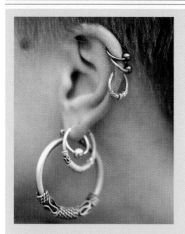

Piercing

These guidelines will help you pick your piercer and piercing studio and can aid you in having a safe piercing experience.

1. *Does the studio seem clean?* A good studio should have five separate areas: counter, waiting room, piercing room, bathroom, and enclosed sterilization room. All areas should be immaculate and staff should be neat and clean.

2. *Ask to see the autoclave (steam sterilizer) and spore tests.* **This is essential.** "Dry heat" and/or chemical soaks are NOT considered adequate for sterilization. A spore test, run regularly, is the only way to know whether the autoclave is working properly.

3. *Does the shop reuse or resterilize needles?* All needles should be sterile, single use and individually packaged, and should be opened while you are present. Make sure your piercer has an approved sharps container and uses it.

4. *See the piercing rooms and set-up.* Ask if you can watch the piercer set up for a piercing. During preparation, the piercer should first wash and glove his or her hands. The equipment should be sealed in individual sterilized packages and placed on a tray. The piercer should change gloves if he or she touches anything in the room other than you and the sterile equipment. If you are not satisfied with the set-up, walk away!

5. *Is the studio using ear-piercing guns?* A number of states have made it illegal to use a gun for body piercings, and with good reason. Most ear guns cannot be sterilized in an autoclave and therefore don't meet the criteria for APP piercers' use of sterile disposable equipment.

6. *Check the studio's jewelry selection.* When referring to size of jewelry, two measurements apply. The width (of a ring) or length (of a bar) is called the "diameter" of the jewelry. The thickness of the jewelry is the "gauge." The smaller the gauge number, the thicker the jewelry. As a general rule, jewelry no thinner than 14 gauge should be used below the neck. Jewelry for initial piercings should be made of material that will not react with the body: implant grade stainless steel and titanium; gold (14K or higher); or platinum. Earring studs should never be used for anything other than earlobes.

7. *Ask questions of the staff and the piercer.* When responding to questions, do they seem knowledgeable? Ask the piercer how long he or she has been piercing and how the piercer learned the trade. Make sure the piercer is well informed. Look at his or her piercings and peruse the piercing photo portfolio. Do you like what you see? If not, leave.

8. *Does the studio have an after-care sheet?* All professional studios should give you an after-care sheet explaining how to take care of your piercing. Read this sheet BEFORE you have the piercing done! If it tells you to clean your piercing with harsh soap, ointment, alcohol or hydrogen peroxide, the studio is not keeping up with the industry standards.

9. *Ask your friends where they got pierced.* Does their piercing look like a piercing you would want? Did they have any problems or infection during healing? Was the staff at the piercing studio able to help them if they had any complications? Would they get pierced there again?

10. *Listen to your instincts.* If you don't feel comfortable with the studio or the piercer, don't get your piercing done by them. Don't feel embarrassed; just leave.

11. *Does the studio have a license to operate?* Many cities and states require that studios and piercers be licensed. In most cases, the license means that the studio meets minimum requirements and has passed some sort of inspection. To find out if your area has established standards and inspections, call your local health department.

12. *Is the piercer recognized by the APP?* Members of the Association of Professional Piercers agree to uphold minimum standards of cleanliness and jewelry quality set forth by the membership of the organization. All APP members will have a membership certificate, usually hanging on the studio wall. It will have an expiration date on it; make sure it is current.

Source: The Association of Professional Piercers, www.safepiercing.org. 2006. Reprinted with permission.

inadequate physical activity, and risky sexual behaviors. Many of them contribute to today's major killers, such as heart disease, cancer, and injuries.

Two especially important aspects of health promotion for adolescents are regular physical activity and good nutrition. There are numerous benefits of regular physical activity, as discussed in Chapter 9. According to the CDC, in 2001, 31%

of high school students did not engage in vigorous physical activity on a regular basis.[21] More than 84% of young people eat too much fat, and more than 91% eat too much saturated fat. Only one in five young people eats the recommended five daily servings of fruits and vegetables. Fifty-one percent of children and adolescents eat less than one daily serving of fruit, and 29% eat less than one daily serving of vegetables that are not fried.[22] In the United States, almost half of high school students are trying to lose weight (43.8%), with girls' rates being almost twice that of boys (59.3% versus 29.1%).[23]

Although all of the essential nutrients are important for good health, the mineral calcium is especially important for young girls. Girls need to consume adequate amounts of calcium to develop good bone health and protect themselves from osteoporosis in their later years. Unfortunately, many adolescent girls become concerned about their widening hips and weight gain, and consequently they follow diets that lack sufficient nutrients. The average calcium intake of adolescent girls is about 800 mg per day, considerably less than the Recommended Dietary Allowance for adolescents of 1,200 mg per day.[24] Even more devastating are the numbers of teenage girls who develop eating disorders as a result of poor body image, unhealthy eating habits, and dangerous purging behaviors (discussed further in Chapters 9 and 12).

Heavy sun exposure during early life has been strongly correlated with an increased lifetime incidence of both **melanoma** and **nonmelanoma** skin cancers. Tanned skin remains fashionable, however, and most teenagers continue to regularly visit beaches or tanning salons. A recent major study of more than 10,000 young people found that sunscreen use was low (about 35%), but was likely to be higher among girls than boys. At least one sunburn during the previous summer was reported in 83% of survey respondents, and three or more sunburns were reported in 36% of survey respondents. About one-tenth of teenagers indicated use of tanning beds. This use was mostly among girls and increased in prevalence as the girls approached age 18.[25]

Generally, adolescence is a period of good health; however, millions of teens suffer from the special health concerns for adolescents mentioned above. The cognitive development occurring during adolescence assists many teenagers in considering the future and understanding the consequences of their present behaviors on their future health. Therefore, it is an excellent time for healthcare providers to provide parents with guidance for encouraging health promotion in their children and to offer adolescents a sense of self-empowerment by encouraging them to make healthy and sensible choices (Table 3.4).

Young Adulthood

As adolescents become adults, they generally become independent of their parents and gain rights that were not afforded to them as children. The age of adulthood is often confusing considering that one can vote and can enlist in the military service at the age of 18, yet cannot legally drink alcohol until age 21. Postsecondary school and the high financial burdens associated with advanced education keep many people dependent on their parents well into their twenties. Nevertheless, as

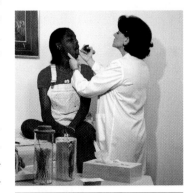
Many young women avoid routine health examinations.

Table 3.4   Secondary Preventive Measures for Adolescents

Pap test three years after onset of sexual activity or by age 21.

Annual STD screening for sexually active adolescents.

HIV screening for high-risk adolescents with their consent.

Annual preventive services visit to screen for depression, risk of suicide, abuse (emotional, physical, and sexual), eating disorders, learning or school problems, and drug use.

Physical exam recommended at least once between ages 11 and 14, once between 15 and 17, and once between 18 and 21.

Annual screening for high blood pressure, cholesterol (if risk factors are present), and tuberculin test (PPD) if risk factors are present.

Annual screening for anemia if any of the following risk factors are present: heavy menstruation, chronic weight loss, nutritional deficit, or excessive athletic activity.

a woman ages, her increased independence and inevitable increase in age bring new health challenges and risks.

For some women, the first stage of young adulthood occurs in college. College can be an extension of adolescence in the sense that many women continue to experiment with new behaviors and explore their sense of self. Other women begin to turn their focus toward choosing a career path. Some find that the freedom of being away from home allows them to engage in behaviors that were not permitted in high school. Young women experience many of the same health threats that affected them as adolescents, including drug and alcohol use, smoking, violence (such as date rape), risky sexual behaviors, poor nutrition, and lack of exercise. For those women who graduate from high school and then directly enter the workforce or begin parenting, as well as for women after graduation from college, different health challenges await.

Specific Health Concerns for Young Adults

Until the age of 24, unintentional injuries, homicide, malignant neoplasms (cancer), suicide, and diseases of the heart are the five leading causes of death for females, in that order. For women ages 25 to 44, cancer tops the list of causes of death, diseases of the heart moves up to third, and HIV is fourth for females of all races.[26] The top causes of death vary significantly by race, however, as seen in Table 3.5. **Chronic diseases,** in contrast to **acute diseases,** are diseases or conditions that are not short-lived. They generally last longer than several weeks and often persist for the remainder of a person's life. Although chronic diseases are generally thought of as afflictions of the elderly, the reality is that they are not limited to any age group. Chronic diseases that affect young adults include cancer, cardiovascular disease, diabetes, and **autoimmune diseases**. Autoimmune diseases that primarily affect women include lupus and multiple sclerosis (MS).

In developing countries, young adult women are at high risk from reproductive health–related disease and infectious disease. The top causes of death for young adult women in developing countries in this age group are six infectious diseases:

Table 3.5 Leading Causes of Death in White, Black, and Hispanic Females, Age 25–44

White Females, 25–34	Black Females, 25–34	Hispanic Females, 25–34
1. Unintentional injuries	1. HIV	1. Unintentional injuries
2. Malignant neoplasms	2. Unintentional injuries	2. Malignant neoplasms
3. Suicide	3. Heart disease	3. Assault
4. Heart disease	4. Malignant neoplasms	4. HIV
5. Assault	5. Assault	5. Heart disease
6. HIV	6. Diabetes	6. Suicide
7. Cerebrovascular disease	7. Cerebrovascular disease	7. Cerebrovascular disease
8. Congenital anomalies	8. Suicide	8. Pregnancy and childbirth
9. Diabetes	9. Anemias	9. Influenza and pneumonia
10. Influenza and pneumonia	10. Pregnancy and childbirth	10. Congenital anomalies

White Females, 35–44	Black Females, 35–44	Hispanic Females, 35–44
1. Malignant neoplasms	1. Malignant neoplasms	1. Malignant neoplasms
2. Unintentional injuries	2. Heart disease	2. Unintentional injuries
3. Heart disease	3. HIV	3. Heart disease
4. Suicide	4. Unintentional injuries	4. HIV
5. Chronic liver disease and cirrhosis	5. Cerebrovascular disease	5. Cerebrovascular disease
6. Cerebrovascular disease	6. Assault	6. Chronic liver disease and cirrhosis
7. Diabetes	7. Diabetes	7. Assault
8. Assault	8. Chronic liver disease and cirrhosis	8. Suicide
9. HIV	9. Septicemia	9. Diabetes
10. Chronic lower respiratory diseases	10. Chronic lower respiratory diseases	10. Septicemia

Source: Anderson, R. N. (2002). Deaths: leading causes for 2000. *National Vital Statistics Reports,* vol. 50, no. 16. Hyattsville, MD: National Center for Health Statistics.

- Pneumonia
- Tuberculosis
- Diarrheal diseases
- Malaria
- Measles
- HIV/AIDS

Young adulthood can be rewarding as well as stressful. During this time, many women are developing or seeking long-term intimate relationships. They may be starting a family and having children. Women may be defining their career path, developing within their career, or still searching for the right career. Many women face obstacles along the way, such as lack of adequate child care and the juggling of family and work responsibilities. Women with disabilities may encounter new

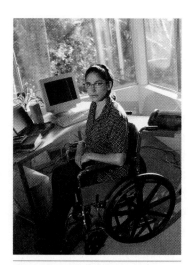

■ Women with disabilities will face many challenges as they enter adulthood and the working world.

challenges as they enter the workforce, including discrimination from employers and employees, lack of accessibility throughout the workplace, and adjustment to new tasks. Some women find it difficult to cope as their friends transition into different stages of life while they feel as if they are standing still. Managing stress and maintaining emotional well-being are important for achieving a healthy perspective.

While women and men report similar levels of stress, causes of stress and coping mechanisms often differ between women and men. A recent study of 1,600 Americans, called *The Tension Tracker 2002*, found that women are more apt to attribute stress to family and health issues than are men. Most women surveyed (52%) were personally concerned about the effect of stress on their health and 30% (versus 24% of men) said that they found it "very challenging" to manage the stress and tension they confront. Men were more likely than women to report watching more television (42% versus 36%) and drinking alcohol (29% versus 18%) as a way of dealing with the stress in their lives. Women report either increased eating of "comfort foods" or decreased contact with the stressor as common strategies of coping.[27]

Alcohol and drug abuse affect the lives of many young women, including women who have children. An estimated 6 million children younger than 18 years of age have a parent who has used illicit drugs in the past month. Marijuana is the drug used most often by parents. Heavy drinking, defined as consumption of five or more drinks at one time on at least three occasions in the past 30 days, was reported by 5.2 million parents (3% of mothers and 14% of fathers).[28]

Young women deal with a host of health-related issues associated with dating and sexual relationships, including sexual violence, STDs, and pregnancy. Consider these statistics:

- Almost 18% of the women in the United States have been the victim of rape or attempted rape that occurred at some point during their lives.
- In college, one in four female students is a rape survivor; experts estimate about 60% of the victims in reported rapes know their assailant.
- Of the estimated 333 million new cases of STDs that occur in the world every year, at least 111 million occur in young people under 25 years of age.
- According to Planned Parenthood International, nearly 4 in 10 pregnancies are unplanned.
- The WHO estimates that between 8 and 30 million unplanned pregnancies result from inconsistent or incorrect use of contraceptive methods, or from method-related failure.

Women who desire to have children may find themselves facing fertility problems or other complications regarding pregnancy or childbearing. Infertility leads to a host of other issues, including physical and emotional stress, financial burdens, and the anxiety and discomfort that often accompany fertility tests and treatment (see Chapter 6). Women with disabilities may face attitudinal barriers from health-care providers as well as friends and family members who feel they should not have children. Lesbians who want to have children may run into opposition while they explore options for sperm donors or adoption agencies.

Preventive Behaviors

Because many chronic diseases can be prevented at least partially by behavioral changes, it is important for a young woman to continue following a healthful diet, participate in regular physical activity, avoid smoking and drug abuse, and moderate her intake of alcohol. Secondary preventive measures, such as screenings for cancer, Pap and HPV tests, and blood pressure screenings, are essential during this time as well (see **It's Your Health**).

As in all stages of life, positive mental well-being is essential for a young woman's overall health. Finding ways to cope with stress and addressing any mental health issues will help to establish a more balanced sense of well-being. Physical activity, healthy relationships with an intimate partner as well as close friends, and participation in enjoyable activities are all effective ways of reducing stress.

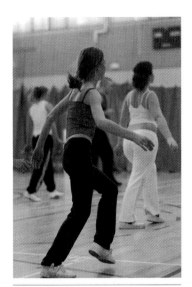

■ Physical activity is important for both physical and mental well-being.

Young adulthood is often a time when women are meeting and dating new people as they try to establish long-term intimate relationships. As such, they must face the extremely difficult challenge of not putting themselves in risky situations, while simultaneously living their lives as independent and open individuals. It is not healthy for women to consider themselves victims or targets for violence at all times, but education about how to avoid compromising situations and how to fight off an attack if it should occur can help women to maintain their independence and peace of mind while dating.

During this period of life, some women may have multiple sexual partners or be sexually involved with someone who has multiple partners. These women are at high risk for contracting STDs if they do not protect themselves by using barrier contraception methods. Most sexually transmitted infections, such as chlamydia and gonorrhea, can cause irritating and often painful symptoms immediately and cause harmful downstream health issues. (See Chapter 7.)

In addition, many women in their twenties and thirties experience pregnancy for the first time. Roughly half of all pregnancies are unplanned, causing a host of anxieties and choices for many women. Whether in a relationship or dealing with a pregnancy on her own, an unplanned pregnancy can be an enormously stressful experience. Seeking advice and counseling from friends, family, healthcare providers, and knowledgeable reproductive health agencies can assist women with their decision-making process.

For a woman who is planning to become pregnant, proper nutrition and consumption of essential vitamins and minerals like folic acid serve as important measures to prevent birth defects. For a woman who is sexually active and does not want to become pregnant, effective birth control becomes a very important preventive health behavior. Other lifestyle choices become significant preventive health choices as well, such as wearing sunblock, reducing unnecessary stress, and making sure that routine medical appointments are made. In the case of skin cancers, routine visits to the dermatologist or primary care physician for full body checks

It's Your Health
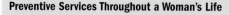

Preventive Services Throughout a Woman's Life

Mammograms. Have a mammogram every one to two years starting at age 40.

Cervical cancer screening. Have a Pap test every one to three years if you have been sexually active or are older than 21. If you are 30 or older, you can have a Pap test and HPV test together.

Cholesterol checks. Have your cholesterol checked regularly starting at age 45. If you smoke, if you have diabetes, or if heart disease runs in your family, start having your cholesterol checked at age 20.

Blood pressure. Have your blood pressure checked at least every two years.

Colorectal cancer tests. Have a test for colorectal cancer starting at age 50. Your doctor can help you decide which test is right for you. If you have a family member who has had colon cancer, you should begin screening earlier and should consult your doctor.

Diabetes tests. Have a test to screen for diabetes if you have high blood pressure or high cholesterol.

Depression. If you've felt "down," sad, or hopeless, and have felt little interest or pleasure in doing things for two weeks straight, talk to your doctor about whether he or she can screen you for depression.

Osteoporosis tests. Have a bone density test at age 65 to screen for osteoporosis (thinning of the bones). If you are between the ages of 60 and 64 and weigh 154 pounds or less, talk to your doctor about whether you should be tested.

Chlamydia tests and tests for other sexually transmitted diseases. Have a test for chlamydia if you are 25 or younger and sexually active. If you are older, talk to your doctor to see whether you should be tested. Also, talk to your doctor to see whether you should be tested for other sexually transmitted diseases.

Immunizations. Stay up-to-date with your immunizations:

- Have a flu shot every year if available.
- Have a tetanus-diphtheria shot every 10 years.
- Talk to your doctor about whether you need hepatitis B shots.

Don't smoke. If you do smoke, talk to your doctor about quitting. You can take medicine and get counseling to help you quit. Make a plan and set a quit date. Tell your family, friends, and co-workers you are quitting. Ask for their support. If you are pregnant and smoke, quitting now will help both you and your baby.

Eat a healthy diet. Eat a variety of foods, including fruits, vegetables, animal or vegetable protein (such as meat, fish, chicken, eggs, beans, lentils, tofu, or tempeh), and grains (such as rice). Limit the amount of saturated fat you eat.

Be physically active. Walk, dance, ride a bike, rake leaves, or do any other physical activity you enjoy. Start small and work up to a total of 20–30 minutes most days of the week.

Stay at a healthy weight. Balance the number of calories you eat with the number you burn off by your activities. Remember to watch portion sizes. Talk to your doctor if you have questions about what or how much to eat.

Drink alcohol only in moderation. If you drink alcohol, one drink a day is safe for women, unless you are pregnant. If you are pregnant, you should avoid alcohol completely. Because researchers don't know how much alcohol will harm a fetus, it's best not to drink any alcohol while you are pregnant.

Source: *Preventive Services.* AHRQ Publication No. APPIP03-0008. Current as of January 2004.

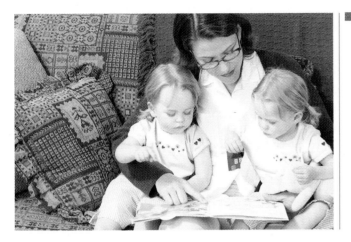

■ Many women no longer choose to begin their families in their twenties.

are important for all women, but vital for women with fair skin or a family history of skin cancer.

Midlife

As women move into their forties, many have completed their families and either remain at home or continue working outside of the home. Some have established productive careers, whereas others struggle to find and maintain a job with decent wages, advancement opportunities, and a satisfactory work environment. Women in this stage of life are often busy raising children, possibly caring for elderly parents, and working to keep their relationships healthy. As they reach their fifties and sixties, many must deal with the mortality of their parents as well as their own aging. Some may be fearful of getting older, whereas others are looking forward to retirement. A scenario that is becoming more common is the raising of grandchildren by grandparents, often women in their fifties and sixties. The parents of these children, for various reasons, have left the responsibility of childrearing with the grandparent, creating a different dimension of aging for these women.

Thanks to trends toward increasing physical fitness and greater access to effective medical treatment, many women discover midlife to be an ideal time to focus on themselves. They realize some of the benefits of the healthier lifestyles they have adopted over the past 20 years and consequently find their retirement years to be filled with physical activity, travel, healthy sexuality, and relaxation.

Specific Health Concerns for Women During Midlife

Between the ages of 45 and 64, the top five causes of death for women are chronic diseases. Cancer, heart disease, cerebrovascular disease, chronic obstructive pulmonary disease, and diabetes are all conditions that benefit from behavioral changes (Table 3.6). In developing countries, the leading causes of death for women in this age group are a mix of infectious diseases, diseases of the reproductive system, and chronic diseases. Chronic diseases such as cancer and heart disease are increasingly dominant causes of death for women in this age group in developing countries as well.

Menopause, the cessation of the menstrual cycle, is a significant transition for women during their midlife years (see Chapter 8). For some women, menopause is a welcome change, eliminating their menstrual cycle and the need for contraception. Other women experience numerous health concerns associated with menopause and have difficulty finding an effective therapy. Women entering menopause today are encountering more confusion than in the past due to recent controversy surrounding hormone replacement therapy (HRT), which has limited the medical options for dealing with the distressing side effects of menopause. Women in perimenopause may find themselves experiencing discomfort during sex or lack of libido.

As women live longer and many postpone marriage, some are finding themselves sandwiched between the demands of their children and their parents. Due

Table 3.6 Leading Causes of Death in White, Black, and Hispanic Women, Age 45–64

White Females, 45–54	Black Females, 45–54	Hispanic Females, 45–54
1. Malignant neoplasms	1. Malignant neoplasms	1. Malignant neoplasms
2. Heart disease	2. Heart disease	2. Heart disease
3. Unintentional injuries	3. Cerebrovascular disease	3. Unintentional injuries
4. Cerebrovascular disease	4. Diabetes	4. Diabetes
5. Diabetes	5. HIV	5. Cerebrovascular disease
6. Chronic liver disease and cirrhosis	6. Unintentional injuries	6. Chronic liver disease and cirrhosis
7. Chronic lower respiratory diseases	7. Chronic lower respiratory diseases	7. HIV
8. Suicide	8. Chronic liver disease and cirrhosis	8. Viral hepatitis
9. Influenza and pneumonia	9. Nephritis	9. Assault
10. Septicemia	10. Septicemia	10. Chronic lower respiratory diseases

White Females, 55–64	Black Females, 55–64	Hispanic Females, 55–64
1. Malignant neoplasms	1. Malignant neoplasms	1. Malignant neoplasms
2. Heart disease	2. Heart disease	2. Heart disease
3. Chronic lower respiratory diseases	3. Diabetes	3. Diabetes
4. Cerebrovascular disease	4. Cerebrovascular disease	4. Cerebrovascular disease
5. Diabetes	5. Nephritis	5. Chronic liver disease and cirrhosis
6. Unintentional injuries	6. Chronic lower respiratory diseases	6. Unintentional injuries
7. Chronic liver disease and cirrhosis	7. Septicemia	7. Nephritis
8. Septicemia	8. Hypertension and hypertensive renal disease	8. Chronic lower respiratory diseases
9. Influenza and pneumonia	9. Unintentional injuries	9. Influenza and pneumonia
10. Nephritis	10. Chronic liver disease and cirrhosis	10. Septicemia

Source: Anderson, R. N. (2002). Deaths: leading causes for 2000. *National Vital Statistics Reports,* vol. 50, no. 16. Hyattsville, MD: National Center for Health Statistics.

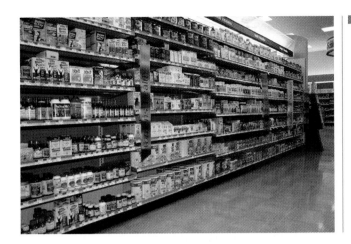

Significant controversy and confusion remain over the use of hormone replacement therapy and dietary supplements for perimenopause and menopause.

to difficult economic times, more children are living at home to attend college, and an increasing number of adult children are returning home after a divorce or loss of job. These "boomerang" children are changing the dynamics of life for many women in their middle years who assumed their children would grow up, leave home, and live as independent, self-supporting adults. Instead, many women must deal with a child at home again precisely at the time when their caregiver roles increase for their own parents.

Preventive Behaviors

Healthful eating, regular physical activity, and avoidance of smoking are all primary preventive measures that should be continued through all stages of life. As a woman ages, secondary preventive measures, such as mammograms and colonoscopies, become extremely important to ensure early detection of disease and, consequently, timely treatment. Methods of prevention are listed in Table 3.7.

As in other stages of life, maintaining mental wellness is of significant importance in midlife. Women who are caregivers for children, elderly relatives, or both often find themselves suffering from severe stress, depression, and anxiety. Many of these women may see the effects spill over from their home life into their work life. Finding support groups, seeking professional help, and establishing time to take care of oneself are effective means for improving the mental health of many women.

Discussing options with a healthcare provider can help improve sexual functioning and desire, if necessary. Many women may still require contraception for preventing pregnancy or STDs if they are not in a mutually monogamous relationship.

The Senior Years

There is significant growth in the elderly population, with women constituting a large sector of the senior population. During the twentieth century, advances

It's Your Health

Contributors to Improved Life Expectancy for Women

Identification, treatment, eradication, and control of some infectious and parasitic diseases.

Better prenatal and antenatal care.

More efficient, effective methods for assisting childbirth.

Greater awareness, identification, and control of threats to health and ways to promote and maximize health.

Improved protection from environmental and workplace toxins and hazards.

Table 3.7 Secondary Preventive Measures for Women During Midlife

Annual screening for high blood pressure.

Periodic height and weight measurement to monitor for overweight and obesity.

Clinical breast examinations yearly.

Periodic screening for high cholesterol levels, at least once every five years.

Behavioral assessment to detect depression and other problems.

Annual fecal occult blood test plus sigmoidoscopy every five years or colonoscopy every 10 years or barium enema every 5-10 years; a digital rectal examination should also be performed at the time of screening—for adults age 40 years and older with a family history of colorectal cancer and all adults age 50 years and older.

Annual mammography for women at high risk beginning at age 35 and for all women after age 50. Some authorities recommend screening mammograms every one to two years for women 40 to 49 years of age.

Annual Pap test or HPV test; after three or more consecutive normal exams, the Pap test may be performed less frequently in low-risk women at the discretion of the patient and clinician.

Counseling about the benefits and risks of postmenopausal hormone replacement therapy.

Bone density measurements for women at risk of osteoporosis.

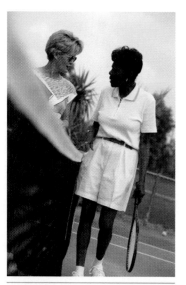

■ Living a healthy life from childhood on may lead to fulfilling and enjoyable senior years.

---

in research, medicine, and public health had a significant positive impact on life expectancy in the United States. In 1900, the average life expectancy at birth for women was 48.3 years. By 2002, it had increased to 79.9 years, compared with 74.5 years for men (Figure 3.5).[29] Life expectancy also has increased for women at age 65 and 85. On average, women who live to age 65 can expect to live to age 84.5; those who live to 85 can anticipate living to age 92.[3] The increase in life expectancy at these ages is partly due to decreased mortality rates, specifically from heart disease and stroke. Despite decreases in mortality rates, heart disease remains the number one killer of women in the United States for women age 65 and older (Figure 3.6).

Life expectancy also varies by race. In 2000, life expectancy at birth was five years longer on average for white women than for black women. These differences become less extreme as women age, however. By age 65, white women live an average of 1.8 years longer than black women; by age 85, life expectancy for black women is nearly equal that for white women; and by age 90, life expectancy for black women is actually higher than that for white women.[29] By 2030, one in four American women will be older than 65.[2] The population over the age of 85 is growing especially quickly and is projected to more than double from nearly 4 million in 1995 to more than 8 million in 2030. In 2050, an estimated 18 million people over the age of 85 will live in the United States, accounting for 4.6% of the U.S. population. The aging of the population presents a unique challenge to society in general and healthcare practitioners in particular, as it creates yet another facet of diversity within the population of women.

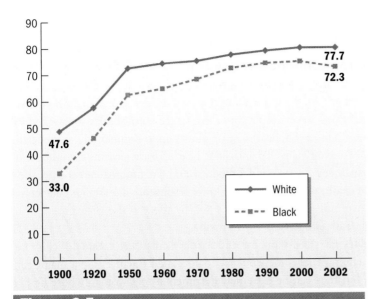

Figure 3.5

Life expectancy for black women and white women, 1900–2002.

Source: National Center for Health Statistics. (2004). *Health, United States 2004 with Chartbook on Trends in the Health of Americans.* Hyattsville, MD.

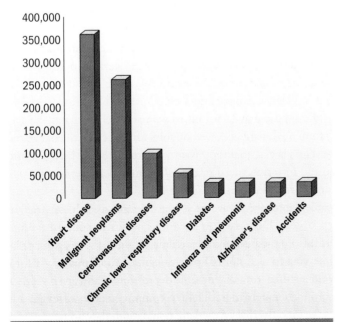

Figure 3.6

Leading causes of death in women in the United States, 2002.

Source: Anderson, R.N. (2002). Deaths: leading causes for 2000. *National Vital Statistics Reports,* vol. 50, no. 16. Hyattsville, MD: National Center for Health Statistics.

Specific Health Concerns During the Senior Years

The years after age 65 represent a wide spectrum of health issues. Many women remain healthy into their nineties and beyond. Other women find themselves struggling with continual health issues as they age. From the age of 65 on, chronic diseases are the leading cause of death for women in the United States.[3] For women age 65–74, the five leading causes of death are malignant **neoplasms,** heart disease, chronic lower respiratory diseases, cerebrovascular disease, and diabetes. For women age 75–84, heart disease moves up to number one as the leading cause of death. For women age 85 and older, heart disease remains the number one killer, but Alzheimer's disease and influenza and pneumonia move into the top five causes of death, surpassing chronic lower respiratory diseases and diabetes. Chronic obstructive lung disease, largely caused by tobacco use or exposure, is a leading cause of death and disability worldwide.

Diseases such as osteoporosis and arthritis may also create difficulty for women in maintaining their independence. Fall-related fractures are a major concern for anyone, but they can be extremely detrimental to a woman whose bone health is suffering (see Chapter 11). Arthritis can make it difficult for a woman to perform daily activities, such as opening jars, lifting objects, bending to pick up an item that has fallen, or lifting herself from the toilet seat. A woman also may begin having problems with vision or hearing, creating new challenges in performing everyday tasks and maintaining independent living.

A major health concern related to aging is the side effects or drug interaction effects that can occur when women take multiple drugs, often for multiple conditions. Healthcare providers are not always aware of harmful drug interactions, and women may find themselves being given additional medications to treat side effects caused by their original medications. Harmful effects of drug interaction may include, but are not limited to, abnormal heart rate and/or rhythm, depression, dizziness and imbalance, constipation, blood pressure increase, and confusion.

The loss of a spouse may factor into a woman's well-being as she ages, too. The number of women who are widowed doubles after the age of 65. Learning to cope with grief and loss is essential for physical and mental well-being. Maintaining independence and fostering social relationships may help women deal with feelings of grief, sadness, and loneliness.

Diagnosable depression, however, is not the same as sadness, grief, or the emotional effects of loss. Depression is a significant health concern for aging women and may result from medication interactions, chronic disease, pain, or loneliness; it should not be viewed as a normal part of aging. An estimated 6% of Americans age 65 and older suffer from diagnosable depression in any given year. Older adults also are disproportionately more likely to commit suicide; although adults age 65 and older make up only 13% of the U.S. population, they accounted for 19% of all suicides in 1997.

Today, women most frequently bear the responsibility of caring for their parents or loved ones when they need help. Women account for more than 80% of the family caregivers for chronically ill elders, and 73% of these women caregivers are

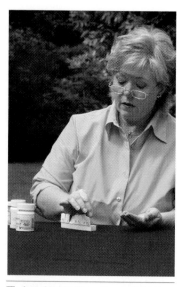

■ A major health concern related to aging is the side effects of taking multiple drugs.

It's Your Health

Evaluating Health Information on the Web

1. **Who runs the site?**
   Any good health-related Web site should make it easy for you to learn who is responsible for the site and its information. Web addresses ending in ".gov" denote a federal government–sponsored site; ".edu" is for educational institutions; ".org" was once limited to nonprofit organizations but now may be used by commercial Web sites.

2. **Who pays for the site?**
   It costs money to run a Web site. The source of a site's funding should be clearly stated or readily apparent. Does it sell advertising? Is it sponsored by a drug company? The source of funding can affect what content is presented, how the content is presented, and what the site owners want to accomplish on the site.

3. **What is the purpose of the site?**
   Check the "About This Site" link, which appears on many sites. The purpose of the site should be clearly stated and should help you evaluate the trustworthiness of the information.

4. **Where does the information come from?**
   Many health/medical sites post information collected from other Web sites or sources. The original source should be clearly labeled and the site should describe the evidence that the material is based on. Medical facts and figures should have references (such as an article in a medical journal). Also, opinions or advice should be clearly set apart from information that is "evidence-based" (that is, based on research results).

5. **How is the information selected?**
   Is there an editorial board? Do people with excellent medical qualifications review the material before it is posted?

6. **How current is the information?**
   Web sites should be reviewed and updated on a regular basis, and a review date should be clearly posted. Even if the information has not changed, you want to know that the site owners have reviewed it recently to ensure that it is still valid.

7. **How does the site choose links to other sites?**
   Web sites usually have a policy about how they establish links to other sites. Some medical sites take a conservative approach and don't link to any other sites; some link to any site that asks or pays for a link; others only link to sites that have met certain criteria.

8. **What information about you does the site collect, and why?**
   Web sites routinely track the paths that visitors take through their sites to determine which pages are being used; however, many health Web sites ask you to "subscribe" or "become a member." Any credible health site asking for personal information should tell you exactly what it will and will not do with your data. Be certain that you read and understand any privacy policy or similar language on the site, and don't sign up for anything that you are not sure you fully understand.

9. **How does the site manage interactions with visitors?**
   There should always be a way for you to contact the site owners with problems, feedback, and questions. If the site hosts chat rooms or other online discussion areas, it should tell visitors what the terms of using this service are. Are chats or discussions moderated? If so, by whom and why? It is always a good idea to spend time reading the discussion without joining in, so you feel comfortable with the environment before becoming a participant.

Source: Adapted from *Ten Things to Know about Evaluating Medical Resources on the Web*, National Cancer Institute, 2002.

65 or older.[30] The value of services provided by caregivers is estimated to be $257 billion per year, which is roughly twice the amount actually spent annually in the United States on home care and nursing home services.[31] Some women may experience cognitive decline, and depression as a result of being the primary caregiver for a partner, relative, or friend. Healthcare providers also need to be aware of the prevalence of abuse within the elderly population and help provide protection when a woman is unable to or afraid to protect herself (see Chapter 14).

As women age, their skin becomes thinner, loses some of its elastic quality, suffers injury more easily, and heals more slowly. Women who have spent a lot of time in the sun during their lives often experience the development of skin cancers at this stage of their lives. Most skin cancers can be removed safely and easily with a simple procedure. If left untreated, however, they can pose a very serious health risk. Proper attention to skin care throughout life can prevent serious consequences as women age.

Sexuality also remains an issue for older women. Although many healthcare providers do not view their patients as sexual beings at this age, many women continue to desire sexual relations and may need advice for maintaining healthy sexuality as they age. A study conducted by the American Association of Retired People (AARP) reported that 44% of women 75 years of age or older believe that "a satisfying sexual relationship" is important to their quality of life.[32] This issue is discussed in more depth in Chapter 4.

Preventive Behaviors

The early senior years can be a time of relaxation and fulfillment for women who are fortunate enough to have achieved financial stability, who have maintained their physical and mental health, and who are surrounded by loving family and friends. Other women may be less fortunate and experience considerable concerns regarding their future. Planning for one's future and maintaining one's health from childhood on may help women to have an easier time in their later years.

■ Flu immunizations significantly reduce the chance of an older woman getting influenza or pneumonia.

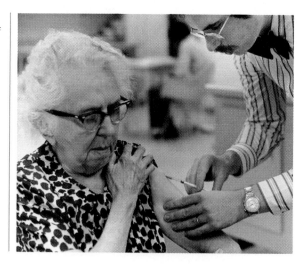

As throughout life, good nutrition, exercise, and avoidance of harmful sub-stances continue to provide protection from harmful diseases in old age. Regular healthcare screening and preventive checkups are essential, as is continual moni-toring for drug interactions and signs or symptoms that may signal a health con-cern. Getting a flu vaccination and paying close attention to colds and minor ill-nesses can help keep a woman safe from pneumonia and influenza (Table 3.8). Women should also take extra special care of their skin as they age, using proper moisturizers and barriers to protect against skin breakdown. In addition, women should get bone density screenings to make sure that they are not at risk for developing osteoporosis.

Informed Decision Making

To take personal responsibility for their own health and wellness, all women should educate themselves about their health status. Integrating primary preven-tion methods into one's daily life can make a significant difference in both present and future health (see Self-Assessment 3.1). By understanding their own sec-ondary prevention needs, such as the appropriate screening methods for women at certain ages, women can better inform their healthcare providers about their health status and demand the healthcare services that they require and deserve.

Table 3.8   Secondary Preventive Measures for Seniors

Annual screening for high blood pressure.

Cholesterol screening every three to five years or as recommended by the healthcare provider.

Periodic height and weight measurement to monitor for overweight and obesity.

Clinical breast examinations yearly or as recommended by one's healthcare provider.

Initial assessment of cognitive function and monitoring of changes as part of a routine preven-tive visit.

Behavioral assessment to detect depression and other problems.

Annual fecal occult blood test plus sigmoidoscopy every 5 years or colonoscopy every 10 years or barium enema every 5 to 10 years; a digital rectal examination should also be performed at the time of screening.

Routine mammography screening as recommended by the healthcare provider.

Pap and HPV test every three years or as recommended by the healthcare provider.

Periodic evaluation for hearing loss and visual acuity.

Thyroid-stimulating hormone test every three to five years.

Bone mineral density test as recommended by the healthcare provider; counseling on fall prevention.

Annual influenza and pneumococcal pneumonia vaccines.

Self-Assessment 3.1

Rate Your Preventive Practices

Answer the following questions:

1. Do you eat a healthful diet consisting of the appropriate servings of fruits and vegetables, grains, protein, vitamins, and minerals?

2. Do you participate in moderate-intensity physical activity at least four days a week?

3. Do you get enough sleep so that you do not feel tired throughout the day?

4. Do you avoid using tobacco products and drugs?

5. If you consume alcohol, do you do so in moderation?

6. If you are sexually active, do you use condoms or other barrier contraceptives to protect against STDs?

7. Do you employ methods to reduce stress, find time to socialize with friends and relax, and maintain an overall sense of mental wellness?

8. Do you practice safe behaviors, such as using seat belts, wearing motorcycle and bicycle helmets, not driving under the influence of alcohol, and not riding with someone under the influence of alcohol?

9. Do you use nonviolent methods of conflict resolution?

10. Do you receive routine preventive care from a healthcare provider?

The more questions to which you answered "yes," the better off you are! If you answered "no" to any questions, try to change that behavior to achieve a better state of overall health.

In recent years, the Internet has evolved into a valuable resource for women who are seeking health information. Yet the quality of health information on Web sites is extremely variable and difficult to assess. Evaluating the information can be a significant challenge, even for an experienced Web user. Being able to identify the validity of the material in a given Web site is crucial, as it could potentially affect health outcomes for millions of people. Most content on the Web is posted without any form of approval or review for accuracy and reliability, or it is posted by a company having a financial stake in the information being communicated (for example, pharmaceutical firms or physicians offering specific surgical procedures). A number of organizations are working to credential health-related Web sites, by providing "stamps of approval" so that consumers can have independent validation that the content is valid; however, this practice is not widespread across cyberspace. In the absence of these content authentication measures, healthcare consumers must often rely on their own common sense and judgment. Following some basic guidelines will help women evaluate the quality of information they find online. In addition, women should understand that open communication with their physicians is their right. Better communication between physicians and patients can improve both the quality of the care women receive and their health promotion knowledge base.

Summary

Primary prevention is the first step toward health promotion and disease prevention for women at all stages of their lives. Many women have already taken the first steps by reclaiming their bodies and taking responsibility for their own health; however, many women remain unable or unwilling to make these changes.

There are different preventive health actions a woman can take at different points in her life. Many tests and behaviors are specifically indicated starting at a given age. Becoming familiar with the appropriate health promotion and prevention activities across a woman's life span is especially valuable. Women can empower themselves by recognizing the central role that proper access to health care

Profiles of Remarkable Women

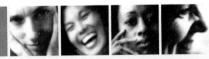

Shirley Temple Black (1928–)

Shirley Temple began life as an actress—the star of more than 40 motion pictures before she turned 12 years old. She exhibited her talents in her song-and-dance routines, most notably in her signature song "On the Good Ship Lollipop," which sold a half million copies and earned Temple an Academy Award. Temple acted in numerous films, including *Little Miss Marker, The Little Colonel* (with Bill "Bojangles" Robinson), *Our Little Girl, Curly Top,* and *The Littlest Rebel.* Working for Fox Studio, Temple became a marketing dream with Shirley-endorsed products ranging from dresses, to cereal, to soup, to dolls. Temple continued acting as a teenager and young adult with well-known actors, but at 21 and already divorced, she decided to leave Hollywood to vacation in Hawaii. There, she met her second husband, Charles Black.

Known throughout her childhood as an ambassador of goodwill, it was a natural progression for her to dedicate her adult life to public service. In 1969, she was appointed by Richard Nixon as the U.S. representative to the United Nations. She also served as a U.S. delegate to many international conferences and summits on cooperative treaties and human environment. In 1972, at the age of 44, Shirley Temple Black found a lump on her breast. She postponed a biopsy to attend government talks in the Soviet Union as the special assistant to the Chairman of the Presidential Council on Environmental Health. After her biopsy showed a malignancy, Black underwent a simple mastectomy. To face her illness, she went public with her disease and received numerous letters of support.

Her breast cancer did not slow her down in terms of her work, however. From 1974 to 1976, Black worked as Ambassador to the Republic of Ghana. In 1976, she became the first female White House Chief of Protocol under Gerald Ford. She later served as a foreign affairs officer in the State Department for Ronald Reagan and as an Ambassador to Czechoslovakia under George H. W. Bush. Her diplomatic skills have made her a success in the political arena as well as in the business sector. She has lent her expertise to major corporations by contributing as a member of the corporate board of directors for such companies as Del Monte, Bancal Tri-State, Fireman's Fund Insurance, and Walt Disney Productions. Her professional activities include numerous board and council memberships, including the Council on Foreign Relations, the Council of American Ambassadors, the World Affairs Council, the United States Commission for UNESCO, and the U.S. Citizen's Space Task Force. She is also the cofounder of the International Federation of Multiple Sclerosis Societies.

Shirley Temple Black has received honorary doctorates from University of Santa Clara and Lehigh University, a Fellowship from College of Notre Dame, and a Chubb Fellowship from Yale University.

for them and their families plays in creating stability in their lives. Around the world, a woman's quality of life is threatened by inequities in access to proper health care, specifically preventive services, medical treatments, surgical interventions, family planning, or proper maternal and child health. These services are essential to women who seek to lead active, healthy, and happy lives at all stages of life.

In addition, across the world, women tend to be the main healthcare observers and resource attainers in the family. Women who are better educated about their and their family's healthcare needs can have a major impact on the well-being of their family and community.

Communities, healthcare providers, workplaces, and educators need to effectively reach underserved women with healthcare services and education. Women must also work to educate one another about the important health-related information that they learn throughout their lives, so as to expand the rich network of communication from which women around the world benefit. By improving access to health care for all women and providing appropriate guidelines for care to both healthcare providers and consumers, women will be better equipped for remaining healthy throughout their life span.

Topics for Discussion

1. How can parents, healthcare providers, and health educators encourage adolescents to follow healthy behaviors? How can they convince adolescents that their present behaviors will have a significant impact on their future health?

2. What are some ways in which you can improve your health? Are there preventive practices from which your parents can benefit that they are not practicing?

3. How do the health needs of women in developing countries differ from those of women in the United States? How are they similar?

4. What are some preventive measures for lesbians? for physically challenged women?

5. Some health behaviors are detrimental to well-being. Should policies such as restricting smoking or mandating bicycle helmets be mandatory or voluntary?

Web Sites

Administration on Aging: http://www.aoa.gov

Administration for Children and Families: http://www.acf.dhhs.gov

Agency for Healthcare Research and Quality: http://www.ahrq.gov

Centers for Disease Control and Prevention: http://www.cdc.gov

Centers for Medicare and Medicaid Services: http://www.cms.hhs.gov

Food and Drug Administration: http://www.fda.gov

Health Resources and Services Administration: http://www.hrsa.gov

Healthy People 2010: http://www.healthypeople.gov

Indian Health Service: http://www.ihs.gov

National Institutes of Health: http://www.nih.gov

Office of the Surgeon General: http://www.surgeongeneral.gov

Substance Abuse and Mental Health Services Administration: http://www.samhsa.gov

U.S. Department of Health and Human Services: http://www.hhs.gov

U.S. Public Health Service Commissioned Corps: http://www.usphs.gov

■ ■ ■ ■

References

1. National Institutes of Health, National Institute of Diabetes, Digestive and Kidney Diseases. Statistics related to overweight and obesity: the economic costs. http://www.niddk.nih.gov/statistics/index.htm.

2. Green, L. W. and Kreuter, M. W. (1991). *Health Promotion Planning: An Educational and Environmental Approach* (2nd ed.). Mountain View, CA: Mayfield Publishing Co.

3. National Center for Health Statistics. (2004). *Health, United States 2004 with Chartbook on Trends in the Health of Americans.* Hyattsville, MD.

4. Solarz, A. L. (ed). (1999). *Lesbian Health: Current Assessment and Directions for the Future.* Committee on Lesbian Health Research Priorities. Institute of Medicine. Washington, DC: National Academy Press.

5. www.movementbuilding.org/prisonhealth/womens.html.2002.

6. Greenfield, L. A., and Snell, T. L. (December 1999). *Women Offenders.* U.S. Department of Justice, Bureau of Justice Statistics Special Report.

7. Weiner, S. (1999). *A Provider's Guide for the Care of Women with Physical Disabilities and Chronic Medical Conditions.* North Carolina Office on Disability and Health.

8. World Health Organization. (2004). *The World Health Report 2004.*

9. World Health Organization. (2002). *AIDS Epidemic Update.*

10. World Health Organization. (1999). *Report on Infectious Disease: Removing Obstacles to Healthy Development.*

11. WHO/RHR/01.5. (2001). *Advancing Safe Motherhood Through Human Rights.*

12. Benderly, B. L., for the Institute of Medicine. (1997). *In Her Own Right: The Institute of Medicine's Guide to Women's Health Issues.* Washington, DC: National Academy Press.

13. Centers for Disease Control and Prevention, National Center for Health Statistics. (1999). *National Vital Statistics System.*

14. Thompson, K. (2000). *Risk in Perspective; "Kids at Risk."* Harvard Center for Risk Analysis.

15. Substance Abuse and Mental Health Services Administration Center for Mental Health Services, in partnership with the National Institute of Mental Health, National Institutes of Health. (1999). *Mental Health: A Report of the Surgeon General.* U.S. Department of Health and Human Services.

16. Kann, L., et al. (2002). Youth Risk Behavior Surveillance—United States, 2001. *Morbidity and Mortality Weekly Report* 51(SS04): 1–64.

17. Ventura, S. J, Mathews, T. J., and Hamilton, B. E. (2002). Teenage births in the United States: trends, 1991–2000, an update. *National Vital Statistics Reports,* vol. 50, no. 9. Hyattsville, MD: National Center for Health Statistics.

18. Centers for Disease Control and Prevention. (2000). *Tracking the Hidden Epidemic: Trends in STDs in the United States 2000.*

19. UNAIDS Global Coalition on Women and AIDS. (2005).

20. World Health Organization. (1997). *Young People and Sexually Transmitted Diseases.* Fact Sheet, No. 186.

21. Centers for Disease Control and Prevention. (2002). *School Health Index for Physical Activity, Healthy Eating, and a Tobacco-Free Lifestyle: A Self-Assessment and Planning Guide.* Middle school/high school version. Atlanta, GA.

22. Centers for Disease Control and Prevention. (2000). *School Health Programs: An Investment in Our Nation's Future.* U.S. Department of Health and Human Services.

23. Centers for Disease Control and Prevention. (2003). *Youth Risk Behavior Surveillance.*

24. Centers for Disease Control and Prevention. (2000). *Promoting Lifelong Healthy Eating: CDC's Guidelines for School Health Programs.* Produced by Division of Adolescent and School Health.

25. Geller, A. C., Colditz, G., Oliveria, S., et al. (2002). Use of sunscreen, sunburning rates, and tanning bed use among more than 10,000 U.S. children and adolescents. *Pediatrics* 109(6): 1009–1014.

26. Anderson, R. N. (2002). Deaths: leading causes for 2000. *National Vital Statistics Report,* vol. 50, no. 16. Hyattsville, MD: National Center for Vital Statistics.

27. *The Tension Tracker 2002.* Based on 1,805 interviews among a representative sample of Americans 18 years or older. Harris Interactive conducted inter-

views from April 29, 2002, to May 8, 2002. http://www.beheadstrong.com/tensiontracker/index.jhtml#article2.

28. *Provisional Report. Summary Health Statistics for U.S. Adults: National Health Interview, 2004 Survey.* (December 2005).

29. National Center for Health Statistics. (2003). *National Vital Statistics Report. Deaths: Preliminary Data for 2001*, vol. 51, no. 5. 45 pp. (PHS) 2003–1120.

30. Hooyman, N. R., and Kiyak, H. A. (1996). *Social Gerontology* (4th ed.). Boston: Allyn and Bacon.

31. Arno. P. S. *Economic Value of Informal Caregiving.* Presented at the American Association of Geriatric Psychiatry, February 24, 2002.

32. AARP/*Modern Maturity.* (1999). *AARP/Modern Maturity Sexuality Survey.*

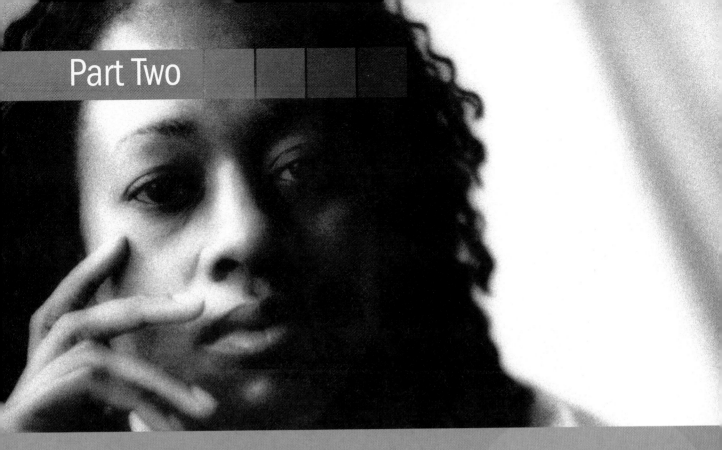

Part Two

Sexual and Reproductive Dimensions of Women's Health

Chapter Four

Sexual Health

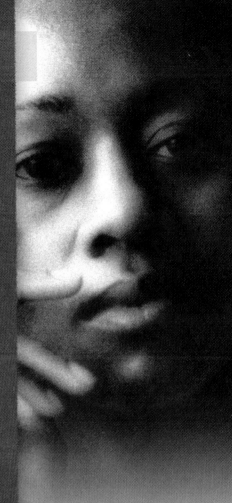

Chapter Objectives

On completion of this chapter, the student should be able to discuss:

1. The ways in which cultural values, stereotypes, and socialization define or influence sexual behavior.

2. The economic, legal, and political dimensions of sexual health.

3. The significance of research on sexual behavior and major contributors to this body of research.

4. The difference between sex and gender and the concepts of gender identity and gender role.

5. Homosexual, heterosexual, and bisexual orientation and issues surrounding homophobia.

6. The location and function of the major external and internal female genital structures.

7. The three phases of the menstrual cycle.

8. The four basic phases of the female sexual response cycle.

9. Several examples of sexual expression.

10. The importance of the gynecological examination and the procedures involved.

11. The major areas of sexual dysfunction in women.

12. The ways in which sexuality is expressed throughout a person's life span.

13. Sexual violence as a public health problem.

14. The significance of communication in intimate relationships and with a woman's healthcare provider.

womenshealth.jbpub.com

Women's Health Online is a great source for supplementary women's health information for both students and instructors. Visit

http://womenshealth.jbpub.com
to find a variety of useful tools for learning, thinking, and teaching.

Introduction

Sexual health refers to the physical, psychological, social, cultural, and emotional facets of human interactions. The World Health Organization defines sexual health as

> . . . a state of physical, emotional, mental and social well-being related to sexuality; it is not merely the absence of disease, dysfunction or infirmity. Sexual health requires a positive and respectful approach to sexuality and sexual relationships, as well as the possibility of having pleasurable and safe sexual experiences, free of coercion, discrimination, and violence. For sexual health to be attained and maintained, the sexual rights of all persons must be respected, protected, and fulfilled.[1]

Sexual health is not limited to an individual's being but extends into that person's relationship with another person. The need for intimacy and physical sharing is a lifelong biological and social theme. Understanding sexual health requires a multifaceted examination from both scientific and psychosocial perspectives. Sexual health entails the need for responsible sexual behavior to avoid sexually transmitted diseases, unintended pregnancy, and sexual abuse, coercion, or violence. Positive sexuality requires thoughtful and respectful discussion of issues that may be difficult or awkward for some people to vocalize. Improving sexual health and acting responsibly in relation to sexuality can be achieved by learning about the physical and emotional aspects of sexuality and by respecting the variations in forms of sexual behavior.

Perspectives on Sexual Health and Sexuality

An underlying assumption throughout history and throughout cultures has been that little boys grow up to be men and do what men do, and little girls grow up to be women and do what women do. Yet when cultures are examined, it becomes readily apparent that no universal standard applies. Because variation in sexual norms exists across cultures, the question arises as to what causes people to assume specific sexual roles and preferences. The biological hypothesis—that sexual behavior is simply a reproductive function—is not substantiated across generations or across cultures.

Cultural and Religious Dimensions

Sexual behavior is often defined by cultural values. Tremendous cultural diversity throughout the world creates considerable diversity regarding a wide spectrum of sexuality issues, including normative sex roles, accepted types of sexual activity, preferences for sexual arousal, and the sanctions and prohibitions on sexual behavior. One consistent theme exists, however—that of "marriage" in some form or another. Within all cultures, marriage provides sanctioned sexual privileges and obligations. Social scientists have recognized that every society

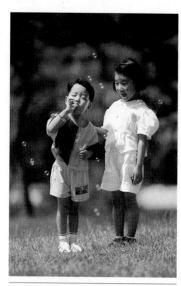

■ Society expects little boys to grow up to be men and do what men do, and little girls to grow up to be women and do what women do.

shapes, structures, or constrains the development and expression of sexuality in all of its members.[2]

Some cultures have strong values that warn against premarital sex; those participating in sexual activity before marriage bring shame to a family and may be ostracized from a community. Other cultures insist on extreme modesty and sexual restraint for females, but have a greater acceptance for male sexual behavior. Many cultures ignore the sexuality and sexual needs of people with disabilities, while stigmatizing people involved in same-sex relationships. Other cultural influences extend into contraception decision making. In some cultures, it is acceptable for a woman to decide what form of birth control to use, as well as to purchase condoms and ask her partner to use them. In other cultures, men take charge of this decision and it would be considered disrespectful of a woman to mention the use of contraception to her partner. The tremendous cultural diversity in the United States results in a spectrum of perspectives, values, and messages to women about sexual practices.

Economic Dimensions

Historically, marriage represented the exchange of property between two families—usually in the form of a daughter. The daughter was either purchased from the maternal family through the exchange of goods or, in some cultures, the father of the girl would offer a dowry to the groom's family to compensate for the financial burden of taking the girl into their house/clan.

Throughout history, and even today in most of the world, the value of a bride often depends on her virginity. A girl who has lost her virginity prior to marriage, either willingly or unwillingly, can lose significant value to both her family and the groom's family she is entering. In the United States and other Western countries, it has become extremely common for young women to have sex prior to marriage.

Sexuality can be viewed within a frame of power and economic dynamics. The less power a woman has, based on either cultural or individual factors, the less able she is to control a given sexual encounter. Significant power imbalances, like those seen between rich and poor, educated and non-educated, and young and old, have been strongly associated with sexual violence and abuse. For example, within the commercial sex industry in Bangkok, Thailand, the highest incidence of sexual violence is documented between Western adult males and native girl sex workers under the age of 12. The ability for women to say "no" to unwanted sexual aggression can be significantly undermined by social and economic factors that give men more power. In contrast, initiatives in the United States and abroad that educate women about how to achieve more parity in the power distribution of their relationships have had a positive effect in reducing sexual violence and empowering women in contraceptive decision making.

A more obvious economic relationship of sexuality occurs between a commercial sex worker, or prostitute, and a sex consumer. In this relationship, sexual acts are delineated and certain price points are attached to them. Many intellectuals have argued that prostitution creates the ultimate power inversion, whereby

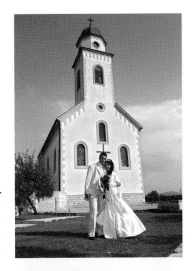

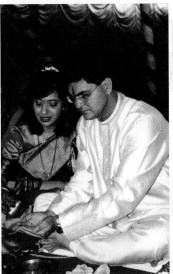

Marriage is a central social underpinning of most societies.

women take control of sexuality and reap the financial rewards of performing sexual acts. They argue that the implicit economics of sex experienced by many people in regular relationships are thrown open in the sex worker/sex consumer relationship, thereby creating a purer interaction. Though each point has some validity, the reality for most sex workers is quite different. The vast majority of sex workers are working under some level of indentured servitude for a male pimp who takes a portion of their earnings in exchange for protection and limiting competition. Pimps are individuals who act as brokers and supposed protectors for sex workers. They often require their sex workers to perform sexual acts on them for free, and they use physical abuse and threats to maintain power in the relationship.

Legal Dimensions

Laws criminalizing sexual intimacy were once in force in all 50 states; they originally were enacted to impose norms on the lives of the nation's citizens and possibly to prevent sexual activity not intended for procreation. Cohabitation and **fornication,** defined as sexual intercourse between unmarried partners, were illegal in most states; currently, 11 states and the District of Columbia retain criminal laws against fornication and a few states have laws against cohabitation. Although these laws exist, they are rarely enforced.

Laws criminalizing **sodomy,** defined as oral and/or anal sex, made it a crime for any unmarried partners—heterosexual, lesbian, or gay—to engage in private, consensual sodomy; some states have exclusively prohibited sodomy between same-sex partners. According to the American Civil Liberties Union, "while most of these laws apply to both straight and gay people, they are primarily used against lesbians and gay men. For example, some courts say sodomy laws justify separating parents from their children."[3] Illinois was the first state to repeal its sodomy law in 1961. In the 1970s and 1980s, 21 states removed the sodomy laws from their books. The laws remained on the books in 13 states and Puerto Rico until a 2003 ruling by the U.S. Supreme Court. The Court struck down state laws that ban sodomy, calling them an unconstitutional violation of privacy.

Same-sex partners also face discrimination when it comes to legalizing their partnership. Same-sex marriages are currently legal in only a few countries around the world; a number of countries and some U.S. states recognize civil unions, which offer some—but not all—of the rights of a civil marriage. A civil union license makes the couple eligible for the same state-provided benefits, protections, and responsibilities that are granted to spouses in a marriage. For example, the couple becomes subject to laws regarding annulment, separation and divorce, child custody and support, and property division and maintenance; however, a civil union does not provide access to federal benefits of marriage, nor does it guarantee recognition of the union outside of the state or country that has granted the union. Likewise, many states ban recognition of marriages of same-sex couples should they be permitted in another state or country.

Political Dimensions

Sex education in school is commonplace these days. Generally, two types of programs exist:

- Abstinence-only programs
- Comprehensive or "abstinence-plus" programs, which include information about abstinence and contraception

Significant controversy surrounds what should be taught in schools, and the guidelines on this issue differ by state. A number of studies show that the majority of Americans favor some form of sexual education in school and believe that birth control information should be made available to adolescents. Although concerns have been voiced that teaching about sex and birth control might lead to an increase in teens having sex, research shows that these types of programs either have no effect on the age of initiation of sexual activity or delay initiation. Some programs also show an increased rate of condom use in teens already engaging in sexual activity.

Despite the support for comprehensive programs, abstinence-only programs have received increased federal funding under the current administration. In 1996, Congress passed a welfare reform bill that included a permanent appropriation of $50 million over five years for abstinence-only education. Not surprisingly, many states with budget problems have turned to abstinence-only education programs, created by businesses and purchased by school districts and states using federal tax dollars. Increases in federal funding for abstinence education have prompted intense debates between supporters of abstinence-only education and supporters of comprehensive sex education.

Sex Research

Sexual behavior, one of the most important of all human activities, is the process by which the species is reproduced, the central behavior around which families are formed, and a way for individuals to express intimacy. Sexual behavior is also central to a number of social and medical problems: marital difficulties and divorce; incest and child molestation; the reproductive issues of infertility, sterility, contraception, unwanted pregnancy, and abortion; and sexually transmitted diseases. Despite its importance, there has been less systematic, scientific research on the sexual behavior of Americans than on most other health and social topics of importance. The AIDS epidemic has improved the accuracy and increased the availability of information on sexual behavior, but the collection of scientific information on sexual matters continues to face much political opposition.

Researchers attempting to understand sexual behavior face many of the same problems that handicap all research into human social behavior. Human subjects cannot be placed in a laboratory-type setting where variables that influence outcome measures can be controlled. Human behavior is infinitely more complex,

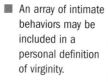 An array of intimate behaviors may be included in a personal definition of virginity.

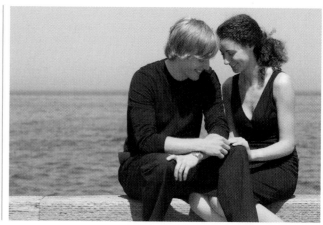

and studies, particularly on human behavior, are prone to many types of contamination and bias. Sex is considered a private arena and as such is even more limited than other areas of behavioral research. Clearly, many problematic issues arise with any attempt to understand the prevalence and nature of contemporary sexual behavior.

Even with these limitations, there are still a number of ways to study sexual behavior—for example, case studies, direct observation, experimental laboratory research, and surveys. What to measure presents another difficulty in sexual research, however. Sexual research could be addressed directly, as in determining the actual prevalence of certain sexual behaviors such as oral-genital sex or types of sexual activity such as the prevalence of homosexual activity. Indirect assessments, such as adolescent pregnancy rates or sexually transmitted disease rates, provide insight into the consequences of sexual behavior.

Definitions create another technical difficulty in research. For example, a frequently quoted statistic in sex research is the number of people in a given category who have engaged in premarital sex. "Premarital sex" has been traditionally defined as penile-vaginal intercourse that takes place before a couple is married. This definition is misleading because it excludes a broad array of noncoital heterosexual and homosexual activities. Heavy petting can include extensive noncoital types of sexual contact, often resulting in orgasm. "Virginity," therefore, may not reflect a lack of sexual activity. The term "premarital" has inherent connotations that may be inappropriate to some individuals, especially given the prevalence of long-term relationships in certain cultures that offer commitments equal to marriage. Not all couples who engage in sexual activity have marital intentions with that partner. Any review of sex studies must take into consideration the inherent limitations of such research.

Well-Known Studies

Several important studies on sexual behavior have been conducted, providing valuable information and insight into sexual practices, behaviors, and attitudes.

- In 1948 and 1953, Kinsey conducted the most comprehensive taxonomic surveys of human sexual behavior to date.[4,5] The 1948 study researched sexual behavior in the human male, and the 1953 study researched sexual behavior in the human female. Both studies aimed at presenting objective data on sexual behavior. The researchers interviewed thousands of people of various socioeconomic status, educational level, marital status, and sex education experiences. The results showed how factors such as age, religious adherence, and gender determined the incidence, frequency, and patterns of sexual behavior.

- Masters and Johnson are perhaps the best-known sex researchers. In 1966, through direct observation techniques, they observed and recorded more than 10,000 completed sexual response cycles.[6] Prior to their work, no significant empirical data had been gathered about male and female sexual arousal. Masters and Johnson were considered pioneers in sexual research for determining that the sexual response cycle consisted of four phases: excitement, plateau, orgasm, and resolution.

- The *Redbook* Survey (1977) was a questionnaire sent to more than 100,000 women that examined sexual behavior and attitudes of American women.[7] This survey was remarkable in that it documented women's sexual fulfillment in respect to their marital status, age at sexual initiation, and sexual fidelity.

- In 1976, the Hite Report, a questionnaire survey on female sexuality, also provided extensive narrative answers to several important questions about the sexual practices of American women.[8]

- Blumstein and Schwartz (1983) elicited excellent information about a variety of sexual and nonsexual components of relationships from a large national sample.[9]

Although each study was criticized for over-representing or under-representing certain population segments, these studies have all provided valuable information and insight into sexual behavior and attitudes. They demonstrate, however, that in evaluating any study of sexual behavior, it is important to consider the quality of the study method and the sampling techniques employed.

In 2001 the Surgeon General's Call to Action to Promote Sexual Health and Responsible Sexual Behavior expanded the research base helping to provide a foundation for promoting sexual health and responsible sexual behavior.[10] The Call to Action is remarkable for being the first time that the promotion of responsible sexual behavior and the improvement of sexual health are being addressed as significant public health challenges (see **It's Your Health**).

Sex and Gender

Gender refers to the economic, social, and cultural attributes and opportunities associated with being male or female. This term should not be confused with the term **sex,** which refers to an individual's biological status as male or female. Issues surrounding sex and gender differences in health have been evolving for the past

---

It's Your Health

Call to Action to Promote Sexual Health and Responsible Sexual Behavior

Individual responsibility includes the following duties:

- Understanding and awareness of one's sexuality and sexual development

- Respect for oneself and one's partner

- Avoidance of physical and emotional harm to oneself or one's partner

- Ensuring that pregnancy occurs only when welcomed

- Recognition and tolerance of the diversity of sexual values within any community

Community responsibility includes assurance that its members have the following characteristics:

- Access to developmentally and culturally appropriate sexuality education as well as sexual and reproductive health care and counseling

- The latitude to make appropriate sexual and reproductive choices

- Respect for diversity

- Freedom from stigmatization and violence on the basis of gender, race, ethnicity, religion, or sexual orientation

Source: *The Surgeon General's Call to Action to Promote Sexual Health and Responsible Sexual Behavior.* (2001). U.S. Department of Health and Human Services.

several decades. The advancement of the women's movement in the 1960s and 1970s gradually culminated in a number of social, political, and scientific actions. The scientific actions, for example, led to a focus on women's health in biomedical research across the globe. This focus, underscored by social and political mandates, increased equity in scientific research and led to significant advances in knowledge of women's health "from womb to tomb."

An intense push by women's health scientists and advocates for more information and greater focus on sex differences resulted in the National Academies of Science's Institute of Medicine being charged with the responsibility of preparing a report on the issue. This report, *Exploring the Biological Considerations of Human Health: Does Sex Matter?*, was published by the Institute of Medicine in 2001.[11] It underscored the importance of understanding sex and gender differences in health and disease across the life span and the myriad factors that influence such differences, from genetics to hormones to the environment. Yet, as expected, the study posed more questions than it answered. The publication resulted in demands to find answers to questions about sex and gender differences, leading to greater funding for research into both sex-based biology and gender-based medicine.

Gender Identity

Gender identity refers to an individual's personal subjective sense of being male or female. Gender identity is clearly influenced by biological sex, which is determined by a complex set of variables; however, a person's gender identity is not necessarily consistent with his or her biological sex.

The genetic material in a fertilized egg is organized within structures known as chromosomes. Chromosomes give rise to the process of sexual differentiation, whereby an individual develops distinct physical male or female characteristics. The physical femaleness or maleness is not simply a result of this chromosome mix, however, but rather the result of processes that occur at various levels of sexual differentiation. Under normal conditions, the prenatal differentiation processes interact to determine biological sex and later gender identity. In early prenatal development, male and female external genitalia are undifferentiated and will remain so unless a specific gene on the Y chromosome involved in sex determination is present and is activated. This gene is necessary for the development of the testis, so it is involved in initiating the male sexing process. Through a series of complex interactions involving gonadal sex hormones, both the internal and the external sex structures differentiate into male or female genitalia. Because the external genitals, gonads, and some of the internal structures of males and females originate from the same embryonic tissues, it is not surprising that they have homologous, or corresponding, parts (Figure 4.1).

Scientists have determined that some important structural and functional differences exist in the brains of males and females and that the process of sex differentiation of human brains occurs largely, if not exclusively, during prenatal devel-

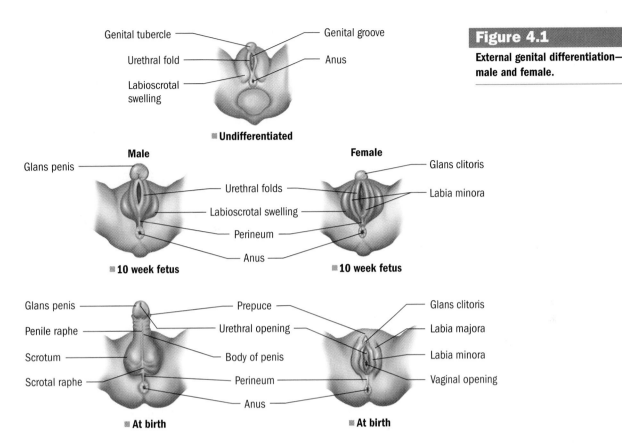

Figure 4.1

External genital differentiation—
male and female.

opment. Sex differences in the brain and the presence of different sex hormones contribute to differences in abilities or processes, such as thinking, remembering, language use, and ability to perceive spatial relationships. Other gender differences such as sensory perception and emotional responses may have significant effects on sexual behaviors. Clearly, these differences also can be significantly influenced by environmental factors and psychosocial factors. It is premature to suggest which factors play the most important role in determining these female–male differences. Some individuals experience considerable confusion and stress in their efforts to establish their gender identity.

Gender Roles

Gender role refers to the public expression of one's gender identity, as well as cultural expectations of male and female behaviors. Behavior thought appropriate for females is termed "feminine"; behavior thought appropriate for males is termed "masculine." Gender-role expectations are culturally defined and vary from society to society. In addition, notions of masculinity and femininity may be era dependent.

Social-learning theory suggests that the identification with either feminine or masculine roles or a combination (androgyny) results primarily from the social and

I used to feel confused about what was feminine or what was masculine. I finally decided that it didn't matter. What mattered is what I wanted to do. I really enjoy nontraditional activities. That really does not make me less of a woman.

18-year-old student

■ Cultural expectations of gender roles and behaviors evolve over time.

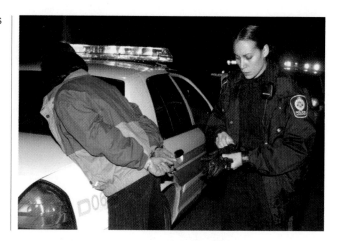

cultural models and influences to which the individual is exposed from birth. Parents typically dress boys and girls differently, for example. Children grow up with "girls' toys" or "boys' toys" and receive reinforcement for gender-expected behaviors. At some point, most children develop a firm sense of being a girl or a boy, as well as a strong desire to adopt behaviors that are considered by society appropriate for their sex. **Socialization** refers to the process whereby society conveys behavioral expectations to the individual. Parents, peer groups, schools, textbooks, and the media frequently help develop and reinforce traditional gender-role assumptions and behaviors. Gender-role conditioning has an impact on all facets of an individual's life, perhaps most importantly in influencing sexuality.

Gender-role expectations and their resulting stereotypes have clearly influenced the ability of women to succeed in traditional male arenas such as sports and professional careers. Stereotyping also influences the sexual health and behavior of women, who naturally find conflict with assumptions and expectations that they be passive, submissive, dependent, emotional, and subordinate. Stereotypical expectations of men and women clearly influence gender-role expectations, for instance. These expectations actually hinder both men and women in maximizing their individual capabilities and in establishing fulfilling relationships. Despite the constraints associated with rigid, stereotypical gender roles, many men and women behave in a manner that is remarkably consistent with the norms that these roles establish (see **It's Your Health**).

Androgyny refers to having characteristics of both sexes. This term is often used to describe flexibility in gender roles. Androgynous individuals have integrated aspects of traditional masculinity and femininity into their lifestyles. Androgyny offers the option of expressing whatever behavior seems appropriate in a given situation instead of limiting responses to those traditionally considered gender appropriate. Androgynous individuals of both sexes are more likely to engage in behavior typically ascribed to the other sex than are gendertyped individuals. Studies have found that androgyny is strongly associated with positive well-being and may be related to successful aging.[12,13]

Transgender

Transgender is an umbrella term that refers to anyone whose behaviors, thoughts, or traits differ from those traditionally ascribed to the person's sex. It is used to describe several groups of people who use other terms to self-identify, including transsexuals and cross-dressers. Like other people, transgender people can be straight, gay, lesbian, or bisexual. That is, transgender is not a sexual orientation. A **transsexual** is a person whose gender identity is opposite to her or his biological sex. A *transsexual* should not be confused with a **transvestite,** an individual who obtains sexual excitement from putting on clothes of the opposite sex. The American Psychiatric Association classifies transsexualism as a gender identity disorder (GID), a mental disorder characterized by strong and persistent cross-gender identification; however, significant controversy exists regarding the classification of transsexuality as a mental disorder.

Gender dysphoria is the overall psychological term used to describe negative or conflicting feelings about one's sex or gender roles. Almost all transgendered people suffer from some degree of gender dysphoria. **Transitioning** is the process in which transsexuals work to change their appearance and societal identity so as to match their gender identity. To acknowledge their transition, transsexuals self-identify as male to female (MTF) or female to male (FTM). Changes are often medical, via surgery and hormones, as well as legal, through name and sex changes on legal documents and forms of identification. Not all transgendered individuals go through transitioning, however. As pointed out by the Human Rights Campaign Foundation, some people "don't feel they fit comfortably identifying as either a man or a woman and instead identify as gender-neutral or simply transgender."[14]

Much literature exists on the characteristics, causes, and treatment of transsexualism. No clear understanding of its nature and causes has yet emerged. Explanations for transsexuality include both biological and social-learning hypotheses. Data support the view that transsexualism may reflect a form of brain hermaphroditism, meaning that structures in the brain are sexually differentiated in a manner opposite to the transsexual's genetic and genital sex.[15] As described by one transgender group, these findings propose "a medical model of transsexuality as an 'obscured' congenital intersex condition in which the genitalia are spared but the brain is not."[16]

Intersexuality refers to the sexual physiology of an individual. A person who is born intersexed is born with sex chromosomes, external genitalia, or internal reproductive organs that are not considered "standard" as male or female. This condition can be manifested as a girl without ovaries, a boy without testes, or a child with genitalia that may appear as neither a vagina nor a penis. Intersex is not simply a gender issue, but encompasses medical ethics and social justice issues. Recent activism has drawn attention to harmful childhood surgeries that are performed to "assign" a sex to an infant; these procedures are referred to as intersex genital mutilation.

■ There is no profile of a lesbian woman. Lesbians may be teenagers, middle-aged, or seniors and of varied socioeconomic status and ethnicity.

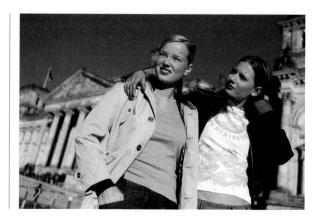

Sexual Orientation

Sexual orientation refers to one's erotic, romantic, and affectional attraction to people of the same sex, to the opposite sex, or to both sexes. **Homosexual orientation** is attraction to same-sex partners, and **heterosexual orientation** is attraction to other-sex partners. A **bisexual** person is attracted to both same-sex and other-sex partners.

Although these concepts imply a clear distinction between the terms, the actual delineation is not so precise. Kinsey described a seven-point continuum that ranged from exclusive contact with and attraction to the other sex to varying degrees of heterosexual and homosexual orientation.[4,5] Although Kinsey's work has been criticized in terms of his methodology and conclusions, the continuum of orientation provides a conceptual model for understanding the variance of sexual orientation in society. The presumption that most people are heterosexual and the idea that heterosexuality and homosexuality represent sharply distinct behaviors are inconsistent with the complex, often unpredictable arena of human behavior.

A homosexual is defined as a person whose primary erotic, psychological, emotional, and social interest is in a member of the same sex. *Gay* is another word often used to describe homosexual men or women as well as social and political concerns related to homosexual orientation.

Homosexual women are often referred to as *lesbians*. There is no profile that fits all lesbian women. Lesbians are of varied socioeconomic status and ethnicity. They may be single, married, divorced, teenagers, middle-aged, or seniors. A large percentage of lesbians exhibit a variety of sexual practices, including heterosexual and bisexual activity. Many misconceptions exist about lesbian sexual expression and lifestyles. The extent to which a lesbian decides to be secretive or open about her sexual orientation has a significant effect on her lifestyle. There are various degrees of being "in the closet" and several steps in the process of "coming out." These steps are usually incremental and include self-acknowledgment, self-acceptance, and disclosure. These steps are particularly difficult because of homophobia.

I am a lesbian. I am still "in the closet." I would like to be more open about my identity, but I am afraid. I hear jokes and comments about homosexuals that really hurt me. I am continually confronted with misunderstandings and fear about homosexuality. If I could erase anything in this world, it would be homophobia.

27-year-old woman

Homophobia is defined as irrational fears of homosexuality, the fear of the possibility of homosexuality in oneself, or self-loathing toward one's own homosexuality. It usually stems from ignorance and popular myths that promote homosexual prejudice. Homophobia may result in activities ranging from verbal assaults to acts of physical aggression or violence. It also may present as attempts to avoid any behavior that might be interpreted as homosexual. It may influence how a woman behaves or responds in lovemaking, what she chooses to wear or not wear, how she embraces other women, or whether she participates in a cause that she may otherwise believe in but avoids because she does not want to be labeled as a lesbian.

Homophobia also leads to discrimination in medical care. More than 50% of physicians from the Gay and Lesbian Medical Association observed colleagues providing substandard care to patients of homosexual orientation.[17] Many healthcare providers, as well as women who identify themselves as lesbians, believe that lesbians are not at risk of sexually transmitted diseases, gynecological infections, or cancers and therefore do not require contraception education, regular cervical cancer screening, or pelvic exams. Some healthcare providers do not address the issue of sexual orientation and assume that any sexually active woman of reproductive age should practice methods of birth control to prevent pregnancy. After encountering physicians who either ignore the facts or respond negatively, many lesbians become hesitant to disclose their sexual orientation or even to visit a healthcare practitioner regularly. By creating awareness among both healthcare providers and lesbians, lesbians should receive better health care and education.[18]

Biological Basis of Sexual Health

Female Sexual Anatomy and Physiology

External Structures

Unfortunately, many women not only harbor misconceptions about their bodies, but also are unfamiliar with their own genitalia. Gaining knowledge and understanding of how her body functions and performs is an important aspect of a woman's sexual health and well-being. One way to begin understanding female sexual anatomy is to examine the vaginal area with a mirror. Some women are afraid to touch themselves. This fear may be an indication of misinformation, cultural or religious beliefs, or insecurity about oneself in a sexual sense.

All women have the same genital structures, but there are individual variances in terms of color, shapes, and textures (Figure 4.2). The **vulva** encompasses all the female external genital structures, including the pubic hair, folds of skin, and urinary and vaginal openings. The **mons veneris,** or "mound of Venus," is the area covering the pubic bone. It consists of pads of fatty tissue between the bone and the skin. Numerous nerve endings in this area are responsible for the pleasure sensations from touch and pressure. At puberty, the mons becomes covered with pubic hair that varies in color, texture, and thickness.

The **labia majora** consist of the outer lips that extend downward from the mons and extend toward each side of the vulva. The color of the labia majora is usually

Figure 4.2

External female sexual anatomy.

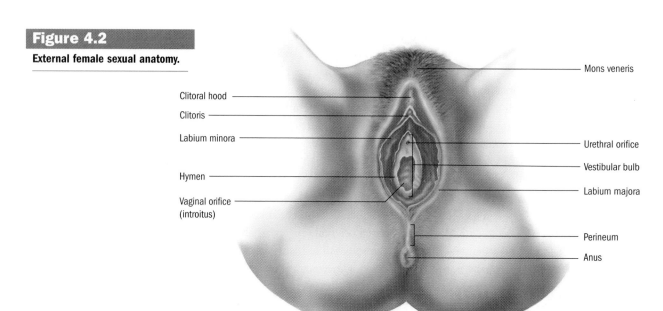

Mons veneris

Clitoral hood

Clitoris

Labium minora

Urethral orifice

Vestibular bulb

Hymen

Labium majora

Vaginal orifice
(introitus)

Perineum

Anus

darker than the color of the thighs. The nerve endings and underlying fatty tissue
are similar to those in the mons. The **labia minora,** or inner lips, are located within
the outer lips and often protrude between them.

The **clitoris** consists of an external shaft and glans and the internal crura; its
function is sexual arousal. The shaft and glans of the clitoris are located just below
the mons area, where the inner lips converge. They are covered by the clitoral
hood, or prepuce. Initially, it may be easier for a woman to locate her clitoris by
touch rather than by sight or location because of its sensitive nerve endings and
small size. The external part of the clitoris, although tiny, has about the same number of nerve endings as the head of the penis.

The vestibule is the area of the vulva inside the labia minora. It is rich in blood
vessels and nerve endings. Its tissues are also sensitive to touch. Both the urinary
and the vaginal openings are located within the vestibule.

The urinary opening is also called the urethral opening. Urine collected in the
bladder passes out through the body via this opening. The **urethra** is the short tube
connecting the bladder to the urinary opening, located between the clitoris and the
vaginal opening.

The vaginal opening, known as the introitus, is located between the urinary
opening and the anus. The **hymen,** a thin piece of tissue, partially covers the introitus. It is typically present at birth and usually remains intact until first penetration, although the vaginal opening is partially open and flexible enough to insert tampons before the hymen has been broken. Although the hymen may serve
to protect the vaginal tissues early in life, it has no other known function. Nevertheless, many cultures have traditionally placed great significance on its presence
or absence. A common misconception is that a woman's virginity can be proved or

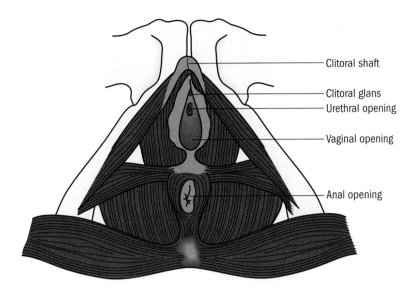

Clitoral shaft

Clitoral glans
Urethral opening

Vaginal opening

Anal opening

It's Your Health

Kegel Exercises

To identify the pelvic floor muscles:

1. Try stopping a flow of urine in midstream while urinating. The muscles that are tightened in this effort are the muscles of the pelvic floor.

2. Tighten the ring of muscles around the rectum, as if trying to stop a bowel movement. The muscles that are tightened in this effort are also muscles of the pelvic floor.

3. While lying down, place a hand over the abdomen. Tighten all of the muscles of the abdomen and pelvis. Notice that the hand will move. These are *not* muscles of the pelvic floor, and they should be relaxed during Kegel exercises. During the first few practice sessions, it is helpful to check with a hand to make sure that the abdominal muscles are relaxed.

To practice Kegel exercises:

1. Take deep breaths—do not forget to breathe.

2. Tighten the anal muscle, pulling inward and outward.

3. Tighten the vaginal muscle, pulling inward and outward.

4. Hold these muscles tight, counting slowly to 10, and then relax.

Do Kegel exercises in sets of 5 to 10 at a time, several times a day. Build up to being able to hold the contraction for 20 seconds at a time.

disproved by the pain or bleeding that may occur with initial coitus. Although discomfort and spotting sometimes occur with first coitus, the hymen can be partial, flexible, or thin enough for there to be no discomfort or bleeding. This very sensitive tissue also may stretch or break while performing activities such as bike riding, horseback riding, and gymnastics.

The **perineum** refers to the area of smooth skin between the vaginal opening and the anus. This tissue is rich with nerve endings and very sensitive to touch.

Internal Structures

Several structures lie along the vaginal opening. The vestibule refers to the area of the vulva inside the labia minora. The vaginal walls are lined with a vast network of bulbs and vessels that engorge with blood during sexual arousal. The vestibular bulbs alongside the vagina also fill with blood during sexual excitement, causing the vagina to increase in length and the vulvar area to become swollen. These bulbs are similar in structure and function to the tissue in the penis that engorges with blood during male sexual arousal and causes penile erection.

The **Bartholin's glands** are located on each side of the vaginal opening. They secrete a liquid that lubricates the tissues at the vaginal opening. The glands are usually not noticeable. Occasionally, the duct from the gland becomes blocked and enlargement results. Medical intervention may be indicated if the condition does not subside within a few days.

In addition to the glands, a complex musculature underlies the genital area. The pelvic floor muscles have a multidirectional design (Figure 4.3) that permits the vaginal opening to expand during childbirth and to contract after delivery. These muscles can lose muscle tone during childbirth or over time. A series of exercises known as **Kegel exercises** can help restore the muscular tone, reduce involuntary urinary incontinence, and enhance sexual sensations (see **It's Your Health**).

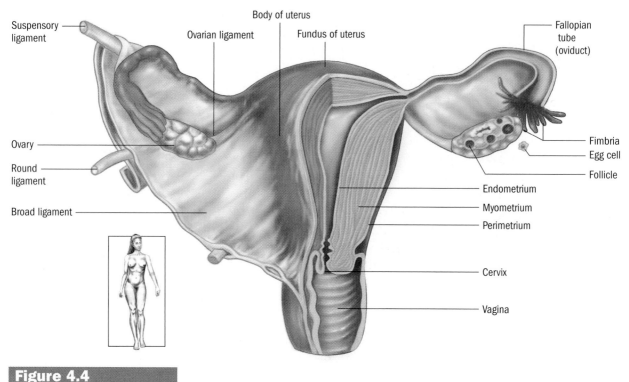

Suspensory ligament

Ovarian ligament

Body of uterus

Fundus of uterus

Fallopian tube (oviduct)

Ovary

Round ligament

Broad ligament

Fimbria

Egg cell

Follicle

Endometrium

Myometrium

Perimetrium

Cervix

Vagina

Figure 4.4

Internal female sexual anatomy.

Internal female sexual anatomy consists of the vagina, cervix, uterus, fallopian tubes, and ovaries (Figure 4.4). The **vagina** opens between the labia minora and extends upward into the body, angling toward the lower back. The vagina is approximately 3 to 5 inches in length when not aroused. The ability of the vagina to expand during sexual arousal and during childbirth is truly amazing. The folded walls of the vagina are known as rugae and form a flat tube. These walls are warm, soft, and moist, and they normally produce secretions that help maintain the chemical balance of the vagina.

The vagina consists of three layers of tissue—mucous, muscle, and fibrous tissue—all of which are richly endowed with blood vessels. The mucosa is a layer of moist membrane inside the vagina. During sexual arousal, lubricating fluid exudes through the mucosa. The muscular tissue is concentrated around the vaginal opening. Fibrous tissue surrounds the muscular layer. This layer aids in vaginal contraction and expansion and also serves as connective tissue to other structures in the pelvic cavity.

The **cervix,** located at the back of the vagina, is the mouth of the uterus and actually looks like a small, pink, glazed doughnut. Glands line the cervical canal and produce a constant downward flow of mucus to protect the uterine cavity from bacterial invasion. The opening in the middle of the cervix, called the os, connects the vagina with the uterine cavity. After childbirth, the os becomes less round and assumes a more horizontal slit position. The cervix is composed of fibrous tissue that is capable of dramatic stretching. During childbirth, the cervical canal is 50 or more times its normal width.

The **uterus,** also known as the womb, is a thick, pear-shaped organ. It is approximately 3 inches long and 2 inches wide in a woman who has never had a child. After a pregnancy, it is somewhat larger. The uterus is suspended within the pelvic cavity by a series of six ligaments. The alignment of these ligaments permits some movement of the uterus within the cavity.

The uterine wall consists of three layers: the endometrium, the myometrium, and the perimetrium. The endometrium is the lining of the uterus, which, in preparation for fertilization, thickens in response to hormone changes during the monthly menstrual cycle. In addition, the endometrium is a source of hormone production. The myometrium, the middle layer, consists of the longitudinal and circular muscle fibers of the uterus. The muscle fibers are interwoven and enable the uterus to expand during pregnancy and contract during labor and childbirth. The myometrium is covered by a thin membrane known as the perimetrium. The perimetrium functions as the external surface of the uterus.

Connecting the uterus with the ovaries are the **fallopian tubes,** which are thin, pale, pink filaments. The outside end of each tube is like a funnel, with fingerlike projections called fimbriae that draw the egg from the ovary into the tube. The **ovaries** are located at the end of the fallopian tubes and are about the size of a small walnut in premenopausal women. They are connected to the pelvic wall and the uterus by ligaments. The ovaries are endocrine glands that produce two classes of sex hormones: estrogens and progesterones. The estrogens influence the development of female physical sex characteristics and help regulate the menstrual cycle. The progesterones help regulate the menstrual cycle and stimulate development of the uterine lining in preparation for pregnancy. During puberty, these hormones play a critical role in the maturation of the reproductive organs and the development of secondary sex characteristics, such as pubic hair and breasts.

The Menstrual Cycle

Women usually begin to menstruate in their early teen years. During the **menstrual cycle,** the uterine lining is prepared for implantation of a fertilized egg. If **conception** does not occur, the lining sloughs off and is discharged as menstrual flow. This menstrual discharge consists of blood, mucus, and endometrial membranes that sometimes present as small clots. The amount of menstrual flow varies, but is usually 6 to 8 ounces in volume per cycle (about half a can of soda). The cycle is often 28 days in length but can vary from 21 to 40 days.

The menstrual cycle (Figure 4.5) is regulated by a complex series of interactions between the hypothalamus and the pituitary gland in the brain, the adrenal glands on top of the kidneys, the ovaries, and the uterus. The hypothalamus produces and secretes hormones and releasing factors that act directly on

Figure 4.5

Female menstrual cycle.

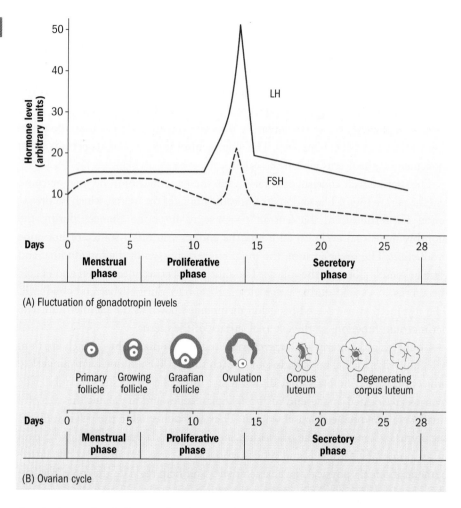

(A) Fluctuation of gonadotropin levels

| Primary follicle | Growing follicle | Graafian follicle | Ovulation | Corpus luteum | Degenerating corpus luteum |

(B) Ovarian cycle

the pituitary gland. One such releasing factor, gonadotropin-releasing hormone (GnRH), is responsible for reproductive hormone control. GnRH varies in amount and frequency during each menstrual cycle. In addition, this hormone is believed to play a role in the timing of puberty. Alterations in the GnRH pulse release may be the mechanism by which stressors such as athletic training or dieting influence menstrual cycles.

■ A wide variety of products are available for use during menustration, including many different styles, sizes, and absorbencies of sanitary napkins or pads, tampons, and menstrual cups.

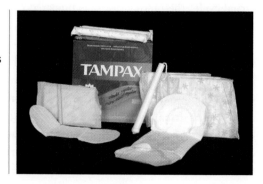

Figure 4.5

(continued)

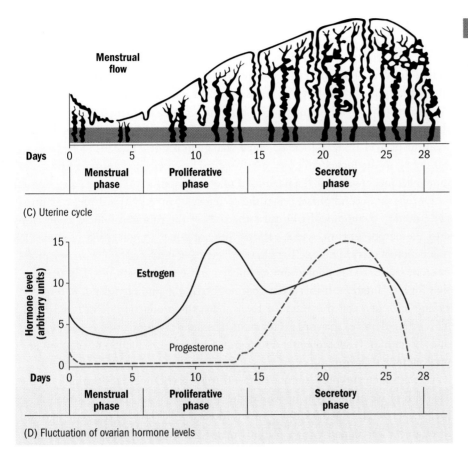

(C) Uterine cycle

(D) Fluctuation of ovarian hormone levels

The menstrual cycle is a self-regulating and dynamic process in which the level of a particular hormone retards or increases the production of the same and other hormones. Throughout the cycle, the hypothalamus monitors the hormone levels in the bloodstream. It sends chemical messages to the pituitary gland, which in turn releases hormones to stimulate the ovaries. These hormones share the general name of gonadotropins because they stimulate the gonads, but they are more specifically known as follicle-stimulating hormone (FSH) and luteinizing hormone (LH). FSH stimulates ovarian production of estrogen and the maturation of the ova and follicles. LH induces the mature ovum to burst from the ovary, and it stimulates the development of the corpus luteum, the portion of the follicle that remains after the egg has matured. The corpus luteum is responsible for producing the hormone progesterone.

These sequenced events are not continuous in nature. Instead, the endometrial menstrual cycle is divided into three stages or phases. Although the menstrual phase is mentioned last in the following discussion, Figure 4.5 illustrates the menstrual phase first to show the development of the primary follicle into an egg (ovum).

In the first phase, known as proliferation, the pituitary gland increases production of FSH, which stimulates the developing follicles to mature and to produce several types of estrogen. Estrogen, in turn, causes the endometrium to thicken. When the level of ovarian estrogen circulating in the bloodstream reaches a peak, the pituitary gland inhibits the release of FSH and stimulates LH production. Approximately 14 days before the onset of the next menstrual cycle, ovulation—the release of the ovum—occurs. The ovum travels into the fallopian tube. Around the time of ovulation, an increase and a change in cervical mucous secretions occur owing to the increased levels of estrogen. The cervical environment becomes more alkaline, enhancing the likelihood of conception.

During the second phase, called the secretory or progestational phase, continued pituitary secretions of LH cause the cells of the ruptured follicle to develop into the corpus luteum, which secretes progesterone. Progesterone inhibits the production of cervical mucus. Together with estrogen produced by the ovaries, progesterone causes the endometrium to thicken and engorge with blood in preparation for implantation. If this event does not occur, the pituitary gland, in response to high estrogen and progesterone levels, halts the production of LH and FSH. This action deprives the corpus luteum of the chemical stimulation needed to produce hormones. It subsequently disintegrates, and the production of estrogen and progesterone decreases.

The estrogen and progesterone drop-off triggers endometrial sloughing during the third phase of the cycle, known as the menstrual phase. The menstrual phase is characterized by the discharge of the thickened inner layer of the endometrium through the cervix and vagina. Various menstrual hygiene products are available for women to use during this time (see Table 4.1). As the hormonal levels continue to fall, the hypothalamus responds to the reduction by stimulating the pituitary to release FSH. The release of the FSH initiates the maturation process of several follicles, and the entire cycle begins again.

Problems with Menstruation

For most women, menstruation creates no medical problems. For others, menstruation brings certain physical and emotional problems. **Dysmenorrhea,** meaning "painful menstrual flow," is a term for what most women call "cramps." It may be caused by the normal production of prostaglandins that produce strong contractions of the uterus (primary dysmenorrhea) or by problems in the uterus, fallopian tubes, or ovaries (secondary dysmenorrhea). Women with primary dysmenorrhea experience pain in the lower abdomen and back, whereas those with secondary dysmenorrhea often feel pain during urination and bowel movements. Relief from primary dysmenorrhea may be found through regular aerobic exercise, stress reduction techniques, adequate sleep, and decreased fat, caffeine, and sodium in the diet. Some women with primary or secondary dysmenorrhea may need anti-inflammatory medications or oral contraceptives to relieve the pain. Secondary dysmenorrhea is treated based on the underlying condition.

Table 4.1	Menstrual Hygiene Products		
Product	**Description**	**Advantages**	**Disadvantages**
Sanitary napkin (pad)	Disposable or washable cloth pad that sticks to inside of underwear; pads come in different shapes, thicknesses, and levels of absorbency	Easy to use	Can become bulky and uncomfortable when wet; some may have an odor after heavy bleeding; cannot use while swimming
Tampon	A "plug" made of rayon/cotton fibers that is inserted into the vagina to absorb the flow of blood; comes with different types of applicators and levels of absorbency	Comfortable for most women and odor-free; allows women to continue with activities such as swimming	Can be difficult for some women to insert and remove; may be uncomfortable for some women
Menstrual cup	A cup that is inserted into the vagina and collects the menstrual flow	Reusable (economical and environmentally friendly); comfortable for many women	Can be messy to empty and clean; may be difficult for women to insert and remove

Premenstrual syndrome (PMS) encompasses a varied set of more than 200 symptoms that present in some women before the menstrual flow and may include tension, increased irritability, depression or anxiety, headaches, and fatigue. Up to 85% of menstruating women have one or more symptoms of PMS, and as many as 10% of women in their childbearing years experience symptoms severe enough to seek treatment.[19,20] Recent studies have shown that estrogen stimulates certain neurotransmitters—specifically, dopamine and serotonin receptors. It has been suggested that the decrease of estrogen prior to the menstrual period causes a fluctuation in the levels of neurotransmitters and consequently produces PMS symptoms.[21] Genetic factors also may play a role.

Women should keep a daily diary to track their premenstrual symptoms over the course of two to three months. Depending on the severity and persistence of the symptoms, women may find the following tips helpful:

- Set a consistent sleep schedule by going to bed and waking up at the same time every day.
- Cut back on sodium and caffeine intake.
- Engage in moderate aerobic exercise.

Over-the-counter products, such as mild diuretics and analgesics, may also be helpful for some women. Although estrogen therapy and oral contraceptives have often been prescribed to women with PMS, there is limited evidence to suggest that these forms of treatment are consistently effective.[22]

An estimated 3–4% of women suffer severe emotional symptoms that interfere with work and social relationships. This form of PMS is called **premenstrual dysphoric disorder (PMDD).** It is believed that women who are susceptible to depression may be more significantly affected by hormonal shifts during the menstrual cycle. Selective serotonin reuptake inhibitors (SSRIs), a type of antidepressant, have proved effective in relieving mood change symptoms in women who experience PMDD.

Amenorrhea is the lack of menstrual flow. Primary amenorrhea occurs in women who have not yet begun menstruation and may result from hormone-related problems or extremely low body fat. Secondary amenorrhea is the lack of blood flow for three or more consecutive months, except during pregnancy, breast-feeding, and perimenopause; it may result from conditions such as anorexia nervosa, ovarian cysts or tumors, substance abuse, stress, or use of oral contraceptives. Healthcare providers will want to work with a woman to first establish the cause of her amenorrhea and then consider options for treatment.

Physical Health and the Gynecological Examination

A gynecological examination usually begins with a medical history and a general physical examination, including a breast examination, and is followed by a pelvic examination. The pelvic exam provides the woman and her clinician with essential basic information about her gynecological health. It should be timed to avoid the menstrual period. It is also advisable to avoid douching at least 24 hours before an examination; some clinicians recommend avoiding vaginal intercourse for at least 48 hours prior to the examination as well. These precautions ensure a more accurate visualization of the cervix and greater likelihood of diagnosing an infection if it is present.

For the pelvic exam, the woman lies on her back with her bottom at the very end of the examining table and her legs supported in foot stirrups. The pelvic examination consists of three phases:

- The first phase is the external examination, in which the clinician inspects the vulva and perineum visually for any evidence of infection or injury.
- The second phase involves the use of a speculum, a device that holds the vaginal walls apart to permit visual inspection of the cervix. The speculum is inserted with the blade closed. Once inside the vagina, the blades are opened and locked into place at the correct width. With the speculum open, the clinician inspects the vaginal walls and cervix for any redness, irritation, unusual discharge, or lesions. Specimens for laboratory tests are collected while the speculum is in place. After the specimens are collected, the speculum is removed.

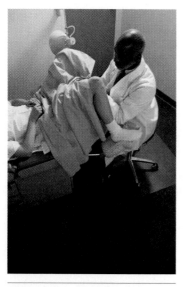

■ The pelvic examination is an important part of a woman's health visit.

- The third phase of the examination is the bimanual examination, which involves the insertion of two gloved fingers of one hand into the vagina while the other hand presses downward on the abdomen. The purpose of this activity is to locate and feel the size, consistency, and shape of the uterus and ovaries and to check for any abdominal masses or tender areas.

A rectal examination also may be performed to evaluate the muscular wall separating the rectum and vagina, the position of the uterus, and any possible masses or tenderness in the area.

A pelvic examination takes only a few minutes, and it provides a starting point to ascertain any gynecological or sexual health concerns. Pelvic examinations should be arranged at regular intervals throughout a woman's adult life (see **It's Your Health**).

Sexual Arousal and Sexual Response

Sexual arousal and response are highly individualized physical, emotional, and mental processes. The female sexual response is not a geographically isolated phenomenon of the vaginal area. Instead, the brain, senses, and hormones all play an integrated role in the response cycle.

The brain plays an important role in sexual arousal by mediating thoughts, emotions, and fantasies that provide the psychological "stage" for the sexual experience. The senses of touch, smell, and sight provide stimuli that can significantly influence the level of sexual arousal. Hormones affect sexual response as well, in addition to performing their primary role of regulating the menstrual cycle. The function of certain hormones in the sexual response cycle—specifically, estrogens and androgens—has been studied extensively for many years. Estrogens promote cell growth and replication in the vaginal cells, increase blood flow in the vagina and urethra, and maintain vaginal lubrication in postmenopausal women. Androgens affect the brain by influencing sexual behavior and libido; when combined with estrogen in postmenopausal women, androgen therapy can bring significant improvements for women in sexual desire and arousal, sensation, energy level, and overall sense of well-being.[23,24] Additional studies are needed to determine the specific roles of estrogen and androgen and the effects of estrogen-androgen therapy on a woman's health.

The sexual response cycle has been described in several ways, most notably by Masters and Johnson.[6] This model is merely a framework for describing physiological sexual response patterns. In reality, tremendous variability and differences are characteristic of sexual response, and these patterns represent only a composite of the physiological reactions. Masters and Johnson reported three variations among women in the sexual response cycle, as shown in Figure 4.6. Pattern #1, which most closely resembles the male pattern, demonstrates that some women are able to have one or more orgasms without dropping below the plateau level of sexual arousal. Pattern #2, a variation of this response, includes an extended plateau with

It's Your Health

Gynecological Examination

A woman should plan to see her clinician once a year for an examination under the following conditions:

Before first coitus

If menarche has not occurred by age 16

At age 20 or earlier for first coitus

Heavy menstrual flow

Menstrual period lasting longer than 10 days

If risk for sexually transmitted diseases is present or if there is a history of abnormal Pap smears or positive HPV test

Any time there is vaginal itching, redness, sores, swelling, unusual odor, or unusual discharge

Painful intercourse

Missed menstrual period if there is a chance of pregnancy

Three missed menstrual periods if there is no chance of pregnancy

Burning or frequency of urination

Sexual partner has a genital infection or sore

Rape

Vaginal or rectal injury

Figure 4.6

Female sexual response cycle.

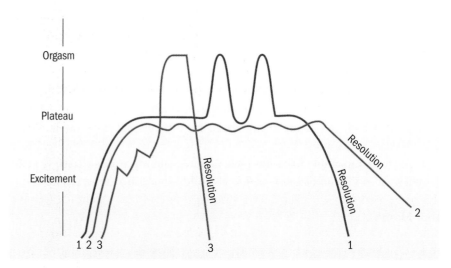

no orgasm. A rapid rise to orgasm with no definitive plateau and a quick resolution pattern is described with Pattern #3.

Each pattern distinguishes four phases: excitement, plateau, orgasm, and resolution. In the excitement phase of the female sexual response cycle, the clitoris swells with blood engorgement. This change ranges from very slight to quite noticeable. The clitoral glans is highly sensitive. Some women find that the entire sexual response cycle can be set into motion and maintained to orgasm by light stimulation of the glans alone. The glans is so sensitive that women usually stimulate the area with the hood covering the clitoris to avoid direct stimulation. In addition to clitoral swelling, the labia majora flatten and separate during the excitement phase. The labia minora increase in size, and lubrication begins.

Lubrication is a unique feature of the vagina and an important aspect of sexual arousal. It is often the first physiological sign of sexual arousal in women. During arousal, a clear, slippery fluid appears on the vaginal mucosa. The lubrication is a result of vasocongestion, the pooling of blood in the pelvic area. During vasocongestion, the extensive network of blood vessels in the tissues surrounding the vagina engorges with blood. Clear fluid seeps from the congested tissues to the inside of the vaginal walls to form the slippery coating of the vagina. Vaginal lubrication serves two primary functions. First, it enhances the possibility of conception by helping to alkalinize the normally acidic vaginal chemical balance. Sperm are able to move more quickly and survive longer in an alkaline environment. Second, vaginal lubrication helps to increase sexual pleasure.

Also during the excitement phase, the uterus elevates and becomes engorged with blood, and the breasts enlarge. Superficial veins in breast tissues may become more visible during this time.

During the plateau phase of the female sexual response cycle, the clitoris withdraws under its hood and shortens in length. The labia majora remain unchanged from the excitement phase, while the labia minora intensify in color. An orgasmic platform develops from further vasocongestion of the outer third of the vagina. Lubrication from the vagina slows, and the uterus is fully elevated in position. Breast tissue remains swollen.

As effective stimulation occurs, many women move from the plateau phase to the orgasmic phase of the sexual response cycle. In contrast to men, who almost always experience orgasm after reaching the plateau level, women may obtain plateau levels without the orgasmic release. Many women cannot reach orgasm by penis insertion alone, and therefore prefer other forms of stimulation in addition to coital stimulation. The "G" spot, or Grafenberg spot, has been identified as a sensitive area that can lead to orgasm when stimulated. It can be felt through the vaginal wall, halfway between the pubic bone and the cervix. The existence of the "G" spot remains controversial, however, with many researchers believing the spot represents the root of the clitoris.[25] Orgasm is the shortest phase of the sexual response cycle, although female orgasms often last slightly longer than male orgasms. It is important to note that orgasmic experiences vary widely in terms of intensity, frequency, and duration among both men and women. The female physiological responses in the orgasmic phase include an elevated blood pressure, heart rate, and breathing pattern. Orgasmic platform contractions are rhythmical, beginning at high intensity and then becoming weaker and slower. The uterus usually contracts at orgasm. These physiological responses are consistent whether they originate from direct clitoral stimulation or from coital stimulation, although women report wide differences in subjective feelings and preferences.[7,9]

The resolution phase is the final phase of the sexual response cycle. During this phase, the sexual systems return to the nonexcited state. If no additional stimulation occurs, the resolution begins immediately after orgasm. Skin coloration quickly subsides, and vital signs return to normal levels. The clitoris, labia majora, and labia minora return to their unaroused sizes and positions.

A significant male–female response difference occurs in the resolution period. After orgasm, the male typically enters a refractory period—a time when no amount of additional stimulation will result in orgasm. This time period has considerable variability among men and depends on a number of physiological and psychological factors. In contrast to men, women generally experience no comparable refractory period. Thus they are physiologically capable of returning to another orgasmic peak during the resolution phase.

The female sexual response cycle described here is simply a framework for understanding the physiological events of sexual response. This model does not attempt to incorporate the emotional, cultural, psychological, and subjective dimensions of the sexual experience, which can significantly influence the experience in dramatically positive or negative directions. The framework is further compromised by not identifying differences between the sexes. In reality, there is considerably more variability in the female sexual response than this model would indicate.

Forms of Sexual Expression

Society has traditionally placed restrictions on the forms of sexual expression that are considered appropriate. One of the most traditional heterosexual positions is known as the "missionary" position (male on top of female). Missionary heterosexual sex is only one of many sexual expression options, however. Women may elect different forms of sexual expression under different circumstances or at different times in their lives.

Masturbation refers to erotic self-stimulation, usually to the point of orgasm. Historical records indicate that masturbation has been practiced since ancient times. Masturbation practices begin early in life with infants exploring their genitals and receiving pleasure from touching them. Often self-stimulation continues throughout life, whether or not the individual is a partner in an intimate relationship. Studies vary greatly regarding masturbation statistics, although all studies show that this practice is more common in boys than girls. By about age 15, 33% of girls report masturbating as compared with 58% of boys. Studies on college students have yielded varied results, showing that from 45% to 56% of women and from 77% to 93% of men had masturbated. Among the people who participated in the studies, men reported masturbating three to four times more frequently than women.[26]

Even though the practice of masturbation is widespread, many women feel ashamed or embarrassed of the practice. Folklore has falsely labeled masturbation as sinful, evil, and even physically or mentally harmful. Such ideas are entirely false, and many therapists and sex experts believe that masturbation can be helpful as a sexual outlet and as a means to become comfortable with one's own body.

Petting is defined as erotic stimulation of a person by a sexual partner, without actual sexual intercourse. It can include kisses, genital caresses, and oral-genital contact. Petting may culminate in orgasm. During adolescence, petting is often a way to experience intense sexual excitement without actually engaging in intercourse. Petting is carried over into adult sexual experiences as foreplay or for sexual variety.

Oral-genital stimulation, also known as oral sex, takes two basic forms. **Cunnilingus** is the act of sucking or licking the vulva, particularly the clitoris. **Fellatio** is the act of sucking or licking the penis and scrotum. A common sexual practice among both heterosexual and homosexual couples, oral sex is often believed to be a "safe" sexual activity. Although the risk is smaller than that with vaginal or anal intercourse, sexually transmitted diseases such as genital herpes, human papillomavirus, gonorrhea, and HIV all can be transmitted through oral-genital sex.

Anal intercourse is another form of sexual expression. Because the anal opening is richly endowed with nerves, this area can be very sensitive and sexually arousing. A couple needs to be careful, however, in performing anal intercourse for many reasons. The anal sphincter tends to be tight and when stimulated can tighten even more, resulting in pain on penetration. In addition, the anal region has no natural lubrication of its own, which increases the possibility of both pain and injury. Usually anal intercourse can be accomplished without discomfort if precautions are taken. A water-based lubricant (not petroleum-based products, which weaken condoms) should be used. Care should be taken to avoid contamination of the vaginal area once anal penetration has occurred. It must be emphasized that anal intercourse is not without risks. This kind of sexual activity has been associated with the transmission of both hepatitis B and HIV as well as most other sexually transmitted diseases. Anyone engaging in anal intercourse should use a latex condom and never use a petroleum-based lubricant. In addition, after anal penetration, the genitals should be washed thoroughly before resuming vaginal or oral sex.

In addition to stimulation with hands or other body parts, many women choose to use sex toys and accessories, either by themselves or with their partner. When used in a mutually comfortable way, these items may enhance the sexual experience of one or both partners. In addition, many women use vibrators to help themselves reach orgasm during masturbation. Other sexual accessories that can enhance arousal include dildos, nipple clamps, and various flavored lotions and oils.

Sexual Dysfunction

Sexual dysfunction is defined as the inability of an individual to function adequately in terms of sexual arousal, orgasm, or in coital situations. According to the U.S. National Health and Social Life Survey, 43% of women suffer from sexual dysfunction:[27]

- One-third of the women lacked sexual interest.
- One-fourth of the women were unable to experience orgasm in menopause.
- One-fifth of the women reported lubrication difficulties.
- One-fifth of the women said they did not find sex pleasurable.

In another study, conducted by Dr. John Bancroft, Director of The Kinsey Institute, 23% of women surveyed reported a sexual problem causing at least moderate distress or worry.[28] In the past, the sexual problems of women were classified under the general label of "frigidity." These problems were severely misunderstood and thought to be symptomatic of a neurosis or some other psychological disorder that required long-term psychiatric therapy. This traditional approach persisted despite the absence of a demonstrated relationship between the treatment and the alleviation of the sexual problem. More recently, however, the pharmaceutical industry has become more interested in understanding and treating female sexual problems with the hopes of uncovering a new market as lucrative as that for male-targeted medications such as Viagra.

Today, four major areas of sexual dysfunction are defined for women: sexual desire disorders, sexual arousal disorders, orgasmic disorders, and sexual pain disorders.

Sexual desire disorders include hypoactive sexual desire disorder and sexual aversion disorder. **Hypoactive sexual desire disorder (HSDD)** appears to be the most common of the sexual dysfunctions. Women experiencing HSDD have a persistent lack of interest in or desire for sex. This disorder often reflects relationship problems but may also be caused by other physical or personal difficulties. Women with HSDD may experience physical symptoms of anxiety when they attempt to engage in sexual activity. Treatment of HSDD is often difficult because the woman may lack insight into the basic motivations of avoidance and hostility that underlie the disorder. The treatment approach most often used seeks to modify the woman's tendency to inhibit erotic feelings and allow them to emerge naturally. Along the way, the woman learns not to fight or suppress the natural tendency to become aroused in sexual situations.

Sexual aversion disorder is persistent anxiety or disgust to sexual stimuli, and thus avoidance of sexual contact with a partner, which causes personal distress. This disorder, which is more common in women than in men, is frequently associated with a history of sexual trauma or abuse. Treatment is difficult and may require working with a psychologist to get to the root of the anxiety or disgust.[29,30]

A woman with sexual arousal disorder is generally nonresponsive and often describes herself as being void of sexual feelings. She experiences little or no erotic pleasure from sexual stimulation. Treatment of general sexual dysfunction is directed primarily at the creation of a nondemanding, relaxed, and sensuous atmosphere in which sexual responsiveness develops. Communication with a partner about her sexual wishes and feelings is encouraged. Other treatment activities for general sexual dysfunction focus on the reduction of sexual anxiety and the unfolding of sexual feelings with sensate focus, genital stimulation, and nondemanding coitus.

Orgasmic disorder refers specifically to the inability to experience the orgasmic component of the sexual response cycle. A woman with an orgasmic disorder may have a strong sex drive, become readily aroused, and develop vasocongestion and lubrication, but the neuromuscular discharge of orgasm is inhibited. Achieving orgasm is not a criterion of sexual competence or normality in women. Nor is orgasmic dysfunction necessarily a symptom of pathology. Orgasm is a physical response that is highly variable among women. Learning effective self-stimulation is often recommended for women who have never experienced orgasm. One advantage of self-stimulation is that a woman without a partner can learn to become orgasmic. For a woman with a sexual partner, becoming orgasmic first by masturbation may help develop a sense of sexual autonomy that can increase the likelihood of satisfaction with a partner later.

Sexual pain disorders include dyspareunia, vaginismus, and noncoital sexual pain disorders.

- **Dyspareunia** relates to painful intercourse and can stem from physical or psychological causes. Painful intercourse may be the result of vaginal irritation or insufficient lubrication. Dyspareunia may also result from very frequent intercourse. Psychological reasons, such as shame, embarrassment, and guilt, may also contribute to painful or uncomfortable intercourse for women.

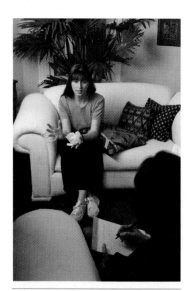

▪ A trained counselor or clinician can often provide valuable assistance for a woman who is experiencing sexual dysfunction.

Self-Evaluation for Sexual Dysfunction

1. Do you experience pain or discomfort during intercourse?
2. Do you lack interest in or desire for sex?
3. Do you feel anxious when you begin to engage in sexual activity?
4. Do you lack pleasure when sexually stimulated?
5. Do you have difficulty achieving orgasm?

Answering yes to one or more of these questions may signify a sexual problem. Communication with one's partner may help resolve some of the issues. If not, women should seek medical attention to rule out any underlying causes and consider therapy to address ways to enhance sexual satisfaction.

- **Vaginismus** is a relatively rare form of sexual difficulty in which a woman experiences involuntary spasmodic contractions of the muscles of the outer third of the vagina. Attempts to achieve coitus are painful and frustrating, and even physical examinations involving vaginal penetration are virtually impossible without anesthesia. Women with vaginismus are often extremely fearful of coital or other penetration and develop high levels of anxiety under such circumstances. Treatment for this problem often begins during a pelvic examination, with the therapist or a consulting physician demonstrating the vaginal spasm reaction to the woman or the woman and her partner. Relaxation and self-awareness techniques are encouraged, along with specific exercises to gradually relax the vaginal muscle spasms.

- Noncoital sexual pain disorders include recurrent or persistent genital pain induced by any type of sexual stimulation other than intercourse. Often, the cause of this type of pain can include vaginal infections, female genital mutilation, or **vestibulitis,** a recurring inflammation and burning sensation around the vaginal opening.

Any form of sexual dysfunction or discomfort with intercourse or sexual stimulation should be evaluated to rule out any underlying pathology (see Self-Assessment 4.1). In addition, the evaluation should include efforts such as counseling or therapy, if needed, to seek resolution of the condition.

Sex Therapy

Professional help may be indicated in those cases in which individualized efforts, couple efforts, or both do not produce the desired effects. Sex therapy has evolved as a legitimate method for understanding sexual problems and increasing sexual satisfaction. In many cases, communication about sexual issues and finding ways to solve problems are critical but often difficult steps toward achieving a satisfying sex life. Sex therapy often can make such communication easier. Strategies with a therapist may range from expanding self-knowledge to sharing more effectively with a partner.

I used to fake orgasms. I am not sure why, but somehow I felt it was necessary. My current partner figured it out, and we have spent a lot of time talking about this. I am seeing a therapist. With a few sessions, I was able to climax with masturbation, and I know that I am much more comfortable with my sexuality. I know that "faking it" was not fair to me or my partner.

35-year-old woman

There are many approaches to sex therapy, and many approaches share common goals. These common goals often relate to permission. That is, a therapist can play an important role in reassuring clients that thoughts, feelings, fantasies, desires, and behaviors that enhance satisfaction are normal, as long as they do not have potentially negative consequences. Often all that is needed is reassurance that clients can appreciate their unique patterns and desires instead of comparing themselves with friends or national averages. In addition, a therapist can be helpful in giving clients permission not to engage in certain behaviors unless they want to.

Providing information is another common activity of therapy. By providing specific accurate and reassuring information, a therapist is often able to address thoughts and feelings that may be interfering with the person's ability to enjoy or respond to sexual activity. A therapist is also able to provide specific activities or homework "assignments" that enable the client to reduce anxiety, enhance communication, and learn new sexually enhancing behavioral techniques. Intensive therapy may be indicated in some situations in which personal emotional difficulties or significant relationship problems interfere with sexual expression.

Sexuality Through the Life Span

In many Western societies, childhood has traditionally been seen as a time of unexpressed sexuality and behavior, and adolescence has been viewed as a time to restrain immature sexual drives. The opinion that adolescent sexual behavior should be curtailed or restricted receives considerable support from multiple sectors of American society. There is also consensus that sexuality and sexual capacity are not "awakenings" that suddenly appear at a definitive time in development, but rather that both male and female infants are born with the capacity for sexual pleasure and response.

Childhood

Considerable variation in sexual development presents among individuals during childhood and adolescence. The pleasures of genital stimulation are generally discovered in the first few years of life. Besides self-stimulation, prepubescent children often engage in play that may be viewed as sexual in nature. The activities may range from exhibition and inspection to simulating intercourse by rubbing genital regions together. Both natural childhood curiosity and curiosity about what is forbidden probably play a role in these behaviors. As children get older, they become more keenly aware of and interested in body changes, particularly those involving the genitals and secondary sex characteristics.

Adolescence

Adolescence, the period from about 12 to 19 years of age, is the most dramatic stage for physiological changes and social role development. Most of the major physical changes actually take place in the first few years of this period, a time known as puberty. In recent years, the average age of puberty appears to have decreased, with some girls seeing physical changes as young as the age of seven. The onset of puberty generally occurs two years earlier in girls than in boys. Secondary sex characteristics appear at this time in response to higher levels of hormones. In females, estrogen levels result in pubic hair growth and breast budding. In one study of 17,000 girls, the mean onset age for breast development was 8.9 years for African American girls and 10.0 years for white girls; pubic hair growth began at age 8.8 years for African American girls and 10.5 years for white girls.[31]

Under the influence of hormone stimulation, additional internal changes occur. Vaginal walls gradually become thicker, and the uterus becomes larger and more muscular. The vaginal pH changes from alkaline to acidic as vaginal and cervical secretions increase in response to the changing hormone status. Eventually, menstruation begins. The first menstrual period is known as menarche. Initial menstrual cycles may be irregular and occur without ovulation. Most girls menstruate at about the age of 12 or 13, but there is considerable variation in this timing. Research has suggested that undernourishment of adolescents can delay menstruation. These findings distinguish circulating energy from stored body energy (fat), emphasizing that the amount of circulating energy within the body is more important than the amount of stored energy. This implies that well-nourished girls will progress through puberty at a normal age even if their percentage of body fat is low.[32] Taller and larger girls, as well as girls who are overweight or obese, tend to have an earlier onset of menstruation. In one study that looked at more than 6,500 girls, overweight prevalence rates were significantly higher in early-maturing adolescents of all racial/ethnic groups but highest among early-maturing black girls. Early maturation nearly doubled the odds of being overweight.[33]

The difficulties of adjusting to new physical characteristics pale in comparison to the psychological adjustments of adolescence. This period is characterized by evolving responsibilities and assimilation of societal expectations. In Western cultures, these expectations include inherent double standards for women. That is, sexual overtones are blasted through the media in everything from ads for jeans to cars, yet the message also prevails for young women to maintain their virginity. In contrast, the expectations for young men are more tolerant of experimentation and overt sexual behavior. On average, men experience first intercourse at 16.9 years of age and women at 17.4 years.[34]

Young to Middle Adulthood

Sexual behavior in adults is influenced by a number of personal and cultural factors. A dramatic shift has occurred, with several factors contributing to the increasing numbers of single, sexually active adults:

- The trend toward marriage at a later age
- An increase in the number of women who never marry
- More women placing career goals before marriage
- An increase in the number of cohabiting couples

It's Your Health

Life Behaviors of a Sexually Healthy Adult

- Appreciate one's own body.
- Seek further information about reproduction as needed.
- Affirm that human development includes sexual development that may or may not include reproduction or genital sexual experience.
- Interact with both genders in respectful and appropriate ways.
- Affirm one's own sexual orientation and respect the sexual orientation of others.
- Express love and intimacy in appropriate ways.
- Develop and maintain meaningful relationships.
- Avoid exploitative or manipulative relationships.
- Make informed choices about family options and lifestyles.
- Exhibit skills that enhance personal relationships.
- Identify and live according to one's values.
- Take responsibility for one's own behavior.
- Practice effective decision making.
- Communicate effectively with family, peers, and partners.
- Enjoy and express one's sexuality throughout life.
- Express one's sexuality in ways congruent with one's values.
- Discriminate between life-enhancing sexual behaviors and those that are harmful to oneself or to others.
- Express one's sexuality while respecting the rights of others.
- Seek new information to enhance one's sexuality.
- Use contraception effectively to avoid unintended pregnancy.
- Prevent sexual abuse.
- Seek early prenatal care.
- Avoid contracting or transmitting a sexually transmitted disease, including HIV.
- Practice health-promoting behaviors, such as regular checkups, breast and testicular self-examinations, and early identification of potential problems.
- Demonstrate tolerance for people with different sexual values and lifestyles.
- Exercise democratic responsibility to influence legislation dealing with sexual issues.
- Assess the impact of family, cultural, religious, media, and societal messages on one's thoughts, feelings, values, and behaviors related to sexuality.
- Promote the rights of all people to obtain accurate sexuality information.
- Avoid behaviors that exhibit prejudice and bigotry.
- Reject stereotypes about the sexuality of diverse populations.

Source: Reprinted with permission from the Sexuality Information and Education Council of the United States (SIECUS), 130 West 42nd Street, Suite 350, New York, NY 10036. http://www.seicus.org.

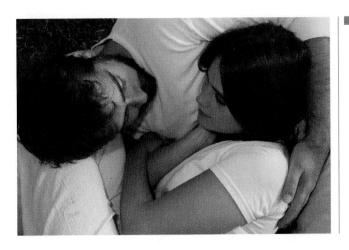

■ Communication contributes greatly to the satisfaction of an intimate relationship.

- A rise in divorce rates
- A greater emphasis on advanced education
- An increase in the number of women who no longer must depend on marriage to ensure their economic stability

It is not appropriate to assume that sexual behavior is always confined to marital arrangements. Instead, contemporary developments and changes in sexual mores and behavior of young adults are often discussed in the context of nonmarital, marital, or extramarital activities. *Extramarital relationship* is a term describing the sexual interaction experienced by a married person with someone other than his or her spouse. These relationships may be further defined as nonconsensual, in which there is no spousal consent for the extramarital relationship, or consensual, in which the spouse is aware of and supports the extramarital involvement. Data evaluating these arrangements are incomplete and biased at best. In the absence of data, it is difficult to draw conclusions about these arrangements.

Regardless of the formal or informal living arrangements, sexual behavior is an important dimension of adult health. One study that examined the relationships between sexual problems, sexual self-disclosure, and sexual satisfaction found that good communication and disclosure of specific sexual likes and dislikes were the strongest factors associated with increased levels of sexual satisfaction.[35] (See **It's Your Health** for more behaviors of a sexually healthy adult.)

Older Adulthood

The term **climacteric** refers to the physiological changes that occur during the transition period from female fertility to infertility. At about age 40, the ovaries begin to slow the production of estrogen and androgens. **Menopause,** one of the climacteric events, refers to the cessation of menstruation and generally occurs at about 45 to 55 years of age (see Chapter 8). The hormonal changes of menopause affect the sexual response of most women. In general, all phases of the response cycle continue but with somewhat decreased intensity. The depletion of hormones

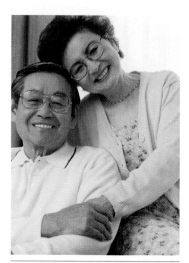

■ Sexuality is an important dimension of aging.

associated with menopause can result in several vaginal changes, including dryness, thinning of the walls, and delayed or absent lubrication during sexual excitement. For many women, hormone replacement therapy may help; however, it is not necessarily a solution for every woman. Other strategies to relieve vaginal dryness include prescription estrogen creams applied directly to the vagina that help prevent dryness and thinning. Water-soluble lubricants and vaginal moisturizers can help solve problems related to dryness. Kegel exercises can help make sex more pleasurable by toning the pelvic floor muscles that support the bladder and uterus, which tend to relax as estrogen declines.

Although the general focus on sexual response in later years tends to highlight a decline in frequency and intensity of sexual activity, in fact the opportunities for sexual expression in a relationship are often increased in later years, as pressures from work, children, and fulfilling life's goals may be reduced and more time becomes available for sharing with a partner. Couples may increasingly emphasize quality rather than quantity of sexual expression. Intimacy may find new and deeper dimensions in later years.

The perception that old age and sex are incompatible is totally erroneous. All too often, women dismiss sexual problems as a consequence of aging. In truth, most people can enjoy an active sex life no matter how old they are. This misconception about aging may have evolved for a number of reasons. The United States is still influenced by the philosophy that equates sexuality with procreation. For older people who are neither capable of nor interested in the reproductive facets of life, this viewpoint offers little sensitivity or insight into their personal needs. Society also sends the message via the media that love, sex, and romance are only for the young and "sexy." The implicit message is that this scenario excludes older individuals.

In addition, there is a pervasive assumption that older people do not have sexual needs. In a large survey of Americans, 65% of women who were 70 years of age or older were "very" or "somewhat" satisfied with their sex life; 49% of women age 70 or older were "more" or "equally" satisfied with their sex life compared to when they were younger.[36] Older people who express interest in sexual activity may be seen as senile or perverted. Elders who are single may meet with disapproval from their family and friends when dating or engaging in sexual relations. People in long-term care facilities also may experience adverse reactions when it comes to sexual behavior. Healthcare providers often feel uncomfortable with sexual activity among the elderly; therefore, many elders may feel deprived of their sexual rights and their rights for privacy to engage in sexual behavior. Studies have found that sexual expression can provide relaxation, reassurance, and companionship and can lead to a decrease in depression and social isolation.[37]

Sexual Violence as a Public Health Problem

Sexual violence against women constitutes a violation of a woman's human rights, fundamental freedoms, and reproductive rights. Rape, female genital mutilation, and forced sterilization are all types of violence that violate a woman's reproductive rights. Sexual violence can occur against young girls, women during midlife, and elderly women. The perpetrator can be a family member or friend, a respected member of the community, a colleague at work, or someone in a health facility or educational institution. Sexual violence can also occur in the highly organized and lucrative form of forced prostitution or trafficking.

Sexual Assault and Rape

Sexual assault and rape are crimes of aggression. **Sexual assault** often refers to forced sexual contact. **Rape** is defined as an event occurring without consent, involving the use of force or the threat of force to sexually penetrate the victim's vagina, mouth, or rectum.[38] Rape may occur among strangers or intimates; it can also happen in a marriage, during a legal separation, or after a divorce. In addition, rape can occur between people of the same sex. Women are disproportionately affected by such sexual violence. One out of every six American women has been the victim of an attempted or completed rape; in 2001, nine out of every 10 people who were raped were female.

Rape and sexual assault crimes occur throughout the world. In the United States, many women who are raped or assaulted blame themselves for the attacks. In some cultures, however, families blame the girl or woman who is raped. Every year, as many as 5,000 women and girls are murdered by members of their own families in honor killings, for the "dishonor" that the rape has brought to the family.[39] More information on sexual violence is found in Chapter 14 of this book.

Female Genital Mutilation

Female genital mutilation (FGM), also known as female circumcision and female genital cutting (FGC), refers to four practices involving the female genitals:

- Type I (clitoridectomy) is the removal of the prepuce (clitoral hood) and/or the tip of the clitoris.
- Type II (excision) is the removal of the prepuce, the entire glans of the clitoris, and the inner labia. The most common form of FGM, it occurs in 80% of all cases.
- Type III (infibulation)—the most extreme form of female circumcision— involves the removal of the clitoris, the labia majora, and the labia minora. The sides of the vulva are then sewn together over the vagina, leaving a small opening to allow for the passage of urine and menstrual blood. Upon marriage, the stitches are cut open to accommodate the penis during intercourse. Type III occurs in 15% of all cases.
- Type IV (unclassified) is pricking, piercing, or incising of the clitoris and/or labia; stretching of the clitoris and/or labia; or cauterization by burning of the clitoris and surrounding tissue.

These practices are undertaken for cultural or religious reasons and are often performed by a nonmedical individual. Girls or infants have no say in the matter and suffer short-term and long-term consequences, including a spectrum of conditions from infection to death. Between 100 million and 130 million women suffered FGM as young girls; every year, an estimated 2 million girls are at risk in Africa, South and East Asia, and in parts of Europe, North America, and Australia. Based on the 1990 U.S. Census, an estimated 168,000 girls and women living in the United States had undergone or were at risk for FGM.[40]

Legislation was passed in 1996 to outlaw these procedures in girls younger than 18 years of age after Congresswoman Patricia Schroeder introduced a bill in 1994 to outlaw FGM in the United States. Some states have outlawed FGM for females of any age. Cultures that continue the practice describe female circumcision as a rite of passage for females, necessary for hygienic purposes, and a requisite to create a marriageable female. Although female circumcision is illegal in many African and Middle Eastern countries, this ban does not prevent the procedure from occurring, especially in remote villages that are somewhat inaccessible to government. Many organizations, including the World Health Organization, are working to reduce FGM and eventually eliminate this dangerous procedure.

Forced Sterilization

Forced sterilization, performed throughout the world for population control and eugenics (the Darwinian notion of producing a "perfect" race of humans), is a violent crime against the reproductive rights of both women and men. People targeted for surgeries may be poor and/or illiterate; they may suffer from alcoholism, chronic disease, or mental and physical challenges. In countries with high rates of poverty, forced sterilization is used to control population growth. Women are often bribed with payments of food, clothing, or money. Women also may be unknowingly sterilized during childbirth or other medical procedures. Forced sterilizations have occurred all over the world and in vast numbers of people, including Nazi-run Germany, Sweden, Japan, Peru, and the United States.

Trafficking

According to the United Nations Crime Commission, **trafficking** is defined as the "recruitment, transportation, transfer, harboring, or receipt of persons, by the threat or use of force . . . or the abuse of power . . . for the purpose of exploitation." An estimated 4 million women and girls are trafficked for sexual exploitation worldwide every year; they are bought and sold either into marriage, prostitution, or slavery.[41] Sex trafficking is highly profitable. Figures from the United Nations indicate that trafficking of women and girls generates nearly $7 billion in profits annually. Many poor women and girls and their families are targeted by traffickers, who lure them with promises of jobs, food, and wealth. Poor families are sometimes persuaded to sell their daughters for small amounts of money. Each year, at least 10,000 girls and women from poorer countries become involved in commercial sex work in Thailand, for example. Nearly 10,000 girls from Nepal are trafficked across the border to Indian brothels each year.[42]

Although the greatest volume of trafficking occurs in Southeast Asia, as many as 50,000 women and children from Asia, Latin America, and Eastern Europe are brought to the United States under false pretenses each year and forced to work as prostitutes, abused laborers, or servants, according to a report by the U.S. Central Intelligence Agency (CIA).[43] Apparently, numerous foreign women respond to advertisements for au pairs, sales clerks, or secretarial jobs in the United States, only to discover that these jobs do not exist. The women are then taken as prisoners and forced into prostitution. The CIA report indicates that the primary sources for traffickers are Thailand, Vietnam, China, Mexico, Russia, and the Czech Republic.[43]

Informed Decision Making

Sexual well-being encompasses far more than sexual arousal and response. It includes effective decision making across the entire spectrum of issues affecting sexual health. A gynecological checkup is a good place to start for guidance in reproductive and sexual health matters, as well as preventive health screening. A woman can maximize the benefits of a gynecological examination by taking the time to carefully select a clinician who is sensitive to her needs. Often that means changing clinicians until the "right" one is found. Even so, it is better to "shop" while feeling well than to wait until a pressing medical problem requires immediate attention.

Understanding personal feelings, thoughts, and symptoms and articulating concerns and questions are essential dimensions of effective personal communication and preventive health. To promote sexual health and responsible sexual behavior, it is important to understand how a woman develops her vocabulary and communication skills and gains sexual knowledge and understanding. Communication is a critical component of sexual behavior and sexual health. Being able to talk about needs, feelings, concerns, and fears is an essential component of a healthy relationship. Sexual communication can contribute greatly to the satisfaction of an intimate relationship. Unfortunately, American language lacks a comfortable sexual vocabulary. Available language seems to be either "clinical" or "medical" in nature, which may be perceived as too cold and unfeeling, or "street language," which may be perceived as too crass or juvenile. Beyond the handicaps imposed by socialization and language limitations, difficulties in sexual communication may be rooted in fears of too much self-exposure. Any sexual communication involves a degree of risk and vulnerability to judgment, criticism, or rejection. The willingness to take risks may be related to the amount of trust that exists within a relationship.

Learning about responsible sexual behavior is essential for promoting positive sexual health. Children look to their parents as a first resource; a healthy, loving, committed relationship can serve as a blueprint for children. Although communication between parents and children can be helpful, many parents find it difficult to discuss sexual health issues. Some parents are unsure of their own knowledge about sexual health and therefore they may not benefit the child by sharing their own experiences and information.

As girls grow up, they begin picking up more information from television and radio, books, magazines, and friends. Although this is a normal healthy behavior, parents should work at creating an open dialogue with their children to ensure that they continue to learn facts and not myths. Although television and radio often suggest sexual behavior, the media typically depict sexual behavior in short-lived romances without the use of contraception. According to the Institute of Medicine's publication *No Time to Lose,* "The Code of Silence has resulted in missed opportunities to use the mass media to encourage healthy sexual behavior."[44] It is important to present negotiation and communication skills, safe sex practices, and healthy and positive relationships.

Healthcare providers also can be a good source of information for adolescent girls and women. It is critical for women to articulate the nature of their doctors' visits and to address questions or concerns specifically. It cannot be assumed the clinician will ask a standard set of questions or that the clinician can ascertain by examination the nature of a sexual concern or automatically detect an underlying fear or anxiety. Insisting that all questions be answered and persisting when answers are not clear are equally important avenues for maximizing the effectiveness of the visit. Women are often eager to please their healthcare providers and will nod as if understanding when in actuality they do not. This behavior results in more confusion and an increased likelihood of problems. Many women find it helpful to write down their questions and concerns and deal with them one by one with the clinician in the office before clothes are removed and the examination begins. Unfortunately, many healthcare providers do not address important topics regarding sexual health and appear uncomfortable when questions are asked of them. Healthcare providers need to find ways to broach the subject in a respectful, culturally sensitive manner.

Summary

Sexuality pervades every aspect of a person's life. It is a continually evolving issue throughout the life span, from the beginnings of sexual urges in girlhood to maintaining a fulfilling sexual life into old age. Consequently, sexual health is an important dimension of women's health. Understanding the biological, psychological, power, and sociological dimensions of sexual health enhances total wellness. Women must understand the unique facets of their own sexuality, from their physiology to their desires. Both positive and negative sexual experiences can affect a woman's overall well-being. Communication and awareness of sexuality are key factors to resolving these experiences in a healthy way. Incorporating open communication and awareness of sexuality into personal relationships, informed decision making, and preventive health care can enhance a woman's sexual health throughout her life span.

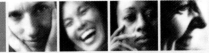

Profiles of Remarkable Women

Eve Ensler (1953–)

Eve Ensler is a playwright and an activist who has devoted her life to stopping violence, envisioning a planet in which women and girls will be free to thrive, rather than merely survive. Her work grows out of her own personal experiences with violence. Ensler's Obie-Award-winning play, *The Vagina Monologues,* is based on her interviews with more than 200 women about their intimate anatomy. The piece celebrates women's sexuality and strength, and exposes the violations that women endure throughout the world. Famous Hollywood actresses, including Glenn Close, Calista Flockhart, and Rosie Perez, are just a few of the women who have performed in *The Vagina Monologues.* The play has been translated into over 45 languages and has been performed in theaters all over the world, including sold-out runs at both Off-Broadway's Westside Theater and on London's West End (2002 Olivier Award nomination, Best Entertainment).

V-Day originated out of Ensler's conversations with women who approached her after early performances of *The Vagina Monologues* to tell her of their own experiences of violence. Ensler began to use performances of the play to raise funds for organizations working to stop violence.

Today, V-Day is a global movement that helps antiviolence organizations throughout the world continue and expand their core work on the ground, while drawing public attention to the larger fight to stop worldwide violence (including rape, battery, incest, female genital mutilation (FGM), and sexual slavery) against women and girls. V-Day stages large-scale benefits and promotes innovative gatherings and programs (The Afghan Women's Summit, The Stop Rape Contest, Indian Country Project, and more) to change social attitudes toward violence against women. In 2001, V-Day was a sellout at Madison Square Garden, a first for a women's event at a major sports arena. In 2006, more than 2,700 V-Day benefit events—produced by local volunteer activists and performed in theaters, community centers, houses of worship, and college campuses—took place around the world, educating millions of people about the reality of violence against women and girls and raising funds for local groups within their communities. In just six years, V-Day has raised over $20 million and was named one of *Worth* magazine's "100 Best Charities" in 2001.

Another of Ensler's plays, *Necessary Targets,* is set in a Bosnian refugee camp and based on a collection of stories from victimized female refugees. The play opened Off-Broadway at the Variety Arts Theater in February 2002, after a hit run at Hartford Stage. Other plays include *Conviction, Lemonade, The Depot, Floating Rhoda and the Glue Man,* and *Extraordinary Measures. The Vagina Monologues* and *Necessary Targets* have both been published by Villard/Random House, as will Ms. Ensler's two newest plays and books, *The Good Body* and *I Am an Emotional Creature.*

Ensler is the recipient of a Guggenheim Fellowship Award in Playwriting, the Berrilla-Kerr Award for Playwriting, the Elliot Norton Award for Outstanding Solo Performance, the Jury Award for Theater at the U.S. Comedy Arts Festival, the 2002 Amnesty International Media Spotlight Award for Leadership, and the Matrix Award (2002). In May 2003, she received an Honorary Doctor of Letters degree from her alma mater, Middlebury College. Ensler is Chair of the Women's Committee of PEN American Center and is an Executive Producer of *What I Want My Words to Do to You,* a documentary about the writing group she has led since 1998 at the Bedford Hills Correctional Facility for Women. The film had its world premiere at the 2003 Sundance Film Festival where it received the Freedom of Expression award; it also premiered nationally on PBS's *P.O.V.* in December 2003 (*P.O.V.*—a cinema term for "point of view"—is public television's annual award-winning showcase for independent nonfiction films.).

Profiles of Remarkable Women

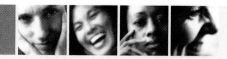

Debra Haffner

Debra W. Haffner is a sexuality education expert and is currently the director of the Religious Institute on Sexual Morality, Justice, and Healing. Haffner served as CEO of the Sexuality Information and Education Council of the United States (SIECUS) from 1988 until 2000; prior to SIECUS, she served as the Director of Education for the Center for Population Options; the Director of Community Services for Planned Parenthood of Metropolitan Washington; a Special Assistant in the U.S. Public Health Service; and the Resource Center Coordinator of the Population Institute. As CEO of SIECUS, Haffner created the Religious Declaration on Sexual Morality, Justice, and Healing; the National Coalition to Support Sexuality Education; the Commission on Adolescent Sexual Health; and the Guidelines for Comprehensive Sexuality Education, Kindergarten–Grade Twelve. Under her leadership, SIECUS tripled in staff size, increased its annual budget revenues more than sixfold, and opened professional offices in New York and Washington, D.C.

Haffner is the author of *From Diapers to Dating: A Parent's Guide to Raising Sexually Healthy Children* and *Beyond the Big Talk: Every Parent's Guide to Raising Sexually Healthy Teens.* Both books have been recognized as valuable resources for parents. She is also the co-author of a college sexuality textbook and *What I've Learned About Sex,* as well as a number of book chapters, journal articles, and pamphlets for the general public. Haffner has been honored for her work by the Yale School of Epidemiology and Public Health, the Robert Wood Johnson Medical School, the Society for the Scientific Study of Sexuality, the Association for the Advancement of Health Education, and the Society for Adolescent Medicine. She received the Connecticut Sexuality Educator of the Year Award in May 2002. Haffner is frequently quoted in the *New York Times* and the *Washington Post,* and has appeared on such programs as *Nightline, PrimeTime Live, 20/20, Dateline, Crossfire, Good Morning America, Oprah,* and *The Today Show.*

Haffner has a Master's of Divinity degree from Union Theological Seminary, a Master's of Public Health degree from the Yale University School of Medicine, and an undergraduate degree from Wesleyan University. In 1996–1997, she was a Research Fellow at the Yale Divinity School. Haffner was ordained as a Unitarian Universalist minister in May 2003.

Topics for Discussion

1. How do the sexual norms of a society restrict individuals? How do they benefit society?

2. Should sex education be taught in the nation's public schools, and if so, what kind of education should be provided? Which topics do you think are appropriate for school-based sex education courses?

3. Explain the terms "gender" and "sex" in your own words. Can a person be of female sex but have a male gender identity?

4. A paradox is that women appear to have a greater capacity for orgasm and can experience orgasm from a wider range of stimulation, yet seem to have more difficulty experiencing orgasm than men. Is this true? If so, which factors may contribute to this paradox?

5. How is homophobia displayed in modern society?

6. In addition to Masters and Johnson's sexual response cycle, a number of other researchers have proposed nonlinear models of sexual response patterns. Identify two of these models.

7. What are ways to maintain healthy relationships while being aware of risks of sexually transmitted disease, pregnancy, and rape?

Web Sites

The Alan Guttmacher Institute: http://www.agi-usa.org

American Civil Liberties Union (ACLU): http://www.aclu.org

American College of Obstetricians and Gynecologists (ACOG): http://www.acog.org

American Society for Reproductive Medicine: http://www.asrm.com

Association of Reproductive Health Professionals (ARHP): http://www.arhp.org

Centre for Development and Population Activities (CEDPA): http://www.cedpa.org

Engender Health: http://www.engenderhealth.org

Gay and Lesbian Alliance Against Defamation (GLAAD): http://www.glaad.org

Go Ask Alice!: http://www.goaskalice.columbia.edu

Human Rights Campaign (HRC): http://www.hrc.org

Intersex Society of North America (ISNA): http://www.isna.org

The Kinsey Institute: http://www.indiana.edu/~kinsey/index.html

National Gay and Lesbian Task Force: http://www.thetaskforce.org

Parents and Friends of Lesbians and Gays (PFLAG): http://www.pflag.org

Sexuality Information and Education Council of the United States (SIECUS): http://www.siecus.org

References

1. World Health Organization. (2002). *Gender and Reproductive Rights Glossary: Draft Working Definition.*

2. Beach, F. (1978). *Human Sexuality in Four Perspectives.* Baltimore: Johns Hopkins University Press.

3. Update on the Status of Sodomy Laws. (August 22, 2001). An ACLU Lesbian and Gay Rights Project Update on the Status of Sodomy Laws. http://www.aclu.org.

4. Kinsey, A., Pomeroy, W., and Martin, C. (1948). *Sexual Behavior in the Human Male.* Philadelphia: W. B. Saunders.

5. Kinsey, A., Pomeroy, W., Martin, C., and Gebhard, P. (1953). *Sexual Behavior in the Human Female*. Philadelphia: W. B. Saunders.

6. Masters, W., and Johnson, V. (1966). *Human Sexual Response*. Boston: Little, Brown.

7. Tavris, C. and Sadd, S. (1977). *The* Redbook *Report on Female Sexuality*. New York: Delacorte Press.

8. Hite, S. (1976). *The Hite Report: A Nationwide Study of Female Sexuality*. New York: Dell Books.

9. Blumstein, P., and Schwartz, P. (1983). *American Couples: Money, Work and Sex*. New York: William Morrow.

10. *The Surgeon General's Call to Action to Promote Sexual Health and Responsible Sexual Behavior.* (2001). U.S. Department of Health and Human Services.

11. Wizemann, T., and Pardue, M. L. (eds.) (2001). *Exploring the Biological Contributions to Human Health: Does Sex Matter?* Washington, DC: National Academy Press.

12. Shimonaka, Y., Nakazato, K., and Homma, A. (1996). Personality, longevity, and successful aging among Tokyo metropolitan centenarians. *International Journal of Aging and Human Development* 42(3): 173–187.

13. Ruffing-Rahal, M. A., Barin, L. J., and Combs, C. J. (1998). Gender role orientation as a correlate of perceived health, health behavior, and qualitative well-being in older women. *Journal of Women Aging* 10(1): 3–19.

14. Human Rights Campaign Foundation. (2003). Transgender 101: An Introduction to Issues Surrounding Gender Identity and Expression. Online at http://www.hrc.org.

15. Kruijver, F. P. M., et al. (2000). Male-to-female transsexuals have female neuron numbers in a limbic nucleus. *Journal of Clinical Endocrinology and Metabolism* 85(5): 2034–2041.

16. Gooren, L. (2001). Gender identity and sexual behavior. In: DeGroot, L. J., et al. (eds.) *Endocrinology,* W. B. Saunders, p. 2039.

17. Carroll, N. M. (1999). Optimal gynecologic and obstetric care for lesbians. *Obstetrics and Gynecology* 93(4): 611–613.

18. Gay and Lesbian Medical Association and LGBT Health Experts. (2001). *Healthy People 2010: Companion Document for Lesbian, Gay, Bisexual, and Transgender (LGBT) Health.* San Francisco: Gay and Lesbian Medical Association.

19. ACOG Practice Bulletin. (April 2000). Clinical management guidelines for obstetricians-gynecologists. Premenstrual syndrome. *Obstetrics and Gynecology* 95: 1–9.

20. Steiner, M., and Born, L. (2002). Diagnosis and treatment of premenstrual dysphoric disorder: an update. *International Clinics of Psychopharmacology* 15(Suppl3): S5–S17.

21. Tiemstra, J. D., and Patel, K. (1998). Hormonal therapy in the management of premenstrual syndrome. *Journal of the American Board of Family Practitioners* 11(5): 378–381.

22. Dickerson, L. M., Mazyck, P. J., and Hunter, M. H. (2005). Premenstrual syndrome, *American Family of Physicians* 67: 1743–1752.

23. Sarrell, P. M. (1999). Psychosexual effects of menopause: role of androgens. *American Journal of Obstetrics and Gynecology* 180(3): S319–S324.

24. Bachmann, G. A. (1999). Androgen co-therapy in menopause: evolving benefits and challenges. *American Journal of Obstetrics and Gynecology* 180(3): S308–S311.

25. Association of Reproductive Health Professionals. (2005). Women's sexual health in midlife and beyond. *Clinical Proceedings* May: 7.

26. Baldwin, J. D., and Baldwin, J. I. (1997). Gender differences in sexual interest. *Archives of Sexual Behavior* 26(2): 181–210.

27. Laumann, E. O., Paik, A., and Rosen, R. C. (1999). Sexual dysfunction in the United States: prevalence and predictors. *Journal of the American Medical Association* 281: 537–544.

28. Bancroft, J. (2000). Sexual well-being of women in heterosexual relationships: a national survey. In: *Female Sexual Function Forum: New Perspectives in the Management of Female Sexual Dysfunction.* Boston University School of Medicine Continuing Medical Education, Department of Urology, p. 17.

29. Kingsberg, S. A., and Janata, J. N. (2003). Sexual aversion disorder. In: Levine S., ed. *Handbook of Clinical Sexuality for Mental Health Professionals.* New York: Brunner-Routledge, pp. 153–166.

30. Anastasiadis, A. G., Salomon, L., Ghafar, M. A., et al. (2002). Female sexual dysfunction: state of the art. *Current Urology Reports* 3: 484–491.

31. Herman-Giddens, M. E., Slora, E. J., Wasserman, R. C., et al. (1997). Secondary sexual characteristics and menses in young girls seen in office practice: a study from the Pediatric Research in Office Settings Network. *Pediatrics* 88(4): 505–512.

32. Cameron, J. L. (1996). Nutritional determinants of puberty. *Nutrition Reviews* 54(2): S17–S22.

33. Adair, L. S., and Gordon-Larsen, P. (2001). Maturational timing and overweight prevalence in U.S. adolescent girls. *American Journal of Public Health* 91: 642–644.

34. The Alan Guttmacher Institute. (2002). *In Their Own Right: Addressing the Sexual and Reproductive Health Needs of American Men.* New York: Alan Guttmacher Institute.

35. MacNeil, S., and Byers, E. S. (1997). The relationships between sexual problems, communication, and sexual satisfaction. *Canadian Journal of Human Sexuality* 9(4): 277–287.

36. Sex and aging [magazine column]. (1998). *Patient Care* 32(20): 14.

37. Calamidas, E. G. (1997). Promoting healthy sexuality among older adults: educational challenges of health professionals. *Journal of Sex Education and Therapy* 22(2): 45–49.

38. Tjaden, P., and Thoennes, N. (1998). *Prevalence, Incidence, and Consequences of Violence Against Women: Findings from the National Violence Against Women Survey.* Washington, DC: National Institute of Justice, Office of Justice Programs, U.S. Department of Justice.

39. *The State of World Population 2000 Report: Lives Together, Worlds Apart: Men and Women in a Time of Change.* (2000). New York: United Nations Population Fund.

40. United States Congress. Report on Female Genital Mutilation as required by Conference Report (H. Rept. 106-997) to Public Law 106-429 (Foreign Operations, Export Financing, and Related Programs Appropriations Act). (2001).

41. Panos Institute. (1998). *The Intimate Enemy: Gender Violence and Reproductive Health*, pp. 1–20. Panos Briefing No. 27. London: Panos Institute.

42. United Nations Children's Fund. (January 20, 2000). UNICEF: child sex trafficking must end. Press release. UNICEF Web site: www.unicef.org.

43. Brinkley, J. Vast trade in forced labor portrayed in C.I.A. report. (April 2, 2000). *The New York Times.*

44. National Institute of Medicine. (2001). *No Time to Lose: Getting More from HIV Prevention.* Washington, DC: National Academies Press.

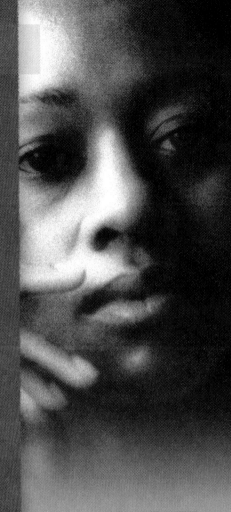

Chapter Five

Contraception
and Abortion

Chapter Objectives

On completion of this chapter, the student should be able to discuss:

1. The four primary mechanisms by which birth control can be accomplished.

2. Contraceptive efforts from a historical perspective.

3. Ways in which sociocultural considerations influence contraceptive decision making.

4. The prevalence of contraceptive use among American women today.

5. Economic issues associated with contraception.

6. The concept of fertility awareness.

7. The mechanisms, risks, benefits, side effects, and contraindications of hormonal, barrier, permanent, and other methods of contraception.

8. The options available for an unplanned pregnancy.

9. The difference between induced and spontaneous abortion.

10. Abortion from a historical perspective.

11. The pro-life, pro-choice, and middle ground positions on abortion.

12. Abortion from an epidemiological perspective.

13. The major types of abortion procedures.

14. Reasons why the assessment of risks, benefits, and contraindications is an integral component of contraceptive decision making.

15. The strategies in effective contraceptive decision making.

16. The importance of careful decision making regarding abortion.

womenshealth.jbpub.com

Women's Health Online is a great source for supplementary women's health information for both students and instructors. Visit

http://womenshealth.jbpub.com
to find a variety of useful tools for learning, thinking, and teaching.

Figure 5.1

Percentage of U.S. women ages 15 to 44 using certain contraceptive methods, 2002, by age group.

Source: Mosher, W.D., Martinez, G.M., Chandra, A., Abma, J.C., and Wilson, S.J. (2004). Use of contraception and use of family planning services in the United States, 1982–2002. *Advance Data from Vital Health Statistics*, no. 350. Hyattsville, MD: National Center for Health Statistics.

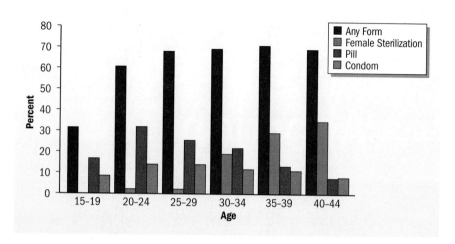

Introduction

A woman's ability to control her reproductive functioning is a necessary component of her health, career preparation, and family growth management. Approximately 70% of reproductive-age women in the United States use some form of birth control. The two most popular forms of birth control are female sterilization and the birth control pill (Figures 5.1 and 5.2). Many methods of **contraception** are available

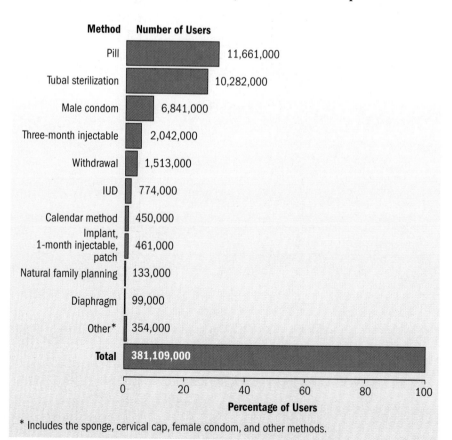

Figure 5.2

Contraceptive method choice among U.S. women using contraception, 2002.

Source: The Alan Guttmacher Institute. (2005). Contraceptive Use: Retrieved online January 16, 2006, from http://www.guttmacher.org/pubs/fb_contr_use.html.

today, and no one method is perfect. Ultimately, contraception is a shared responsibility. The best method is one that a woman and her partner feel comfortable using and one that they will use correctly and consistently. The risk for sexually transmitted diseases, including HIV, should also play an essential part in a couple's decision.

Choosing the right contraception is a decision that couples should make together.

Perspectives on Contraception

Although the terms "birth control" and "contraception" are often used interchangeably, each conveys a slightly different perspective on **fertility** control. *Contraception* is a specific term for any procedure used to prevent fertilization of an ovum. *Birth control* is an umbrella term that refers to procedures that prevent the birth of a baby, so it would include all available contraceptive measures as well as sterilization, the **intrauterine device** (IUD), and abortion procedures. Contraceptive methods do not necessarily provide protection from sexually transmitted diseases.

There are four primary mechanisms by which birth control can be accomplished:

1. Preventing sperm from entering the female reproductive system. Strategies that use this mechanism include abstinence, withdrawal, the condom, and male sterilization.

2. Preventing sperm from fertilizing an ovum once it has entered the female reproductive system. Strategies that use this mechanism include the diaphragm, cervical cap, contraceptive sponge, and spermicides.

3. Preventing ovulation and/or preventing the ovum from reaching the sperm. Strategies that use this mechanism include oral contraceptives, hormone implants, hormone injectables, hormone patch, vaginal ring, and female sterilization.

4. Preventing progression of a fertilized egg. Strategies that use this mechanism include the IUD, some forms of oral contraceptives, emergency birth control, and abortion.

Not all forms of sexual activity require contraceptive measures. For example, sexual gratification and excitement may occur with handholding, hugging, petting, kissing, and mutual masturbation. These forms of sexual activity do not require contraception. Ejaculation on, next to, or inside the vaginal opening has inherent risks for pregnancy and requires contraception if pregnancy is not desired.

Contraceptive decision making is not easy. Couples are often faced with a choice between highly effective contraceptive methods that have a number of side effects and other methods that have few side effects but may detract from sexual enjoyment and may have a higher failure rate.

Historical Overview

Throughout history, women have attempted to control their fertility status by using many different methods. Egyptian records indicate that women made primitive diaphragms by inserting paste-like mixtures into their vaginas. Early Greeks followed the same plan but used different recipes. Women from many ages and cultures have consumed various teas and septic solutions with the hopes that they would prevent unwanted pregnancy. Early IUDs consisted of stones that were placed in the uterus of camels to protect from pregnancy on desert treks. Women followed this example, placing various foreign objects in the vagina with hopes of similar results. Early attempts at spermicidal agents included mixtures of acid, juice, honey, alcohol, opium, and vinegar.

Until the introduction of the birth control pill in 1960, diaphragms and condoms were the primary forms of contraception. Early condoms were probably made from linen sheaths. The cervical cap was introduced in the early 1800s, and the diaphragm was introduced later in the same century. In the mid-nineteenth century, feminists in the United States began a birth control campaign associated with the slogan "Voluntary Motherhood." This campaign advocated birth control by abstinence. Margaret Sanger (1879–1966) and Mary Coffin Dennett (1872–1947) were early promoters of contraceptive birth control (sexual intercourse without pregnancy) in the United States, although the two advocated different means to achieve their goals (see the **Profiles of Remarkable Women** at the end of this chapter).

Birth control remained at the center of national attention for many years. "Race suicide" was an antifeminist theory developed between 1905 and 1910 in reaction to the lower birth rates and changes in family structure that were attributed to the birth control movement. Proponents of this theory, including President Theodore Roosevelt, believed that upper-class, educated women were failing society by not having large families and that they were allowing the upper classes to be overtaken by immigrants and the poor.

Although women today take the availability of birth control devices and information for granted, only in recent years has it been legal to use them. Just four decades ago, birth control pills were illegal in some states. That changed in 1965 with the Supreme Court's landmark decision, *Griswold v. Connecticut*, which struck down a statute that made the use of birth control illegal and criminalized spreading information about its use. Justice William Orville Douglas found the strength for the decision in the fact that the case involved "the intimate relationship of husband and wife" and contraceptives were a logical extension of the marital relationship. In 1972, the Court invalidated a Massachusetts law that had made it a felony to give contraceptives to anyone other than a married person.

Recent legal victories in the contraceptive movement have mandated increased women's access to contraception through their health insurers. Federal employees won mandated coverage for contraception via an act of Congress in 1998.[1] More recently, women's advocacy groups have pressured insurers and employers to include oral contraception in covered prescription drug benefits. More than two-thirds of women age 18–44 rely on private insurance. Until recently, many insurers did not offer reimbursement for oral contraception, leaving many women to pay for their "pill" out of pocket. In contrast, the majority of payers cover surgical sterilization for both men and women. Although the coverage is not universal, many health plans that offer a prescription drug benefit now cover some oral contraceptives.[2] Conversely, other forms of birth control, such as condoms, are usually not covered. Coverage for diaphragms, IUDs, and injectables varies widely among payers. As of 2006, 23 states require health insurance companies that already provide prescription drug benefits to provide full coverage of FDA-approved contraceptives; 21 of these states require emergency contraception to be included.[2]

Federal restrictions on contraceptive development have resulted in the United States lagging behind many countries in this arena, leaving U.S. couples with fewer contraceptive options than couples in other developed nations. American women have a responsibility to stay informed as contraceptive technology continues to evolve and to stay aware of the political and economic forces that might facilitate or impede the availability of these devices or agents.

Sociocultural Considerations

Birth control attitudes and practices vary widely among social classes. In some cultures, motherhood has the ultimate status and is considered a personal achievement. In male-dominated relationships and marriages, a woman may have considerable difficulty in expressing and asserting her concerns and needs for contraception.

Religious beliefs also may play a significant role in influencing a woman's attitudes and practices about contraception. Many Protestant denominations endorse birth control as a marital option, although a growing number of ultraconservative Protestant denominations are espousing limiting its use. Conservative and Reform Judaism teachings emphasize the individual choice of the married couple, with couples able to limit their family size for either health or social reasons. Orthodox Jews may practice contraception under special health circumstances by consulting with medical and rabbinical authorities. The Roman Catholic Church traditionally and still officially accepts only rhythm methods of contraception. According to its teachings, the primary purpose of sexual intercourse is procreation, and any interference with procreation is considered to be a violation of natural law. Studies show that significant numbers of Catholics do use contraceptives, but this practice in violation of church teachings creates emotional difficulties for some Catholic women. Women who describe themselves as fundamentalist Protestants are most likely to use female sterilization as a contraceptive method, while Catholic and other protestant women are most likely to use the pill.[3] The Muslim faith also forbids contraception, because reproduction is seen as both a sacred duty and a gift. Although Muslims, on average, have the highest birth rates in the world, there is some variation among individuals as to whether they choose to use contraception.

Use of family planning services has increased in recent years from 33% in 1995 to 42% in 2002. The National Survey of Family Growth, conducted by the U.S. federal government, revealed that in 2002, white nonHispanic women were about as likely as Hispanic or black non-Hispanic women to receive family planning services

I am really concerned about birth control. My family expects me to be a virgin when I marry. But we aren't ready to get married yet and I am not a virgin. I am afraid that my family will not understand this problem.

20-year-old Hispanic American woman

Figure 5.3

Percentage of U.S. women, ages 15 to 44 years, using certain methods of contraception, distributed by ethnicity/race, 2002.

Source: Mosher, W.D., Martinez, G.M., Chandra, A., Abma, J.C., and Wilson, S.J. (2004). Use of contraception and use of family planning services in the United States, 1982–2002. *Advance Data from Vital and Health Statistics,* no. 350. Hyattsville, MD: National Center for Health Statistics.

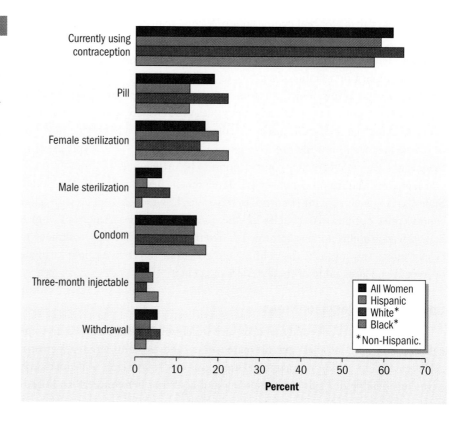

We are happily married, and someday we wish to have children, but right now our goals are to establish our careers. It would be really difficult for me to establish myself professionally if I become pregnant during the next three years.

26-year-old attorney

in the past year. However, white non-Hispanic women were more likely to receive family planning from private doctors or HMOs and less likely to receive their family planning from clinics, which deliver services to people with lower incomes and often have fewer resources.[4] The underlying reasons for these differences are complex, but may in part be because black and Hispanic women are less likely than white women to have health insurance coverage or sufficient monetary means to pay private practitioners. The geographical distribution of clinics and private practitioners' offices may also help explain disparities in contraceptive use.

The same study compared specific contraceptive behaviors among these three groups of women. It found that white non-Hispanic women were more likely to use some form of contraception than black or Hispanic women (64.5% versus 57.4% and 59.0%, respectively). The most commonly used contraceptive method also differed between racial and ethnic groups. White women were most likely to rely on birth control pills, while black and Hispanic women were most likely to rely on female sterilization. However, male sterilization was much more common among white couples than it was among black or Hispanic couples (Figure 5.3).

Economic Perspective

People using birth control often incur significant out-of-pocket expenses. Whether using condoms, birth control pills, the sponge, or spermicide, protection

Table 5.1 Contraceptive Costs

Method	Cost	Associated Costs
Female sterilization	$1,450–$2,004	
Male sterilization	$430–$920	
Oral contraceptives	$22–$26	Annual GYN exam
Male condom	$0.40–$1.26	
Injectable	$37	Quarterly office visits
Diaphragm	$18–$22	Office visit for fitting; spermicides
IUD	$99–$224 depending on type	$75–$250 for insertion and $13–$85 for removal; office visit
Female condom	$1.50–$4.50/condom	
Spermicides	$10.75–$14.61/approx. 12 applications	
Sponge	$1–$1.80/sponge	
Cervical cap	$23–$38	Office visit for fitting; spermicides
Evra patch	Similar to OCs	
NuvaRing	$36–$43/month	Office visit

Source: Hatcher, R. A., et al. (1998). *Contraceptive Technology,* 17th ed. New York: Ardent Media. Adjusted for inflation for 2006.

from pregnancy is rarely free. This is true even for people with good health insurance. Table 5.1 lists the major contraceptive methods and their costs.

Sterilization is often covered by health insurance. Methods such as condoms and sponges are rarely covered, however, so the individual is responsible for paying their entire cost. Birth control pills lie somewhere in between these two extremes—some health insurers pay for a large portion of their cost, others do not. Some states have mandated coverage for contraceptives by public and private health insurers, though the majority of states do not have such legislation in place (see Figure 5.4). None of these options, however, are available to the 20% of women in the United States who lack health insurance.

Epidemiology of Contraceptives

Contraceptive Use

National data indicate that 62% of reproductive-age women (15 to 44 years) use some method of birth control.[5] Oral contraceptives, sterilization of the male or female, and the male condom are the most popular methods in the United States. **Oral contraceptive** use has increased slightly, from 27% of total contraceptive users in 1995 to 31% in 2002. IUD use has also increased slightly, from

Figure 5.4

State-mandated benefits: Contraceptives, 2006.

Source: "State Mandated Benefits: Contraceptives, as of June 1, 2006," The Henry J. Kaiser Foundation (http://www.statehealthfacts.org). This information was reprinted with permission of the Henry J. Kaiser Family Foundation of Menlo Park, California. The Kaiser Family Foundation is an independent healthcare philanthropy and is not associated with Kaiser Permanente or Kaiser Industries.

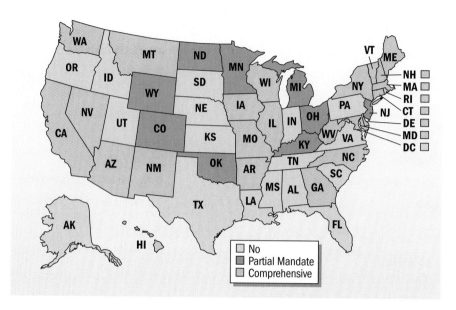

less than 1% of contraceptive users in 1995 to 2% in 2002. Diaphragm use, however, has sharply declined, from 6% in 1988 to 2% in 1995, to close to zero in 2002. Currently 15% of women using contraceptives use two methods at once, usually a male latex condom and another method.[5] The 38% of women who do not use birth control include, among others, women who are pregnant, women who are not sexually active, women who are sterile for noncontraceptive reasons, and women who have never had intercourse.

According to a study conducted by the Kaiser Family Foundation, women consider the following characteristics to be "very important" when choosing a contraceptive method:[6]

- Effectively prevents pregnancy (90%)
- Effectively protects against sexually transmitted diseases (77%)
- Provides no health risk (77%)
- Is easy to use (51%)
- Requires no advance planning (45%)

Together these factors influence which contraception is chosen, how regularly it is used, and ultimately how effective a contraceptive strategy will be for a woman.

Contraceptive Failure

Contraceptive failure rates provide important information in the selection of a birth control method. Failure rates are determined by following large groups of couples who use specific methods of birth control for a specified time and then counting the number of pregnancies that occur. The larger the number of study

Table 5.2 Birth Control Failure Rates

Method	Percentage of Women Experiencing an Accidental Pregnancy in the First Year of Use	
	Perfect Use	Typical Use
Pill (combined)	0.3	8.0
Tubal sterilization	0.5	0.7
Male condom	2.0	15.0
Vasectomy	0.1	0.2
Three-month injectable	0.3	3.0
Withdrawal	4.0	27.0
IUD (copper-T)	0.6	1.0
IUD (Merena)	0.1	0.1
Periodic abstinence (fertility awareness)	1.0–9.0	25.0
One-month injectable	0.05	3.0
Implant	0.05	1.0
Patch	0.3	8.0
Diaphragm	6.0	16.0
Sponge	15.0	25.0
Cervical cap	18.0	24.0
Female condom	5.0	27.0
Spermicides (alone)	18.0	29.0
No method	85.0	85.0

Source: The Alan Guttmacher Institute. (2005). Contraceptive Use: Facts in Brief. Retrieved online January 16, 2006, from http://www.guttmacher.org/pubs/fb_contr_use.html.

participants, the more reliable the study results. A failure rate of 2% means 2 pregnancies per 100 women per year studied.

Two types of failure rates exist:

- The lowest observed failure rate represents a method's absolute top performance, the highest efficacy ever achieved in a reputable clinical trial. This rate is often referred to as the failure rate with perfect use.
- The failure rate for typical users is an average rate based on an analysis of a range of reputable studies. The failure rate for typical users is usually lower than the best observed failure rates (Table 5.2).

Age influences the efficacy of the birth control method, with married older women generally being more successful contraceptors than unmarried younger

Table 5.3 Percentage of Women Experiencing Contraceptive Failure During the First 12 Months of Use, by Method, According to Marital Status, Age

| Demographic Characteristics | Method of Birth Control[a] | |
Marital Status and Age	Pill	Condom
Married		
Age < 20	7.6	13.9
Age 20-24	6.7	12.3
Age 25-29	5.3	9.8
Age ≥ 30	3.3	6.2
Unmarried, not cohabiting		
Age < 20	7.6	14.0
Age 20-24	7.4	13.7
Age 25-29	7.7	14.3
Age ≥ 30	4.7	8.8
Cohabiting		
Age < 20	31.4	51.3
Age 20-24	14.7	26.1
Age 25-29	7.8	14.3
Age ≥ 30	6.3	11.7

[a]Percentage of women experiencing contraceptive failure during the first 12 months of method use, after correction for abortion underreporting, by characteristic, according to method.

Source: Reprinted with permission of the Alan Guttmacher Institute from Fu, H., Darroch, J. E., Hass, T., and Ranjit, N. (1999). Contraceptive failure rates: new estimates from the 1996 national survey of family growth. *Family Planning Perspectives* 31(2): 56-63.

women (Table 5.3). The reasons for this discrepancy are not totally understood. It may be that younger women are less experienced with careful planning, are less likely to follow a routine, may be more fertile, may have intercourse more often, or may experience a combination of these factors. At any rate, young women who wish to avoid pregnancy need to take extra care with contraception.

Several methods of contraception have demonstrated high levels of effectiveness, defined as a failure rate of two or fewer pregnancies per 100 couples per year. These methods include pills (oral contraceptives), Norplant (hormone implants), Depo-Provera and Lunelle (hormone injectables), IUDs, spermicidal condoms (if used correctly), NuvaRing (vaginal hormone ring), Ortho Evra (hormone patch), and sterilization. Methods that have lower rates of effectiveness include diaphragms, cervical caps, sponges, and spermicidal agents, such as foams, creams, gels, suppositories, and vaginal contraceptive film. The effectiveness of a birth control method depends in large part on how carefully and consistently it is used. A diaphragm does not work when it is left in a drawer, pills may be forgotten, and condoms may break or leak.

Special Population: Adolescents

Teenage girls tend to rely on their male partners for contraceptive implementation (withdrawal and use of condoms) during early sexual intercourse experiences and later adopt prescription methods. The average delay between first intercourse and the first visit for medical consultation is about one year, and this visit is often motivated by a pregnancy scare. Among single female adolescents using contraceptives, however, the pill and condom are the most popular methods (see Table 5.4).

Table 5.4 Adolescents and Young Adults: Contraceptive Use

Percentage of sexually active adolescents and young adults who report the following experiences with birth control and protection

| | Total 15–24 | Age | | Gender | | Race/Ethnicity | | | |
		15–17	18–24	Male	Female	White	African American	Latino	Asian
Use birth control or protection									
All of the time	60%	70%	57%	53%	67%	62%	59%	52%	62%
Most of the time	23%	21%	23%	27%	18%	23%	20%	23%	22%
Some of the time	11%	5%	12%	13%	7%	9%	15%	15%	5%
Never	6%	4%	7%	5%	8%	6%	4%	10%	8%
Specific Contraceptive Use									
Report using condoms									
Ever	90%	94%	89%	91%	89%	90%	93%	89%	85%
Regularly	60%	79%	55%	67%	52%	58%	72%	55%	57%
Ever had sex without a condom	63%	38%	68%	62%	63%	67%	57%	58%	49%
Used a condom the last time had sexual intercourse	58%	80%	52%	64%	50%	56%	67%	52%	62%
Report using birth control pills									
Ever	62%	40%	67%	59%	66%	67%	53%	53%	46%
Regularly	44%	30%	48%	39%	51%	50%	33%	35%	35%
Report using withdrawal or pulling out									
Ever	42%	40%	43%	45%	39%	41%	48%	42%	45%
Regularly	12%	13%	12%	13%	11%	11%	17%	15%	5%
Report using the rhythm or calendar method									
Ever	8%	7%	8%	10%	6%	6%	5%	11%	13%
Regularly	2%	2%	2%	2%	2%	2%	2%	4%	
Total number of respondents	943	185	758	478	465	440	188	200	74

Note: Among those 18–24 who are not currently pregnant or trying to become pregnant.

Source: National Survey of Adolescents and Young Adults, Sexual Health Knowledge, Attitudes and Experiences. Kaiser Family Foundation 2003. This information was reprinted with permission of the Henry J. Kaiser Family Foundation of Menlo Park, California. The Kaiser Family Foundation is an independent healthcare philanthropy and is not associated with Kaiser Permanente or Kaiser Industries.

Teen contraceptive use does appear to be improving. Compared to teenagers in 1995, teenagers in 2002 were more likely to use contraception the first time they had intercourse. Teenagers in 2002 were also more likely to have used condoms or injectable methods of birth control and were less likely to use no method of contraception at all.[3] Adolescent sexual activity poses a risk not only for unintended pregnancy, but also for sexually transmitted disease (see Chapter 7).

Contraceptive Methods

Fertility Awareness Methods

Methods of fertility awareness include the calendar method, basal body temperature, and cervical mucus or ovulation method. These methods are based on avoidance of sexual intercourse during a woman's fertile time of the month, which includes the days previous to, during, and immediately following ovulation. An understanding of the female menstrual cycle is essential as a foundation for using fertility awareness methods. Couples using fertility awareness tend to have more accidental pregnancies than couples using most other contraceptive methods (Table 5.2).

One of the most important changes during the menstrual cycle is the cyclical variations of hormones from the anterior pituitary and the ovaries. The cyclical variations in these hormones cause biological alterations throughout the cycle. These cyclical hormones cause fluctuations in basal temperature patterns and variations in the type of cervical mucus produced. Many women are able to feel these changes during their fertility cycles and use methods of fertility awareness as either contraceptive techniques or methods for contraception.

The calendar method requires determining when ovulation occurs by calculating the length of consecutive menstrual cycles. It is not reliability effective, especially for women who do not have regular menstrual cycles. Measuring the body's daily temperature (basal body temperature) is another way to determine that ovulation has occurred. When progesterone is released immediately after ovulation, the body's temperature increases a small amount; however, women need to be certain that other factors, such as sexual activity, illness, or infection, are not causing these temperature fluctuations. Women also may determine the most fertile phase of the menstrual cycle by monitoring the change in the quality of the cervical mucus. During the fertile phase, women experience an increase in discharge and change in color and consistency of the mucus.

Advantages of fertility awareness methods are that they have no side effects, and anyone can use them. Also, a couple using fertility awareness with another contraception method has a lower risk of unintended pregnancy than a couple using either method alone. These methods have many drawbacks, however, including limited effectiveness, the need to abstain from sexual intercourse during many days of the month, and the lack of protection against sexually transmitted diseases. For a woman who absolutely does not wish to become pregnant, fertility awareness methods for contraception have inherent liabilities. The overall effectiveness

Well, I am proof that you need to follow directions. I thought that using a diaphragm was enough. I don't like that spermicidal stuff, and I thought a diaphragm alone was good protection. So I am pregnant. I can't believe that this is because I didn't follow directions.

21-year-old pregnant woman

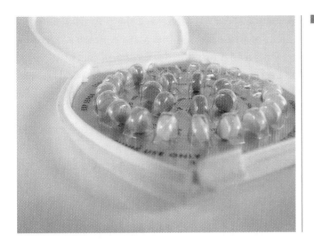

One type of birth control pills.

of these methods may improve as technological advances evolve and better prediction of ovulation becomes possible. Of course, timing of ovulation is not the only critical dimension of fertility awareness. Because sperm are able to survive 48 to 72 hours in the female reproductive tract, intercourse before ovulation is not necessarily free from pregnancy risk.

Hormonal Methods

Oral Contraceptives

Currently about 19% of women 15 to 44 years of age who use contraception take oral contraceptives, or birth control pills, making them the most commonly used nonsurgical method of birth control (see Figures 5.1 through 5.3). Since its introduction in the United States in the 1960s, the birth control pill has been one of the most extensively studied pharmacological preparations. The pill has changed considerably since its initial launch into the marketplace. Although the specific hormones are the same or similar, the dosages and formulations have undergone tremendous changes.

Birth control pills offer many benefits, in addition to contraception, for women. Oral contraceptives are associated with lighter and less painful periods, decreased symptoms of premenstrual syndrome (PMS), and improved skin conditions. They may also provide some protection against benign breast disease, ovarian cysts, pelvic inflammatory disease (PID), ovarian cancer, and endometrial cancer. Long-term use of oral contraceptives also increases a woman's bone density, thereby protecting her against osteoporosis. Many perimenopausal women also receive benefits from oral contraceptives, such as decreased complaints associated with menopause. Although generally safe, birth control pills may be a health risk for some women, primarily smokers or women at risk for high blood presure.

With birth control pills, the woman's own reproductive hormone cycle is generally suppressed, and the synthetic estrogen and progestin of the pill produce an artificial cycle to replace it. Without the natural signals, the egg follicle in the ovary cannot mature, and ovulation cannot occur. Another way the pill prevents pregnancy is by inducing development of thick cervical mucus, in contrast to the profuse, slippery mucus associated with ovulation. The thick cervical mucus serves to impede sperm movement through the cervical canal and inhibits chemical changes in sperm cells that would permit them to penetrate the outer layer of the egg. The pill also acts as a contraceptive by preventing the uterine lining from thickening as it normally does in the menstrual cycle. Thus, even if ovulation and conception did manage to occur, successful implantation would be quite unlikely.

Overall, birth control pills are highly effective in preventing pregnancy. Effectiveness rates of 99% can be expected when they are taken properly.

Side Effects

Several side effects have been associated with birth control pills. They may include both negative and positive changes:

1. Shorter, lighter, and more regular menstrual periods. The reduced amount of uterine lining results in less uterine shedding.

2. Reduction or elimination of menstrual cramps. Cramping is often associated with ovulation; because ovulation does not occur with use of birth control pills, cramping is reduced or eliminated. When menstrual bleeding begins, endometrial cells release prostaglandin as the cells shed from the uterine lining. Women who have severe cramps have significantly higher levels of prostaglandin in their menstrual fluid than do women who do not have cramps. Steady progestin exposure with birth control pills tends to reduce or eliminate cramps.

3. Mood changes. Some women may experience diverse reactions to birth control pills, such as irritability, depression, or mood swings. Some women, particularly those with a history of depression or premenstrual syndrome (PMS), may find these mood-related changes intolerable and choose to discontinue the pill.

4. Reduction or elimination of premenstrual symptoms. In many women, PMS tends to be significantly reduced or eliminated with birth control pills.

5. Decreased libido. For some women, birth control pills may increase sex drive by reducing anxiety about pregnancy and alleviating discomfort or distaste at having to "get ready" for sex. From a biochemical perspective, however, some women may experience adverse reactions to birth control pills and experience a decrease in sex drive, depression, irritability, or mood swings.

6. Spotting or bleeding between periods. The estrogen level maintained in the body by the pill is often lower than the natural level produced by the ovaries. This lower level may trigger slight uterine bleeding, which is generally referred to as "breakthrough bleeding." Such bleeding is more likely to occur when a pill is taken late or forgotten.

7. Weight changes. Some birth control pill users gain weight with the pill; others lose weight with its use.

8. Acne improvement. Most women who have acne notice significant improvement when they take birth control pills. Birth control pills may cause chloasma, however. Chloasma is the darkening of skin pigment on the upper lip, under the eyes, and on the forehead. It is not common and disappears when use of the birth control pills is discontinued.

Other effects associated with birth control pills include nausea, tender or larger breasts, headaches, and fluid retention.

Risks and Complications

Risks and complications are a major concern for oral contraceptive users, although many of these fears are unfounded. Safety issues concerning oral contraceptives are mainly based on the use of pills with high levels of hormones (current brands contain less than 50 micrograms of estrogen) and the risks associated with smoking and use of oral contraceptives.

One concern about oral contraceptives has been that they may increase the risk of venous thromboembolism, or the formation of abnormal blood clots. Current evidence indicates that this increased risk, if it exists, is very small. In a recent meta-analysis study, only 10 of 16 studies examining oral contraceptives' influence on venous thromboembolism found "good" evidence for an increased risk.[7]

An increased risk of high blood pressure, especially for older women and obese women, also has been associated with use of birth control pills. Other concerns identified by earlier studies of high-dose oral contraceptives include an increased risk of stroke and heart attack. Recent studies show that there is no increased risk for either condition in women who have no preexisting risk factors, regardless of age. There is, however, an increased risk if the woman is a smoker or has hypertension. For women with cardiovascular risk factors or for women who smoke, nonhormonal methods of birth control may be the best option.[8]

Cancer is another area of tremendous concern and discussion with the pill. Studies to date have shown important cancer-related benefits of the pill, which can significantly affect women's health. For example, modern birth control pills have been shown to reduce a woman's risk for endometrial and ovarian cancer.[9] Use of the pill for 10 to 20 years is associated with a 50% to 80% reduction in occurrence of these cancers, and this protection may last as long as 10 to 15 years after the pills have been discontinued.[10]

Some evidence has shown that long-term use of birth control pills is associated with changes in the surface of the cervix. These changes may make pill users more vulnerable to cervical cancer and sexually transmitted diseases of the cervix, particularly chlamydia. Confounding factors, however, make it very difficult to draw conclusions based on this evidence. Contradictory studies have shown no significant alterations of the cervix that would lead to associated risks. Women who have more than one sexual partner or who are at risk of transmission of sexually transmitted diseases should consider using condoms in combination with birth control pills.

While some small studies have suggested a relationship between breast cancer and oral contraceptives, others have not. A recent international review by the World Health Organization's International Agency for Research and Cancer (IARC) classified combined hormone contraception and menopausal therapy as "carcinogenic in humans." These conclusions were regarded as highly controversial in that no proof was presented for a causal relationship of estrogens with reproductive cancer. International clinicians reported no new reasons to change management principles with combined hormone contraception and therapies.[11] In a recent large U.S. population-based, case-control study, among women 35 to 64 years of age, current or former oral contraceptive use was not associated with a significantly increased risk of breast cancer. Relative risk did not increase consistently with longer periods of use or with higher doses of estrogen. The results were similar among white and black women. Use of oral contraceptives by women with a family history of breast cancer was not associated with an increased risk of breast cancer, nor was the initiation of oral contraceptive use at a young age. [12]

Several drugs can reduce the contraceptive effectiveness of the pill and increase the risk of bleeding between periods. These drugs include barbiturates, some anticonvulsants, antifungal medications, phenytoin (Dilantin), and certain antibiotics such as isoniazid, rifampin, and possibly tetracycline. It is probably wise for any woman using birth control pills to employ a backup form of contraception while taking any of these medications. Oral contraceptives also may prolong the effects of caffeine, theophylline, and benzodiazepines (e.g., Librium, Valium, and Xanax).

Advantages

Birth control pills provide the maximum protection possible with a temporary contraceptive method. They do not require any additional supplies or equipment, and they do not interfere with the spontaneity of lovemaking. Also, they provide freedom from heavy menstrual cramps and excessive menstrual bleeding, and often relieve premenstrual symptoms. Menstrual periods become regular and predictable. As noted earlier, birth control pills provide benefits in addition to pregnancy prevention. For example, women who take birth control pills have a lower prevalence of ovarian and endometrial cancers, and benign breast disease and ovarian cysts are less common in them. Women who take the pill also may be at lower risk for developing PID, iron-deficiency anemia, and osteoporosis.

Contraindications

A contraindication is a medical condition that renders a treatment or procedure that otherwise might be recommended inadvisable or unsafe. Women who are contemplating use of birth control pills should carefully review and evaluate the contraindications before deciding to proceed with them. Absolute contraindications—meaning that the pills absolutely should not be taken—specified by the FDA include the following conditions:

- Known cardiovascular disorder, now or in the past, such as thrombophlebitis, stroke, heart attack, coronary artery disease, or angina pectoris

- Impaired liver function
- Known or suspected cancer of the breast, uterus, cervix, or vagina
- Known or suspected estrogen-dependent neoplasia (abnormal tissue growth)
- Current or suspected pregnancy
- Abnormal vaginal bleeding
- Jaundice during previous pill use or pregnancy
- Malignant melanoma, now or in the past
- Smoking in women older than 35 years of age

Oral contraceptive use when breastfeeding has generated concern for infant safety. Studies are limited and while there is no evidence of harm, the question cannot be definitively answered. The American Academy of Family Physicians noted that the existing low-quality research evidence suggests that combined oral contraceptives may reduce the volume of breast milk but does not affect infant growth.[12]

Types of Birth Control Pills

There are currently more than 30 birth control pill brands available in monophasic (each cycle provides 21 identical hormone-containing pills), biphasic (two-phase), and triphasic (three-phase) formulations. Triphasic pills, the most recently introduced combination pills, contain three different **progestin** doses for different parts of each pill cycle. The primary advantage of triphasic pills is that the overall amount of progestin in a cycle is lower than it is with regular, identical-dose pills.

Traditionally, oral contraceptives have been prescribed in 21-day cycles of active hormone pills followed by a 7-day placebo or pill-free interval that produces predictable withdrawal bleeding in most users. Some women who follow this regimen, however, experience nuisance breakthrough bleeding, spotting, or amenorrhea. New formulations of continuous oral contraceptive therapy provide continuous hormonal dosing without periods of menstrual flow. The most commonly prescribed regimen for extended therapy is 84 days of active pill use followed by a 7-day hormone-free interval. Patient satisfaction studies indicate that many women prefer continuous therapy, as it provides fewer and lighter bleeding days and less bloating and menstrual pain.[14] Most clinicians do not feel that prescribed withdrawal bleeding has benefits or is necessary.[15]

Estrogen dose is generally considered to be the single most important factor in selecting a pill. Side effects and complications are reduced with lower estrogen doses. Minipills are estrogen-free birth control pills that provide a continuous, low dose of progestin. They are slightly less effective than the phasic pills and often cause irregular menstrual patterns. Minipills do not totally suppress hormone production. Natural estrogen and progesterone production usually remains sufficient to trigger menstrual periods. There is less margin of error with these oral contraceptives, however. The likelihood of pregnancy increases substantially with just one or two missed tablets. Although menstrual periods tend to be less predictable with the minipills, women who use them generally experience fewer premenstrual

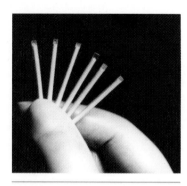

■ Norplant is inserted in the inside part of the upper arm. It consists of flexible rods that contain hormones.

symptoms, lighter or absent menstrual periods, decreased menstrual cramps, and less pain during ovulation.

An advantage of the minipill is that it can be used by smokers, women older than age 35, breastfeeding women, and women with histories of blood clots. In fact, minipills are believed to be nearly 100% effective in breastfeeding women owing to the added effect of lactation.[16] The progestin does not alter the quantity of breast milk produced. Because minipills do not contain estrogen, they are associated with fewer side effects. Women who have difficulty taking estrogen find progestin-only minipills to be a good alternative method of contraception. Like combination oral contraceptives, progestin-only minipills seem to offer protection against endometrial and ovarian cancer, as well as PID. They may also be helpful in managing pain associated with endometriosis. Because data on minipills are relatively scarce, information on their risks and benefits is somewhat limited.

Hormonal Implants

Hormonal implants are the newest approach to contraception since the birth control pill. Like the minipill, hormonal implants work by releasing progestin. They consist of one or two rods that are inserted under the skin of the upper arm and provide contraception from three to five years. Although many women have voiced concerns about the possible pain of insertion, most women who received the implant reported either slight or no discomfort during the insertion procedure.

Menstrual irregularities (prolonged bleeding, spotting, amenorrhea, and an increase in spotting/bleeding days) have been the primary adverse effects reported with the implants. Headache, acne, mood changes, and changes in weight also have been reported as side effects of the implants. Another possible side effect relates to difficulty in removing the implants. This procedure often takes a little longer than insertion. Once again, a local anesthetic is used and a small dressing is applied to the site. Fertility is not affected after the implant is removed. Benefits, cautions, and contraindications for implant use are similar to the minipill. If implants remain in longer than five years, their presence is associated with a significant risk of ectopic pregnancy.[17]

Candidates for hormonal implants include those women who do not desire children for at least three to five years and who are seeking an effective, convenient form of birth control. Women for whom other methods may be contraindicated or who have experienced difficulty complying with other methods also may be candidates for implants. When total costs are considered for a five-year period, the implant is less expensive than oral contraceptives, although the initial cost is high.

Safety concerns about Norplant emerged in the late 1990s. Women took Norplant's makers to court in 1998 alleging that the company failed to properly and adequately warn them about the severity of implant-associated side effects such as nausea, headaches, irregular menstrual bleeding, ovarian cysts, weight gain, removal problems, and depression. Although the makers of Norplant initially settled these claims with more than 36,000 women and continued to market the product, problems arose with the effectiveness of some lots of the implants in late 1999 and 2000, which eventually led to the recall of the contraceptive in 2003. As of January 2006, hormonal implants are not available to women in the United States. Because the implants have a five-year lifetime, some women may still be using the Norplant system for birth control. These women will need to seek other contraceptive options as the implants expire. Two other forms of hormonal implants, Jadelle, the second generation of Norplant, and Implanon, may be available to women in the near future.

Hormone Delivery Methods: Injectables, Patches, and Vaginal Rings

Another form of hormonal contraceptives is the birth control shot. Medroxy-progesterone (Depo-Provera) is the most common of the injectable progestins. The long-acting progestin injection, which is given as an intramuscular injection every three to four months, has a theoretical and actual-use effectiveness of almost 100%. Injectables work similarly to other forms of hormonal contraceptives—by preventing ovulation and thickening the cervical mucus. Menstrual irregularities such as breakthrough bleeding, or heavy or continuous bleeding, have been reported mainly in the first year of use. Some women become amenorrheic during the first year of use. Weight gain, fluid retention, headaches, and mood changes are just some of the other side effects that may occur with use of Depo-Provera. Some women may experience a delayed return to fertility after discontinuing the injections. Women who cannot take estrogen or are breastfeeding are good candidates for this form of contraception. Benefits, contraindications, and cautions are similar to those noted with the minipill and implants. Depo-Provera may increase a woman's risk of acquiring an STD if she has an exposure. One study found that women using Depo-Provera were more likely to develop gonorrhea or chlamydia than otherwise equal women who were taking oral contraceptives or other forms of birth control.[18] Women who use injectable contraceptives and who have multiple sex partners may wish to use condoms during sex to reduce risk of infection.[15]

Lunelle, an estrogen and progestin hormone injectable given once a month, was also briefly available to women. In 2002, concerns about high contraceptive failure rates led the manufacturer to recall the device.

Another method of administration of birth control is the patch. Ortho Evra, for example, is a highly effective weekly hormonal birth control patch that is worn on the skin for one week and replaced on the same day of the week for three consecutive weeks, with the fourth week being "patch free." The patch prevents pregnancy in the same way as birth control pills. That is, it works primarily by preventing ovulation and by causing changes to the cervical mucus (making it more difficult for sperm to enter the uterus). In November 2005, the FDA added a warning to all labels of Ortho Evra after it was discovered that women taking the contraceptive were exposed to more estrogen than originally estimated. Although the side effects of this additional small dose of estrogen are not yet known, high dosages of estrogen are linked to blood clots in the arms and legs, strokes, and heart attacks. Women who already have high blood pressure or who are at risk for

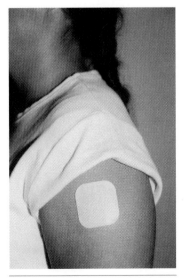

The patch is worn on the skin for one week and replaced on the same day of the week for three consecutive weeks.

heart attack or stroke may wish to consult their physicians before taking Ortho Evra.[19]

Vaginal rings are also available as a contraceptive choice for women. One vaginal ring, the NuvaRing, is inserted in the vagina for three weeks and then removed for the week of menstruation. It releases hormones and prevents pregnancy in a similar way to the patch. After menstruation, a new ring is inserted.

Barrier Methods

Barrier methods of contraception were the primary forms of contraception before the pill and IUD. After the introduction of the latter "high-tech" birth control measures, barrier methods were seen as messy, unromantic, and less sophisticated. Barrier methods do offer several advantages over other contraceptives. Some feminists and health advocates have objected to the pill on the grounds that it introduces unknown chemicals into the body and its long-term effects are unknown. The condom has reemerged, particularly as a result of the AIDS epidemic, as a major form of protection against HIV infection as well as other sexually transmitted diseases, such as herpes and gonorrhea. In addition, the diligent and proper use of condoms has demonstrated pregnancy protection rates fairly comparable to those seen with the pill and IUD. Another major compelling reason for the return to barrier methods is that they have virtually no associated health risks, with the exception of rare allergic responses or localized irritation.

Barrier methods, as the name implies, provide a physical or chemical barrier that prevents sperm from fertilizing eggs. All barrier methods (except plain condoms) are used with **spermicide,** a chemical that breaks down the cell membranes of sperm. Most barrier methods are used inside the vagina to cover the cervix and prevent sperm from entering the uterus. Male condoms are protective sheaths that enclose the penis during intercourse and ejaculation. Female condoms will be discussed later in this chapter.

Barrier methods are very safe for the user, and problems and risks tend to be rare. One rare but important risk from barrier methods is toxic shock syndrome (TSS), which may be associated with the diaphragm, cap, and sponge. Although the TSS risk is small, it is recommended that the diaphragm, sponge, or cervical cap not be used during a menstrual period or when any type of vaginal bleeding occurs. Further recommendations include delaying using these devices four to six weeks after having a baby or until all postpartum bleeding completely stops. TSS risk also can be minimized by not leaving the devices in place in the vagina for longer than the recommended time period.

Vaginal birth control devices are also associated with some other complications. A **diaphragm,** sponge, or **cervical cap** may cause a vaginal bacterial infection if it is left in place for more than 24 hours. A foul-smelling discharge is an indication of such an infection and should be evaluated by a clinician. The diaphragm and cervical cap also may increase the risk of urinary tract infections, indicated by painful and frequent urination.

Barrier methods have several advantages. Overall, these contraceptive methods are very safe. Although the diaphragm and cervical cap require fitting by a clinician, the other barrier methods may be conveniently purchased in pharmacies. With the exception of abstinence, condoms are the only contraceptive method that can reduce the risk of transmission of sexually transmitted diseases, including HIV. Barrier methods are seen as noninvasive contraceptive measures by those women who do not want to have an IUD inside their uterus and who do not want to manipulate their hormonal system. They may also be used as backup contraceptive measures for a woman who as forgotten a pill or who questions an IUD's effectiveness. Some couples have intercourse sporadically or infrequently and find that barrier methods are appealing because they are effective but have to be used only when necessary. Older women and careful users find barrier methods to be more effective than do younger women, women who have frequent intercourse, and those who are not careful users.

Spermicides

Spermicidal agents are sold as creams, foams, films, suppositories, or gels (Figure 5.5). They are available without prescription, and most contain detailed printed materials on their use. Spermicides provide some protection as a mechanical barrier, by spreading over the surface of the cervix and blocking access to the cervical opening. More importantly, however, they inactivate sperm by breaking down the surface of the sperm cells on contact. The spermicide should be inserted deep into the vagina.

Spermicidal agents have the advantage of being effective immediately upon use, but they do have time limits for their effectiveness. It is important to read the printed sheet available with each product and know the range of time for its effectiveness. An additional application is needed for each round of lovemaking, and the product should be left in place, with no douching, for at least six hours after the last round.

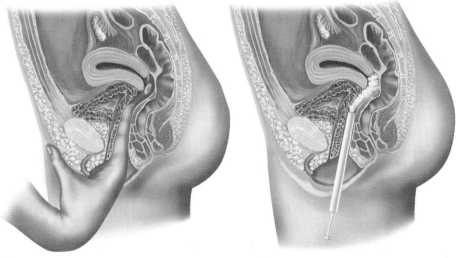

(a)   (b)

Figure 5.5

Spermicidal agents.
Hints: (1) Woman should lie down after insertion; spermicide will leak out and have reduced effectiveness if she is in a vertical position. (2) No douching for 8 hours. (3) Keep extra supplies available—it is not possible to measure residual amounts of foam in containers. (4) Repeat intercourse requires repeat application of spermicide. (5) Wash reusable applicators with soap and water after use. Follow directions carefully for amounts and frequency of use.

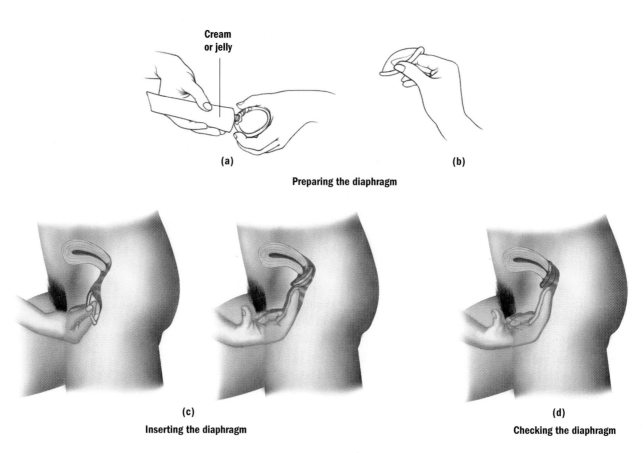

Cream or jelly

(a)   (b)

Preparing the diaphragm

(c)   (d)

Inserting the diaphragm   **Checking the diaphragm**

Figure 5.6

Diaphragm. *Hints:* (1) Apply 1 to 2 tsp of spermicide to diaphragm rim and inside dome. (2) Insert the diaphragm by holding it in one hand, squeezing rim together in center. With other hand, spread labia and insert diaphragm. (3) Diaphragm is inserted deep into vagina with the anterior rim tucked into place last. (4) Check for proper placement of the diaphragm. Cervix is felt through dome—feels like tip of the nose. (5) To remove the diaphragm, assume the squatting position and break the suction by placing index finger between diaphragm and pubic bone. Hook finger behind anterior rim, bear down, and remove.

Foams, creams, and jellies are inserted via an applicator. Suppositories are capsules inserted into the vagina that melt into a thick spermicidal liquid. Contraceptive film is contained in a small thin sheet of glycerine, which is placed over the cervix before intercourse. Its effect is similar to that of contraceptive suppositories: as the sheet dissolves, the spermicide is released.

Diaphragm

A diaphragm is a dome-shaped latex cup rimmed with a firm but flexible band or spring (Figure 5.6). It must be first coated with a spermicidal agent before being inserted into the vagina before intercourse. The spermicidal agent is important because it creates a tighter seal around the cervix and kills sperm on contact. The musculature of the inner vaginal walls holds the diaphragm in place. Because the diaphragm must fit the cervix it is to cover, this contraceptive method requires clinician examination, fitting, and prescription. During the fitting, it is important to evaluate the comfort of the diaphragm as well as to practice its insertion and removal.

Diaphragm effectiveness depends on proper fit and diligent use. A diaphragm that is too small may not stay in place and slip off the cervix; one that is too large may press on the urethra and cause a urinary tract infection. Application of the spermicidal cream or gel and insertion of the diaphragm can occur as long as six hours before intercourse. If intercourse occurs more than once, it is important to use an additional application of spermicide for each event, regardless of how short a time the diaphragm has been in place. The diaphragm should not be removed or dislodged to add the cream or gel for a follow-up round of lovemaking; spermicide can be inserted directly into the vagina.

The diaphragm may be inserted in a standing, squatting, or lying-down position. For insertion, the diaphragm should be held with dome down (spermicide inside the dome) in one hand. The opposite sides of the rim should be pressed together so that the diaphragm folds. The other hand should spread the lips of the vagina to facilitate insertion. The diaphragm should be inserted into the vagina toward the small of the back as far as it will go. A finger can tuck the rim behind the firm bulge in the roof of the vagina that covers the pubic bone. Once the diaphragm is in place, the woman should not be able to feel it except with her fingers. If it is uncomfortable, it should be removed and reinserted. It is a good idea to check the position of the diaphragm before having intercourse. This can be done by the woman or her partner. The back rim should be below and behind the cervix, and the front rim should be tucked up behind the pubic bone. It should be possible to feel the cervix through the soft rubber dome of the diaphragm.

Like the cervical cap, the diaphragm may be inserted as long as six hours before intercourse and need not interrupt or interfere with lovemaking. It should be left in place for a minimum of six hours after intercourse to allow the spermicide to kill all of the sperm. Douching should not occur during that time.

The diaphragm should not remain in place longer than 24 hours. It may be removed by reaching up inside the vagina with an index finger or thumb and grabbing the front rim of the diaphragm. It then can be pulled down and out of the vagina. A squatting position facilitates removal of the diaphragm for some women. After removal, the diaphragm should be washed with warm water and soap, rinsed, and dried with a towel. It is a good idea to inspect the diaphragm for defects or holes. Petroleum jelly or oil-based lubricants should not be used with a diaphragm for lubrication because they will weaken the latex. If additional lubrication is desired, a water-soluble lubricant, such as K-Y Jelly® or Astroglide®, may be used.

Side effects with the diaphragm are infrequent. An allergic response to the latex of the diaphragm or to the spermicide is possible but rare. Symptoms of an allergic response may include burning, itching, swelling, or blistering. Urinary tract infections are another possible side effect of the diaphragm; they may take the form of either cystitis (infection of the bladder) or urethritis (inflammation of the urinary opening). Some diaphragm users feel bladder pressure, rectal pressure, or cramps when the diaphragm is left in place six hours after intercourse. A smaller diaphragm or a different rim type might help relieve this side effect. Women with poor muscle tone of the vagina, a vaginal or cervical infection, vaginal bleeding, or a history of toxic shock syndrome should not use a diaphragm. After childbirth, weight loss or gain of more than 10 pounds, pelvic surgery, or a miscarriage or abortion, women should have their diaphragms refitted to ensure proper size.

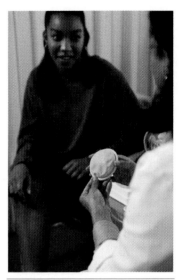

■ A diaphragm is a dome-shaped latex cup rimmed with a firm but flexible band or spring.

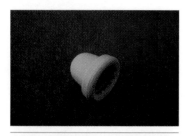

■ The cervical cap looks and works much like a small, deep diaphragm; it is made of latex and is used with a spermicidal agent.

Cervical Cap

The cervical cap (Figure 5.7) looks and works much like a small, deep diaphragm. It is made of latex and is used with a spermicidal agent such as cream or jelly. The cap fits snugly over the cervix and is held in place by suction. Caps require a clinician's examination, fitting, and prescription. Not every woman can be properly fitted, and some women find that insertion and removal of the cap are more frustrating than with the diaphragm.

The cervical cap's effectiveness depends on proper fitting and placement. The cap is inserted in a manner similar to the diaphragm. Like the diaphragm, the cap may be inserted as long as six hours before having sex, so it need not interrupt activity. It must be inserted at least 20 to 30 minutes before sex, however, to allow a tight seal to form between the cap and the cervix. The most common reason for the cap's failure is dislodgement from over the cervix. Women should check the seal before and after sex, and move the cap back in place if necessary. If the cap has moved during sex, more spermicide should be inserted into the vagina. Otherwise, additional spermicide is unnecessary once the cap has been inserted, allowing more sexual spontaneity than the diaphragm.

The cervical cap, unlike the diaphragm, may be left in up to 48 hours. It must remain in place for a minimum of 8 hours after intercourse; women should not douche during this time. The cap is removed in a manner similar to the diaphragm, but removal is more difficult for some women.

Figure 5.7

Cervical cap. *Hints:* (1) Fill cap approximately two-thirds full of spermicide. (2) Insert the cap by holding it in one hand, squeezing rim together in center. With other hand, spread labia and insert cap. (3) Cap is inserted deep into vagina. Use the index finger to press cap around the cervix until dome covers the cervix. (4) To avoid odor and reduce the risk of complications, remove within recommended time. (5) To remove the cap, break the suction by placing index finger between cap and pubic bone. Grasp dome and pull down and out.

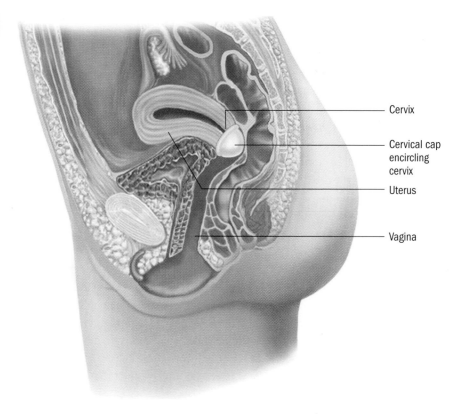

Cervix

Cervical cap encircling cervix

Uterus

Vagina

Side effects of the cap are rare but include an allergic reaction to the latex or spermicide or an unpleasant vaginal odor. After childbirth, weight loss or gain of more than 10 pounds, pelvic surgery, or a miscarriage or abortion, women should have their cervical caps refitted to ensure proper size. Women should not use the cap if they have a history of toxic shock syndrome or an infection of the reproductive tract. Unlike with the diaphragm, women with poor muscle tone of the vagina or a history of urinary tract infections can use a cervical cap.

Condom

Condoms (Figure 5.8) recently have resurfaced as a popular barrier contraceptive. Women are now responsible for nearly 40% of total condom sales, and these contraceptive methods are advertised in women's magazines. Condoms are available with lubricants and spermicides and come in a variety of colors and textures.

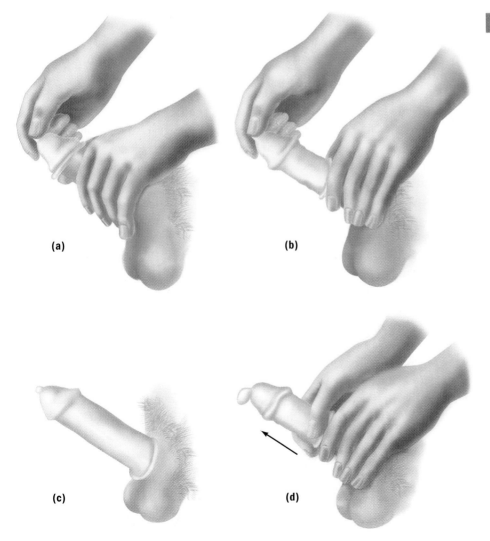

(a)

(b)

(c)

(d)

Figure 5.8

Condom use. *Hints:* (1) Avoid prolonged heat or pressure—condoms should not be stored in glove compartments or wallets. (2) Use only once and throw away. (3) If condom should break, use an extra dose of spermicide. (4) Put condom on an erect penis *before* it comes into contact with the vagina, pinching the tip of the condom to prevent air from becoming trapped. (5) Hold onto the rim of the condom as the penis is withdrawn from the vagina. (6) Do not use petroleum-based lubricants with condoms. (7) Latex condoms are more impermeable to the AIDS virus.

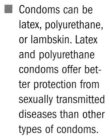 Condoms can be latex, polyurethane, or lambskin. Latex and polyurethane condoms offer better protection from sexually transmitted diseases than other types of condoms.

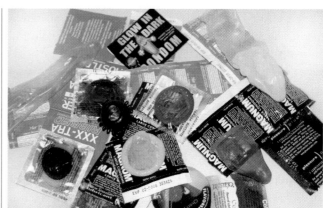

Condoms are portable, disposable, and easy to purchase. They may be discreetly carried and are, therefore, easily available when necessary. Women do not experience any post-intercourse vaginal leaking, and condoms permit the male partner to take an active role in birth control. Latex and polyurethane condoms are also the only methods that effectively prevent sexually transmitted diseases, including HIV infection. For couples who want to be especially diligent in their birth control efforts, condom use can supplement other forms of contraception.

Condoms should be stored in a cool, dry place, as storage in a heated unit (such as a glove compartment) can result in their deterioration. Latex condoms should not be lubricated with an oil-based lubricant (such as Vaseline®), which can weaken the latex. If extra lubrication is desired, a water-soluble lubricant (such as K-Y Jelly®) or prelubricated condoms can be used. Prelubricated condoms may also help to reduce friction during intercourse and reduce the risk of vaginal or penile irritation.

If a couple selects condoms as their method of birth control, it is essential that a condom be used for every lovemaking event. Effective use of this contraceptive method requires commitment and discipline. A spermicide-coated condom affords the most effective birth control protection and offers additional protection from sexually transmitted diseases. The clear fluid that collects on the end of an erect penis may contain living sperm, so the condom should be placed on the penis before the penis comes near the vagina. It is important that room be left at the end of the condom to collect the semen. A person should pinch the tip of the condom before putting it on; this will ensure that there is room for the semen and will prevent air bubbles, which increase the risk for breakage, from forming. A condom that is stretched very tightly over the head of the penis is more likely to break or to force the seminal fluid along the shaft of the penis and out the upper end of the condom. The penis should be withdrawn from the vagina before the erection subsides, and the condom should be held during this withdrawal of the penis. As the penis begins to lose its erection, the condom will collapse and the contents of the condom may spill within the vagina. A quick visual inspection to ensure that the contents are inside and that no spill or leakage has occurred is a good idea.

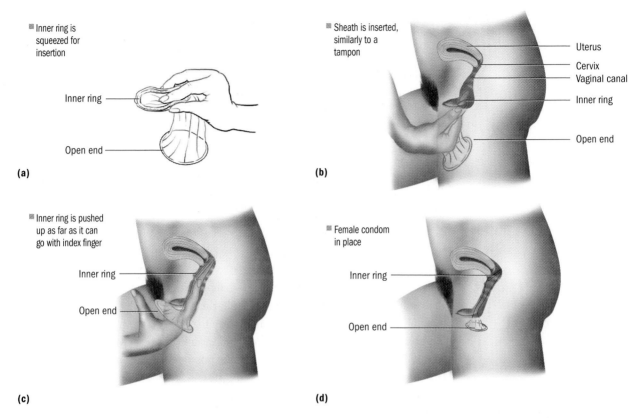

- Inner ring is squeezed for insertion

Inner ring

Open end

(a)

- Sheath is inserted, similarly to a tampon

Uterus

Cervix

Vaginal canal

Inner ring

Open end

(b)

- Inner ring is pushed up as far as it can go with index finger

Inner ring

Open end

(c)

- Female condom in place

Inner ring

Open end

(d)

Figure 5.9

The female condom.

Couples should use condoms both during and after treatment for any reproductive tract infection as a precaution against reinfection. Use of a latex or polyurethane condom is encouraged for women who are at risk for sexually transmitted diseases—even for those who are using an effective form of birth control, such as the pill. Lambskin and novelty condoms do not protect against diseases. Condoms also should be used on any items that are used during sexual activity that penetrate both partners. Examples would include shared sex toys, such as vibrators and dildos. In such cases, condoms should be changed between insertions if penetrating both vaginal and anal regions.

Female Condom

The FDA approved the female condom, another form of barrier contraceptives, in 1993 (Figure 5.9). The condom lines the entire vagina, preventing the penis and semen from coming in direct physical contact with the vagina. It also covers part of the external genitals, providing extra protection from semen leakage and sexually transmitted diseases. The female condom consists of a polyurethane sheath with a closed ring at one end and an open ring at the other. Although lubricant is contained inside the condom, additional lubricant is provided with the condom and should be used. Unlike the male condom, the female condom can be inserted as long as eight hours before sex; however, because of the awkwardness of its shape, most women insert the condom immediately before intercourse.

■ The female condom works by lining the entire vagina, thereby preventing the penis and semen from coming in direct physical contact with the vagina.

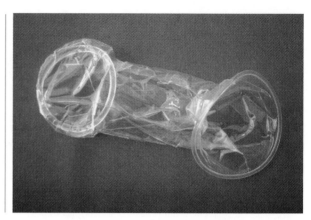

Before insertion, the sides of the female condom should be rubbed together to evenly distribute the lubrication inside the pouch. With the open end of the pouch hanging down, the closed ring at the end of the condom should be squeezed between the middle finger and thumb and inserted into the vagina. The condom should be pushed as far into the vagina as possible. Insertion is often tricky the first time due to the slipperiness of the condom. The condom should be straight (not twisted) within the vaginal canal, and the outer ring should remain outside the body. During intercourse, women should ensure that the penis enters inside the condom and that about 1 inch will cover the external genitals. Upon removal, the end of the condom should be squeezed and twisted to prevent leakage of semen.

Like the male condom, the female condom can be used only once and should be stored in a cool, dry place. The male and female condoms should not be used together. Likewise, the female condom should not be used with the diaphragm, cervical cap, or sponge. The only side effect of the female condom is possible allergy to the lubricant. Although the popularity of the female condom has not grown as hoped, it remains a promising method of contraception because it is a woman-controlled method of protecting against sexually transmitted diseases.

Contraceptive Sponge

The **contraceptive sponge** is a modern version of a historical form of birth control. Centuries ago, women soaked small sea sponges in solutions and placed them inside their vaginas to prevent conception. The sponge acts as both a cervical barrier and a source of spermicide, and it absorbs the ejaculated semen. One side of the sponge has a dimple in it that fits against the cervix; the other side has a nylon loop for easy removal. This contraceptive method is available without fitting or prescription. Sponge effectiveness depends somewhat on a woman's previous pregnancy history—this product is less effective for women who have previously completed a full-term pregnancy and delivery than in women who have not done so. The sponge was taken off the market in 1995 due to the problems in the

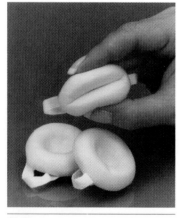

■ The contraceptive sponge acts as both a cervical barrier and a source of spermicide. It absorbs ejaculated semen.

manufacturer's factory and a lack of funds for fixing those problems. Today, the sponge is once again available for purchase over the counter.

The contraceptive sponge has the advantage of being portable and disposable. It can be inserted as long as 24 hours before intercourse and need not interrupt lovemaking. It does not require a repeat application of spermicide for a second round of lovemaking, and it is less messy than other spermicidal agents.

Before inserting the sponge, a woman should moisten it with a small amount of tap water. The sponge is held between two fingers and inserted into the vagina with the dimple side against the cervix. It is a good idea to check for proper placement by feeling the cervix through the sponge. Because it can absorb vaginal lubrication, some women use an additional lubricant such as K-Y Jelly® or spermicidal jelly after the sponge is in place.

The sponge is designed for 24 hours of use and should remain in place for 6 hours after the last round of intercourse. Care should be taken to ensure that it is not left in place longer than necessary. Before discarding a used sponge, it is wise to check to make sure that it is intact. If the sponge is not intact, the woman must check the vagina for fragments.

Permanent Methods

Healthy women and men usually have many years of fertility after they have completed their childbearing. Surgical sterilization offers permanent birth control for those individuals who do not wish to have any more children. Female sterilization is second only to birth control pills in overall popularity as a method of birth control and is the most popular method among minorities (see Figures 5.1 and 5.3). Advantages of **sterilization** include a high rate of effectiveness and relatively quick, simple procedures that have minimal complications and side effects.

Female Sterilization (Tubal Ligation)

Trends among contracepting older reproductive-age U.S. women show a dramatic increase in sterilization rates. Sterilization of women has been made much easier in recent years by the development of new instruments and new techniques that have replaced laparotomy, which involves surgically opening the abdomen and tying off the fallopian tubes. Because a significant number of unwanted subsequent pregnancies occurred with this procedure, newer techniques were developed that add destruction or removal of part of the fallopian tube.

Laparoscopic sterilization, also known as "band-aid" surgery, is one of these techniques. A laparoscope, a tube equipped with light and magnification lenses (see Figure 5.10), is inserted into the abdomen to provide a view of the uterus and tubes. The doctor uses a cauterizing instrument, rings, or clips to seal the fallopian tubes.

Minilaparotomy is the latest technique for tubal ligation. It requires a small abdominal incision and is performed under local or general anesthesia. The fallopian tubes are lifted out through the incision, cut, sealed, and replaced. The entire procedure takes a few minutes; the woman is able to go home after a few hours of recovery and observation.

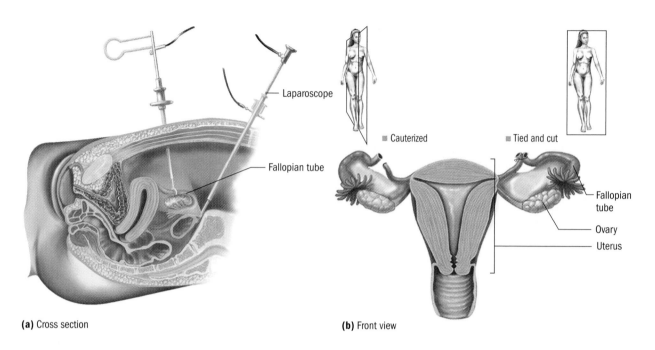

(a) Cross section   **(b)** Front view

Figure 5.10

Female sterilization. *Hints:*
(1) Resume normal activity slowly after procedure. (2) Most sutures are dissolvable. (3) Take mild analgesic for discomfort. (4) Resume sexual activity when comfortable. (5) Seek medical attention if temperature rises above 100°F, or if acute pain, discharge from incision, or bleeding is experienced.

We have three children and that is our family. The decision for sterilization was not difficult once we realized that we did not wish to become pregnant again. Our sex lives have improved—there is no need to worry about birth control anymore.

35-year-old woman

Sterilization should be undertaken with the expectation that the procedure will not be reversible. Some reversal procedures, however, have been successful. The chances of repairing the tubes for future pregnancy depend on the amount of fallopian tube that was destroyed at the time of the sterilization procedure. A new outpatient reversal technique, named Essure, takes less time to perform and requires less recovery time than previously used reversal procedures. Sufficient data comparing the procedures' rates of effectiveness are not yet available, but preliminary results indicate that it is 99.8% effective.[20]

Male Sterilization (Vasectomy)

A **vasectomy,** a surgical procedure usually performed under local anesthesia in a physician's office, can permanently sterilize a man. In most cases, one or two small incisions are made just through the skin of the scrotum. The vas deferens is lifted through the incision and the two ends are tied or cauterized to seal them. Most men are able to return to work and normal activities the day after surgery but are advised to avoid strenuous activities, such as straining and lifting, for the first week after surgery.

Vasectomy does not provide immediate contraceptive protection. Live sperm may remain in semen temporarily because mature sperm are stored in the vas deferens above the surgical site. As a consequence, men often are advised to use backup contraception for approximately 15 to 20 ejaculations.

Vasectomy offers several advantages. It is extremely effective as a permanent form of birth control and has a very low risk of complications compared to temporary forms of birth control or tubal ligation for women. Vasectomy does not cause any change in hormone levels or in the appearance or volume of semen. It also permits the male partner to take an active role in contraceptive responsibility.

Other Forms of Contraception

Not all contraceptive methods are appropriate for general use. Some methods are valid approaches to birth control, yet are associated with fairly high failure rates. **Abstinence** refers to no penis-in-vagina intercourse and depends on a couple's sustained willpower. Some couples consider oral sex or mutual masturbation, which do not result in pregnancy, a form of abstinence. In theory, abstinence is 100% effective; unfortunately, this method requires considerable sacrifice and has a high rate of failure in practice.

Withdrawal, also known as coitus interruptus, refers to interrupting lovemaking before ejaculation of semen. Although it may seem logical that conception requires semen and therefore requires ejaculation, withdrawal often fails as a form of birth control when the man is unable to remove his penis in time or because some sperm are released before ejaculation. The failure rate for withdrawal as a form of birth control is fairly high because it is difficult for a man to know exactly when ejaculation will occur. It also is mentally and physically difficult to suddenly stop in the midst of lovemaking.

Other methods of contraception, such as the lactational amenorrhea method (during breastfeeding) and the intrauterine device (IUD), can be effective for birth control but are not for everyone.

Lactational Amenorrhea Method

Breastfeeding women may use the lactational amenorrhea method, alone or with other forms of contraception, for the first six months postpartum. For this method to be effective, the woman must be breastfeeding exclusively on demand, be amenorrheic (no vaginal bleeding after eight weeks postpartum), and have an infant younger than six months. The failure rate of this contraceptive method is reported to be less than 2% if these criteria are met.[21]

Intrauterine Device

An intrauterine device (IUD) is a small plastic object that is placed in the uterus through the cervix and remains there for 1 to 10 years. The IUD kills sperm before they reach the ovum and alters the cervical mucus. There are two kinds of IUDs: Mirena, which releases a synthetic version of the female hormone progesterone, and ParaGard, which uses copper as a spermicidal agent.

The IUD was a popular form of birth control in the 1970s. Since then, its popularity has declined in the United States, but this contraceptive method remains very popular in Europe. Medical problems and lawsuits against the manufacturers of certain types of IUDs (mainly the Dalkon shield) have led to decreased production and use of such devices as a form of contraception.

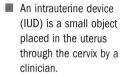
■ An intrauterine device (IUD) is a small object placed in the uterus through the cervix by a clinician.

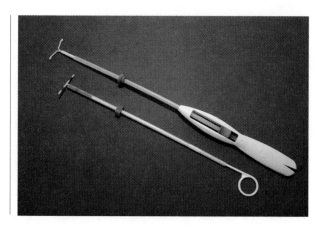

An IUD is inserted by a clinician into the uterus via the cervix with special instruments. A string attached to the IUD permits identification and removal of the device. Insertion may be painful and carries a high risk of infection.

PID was previously considered to be an associated risk of the IUD. New data suggest that this risk is no longer apparent.[22]

Some women should not have an IUD inserted. Anyone who has an active pelvic infection, including gonorrhea, or who is pregnant should never have an IUD placed in her uterus. Insertion of an IUD is strongly contraindicated if a woman has had recent or recurrent pelvic infections, inflammation of the cervix or vagina, history of ectopic pregnancies, valvular heart disease, abnormal Pap smears, cancer of the reproductive organs, immune diseases, or unexplained vaginal bleeding.

Advantages of the IUD include no supplies or equipment for lovemaking, no manipulation of normal hormonal cycles, and high rates of effectiveness as a form of contraception. The IUD also decreases menstrual cramps and bleeding. Newly approved low-dose progesterone IUDs are highly effective for as long as five years.

The IUD has two main disadvantages: expulsion and rare but potentially serious complications from pelvic infections or prenancies. In about 5% of women who have an IUD inserted, the IUD will be expelled from the uterus, doing no major harm to the woman but rendering the IUD ineffective as a contraceptive. Pelvic infections in women who have IUDs may also be more difficult to cure than those in women who do not have IUDs. If a woman becomes pregnant with an IUD in place, the pregnancy may be ectopic. The IUD should be removed immediately to avoid a serious infection, miscarriage, or premature delivery. Removal of the IUD, however, may result in a miscarriage. The total amount of menstrual bleeding tends to increase with the IUD, and spotting between periods commonly occurs. Nevertheless, the IUD remains a valid birth control choice for a woman who has finished childbearing and whose risk of infection is very low.

Emergency Birth Control

A woman who engages in unprotected sexual activity runs the risk of both sexually transmitted diseases and pregnancy. Birth control measures must be used in accordance with the manufacturer's guidelines to ensure their maximum effectiveness. Removing a diaphragm too early, failing to use a spermicidal agent with a diaphragm, and using too little foam are all problems that may increase the risk of an unplanned pregnancy. Occasionally, accidents happen. A condom may tear or slide off, or a diaphragm may dislodge from the cervix. In these situations, one convenient but unreliable option is to use a spermicidal agent immediately. Foam or cream would be more immediately effective than a vaginal suppository, which takes time to dissolve. There are no guarantees, but the spermicide may help reduce the risk of an unplanned sperm/egg union. Contrary to popular belief, postcoital douches are not effective as birth control. They actually may push sperm further into the vagina, increasing one's chance of pregnancy.

One form of emergency birth control (EBC) involves the use of high-dose oral contraceptive pills. Often called the "morning-after" pill, this kind of EBC can actually be taken as many as three days after having unprotected sex. EBC pills are not the same as RU-486—they do not cause an abortion. Emergency contraceptive pills have been presented in a variety of forms and doses, including the more common dose called the Yuzpe regimen. This regimen consists of estrogen and progestin taken in two doses—the first dose within 72 hours of unprotected intercourse, and the second dose 12 hours later. The risks associated with emergency contraceptive pills are similar to those linked to oral contraceptives, and the most common side effects are nausea and vomiting.

For many years, few women knew that the "morning-after" pill existed. In 1997, the FDA approved the marketing of such pills for the sole purpose of preventing pregnancy after intercourse has occurred. Ovral and Alesse are two brands of pills that are commercially available in the correct dose for emergency purposes. In late 1998, the FDA approved an emergency contraception kit, called Preven, which is available by prescription. It contains a patient information book, a urine pregnancy test, and four emergency contraceptive pills. In 1999, the FDA approved Plan B, the first progestin-only pill intended for use as emergency contraception. Progestin-only pills may be safer and more effective, and they produce fewer side effects than some of the other older regimens.

Access is an essential component of emergency contraception. Some socially conservative groups strongly oppose increasing access to emergency contraception, believing that it will encourage teenagers to engage in unsafe sexual behaviors and ultimately lead to higher rates of teenage pregnancy and sexually transmitted diseases. The administration of President George W. Bush has been one of emergency contraception's strongest opponents. The FDA, under leadership appointed by Bush, has repeatedly delayed making Plan B contraception available to women without a prescription. In so doing it overruled both its own staff and the unanimous recommendation of outside experts. However, a recent large-scale study found that easing access to emergency contraception resulted in preventing many unwanted pregnancies without causing significant sexual behavior change.[23]

The success rate of postcoital contraception is approximately 80%. This means that women who use emergency contraception are 80% less likely to become pregnant than women who do not. In general, about 8 of 100 women will become pregnant after one act of unprotected intercourse in the second or third week of their menstrual cycles. If all 8 of those women used an emergency contraceptive pill, on average 2 of them would become pregnant.

An IUD also may be used after unprotected intercourse. For up to seven days after unsafe sex, women can have an IUD inserted, which guarantees them an effectiveness rate of greater than 99%. This method, however, will not protect a woman from exposure to a sexually transmitted disease. Emergency birth control should not be used as a routine form of contraception.

Handling an Unplanned Pregnancy

Women who experience an unplanned pregnancy must face a difficult decision. They may decide to terminate the pregnancy, to carry the baby to term and keep the child, or to carry the baby to term and have the child adopted. A woman must consider the implications of each decision and feel comfortable with her choice. Having a baby brings major changes to a woman's life, and it may cause many difficulties for a woman who is young and single. Plans for future education, careers, or relationships may have to be sacrificed to raise a child. All of these issues must be considered so that a woman does not resent her child based on a decision she has made. A woman may be concerned about financial and emotional support during the pregnancy, especially if she does not have support from the baby's father or from family and friends. Many family planning clinics, crisis pregnancy centers, and health departments have programs set up to meet the needs of these women.

Unplanned pregnancies are not always unwanted pregnancies. Often, a couple is not planning to have a child at the time that they become pregnant, but they want a child and happily decide to proceed with the pregnancy.

If a woman decides that she would like to carry the baby to term but not raise the child, she should look into adoption. Adoption can be "open," where the birth mother has some role in the child's future, or "closed," where the whole process remains confidential. Both public and private adoption services are available. Public adoption services are usually less costly but may be very competitive and require long waits. Parents often have to be more flexible about the age or race of child they are willing to take. Private adoptions usually involve a financial arrangement negotiated by an agency or lawyer between the adoptive parents and the birth mother. Private adoptions can be faster and allow adoptive parents and birth mothers to have more options in selecting each other. Adoptions also can be domestic or international, though adoption laws vary from country to country. In all adoptions, a host of legal and ethical factors must be considered by all parties involved. Many adoption agencies can help match the child with an adoptive family and may be able to arrange for the adoptive parents to pay for the mother's healthcare costs during the pregnancy.

Other women choose to terminate their pregnancies. In these cases, a decision should be made as early as possible to ensure a safe abortion.

Perspectives on Abortion

Abortion may be defined as the spontaneous or induced expulsion of an embryo or fetus before it is viable or can survive on its own. This can occur without human interference if natural complications of fetal development, perhaps due to genetic, medical, or hormonal problems, result in the spontaneous termination of the pregnancy. This termination of pregnancy is called a miscarriage or a spontaneous abortion (see Chapter 6). In contrast to a spontaneous abortion, an induced abortion involves a decision to terminate a pregnancy by medical procedures.

Abortions are a critical facet of women's health. Each year, more than 6 million American women become pregnant, and half of these pregnancies are unintended. Approximately 1.3 million women terminate their unintended pregnancy through abortion each year.[24]

Historical Overview

Induced abortion has been both controversial and widely practiced for centuries. Anthropological studies reveal that abortion was a widespread practice in ancient and preindustrial societies. In the Western world before Christianity, Greeks and Romans considered it to be acceptable during the early stages of pregnancy, though they did not allow women active roles in family planning. A prescription for abortion has been found in the Hippocratic oath taken by Greek physicians. Until the late 1800s, women healers in Western Europe and the United States provided abortions and trained other women to do so, without legal prohibitions.

The movement to establish abortion as both criminal and sinful was led by male physicians as part of a crusade from 1860 to 1880 to outlaw all forms of contraception. By 1910, many U.S. states had passed legislation prohibiting abortion during all stages of pregnancy, with the exception of pregnancy causing a threat to the mother's health. During this time, the issue of equity emerged as an abortion public policy consideration. Women with greater personal financial resources were able to arrange for safer, more "legal" abortions by traveling to less rigid jurisdictions or by persuading physicians to make therapeutic exceptions. Women with fewer financial resources were more likely to suffer from unsafe abortions and incompetent abortionists. Legal prohibition did not have its intended effect of reducing the incidence of abortions, however. Estimates of the number of illegal abortions performed annually in the 1950s and 1960s range from 200,000 to 1.2 million.

In the early 1970s, many prohibitions of a woman's right to receive an abortion were struck down. Abortion was legalized in the United States on January 22, 1973, through the landmark Supreme Court decision *Roe v. Wade*. This decision declared unconstitutional all state laws that prohibited or restricted abortion during the first trimester of pregnancy. The decision stated that the "right of privacy . . . founded on the Fourteenth Amendment's concept of personal liberty . . . is broad enough to encompass a woman's decision whether or not to terminate her

I am an organized and responsible person. I was a victim of contraceptive failure. It was impossible for me to have a child at that time in my life. It would have destroyed everything that I had worked years for. So I had an abortion. I am not proud of it, but I am grateful that I was able to go to a safe facility.

32-year-old woman

pregnancy." The ruling also limited state interventions in second-trimester abortions and left the issue of third-trimester abortions up to each individual state.

Socially conservative groups quickly rallied against the decision. The "right-to-life" movement was originally a creation of the Family Life division of the National Conference of Catholic Bishops (NCCB), the directive body of the Catholic Church in the United States. Immediately following the Supreme Court decision, the NCCB Pro-Life Affairs Committee declared that it would not accept the Court's judgment and called for a major legal and educational battle against abortion. A religious pro-choice group, the Religious Coalition for Abortion Rights, was formed in 1973 to support the Supreme Court decision and preserve the right of women, regardless of income, to have their choice of legal abortions.

In 1974 and 1975, some states sought to restrict the Supreme Court's ruling by requiring teenagers seeking abortions to have parental permission. This legislation, however, was declared unconstitutional by the Supreme Court in 1976. The Court's decision stated that a minor should have free access to sex-related health care and that a third party such as a parent could not veto a decision made by the physician and the patient to terminate the patient's pregnancy.

In 1976, Congress introduced and passed the Hyde Amendment, a major setback for the abortion movement. This legislation banned Medicaid funding for abortion unless a woman's life was in danger. Regardless of its original intent, this amendment disproportionately affected low-income women. A temporary injunction stalled the implementation of the Hyde Amendment for a year. Meanwhile, in June 1977, the Supreme Court ruled that states did not have to fund what they considered "medically unnecessary" abortions. In December 1977, a compromise version of the Hyde Amendment added exceptions for promptly reported rape and incest cases in which two physicians would testify that the woman's health would be seriously impaired by maintaining the pregnancy. Many groups fought against the Hyde Amendment, but the Supreme Court ultimately upheld it in the 1980 *Harris v. McRae* decision. Although the Supreme Court reaffirmed the central holding of *Roe v. Wade* in 1986, a newly constituted Court agreed to hear the case *Webster v. Reproductive Health Services* in 1989. Its decision on the *Webster* case returned to the states the authority to limit a woman's right to a legal abortion.

The 1991 case of *Rust v. Sullivan* upheld the constitutionality of the "gag rule," which prohibited federally funded clinics from providing information about and referrals for abortion. In 1992, the Court's ruling in the case of *Planned Parenthood of Southeastern Pennsylvania v. Casey* reaffirmed the central holdings of *Roe v. Wade*, but allowed states to restrict abortion access. This decision prompted many states to require parental consent and waiting periods.

Laws have also limited antiabortion demonstrators' proximity to abortion clinics. These laws were instituted to ensure the safety and privacy of women seeking abortions after many attacks on abortion clinics, women seeking abortions, and abortion providers took place.

Legal questions about abortion and people's rights to demonstrate for or against it abound, filling the courts. Many legal challenges seek to establish the legal status of a fetus, thereby setting the stage for eventually outlawing abortions. A rising tide of conservatism in the United States has created an environment that puts into question the future of women's right to choose. This saga continues with an ever-growing intensity as people on both sides of the issue become more entrenched in their determination and steadfast approach to the issue.

Current Perspectives

Abortion is one of the United States' most passionately debated and controversial topics. People who believe abortion should be illegal describe themselves as "pro-life," while people who believe that a woman should be able to choose an abortion describe themselves as "pro-choice." Millions of Americans have opinions that fall somewhere between these two absolutes. Journalists, who wish to appear neutral and not imply that either group is against life or choice, use the terms "antiabortion" and "abortion rights" to describe activists on either side.

Recently, abortion took a center stage in the confirmation hearings for two Supreme Court vacancies. On the state level, more states are actively passing legislation restricting access to abortion, creating more waiting periods or consent requirements, and mandating certain information be distributed to a woman prior to a procedure.

Pro-Life

Pro-life advocates argue that the human fertilized ovum is a human being that should be afforded legal protection. Pro-life efforts to overturn abortion public policy have taken three major approaches: human life amendments to the U.S. Constitution, human life statutes and governmental action through legislation, and other means to restrict access to abortion services. Antiabortion groups have been lobbying for legislation and raising revenue for electoral campaigns targeting pro-choice electoral candidates. The National Right to Life Committee, which includes most pro-life groups, has chapters in all 50 states and tens of millions of members along with a $12 million annual budget.

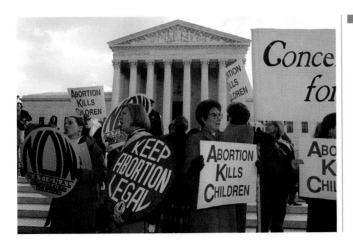

Abortion continues to be one of the greatest debates in American society.

Recently, pro-life groups have adopted the strategy for lobbying for laws that establish a fetus as a human being with legal rights. Pro-life activists have sought to provide fetuses with rights to state health insurance coverage and to increase sentences for people convicted of attacking or murdering pregnant women. Additionally, in many states, a woman who takes drugs during her pregnancy can now be convicted of child abuse.

Pro-Choice

Pro-choice advocates favor legalization and ready availability of abortions. They believe that an abortion is a personal medical decision that should be made between a woman and her doctor. From their perspective, for women in one of the most industrialized countries in the world to have a personal issue played out in a political arena is deplorable. They believe that a woman has the right to exercise control over her own body and, therefore, that a pregnant woman has the right to freedom of choice as to whether she will terminate an unwanted pregnancy. Many also believe that a fertilized ovum is not yet "human." Many members of the pro-choice movement distinguish between whether on a personal level they would choose to have an abortion, and the belief that women as a group should have the choice to have an abortion.

Middle Ground

Unfortunately, the polarization of the abortion issue by the pro-life and pro-choice positions prohibits dialogue and an opportunity to find common ground of interest and concern. One group that is working to change this situation is the Common Ground Network for Life and Choice. This national organization is made up of pro-choice and pro-life supporters who support the goal of finding new approaches to resolve the abortion conflict. The group has agreed to disagree, and advocates of each side have worked through facilitated discussions to achieve understanding of the other's views and express shared concerns. Without changing their individual positions on abortions, the members are able to work together on issues such as reducing teen pregnancy rates and improving social conditions for women and children. The goals of such efforts are to prevent unwanted pregnancies, thereby avoiding the need for abortions.

Epidemiology

Abortions have been legal throughout the United States since 1973. Data on pre-1973, illegal abortions are not valid or reliable indications of actual prevalence. After an initial rise in the 1970s following legalization, the number of induced abortions stabilized in the 1980s at about 1.6 million per year.[24] Figure 5.11 depicts the rate of abortions around the country.

Abortion rates dropped throughout the 1990s (Figure 5.12). This decline slowed but continued into the first few years of the twenty-first century.[21] Several factors have played a part in this decline. Changes in U.S. demographics meant that a lower pro-

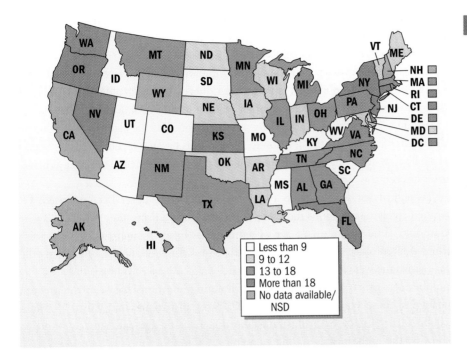

Figure 5.11

Rate of legal abortions per 1,000 women of reproductive age by state of occurrence, 2001.

Source: Centers for Disease Control and Prevention. (November 2004). Kaiser Family Foundation via Abortion Surveillance—United States, 2001. Table 3. *Morbidity and Mortality Weekly Report* 53, No. SS-9. Available at http://www.cdc.gov/mmwr/PDF/ss/ss5309.pdf.

portion of the female population was of childbearing age and at risk for having to consider abortion. The drive to educate girls about teen pregnancy and contraceptive options has also played a significant role in decreasing teen pregnancies. Other factors affecting this decline may include reduced access to abortion services, changing attitudes toward abortion, or continuation of unplanned pregnancies.

The profile of the typical abortion seeker has also changed in the last 20 years. In addition to young women who experience an unintended pregnancy, the growing

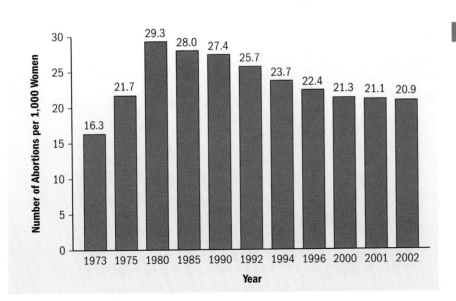

Figure 5.12

The number of abortions in the United States per 1,000 women aged 15–44, by year.

Source: The Alan Guttmacher Institute. (2006). Induced Abortion: Retrieved online from http://www.guttmacher.org/pubs/fb_induced_abortion.html.

number of women who get pregnant over the age of 35 has led to an increase in women who find out that their developing babies are at very high risk of birth defects or have a chromosomal abnormality like trisomy 18. This trend adds new dimensions to the ethics of abortion in the United States. A perspective that places a high value on social equity and reproductive rights dictates that older women should have the same rights and access as other women to receive abortions if they decide to terminate a pregnancy. At the same time, a perspective that places a high value on all human life could see the decision to abort a fetus because of a birth defect as part of a "slippery slope" that leads to abortions based on minor mental or physical handicaps or even the "wrong" gender.

Two-thirds of women who receive abortions have never been married. Of women receiving abortions in 2000–2001, 42.8% were Protestant and 27.4% were Catholic.[25] The predominant age of patients has been changing since 1980, with more women older than age 25 having abortions. In 1980, 64.7% of women who had abortions were age 24 or younger; in 1996, 52.2% were younger than 24. The number of women age 19 or younger obtaining abortions has seen the greatest change in these years, dropping from 29.2% of all patients in 1980 to 19.3% in 2000–2001.[25] Figure 5.13 illustrates abortion rates by age and by race/ethnicity, showing the highest rates among women age 20 to 29.

Adolescent females are a special population of concern with abortions. Factors contributing to adolescent pregnancies and decisions about keeping or terminating the pregnancy depend on a variety of socioeconomic considerations. Data indicate that girls age 19 and younger account for 20% of all abortions in the United States.[25] One study found that 61% of the adolescents indicated that one or both parents knew about the abortion.[26] Studies also have found that a teen's decision to have an abortion is based on concerns about how a baby would change her life and feelings that she is not mature enough or financially capable to raise a child.[26]

Figure 5.13

Percentage of total abortions in the United States, by age and race/ethnicity, 2000–2001.

Source: Jones, R.K., Darroch, J.E., and Henshaw, S.K. (2002). Patterns in the socioeconomic characteristics of women obtaining abortions in 2000-2001. *Perspectives on Sexual and Reproductive Health* 34(5): Table 1. Reprinted with permission from The Guttmacher Institute.

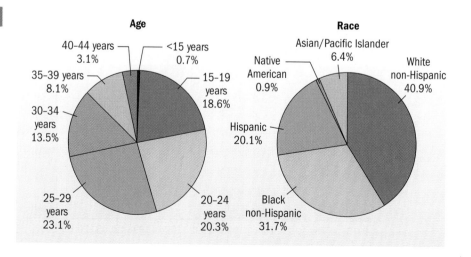

Abortion Procedures

Surgical Abortion

Vacuum curettage is the most widely used abortion technique in the United States. This procedure is performed while the woman is under local anesthesia. More than 91% of all legal abortions done in the United States use vacuum curettage.[27] It involves dilating the cervix and then inserting a vacuum curette—an instrument consisting of a tube with a scoop attached for scraping away tissue—through the cervix into the uterus. The other end of the tube is attached to a suction-producing apparatus, and the contents of the uterus are aspirated into a collection vessel. Vacuum curettage is usually performed during the first trimester of pregnancy, or until 13 weeks, but can be done up to 20 weeks following conception. The length of pregnancy is determined from the onset of the last menstrual flow or the last missed period. Through 13 weeks of pregnancy, this procedure can be performed in a clinical office setting with appropriate backup facilities for unexpected medical problems.

Dilation and curettage (D&C) is a technique used for many gynecological procedures but rarely in abortions. A sharp curette is used to scrape out the contents of the uterus. The procedure requires that the woman be under general anesthesia. D&C is rarely used in abortions in the United States because it is more painful than the vacuum curettage method, causes more blood loss, and requires larger cervical dilation.

Dilation and evacuation is a procedure that combines the D&C and vacuum curettage approaches. It is usually done between 13 and 15 weeks' gestation, but may be done through week 22. At this time, the cervix needs to be dilated to a greater extent because the products of conception are larger. This procedure is performed in the operating room of a clinic or hospital.

Nonsurgical methods also can be used to terminate a pregnancy. The use of prostaglandins—potent biochemical compounds produced naturally by both males and females—to terminate pregnancies has increased in recent years. The prostaglandin compounds may be used intra-amniotically, injected into the amniotic sac that surrounds the uterus, or inserted into the vagina as suppositories. They are used in second-trimester pregnancies (14 to 24 weeks of gestation). Prostaglandins cause the uterus to expel the fetus.

Hypertonic saline, a concentrated salt solution, may be used in second-trimester abortions as well. In such instances, the saline is infused slowly into the amniotic cavity through a needle in the abdomen. It causes fetal death, and a substance called oxytocin then causes expulsion of the fetus from the uterus. A hypertonic solution of urea also may be used to induce abortions; it is infused into the amniotic cavity and works in the same manner as the saline solution.

In some abortions, laminaria, a type of seaweed, is used to dilate the cervix. In a few hours, the laminaria dilates the cervix sufficiently to permit implementation of the abortion procedure.

Oxytocin, a product produced in the posterior pituitary and also commercially manufactured, is often used to facilitate uterine contractions. It is commonly used with the D&C method and with hypertonic saline during second-trimester abortions.

As with all medical procedures, abortions carry some health risks. Abortion-related health risks are greatly reduced if the pregnancy is terminated as early as possible, the woman is healthy, the clinician is skilled, and the woman is confident in her decision to have an abortion.[8] The risk of death or serious complications increases dramatically as the gestation period increases; however, a woman is 11 times more likely to die during childbirth than from a legal abortion.[28] The most common post-abortion problems include infection, retained products of conception in the uterus, continuing pregnancy, cervical or uterine trauma, and bleeding.

Medical Abortion

Medications permit some abortions to be performed without surgery. Methotrexate and mifepristone, along with misoprostol, can end a pregnancy.

Methotrexate has been used for years to treat certain types of cancer as well as other chronic conditions. It is currently available for "off-label" use for medical abortions, referring to the legal use of a drug approved for another purpose. To induce abortion, methotrexate is injected in the buttocks to cease embryonic development. A misoprostol suppository is then inserted into the vagina five to seven days later to cause contractions of the uterus.

Mifepristone, formerly known as RU-486, is a hormone pill that blocks the action of progesterone, which is necessary for maintaining a pregnancy. In September 2000, after more than a decade of delays, mifepristone received final approval from the FDA to be used as a safe and effective alternative to surgical abortion in the United States. This drug has been available to women in Europe for more than a decade. After taking mifepristone, a woman's uterine lining begins to break down. Days later, misoprostol is used to induce contractions and expel the fetal tissue.

Medical abortions must be administered by a woman's doctor. In both the methotrexate and mifepristone procedures, heavy bleeding and cramping ensue as a result of the misoprostol. These symptoms may last from a few hours to two weeks. The entire abortion is therefore considered to take anywhere from a few days to a few weeks and requires several visits to the healthcare provider's office. Possible side effects may include nausea, vomiting, diarrhea, headaches, hot flushes, and mouth sores.

Medical abortions may be performed as soon as a pregnancy is confirmed, and they must be performed within seven weeks after a woman's last menstrual period. Women who are older than 35 years of age or who smoke should not use methotrexate or mifepristone. Other conditions that may preclude a woman from having a medical abortion include history of asthma, cardiovascular disease, uncontrolled hypertension, diabetes, ovarian cysts or tumors, and severe anemia.

Currently, lawmakers in many states are moving to restrict medical abortion. At both the federal and state levels, some have proposed legislation designed to curtail the availability of mifepristone and limit the number of doctors who can prescribe it.

Other Abortion Techniques

Terms such as "menstrual induction," "menstrual extraction," and "aspiration without dilation" have been used in the past to refer to vacuum procedures performed very early in pregnancy before a routine urine pregnancy test could confirm pregnancy. These procedures were used and taught by certain groups as "do-it-yourself" methods. The technique for menstrual induction or extraction is identical to that for early vacuum abortion. Because it is now possible to confirm pregnancy as early as one week after conception, these terms are no longer meaningful. A woman who requests "menstrual induction" because her period is a few days late can now find out for certain whether she is pregnant. If her pregnancy test is positive, the vacuum procedure can be done. If the test is negative, there is no need for the procedure.

A major area of concern is in the preparation, training, and skill of the person performing a "menstrual extraction." A lack of training and nonavailability of emergency medical backup in the event of a problem are potentially life-threatening conditions.

A ban on a rare abortion technique, commonly referred to as the "partial-birth abortion" ban, has been at the center of a debate over a woman's reproductive rights. Former President Bill Clinton twice vetoed national laws calling for a "partial-birth" ban, and in the 2000 case *Stenberg v. Carhart,* the Supreme Court declared a "partial-birth" ban in Nebraska unconstitutional because it did not allow exceptions to protect the mother's health. Despite this ruling, in 2003, a Republican Congress approved, and President George W. Bush signed into law, the Partial-Birth Abortion Ban Act. As of January 2006, legal challenges have prevented this Act from taking effect. Although partial-birth abortion is not a medically accepted term, it is described in the ban as a case in which the entire fetal head is outside the body of the mother or, in the event of a breech delivery, if "any part of the fetal trunk past the navel is outside the body of the mother." Opponents of the bill banning the procedure state that the ban is unconstitutional, as it lacks any provision that protects the mother in cases where the pregnancy endangers her health. They say that second and third trimester abortions can be necessary to protect the health and future fertility of a woman. Critics see the "partial-birth" ban as a part of a larger agenda to undermine a woman's right to end a pregnancy. There is also confusion as to what procedure the ban corresponds to and when in pregnancy the ban would apply. Supporters of the ban state that this type of abortion is never needed to protect a woman's health. More information on the "partial-birth abortion" ban can be found in the Web sites listed at the end of this chapter.

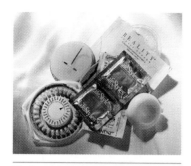

■ Several contraceptive choices are available today.

■■■■

Informed Decision Making

Contraception

Many effective, yet imperfect, birth control methods are available to women today. The decision-making challenge is to determine which method or combination of methods best meets each woman's unique needs. Safety and reliability are always the first concern. Other factors, such as health status, lifestyle, financial considerations, and patterns in sexual activity, also determine which method is best suited to meet a woman's needs. Many women will decide to change to a different birth control method as factors change. Communication is an essential component of contraceptive decision making. It is important that couples talk about their feelings, needs, and fears.

Determining Personal Needs

Sexual urges and sexual activity are normal, but a very real possible consequence of heterosexual intercourse is pregnancy. Both homosexual and heterosexual relationships also carry the risk of sexually transmitted diseases, including HIV. For both technological and sociological reasons, women have traditionally shouldered the major responsibility for contraception. This has been both unfair and unreasonable for women. Although most of the current contraceptives require primary use by women, couples can share the responsibility for contraception in many ways. Open and honest communication, sensitivity to each other's needs and feelings, and awareness of each method's strengths and weaknesses are essential components for effective decision making.

Specific strategies for informed contraceptive decision making include the following (Self-Assessment 5.1):

1. Review needs.

   · It is important to consider when or if pregnancy may be desired. If never, perhaps sterilization is a more logical option. If pregnancy is desired in a few years, the more effective hormonal methods may be preferable. If pregnancy is desired later within the year, one of the barrier methods may be a better choice. If a woman does not want to become pregnant and an abortion is out of the question, she may wish to consider a combination of two good birth control methods, such as foam and condoms, or pills and condoms.

   · Frequency of intercourse is another major consideration to review. If intercourse occurs frequently, barrier methods may prove to be inconvenient.

   · Number of partners should be considered. If a woman has more than one partner, or if her partner has another partner, she is at a greater risk for infection. In this case, a condom with spermicide in addition to birth control pills would provide the best protection against both sexually transmitted diseases and pregnancy.

Strategies for Contraceptive Decision Making

Contraceptive decision making is a personal and private decision between a woman and her partner. Several factors should be carefully considered when making the decision.

1. **Evaluate needs:**
   When/if pregnancy will be desired
   How disruptive an unplanned pregnancy would be
   Frequency of intercourse
   Number of partners
   Risk of STDs
   Personal preferences for lovemaking
   Level of partner cooperation
   Significance of spontaneity
   Comfort with touching one's own body
   Manual dexterity for certain methods

2. **Review medical history:**
   Cardiovascular risk factors
   History of cancer
   Vaginal or cervical infections
   Certain disabilities or chronic conditions
   Smoking status
   Allergies
   Circulatory disorders

3. **Put risks and benefits of methods in perspective:**
   Weigh all the advantages and disadvantages of each method in a personal perspective

4. **Reevaluate decision periodically:**
   Assess level of compliance
   Assess level of satisfaction

- Emotional, behavioral, and psychological needs should be considered. Even though a method may appear perfectly logical from a medical point of view, if it is distasteful or undesirable, chances are that compliance with that method will be poor. The degree of partner cooperation is another important consideration, because barrier methods are more likely to be successful if there is partner cooperation and support.

- Couples should be honest and realistic when deciding which kinds of contraception they will use. Couples who are unable or unwilling to use condoms every time they have sexual intercourse may wish to consider another form of contraception to supplement or replace condoms. Birth control pills will not be effective unless a woman remembers to take them every day.

- Perhaps one of the most important considerations is an evaluation of partner feelings and support. Ideally, the contraceptive choice will be a joint decision made by a couple following open, honest discussion of all the considerations and issues. In a less than ideal situation, a woman would be unwise to depend on her partner for contraceptive decision making or use.

2. Consider medical factors. Risk factors for cardiovascular disease, smoking status, circulatory disorders, and other medical factors must be carefully reviewed before deciding on birth control pills. A history of vaginal or cervical infections may rule out the use of diaphragms or cervical caps.

3. Review failure rates. The higher the failure rate, the greater the risk of an unwanted pregnancy. The difference in failure rates between "typical" and "perfect" use provides an estimate of the role human error plays for most couples. Some contraceptive methods, such as sterilization, are effective for virtually all couples; for other methods, failure rates for the average couple may be several times higher than for a consistent and diligent couple. Remember that typical failure rates are only an average, and that failure rates for couples who are less than diligent may be even higher.

4. Put the risks and benefits of the various methods in perspective. It is important to weigh all dimensions and issues of the relationship carefully against the advantages and disadvantages of each birth control method. The risks and benefits of each method need to be carefully assessed in terms of the individuals involved and their relationship. Some couples find that they can use a numerical rating scheme to determine the best contraceptive that meets their unique needs.

5. Periodically reevaluate the decision. At regular intervals, contracepting couples need to reexamine the level of effectiveness and their individual levels of satisfaction with the selected method. Reevaluation requires review of each of these steps and consideration of any new contraceptive developments, possible medical contraindications, and a current assessment of the couple's needs, feelings, and family planning goals.

When to See a Healthcare Provider

It is necessary to see a clinician for prescription of the diaphragm, cervical cap, any hormonal methods, IUD, or sterilization. Other forms of birth control do not require a clinician's prescription, but conditions associated with these forms may warrant a clinic visit. In general, a clinician should be consulted any time that a woman experiences pain during intercourse or any unusual bleeding, spotting, discharge, or odor. Any burning or itching associated with spermicide use may be an indication of an allergy to the agent.

With a diaphragm, it is wise to check with a clinician any time that the diaphragm does not seem to be fitting properly or there is discomfort, pain, or recurring bladder infections. After having a baby, it may be necessary to be refitted for a different-sized diaphragm because vaginal depth and muscle tone are usually altered by full-term pregnancy.

Abortion

Decisions regarding an unwanted pregnancy are private, personal, and difficult. They should not be rushed, and all options should be carefully weighed. Being able to talk through the process with a trusted person is essential. Options include terminating the pregnancy, continuing the pregnancy and raising the child, or continuing the pregnancy and relinquishing the child for adoption. Many supportive services are available for each of these options.

If a woman elects to have an abortion and is confident in her decision, she can reduce her risk of medical complications from the procedure by making arrangements in a timely fashion. In selecting an abortion facility, a primary concern should be the availability of around-the-clock emergency care services. Infection, bleeding, and other complications can almost always be treated successfully if treatment begins promptly. Other ways to minimize risks from an abortion include making sure that the surgeon who performs the procedure is well trained and experienced and verifying that the facility provides comprehensive care including postoperative instructions, education, and supportive services. Abortion counseling services are perhaps one of the most important features of a comprehensive facility.

Summary

Being able to control reproductive functioning is a necessary component of women's health, career preparation, and family growth management. Many methods of contraception are available today, and no one method is perfect. Table 5.5 compares the methods discussed in this chapter. Ultimately, contraception is a shared responsibility. The best method is one that a woman and her partner feel comfortable using, and one that they will use correctly and consistently. While ideally contraception is a shared responsibility between both partners, in today's world a woman is likely to bear the burden of an unexpected pregnancy. All women in relationships where there is the possibility of pregnancy should therefore make informed, well-thought-out decisions regarding contraception.

Abortion is something that no woman wants to face, but it is something that many women facing unwanted pregancies will have to consider. Whether a woman is pro-life or pro-choice, she should be sensitive to the difficulty that is caused by facing the possibility of abortion. Abortion is not just an issue for young, unmarried women; many women who have planned a pregnancy turn to abortion when they discover their developing fetus has a serious birth defect or chromosomal abnormality. Questions around abortion continue to be a focus for much of the women's health and women's rights movements, as well as for conservative and religious political movements.

Table 5.5 Comparison Issues: Contraceptives

	Birth Control Pills	Intrauterine Device (IUD)
"Perfect Use" Effectiveness	99.7%	99.4–99.9%
Typical Effectiveness	92%	99–99.9%
How It Works	Prevents the release of eggs from the ovaries; thickens cervical mucus	Kills sperm before reaches ovum and affects cervical mucus
Advantages	Most effective temporary form of contraception; lighter and more regular periods; protective factor for ovarian and uterine cancer; decreases risk of PID, fibrocystic breast disease, and benign ovarian cysts; does not interfere with sexual activity	Once inserted, remains in place; remains effective while in place; does not interfere with sexual activity
Disadvantages	Contraindicated for women with cardiovascular risk; some women experience minor side effects during first 3 months of use; major complications occur in women who are over 35 and who smoke; must be taken daily	May cause bleeding and cramping; increased risk of PID; increased risk of ectopic pregnancy and possibly infertility
Availability	By clinician examination and prescription only	Limited availability—by examination and fitting only
Comments	Combination pills contain both synthetic estrogen and progesterone. Minipill contains only progesterone and may produce irregular bleeding	Better for those women who do not desire future pregnancies
	Condoms (Latex or Polyurethane)	**Cervical Cap**
"Perfect Use" Effectiveness	98.7% (male) 95% (female)	82%
Typical Effectiveness	85% (male) 73% (female)	76%
How It Works	Prevents sperm from entering the vagina	Blocks sperm from reaching egg; spermicide kills sperm
Advantages	Protects against STDs, including AIDS and herpes; may help reduce risk of cervical cancer; can be used as a backup device for other methods; no hormonal or systemic effects; easy to use	Smaller than a diaphragm; may be left in place longer than diaphragm; does not require additional spermicide for repeated intercourse as does the diaphragm
Disadvantages	Male Condom: must be applied in midst of lovemaking; rare cases of allergy to latex; may break or cause diminished sensation Female Condom: may feel awkward during first few times of use	More difficult to position properly; may become dislodged during intercourse; may increase risk of urinary tract infections
Availability	Widely available in over-the-counter purchase	Must be fitted by clinician; not widely used in the United States
Comments	More effective when used with a spermicide	Must be used with a spermicide

(continued)

Table 5.5 Comparison Issues: Contraceptives *(continued)*

	Vaginal Spermicide (Used Alone)	Diaphragm
"Perfect Use" Effectiveness	82%	94%
Typical Effectiveness	71%	84%
How It Works	Kills sperm	Blocks sperm from reaching egg; spermicide kills sperm
Advantages	Able to use it only as needed; few side effects and contraindications; may protect against some STDs; provides additional lubrication	No side effects (rare allergies to latex or spermicide); can be inserted up to 6 hours before intercourse
Disadvantages	Messy; must be applied just before intercourse; effective for only 30–60 min; may be awkward or embarrassing to use	Must be used with a spermicide; proper fit is essential; may be awkward or inconvenient to use; may increase risk of urinary tract infections
Availability	Available over-the-counter as foam, jelly, cream, film, or suppository	Clinician examination and fitting required
Comments	Best results when used with a barrier method such as condom or diaphragm	Requires repeat application of spermicide with repeat intercourse
	Contraceptive Sponge	**Withdrawal**
"Perfect Use" Effectiveness	85%	96%
Typical Effectiveness	75%	73%
How It Works	Kills sperm; absorbs ejaculate; blocks sperm from entering vaginal tract	Keeps sperm from reaching egg
Advantages	Easy to use—spermicide is contained in sponge; may be inserted up to 24 hours before intercourse; continuous protection for 24 hours	Free; causes no health problems—no side effects or contraindications; no supplies or advance preparation; shared responsibility by male
Disadvantages	May be difficult to remove; may fragment; may cause irritation to vaginal lining; cannot be used during period	Unreliable; requires considerable control, discipline, and commitment from each other; may decrease pleasure
Availability	Available over the counter; relatively expensive	No purchase required
Comments	Must be left in place for 6 hours after intercourse; must be moistened before use	Not reliable form of contraception

(continued)

Table 5.5 Comparison Issues: Contraceptives *(continued)*

	Tubal Ligation (Female Sterilization)	Vasectomy (Male Sterilization)
Estimated Effectiveness	99.9%	99.9%
Typical Effectiveness	—	—
How It Works	Prevents egg from traveling into uterus	Prevents sperm from being in ejaculate
Advantages	Permanent; removes fear of pregnancy; no interruption of lovemaking	Permanent; removes fear of pregnancy; no interruption of lovemaking; shared responsibility by male
Disadvantages	Surgery-related risks; irreversible	Irreversible
Availability	Surgical expense	Surgical expense
	Progestin Implants (not available in U.S.)	**Depo-Provera**
Estimated Effectiveness	99.9%	99.7%
Typical Effectiveness	99%	99.7%
How It Works	Prevents the release of eggs from the ovaries and thickens the cervical mucus	Prevents the release of eggs from the ovaries and thickens the cervical mucus
Advantages	Most effective form of contraception, other than sterilization; can be left in place for up to 5 years	Very effective form of contraception; requires only an injection once every 3 months
Disadvantages	Must undergo surgical procedure; is slightly visible under skin	Once shot is received, patient experiences any side effects until shot wears off; may have a waiting period before returning to fertility
Availability	By clinician examination and surgical procedure only	By clinician examination and prescription only
Comments	Hormonal implants contain progestin only. Therefore, it is a good method for those who cannot use estrogen and who want long-term protection	Depo-Provera contains progestin only. Therefore, it is a good method for those who cannot use estrogen and who do not want the daily pill taking
	Note: Norplant is no longer available for use. Other implants currently available in Europe and other countries may soon be made available in the U.S.	

Profiles of Remarkable Women

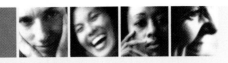

Margaret Sanger (1879–1966) and Mary Coffin Dennett (1872–1947)

Margaret Sanger and Mary Coffin Dennett were pioneers in the birth control movement.

Margaret Sanger began her career by attending the nursing program at White Plains Hospital in New York in 1900. She and her husband became involved in the pre-war radical bohemian culture in New York City and spent time with intellectuals, activists, and artists of the era. Sanger also joined the Women's Committee of the New York Socialist Party and took part in labor actions led by the Industrial Workers of the World.

As a nurse, Sanger began focusing on women's health and sex education. In 1912, she wrote a column on sex education for a New York publication, which was censored when she wrote about venereal disease. Upon seeing poor women suffering from miscarriages, abortions, and lack of effective birth control, Sanger began promoting the need to free women from unwanted pregnancies. Sanger published *Family Limitation,* a pamphlet that provided clear and frank descriptions of birth control methods and devices. The distribution of diaphragms and her publication were hampered by the Comstock Laws, which had been enacted by Congress in 1873, restricting the circulation of obscene materials—specifically birth control information—in the mail.

In 1916, Sanger opened the first birth control clinic in Brooklyn, New York. Although the clinic was raided and the staff was arrested shortly after its opening, the publicity brought supporters who helped to build a movement for birth control reform. Sanger founded the American Birth Control League (ABCL) in 1921 to promote the establishment of birth control clinics and the cause of fertility control. The ABCL set up its own clinic and dispensed diaphragms and lactic acid jelly for contraception. In 1942, the ABCL became the Planned Parenthood Federation of America.

Sanger continued fighting for the right to legally disseminate contraceptives. She met with much opposition due to her focus on radical feminism; in fact, she was even viewed as too radical for the birth control movement that she herself had launched. Ultimately, Sanger resigned from her position with ABCL and took respite from the birth control movement for many years.

After World War II, Sanger worked with family planning leaders in Europe and Asia to help establish the International Planned Parenthood Federation in 1952. She served as the organization's president until 1959. During this time, Sanger was instrumental in securing funding that helped make the development of birth control possible. Sanger died a few months after the Supreme Court decision *Griswold v. Connecticut* made birth control legal for married couples.

Mary Coffin Dennett attended the school of the Boston Museum of Fine Arts and taught design at Drexel University in Philadelphia from 1894 to 1897. She later became co-owner of a handicraft shop in Boston. Her interest in the suffrage movement began when Dennett worked first for the Massachusetts Woman Suffrage Association from 1903 to 1910 and then for the National American Woman Suffrage Association from 1910 to 1914. She advocated for pacifist beliefs and became a co-founder of the People's Council, an antiwar organization.

Dennett also became dedicated to reforming birth control laws. Opposing the radical, confrontational tactics espoused by Margaret Sanger, she focused her efforts on lobbying for legislative reform that would allow for the transmission of contraceptive information. Through her efforts to challenge the definition of legal obscenity, Dennett became one of the nation's most effective defenders of civil liberties. Along the way, she established the Voluntary Parenthood League. Unlike Sanger, who promoted the diaphragm, which only physicians could prescribe, Dennett stressed that ordinary people should be able to get birth control information without having to rely on medical experts.

Dennett was arrested during her career for mailing publications that were deemed obscene by the postal service. Throughout her life, she continued to press for women to become informed consumers and to gain direct access to birth control information. Dennett published a newspaper called the *Birth Control Herald* from 1922 to 1925 and several books, including *Birth Control Laws* (1926), *Who's Obscene* (1930), and *The Sex Education of Children* (1931).

Preventing unwanted pregnancy is a primary responsibility of all sexually active couples. In the event of an unwanted pregnancy, understanding all options and risks is a critical prerequisite for effective decision making.

■■■■

Topics for Discussion

1. What are some explanations for the higher contraceptive failure rate among younger women compared with older women?

2. What are some of the common reasons for using birth control?

3. What are some reasons that couples fail to use contraceptives or fail to use them correctly?

4. How can couples share in the responsibilities associated with contraception?

5. When are contraceptive "risky" times likely to occur in a relationship?

6. How can a couple improve their communication about sexuality issues, including contraception?

7. How may sociocultural beliefs and practices influence contraceptive decision making?

■■■■

Web Sites

The Alan Guttmacher Institute: http://www.agi-usa.org

The Association of Reproductive Health Professionals: http://www.arhp.org

Center for Reproductive Rights: http://www.crlp.org

The Emergency Contraception Website: http://www.not-2-late.com

Engender Health: http://www.engenderhealth.org

International Planned Parenthood Federation: http://www.ippf.org

The Henry J. Kaiser Family Foundation: http://www.kff.org

NARAL Pro-Choice America: http://www.naral.org

Planned Parenthood Federation of America: http://www.plannedparenthood.org

Public Agenda Issues Guide on Abortion: http://www.publicagenda.org

■■■■

References

1. Center for Reproductive Rights. (2003). Contraceptive converage in the Federal Employee Health Benefit Program. Available online at http://www.crip.org.

2. The Alan Guttmacher Institute. (2006). State Policies in Brief: Health Insurance Coverage of Contraceptions. Retrieved January 20, 2006, from http://www.agi-usa.org/sections/contraception.php.

3. Mosher, W. D., Martinez, G. M., Chandra, A., Abma, J. C., and Wilson, S. J. (2004). Use of contraception and use of family planning services in the United States, 1982–2002. *Advance Data from Vital and Health Statistics,* no. 350. Hyattsville, MD: National Center for Health Statistics.

4. U.S. Department of Health and Human Services. (December 2005). *Fertility, family planning and reproductive health of U.S. women: data from the 2002 National Survey of Family Growth.* Hyattsville, MD: National Center for Health Statistics.

5. The Alan Guttmacher Institute. (2005). Contraceptive Use: Facts in Brief. Retrieved January 20, 2006, from http://www.agi-usa.org/statecenter/contraception.html.

6. Grady, W., Klepinger, D., and Nelson-Wally, A. (1999). Contraceptive characteristics: the perceptions and priorities of women and men. *Family Planning Perspectives* 31(4): 168–175.

7. Mohllajee, A. P., Curtis, K. M., Martins, S. L., and Peterson, H. B. (2006). Does use of hormonal contraceptives among women with thrombogenic mutations increase their risk of venous thromboembolism? A systematic review. *Contraception* 73(2): 166–178.

8. Curtis, K. M., Mohllajee, A. P., Martins, S. L., and Peterson, H. B. (2006). Combined oral contraceptive use among women with hypertension: a systematic review. *Contraception* 73(2): 179–188.

9. Hanna, L., and Adams, M. (2006). Prevention of ovarian cancer. *Best Practice and Research Clinical and Obstetrical Gynecology* 20(2): 339–362.

10. Shulman, L. P. (1999). Oral contraception: safety issues re-examined. *International Journal of Fertility* 44(2): 78–82.

11. Schneider, H. P., Mueck, A. O., and Kuhl, H. (2005). IARC monographs on carcinogenicity of combined hormonal contraceptives and menopausal therapy. *Climacteric* 8(4): 311–316.

12. Marchbanks, P. A., McDonald, J. A. A.,Wilson, H. G., Folger, S. G., et al. (2002). Oral contraceptives and the risk of breast cancer. *New England Journal of Medicine* 346(26): 2025–2032.

13. Guthmann, R. A., Bang, J. and Nashelsky, J. (2005). Combined oral contraceptives for mothers who are breastfeeding. *American Family Physician* 72(7): 1303–1304.

14. Kwiecien, M., Edelman, A., Nichols, M. D., and Jensen, J. T. (2003). Bleeding patterns and patient acceptability of standard or continuous dosing regimes of a low-dose oral contraceptive: a randomized trial. *Contraception* 67(1): 9–13.

15. Sulak, P. J., Buckley, T., and Kuehl, T. J. (2006). Attitudes and prescribing preferences of health care professionals in the United States regarding use of extended-cycle oral contraceptives. *Contraception* 73(1): 41–45.

16. Hatcher, R. A., et al. (1998). *Contraceptive Technology,* 17th rev. ed. New York: Ardent Media.

17. USAID/WHO. (1996). Family planning methods: new guidance. *Population Reports* 4(XXIV): 1–48.

18. Morrison, C. S., et al. (2004). Hormonal contraceptive use, cervical ectopy, and the acquisition of cervical infections. *Sexually Transmitted Diseases* 31(9): 561–567.

19. U.S. Food and Drug Administration. (2005). Questions and Answers about Ortho Evra (Norelgestromin/Ethinyl Estradiol). Retrieved January 6, 2006, from http://fda.gov/cder/drug/infopage/orthoevra/qa.htm.

20. Women's Health: Essure. (2005). Retrieved January 21, 2006, from http://www.mayoclinic.com/health/essure/W000061.

21. Blenning, C. E., and Paladine, H. (2005). An approach to the postpartum office visit. *American Family Physician*. 72(12): 2443–2444.

22. Women's Health: Intrauterine Devices (IUDs). (2005). Retrieved January 20, 2006, from http://www.mayoclinic.com/health/iuds/W000087.

23. Raine, T. R., Harper, C. C., Rocca, C. H., et al. (2005). Direct access to emergency contraception through pharmacies and effect on unintended pregnancies and STIs: a randomized controlled trial. *Journal of the American Medical Association* 293: 54–62.

24. The Alan Guttmacher Institute. (May 18, 2005). Induced Abortions: Facts in Brief. Retrieved January 16, 2006, from http://www.agiusa.org/statecenter/contraception.html.

25. Jones, R. K., Darroch, J. E., and Henshaw, S. K. (2002). Patterns in the socioeconomic characteristics of women obtaining abortions in 2000–2001. *Perspectives on Sexual and Reproductive Health* 34(5): 226–235.

26. Koonin, L. M., et al. (1998). Abortion surveillance—United States, 1995. *Morbidity and Mortality Weekly Report* 47(SS-2): 31–68.

27. Strauss, L. T., Herndon, J., Chang, J., Parker, W. Y., Bowens, S. V., and Berg, C. J. (2005). Abortion surveillance—United States, 2002. *Morbidity and Mortality Weekly Report* 54(SS07): 1–31.

28. Bartlett, L. A., et al. (2004). Risk factors for legal induced abortion-related mortality in the United States. *Obstetrics and Gynecology* 103(4): 729–737.

Chapter Six

Pregnancy
and Childbirth

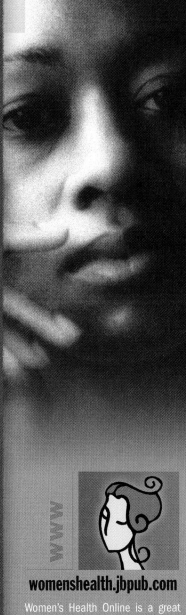

Chapter Objectives

On completion of this chapter, the student should be able to discuss:

1. Historical dimensions of pregnancy, childbirth, and breastfeeding.

2. Conception and the process of cell division after fertilization.

3. Hormonal changes and fetal changes during pregnancy.

4. Nutritional and weight gain recommendations for pregnancy and exercise concerns with pregnancy.

5. Detrimental effects of smoking, alcohol, drugs, and various environmental risks on pregnancy.

6. Techniques for prenatal testing and complications of pregnancy.

7. The significant issues surrounding childbirth preparation, labor and delivery, cesarean section, and vaginal birth after cesarean section.

8. Physiological changes of the breast for breastfeeding.

9. Benefits and complications associated with breastfeeding.

10. The concepts of fecundity and infertility.

11. Causes and diagnoses of infertility.

12. Treatment of infertility, including assisted reproductive technologies.

13. Emotional effects of infertility.

14. Trends in breastfeeding.

15. Prevalence of infertility, its major causes, and the types of treatment used.

womenshealth.jbpub.com

Women's Health Online is a great source for supplementary women's health information for both students and instructors. Visit

http://womenshealth.jbpub.com

to find a variety of useful tools for learning, thinking, and teaching.

There is a realization that women's attitudes toward and behavior during birth are shaped and conditioned by the demands and expectations of family, peers, community, and often religion. What a woman expects from her childbirth experience, what she will do, what she will fear and not fear, how she will interpret what is happening to her, and what in fact will happen when she gives birth, depend in large measure upon how her society defines what birth should be and where she fits in the various hierarchies of that society.

Janet Carlisle Bogdan (1990). Childbirth in America, 1650 to 1990. In R. D. Apple (ed.), *Women, Health in Medicine in America.*

Introduction

Pregnancy and childbirth are exciting and complex facets of women's health. In addition to the obvious biological aspects, pregnancy and childbirth are greatly influenced by social, cultural, historical, legal, and ethical dimensions. This chapter provides an overview of pregnancy, childbirth, breastfeeding, and infertility.

Historical Dimensions

The academic examination of childbirth as a social phenomenon did not really begin until the 1960s. Before that time, knowledge about childbirth had been derived principally from the writings of medical historians who stressed the progressive history of scientific advances in obstetrics. This medical and historical account provided little insight into how the management of pregnancy or birthing affected women's experiences of birth or about women's reactions to and participation in such changes. The accounts also failed to document how the birth experience felt to the woman.

Today there is considerably more focus and investigation on the social, racial, economic, and ethnic spectrum of childbirth. Childbirth history is now studied in a variety of contexts—medical, demographic, cultural, social, economic, professional, and symbolic, among others. The term "childbirth," however, generally evokes an image of a medical environment, with physicians and nurses, surgical drapes, intravenous poles, and fetal monitors. In contrast, in the early United States, childbirth did not have an association with medical personnel or equipment except when a woman's life was threatened. Childbirth was considered to be part of a woman's domestic responsibilities, among both immigrants and native populations.[1] Although specific cultural and ethnic variations existed in the management of the birthing process, all shared the tradition that only women attended other women. Women were the experts on birthing.[1]

■ The twentieth century brought medicalization and hospitalization to the childbirth experience.

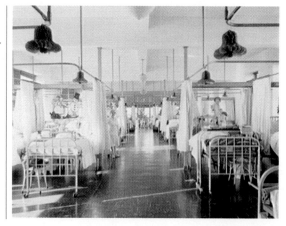

During the mid-eighteenth century, the expertise of women in birthing began to be questioned. Women in France were beginning to deliver babies in hospitals under the watchful eyes of not only traditional midwives, but also physicians. Although physicians had previously witnessed or participated in abnormal deliveries, the hospitalization practices enabled them to study and understand the normal childbirth process. Through close observation, measurements, and recordings, French physicians attempted to explain the mysterious process of childbirth.[2] During the same period, the English medical establishment became more oriented to surgical techniques—specifically, the development of instruments known as **forceps** to assist in the extraction of the fetus from the woman. The European obstetrical knowledge quickly crossed the Atlantic, and American physicians began appearing at the births of middle- and upper-class urban women. At first, physicians attended along with traditional midwives, but soon physicians replaced midwives in the birthing process. Medical schools began to certify men as birth attendants, leading to a decline in traditional midwifery. By the end of the eighteenth century, physicians had established roles in managing childbirth experiences throughout urban areas, including those for poor women.

With the medical presence during childbirth came a widening array of interventions, including medications, anesthesia, and birthing instruments. Accompanying the newly introduced technologies were additional problems of birth accidents, including tears and infections. Physician attitudes had changed from observing and learning to affecting and controlling. Women continued to actively participate in determining the terms of their childbirths only as long as the home was the birthing environment. Once birthing moved to the hospital, however, women lost this power.[3] The American medical management of childbirth originated in urban northeastern areas. In the South and in some religious communities, childbirth retained much of its traditional aspects during the nineteenth and early twentieth centuries. Immigrant groups also were more likely to continue with traditional practices.

The twentieth century brought additional medicalization and hospitalization to the childbirth experience. Midwives remained in the more inaccessible portions of the United States. Despite the increased technology and promises of greater safety, women were exposed to greater mystification of childbirth than they had ever known.[3] This trend was in some ways ironic because women were electing to control their fertility and have fewer children, thereby increasing the significance of the childbirth experience. At the same time, they understood less about the process and were less in control of birthing than their grandmothers had been. This trend continued until the late 1950s and 1960s, when women began to openly express their dissatisfaction with medicalized births. Europe again was the leader in a new trend of childbirth experiences that suggested that childbirth should be anticipated with joy and knowledge, not fear and ignorance, and could be accomplished with less pain, less medication, and less of the medical and surgical control typical of American births. These natural-birth relaxation techniques are the foundation of modern efforts toward "prepared childbirth."

Breastfeeding also has seen many changes over the years. The first variation on the practice of breastfeeding was the substitution of the mother's breast with that of a "wet nurse"—another woman who was able and willing to breastfeed for the mother. In the 1700s, "dry nursing," the mixing of flour, bread, or cereal with broth or water, became popular. This early form of infant formula was a cheaper option than "wet nursing." As women entered the workforce during the Industrial Revolution, substitutes for milk were produced, resulting in a decline in the practice of breastfeeding.[4] Formula substitutes remained popular for those women who could afford them, until reports surfaced on the benefits of breastfeeding in the 1970s. Since that time, breastfeeding rates have again fallen and risen as a result of various factors, ranging from a woman's place of employment to her personal finances, from her religious beliefs to her network of social support, and from her comfort with her own body to medical contraindications.

Pregnancy

Pregnancy lasts an average of 266 days from the time of fertilization or 280 days from the first day of the last menstrual period (often referred to as LMP). The gestational period is divided into three phases or trimesters of approximately three months each. Not all women have 28-day menstrual cycles, so due dates cannot be precisely determined (see **It's Your Health**).

Conception

Conception, also known as **fertilization,** is the union of the male sperm cell and the female egg cell. Before conception is possible, certain changes must take place within the sperm cells. Namely, they must mature in the male reproductive tract before ejaculation and undergo more biological changes in the female reproductive tract before they can fertilize the egg. The sperm cell is one of the smallest cells in the body and is produced in enormous quantities: approximately 50 million each day by a healthy male. Sperm production is a continuous, lifelong process. Sperm are produced in the testicles; they are then moved through the epididymis to the seminal vesicles, where the sperm mature into motile sperm and are stored until they are needed in the semen. Mature sperm cells swim like miniature tadpoles with an undulating movement of a threadlike tail. During the process of ejaculation, these cells are combined with secretions from the male reproductive tract to form semen. If ejaculation occurs into or around the entrance of the vagina, fertilization is possible. It has been estimated that as many as 300 million sperm are deposited with ejaculation, but fewer than 20 actually arrive anywhere near the unfertilized egg.[5]

The human egg, or ovum, is far rarer than the sperm. Each woman is born with a supply of approximately 1 million egg cells. Only about 300,000 eggs remain by the time a girl reaches puberty. One mature egg is released from a woman's ovaries each month during ovulation, usually resulting in 300 to 500 eggs being released during a woman's lifetime.

After the sperm separates from the seminal fluid, it becomes more mobile as it travels toward the egg. If the woman is in the early or middle segment of her menstrual cycle, the cervical mucus is of a consistency to allow the sperm to pass into the uterus. If progesterone is the dominant hormone, as in the late segment of the menstrual cycle, the cervical mucus inhibits sperm penetration past the cervix. Conception usually takes place in the upper third of the fallopian tube. In a process called the acrosome reaction, the sperm releases an enzyme called hyaluronidase, which works to dissolve the outer layer of the egg cell and allows the sperm cell to advance toward the center of the egg to join with its nucleus.[6] Only one sperm is able to penetrate the protective coating of the egg.

Two offspring born of the same pregnancy are called twins.

- **Dizygotic twins** (also known as fraternal twins) result when two eggs are released from the ovary in one menstrual cycle and fertilized at the same time. Fraternal twins may be of the same or opposite sex, have different genetic traits and therefore different physical appearances, and are sustained through separate placentas and membranes.

- **Monozygotic twins,** also referred to as identical twins, result from a single fertilized egg splitting into equal halves. If both eggs become implanted within the uterus, two babies with identical genetic information will develop. Identical twins may share or have separate placentas and membranes.

At fertilization, the 23 **chromosomes** from the sperm combine with the 23 chromosomes of the egg to form the **zygote.** The zygote, or fertilized egg, contains the full complement of 46 chromosomes. This genetic information determines the unique characteristics of the individual, including eye and hair color, height, and all the other physical characteristics that are passed from one generation to the next. One pair of chromosomes determines the sex of the individual, with the usual arrangement of males having one X and one Y chromosome and females having two X chromosomes; however, chromosomal abnormalities can occur. Among the most common chromosomal abnormalities are those that involve missing or extra sex chromosomes. Abnormalities involving the X or Y chromosome can affect sexual development and may cause infertility, growth abnormalities, and other problems. (See Table 6.1.)

Cell division of the zygote usually occurs within 36 hours of fertilization and continues as the dividing cell mass is propelled by the cilia in the fallopian tubes toward the uterus. It generally takes three to five days to reach the uterus; at this stage, the cell mass is known as a **blastocyst.** The blastocyst freely floats within the uterus for one to two days before implanting itself into the lining of the uterus. **Implantation** is often the marker for the beginning of a pregnancy. The products of conception are generally referred to as the **conceptus.** For the first eight weeks of gestation, the material is known as an **embryo;** from week nine until birth, it is known as a **fetus.**

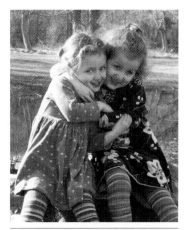

Dizygotic twins (fraternal twins) have different genetic traits and therefore different physical appearances.

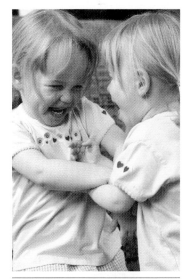

Monozygotic twins (identical twins) result from a single fertilized egg splitting into equal halves. As a result, these babies have identical genetic information.

Table 6.1   Selected Sex Chromosome Abnormalities

Chromosomal Arrangement for Girls	Description
Turner syndrome (monosomy X; XO)	▪ Short stature and may have certain physical features such as a webbed neck
	▪ Lack ovarian development and are infertile
	▪ May be born with heart or kidney abnormalities
	▪ Intelligence may be impaired
Triple X (XXX)	▪ Girls tend to be taller than expected but otherwise normal in appearance
	▪ Normal fertility
	▪ At risk for language and motor delay
Chromosomal Arrangement for Boys	**Description**
Klinefelter syndrome (trisomy XXY)	▪ Boys tend to be taller than expected and effeminate but otherwise normal in appearance
	▪ Decreased testicular size, normal sex function, but usually infertile
	▪ May have slight breast development during adolescence
	▪ At risk for learning disabilities
XYY male	▪ Boys tend to be taller than expected but otherwise normal in appearance
	▪ Sexual function, genitalia, and fertility are normal
	▪ Increased risk for motor delay, developmental delay, and learning disabilities

Confirming Pregnancy

The benefits of early diagnosis of pregnancy are immeasurable. When pregnancy is desired, good prenatal care can begin immediately, and extra efforts can be made to protect the vulnerable embryo from chemical and physical agents. When pregnancy is not desired, early detection permits early decision making; if the woman elects to have an abortion, risks of complications are reduced at this stage.

Several symptoms often occur in the first six weeks of pregnancy (see **It's Your Health**). Most women begin to have symptoms two or three weeks after conception. An overdue period is usually the first definitive sign of pregnancy, although it is important to note that there are many reasons for missed periods other than pregnancy. The bottom line is that some women do not always miss periods when they are pregnant, and missed periods do not always signal a pregnancy.

Confirming a pregnancy involves a pregnancy test and a pelvic examination. **Human chorionic gonadotropin (hCG),** a hormone specific to pregnancy, is easily

It's Your Health

Early Signs of Pregnancy

Symptoms of pregnancy that often occur in the first six weeks:

Missed period(s)

Breast swelling and tenderness

Fatigue

Queasiness or nausea, vomiting

Slightly elevated body temperature

Mood swings

Need to urinate frequently

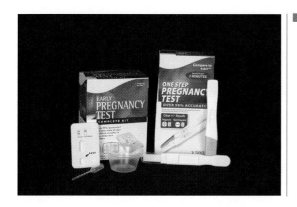

Home pregnancy tests are fairly expensive but quite simple to use.

detectable in blood and urine throughout the first three months of pregnancy. All pregnancy tests use chemical procedures to detect its presence.

Home pregnancy tests can be purchased without a prescription. Such tests are fairly expensive but quite simple to use. It is important to follow the directions carefully to ensure accurate results. If an initial test is negative and the menstrual period has still not started, it is often a good idea to repeat the test in a week or so. Tests give the most reliable results when the urine is highly concentrated; hence, women are advised to use early morning urine as the testing sample.

Although home pregnancy tests are valuable sources of information, they are merely the beginning. If the findings are positive, it is important to set up an appointment for a pelvic examination. If the findings are negative, there is a need to determine why the menstrual period is late or missed. Urine or blood tests performed in a doctor's office are virtually 100% accurate and can be used to validate the pregnancy.

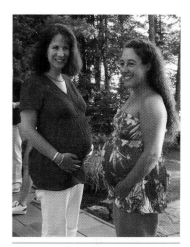

A woman's body experiences significant changes throughout pregnancy.

Hormonal Changes During Pregnancy

During pregnancy, a woman's body undergoes dramatic changes in hormone levels and physical alterations. The secretion of certain hormones, such as follicle-stimulating hormone (FSH) and luteinizing hormone (LH) produced by the anterior pituitary gland, is suppressed throughout pregnancy. Pregnancy-specific hormones, such as hCG and human placental lactogen (HPL), are responsible for influencing the course of the pregnancy. Likewise, the production of estrogen and progesterone is important for pregnancy.

Shortly after implantation, specific cells in the outer portion of the developing embryo secrete hCG. The presence of this hormone in the woman's system produces a positive pregnancy test result because, as noted earlier, hCG can be detected in the woman's blood and urine. Large amounts of hCG are produced during the first trimester to stimulate the **corpus luteum,** a structure formed on the wall of the ovary that secretes estrogen and progesterone to prepare the body for pregnancy. The corpus luteum is essential for the maintenance of early pregnancy. If it regresses, a spontaneous abortion, or miscarriage, results.

After the first three months of pregnancy, the corpus luteum is no longer essential to maintain the pregnancy and hCG levels drop off. This change occurs because the placenta begins producing large amounts of estrogen and progesterone. The fetus also plays a role in maintaining the pregnancy. The fetal adrenal glands produce a precursor hormone during the first three months of pregnancy that is converted to estrogen in the placenta. The growing fetus and placenta contribute increasing quantities of estrogen and progesterone to the maternal blood system as the pregnancy progresses; the levels of both hormones rapidly decline at birth. Estrogen helps to regulate progesterone, thereby protecting the pregnancy, and initiates one of the major processes of fetal maturation; without estrogen, fetal lungs, liver, and other organs and tissues cannot mature. Estrogen also promotes the growth of ducts in the breast to prepare for lactation. Progesterone suppresses uterine contractions during pregnancy and stimulates the alveoli of the breasts.

Another hormone unique to pregnancy, HPL, is believed to stimulate breast growth during pregnancy and to prepare the breasts for lactation. HPL also has growth-promoting properties and may be responsible for the physical changes that occur in the maternal system to accommodate the growing fetus. HPL levels rise throughout the pregnancy; as birth approaches, the levels decline.

Physical and Emotional Symptoms

A woman's body experiences significant changes throughout pregnancy, with each trimester bringing new physical and emotional symptoms. Figure 6.1 shows many of the physical changes that occur during pregnancy. The first trimester is characterized by enlarged and tender breasts and, for many women, nausea and vomiting (commonly referred to as morning sickness). Women also may experience extreme fatigue, decreased interest in sex, moodiness and irritability, and skin changes such as darkening of the nipple and areola.

During the second trimester, morning sickness usually subsides, but is replaced for many women with other gastrointestinal problems such as heartburn, gas, and constipation. The second trimester also is the period in which women gain most of their weight, usually between 12 and 14 pounds. The growing fetus can lead to breathing problems, due to pressure of the uterus and fetus on the bottom of the rib cage, and backache, caused by changes in posture to accommodate the growing fetus. Some women experience muscle and leg cramps, numbness and tingling of the hands, swollen or bleeding gums, and **Braxton-Hicks contractions** (false labor). Swelling of the feet, ankles, and hands is common and is caused by the increased weight of the uterus slowing down blood and fluid circulation. Many women have significant changes in their skin's appearance during the second trimester. Striae gravidarum (known as stretch marks) begin to appear on the abdomen, breasts, and thighs; for some women, varicose veins appear in the legs. Other skin changes may include chloasma (brown patches on the face or neck) and linea nigra (a dark line from the belly to the pubic area) due to increases in melanocyte-stimulating hor-

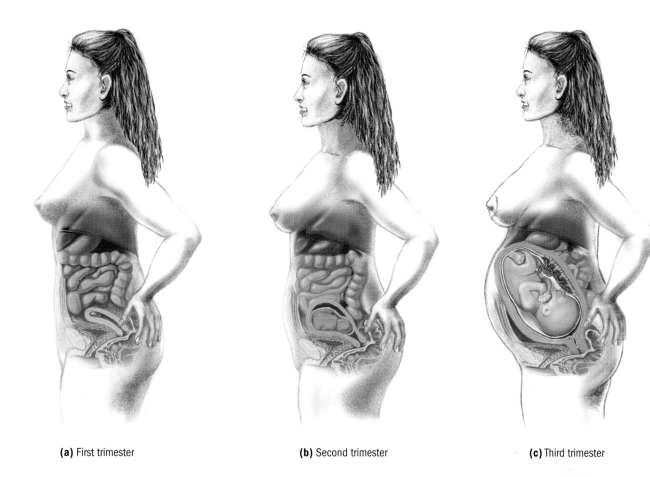

(a) First trimester   **(b)** Second trimester   **(c)** Third trimester

Figure 6.1

Changes in a woman's body during pregnancy. Through the three trimesters, the shape of the pregnant woman's body changes dramatically.

mone. Changes in estrogen levels may cause redness of palms and red spots on the upper body. The second trimester also may be a time of renewed interest in sex.

In the third trimester, many of these symptoms—for example, heartburn and constipation, leg cramps, backache, breathlessness, and Braxton-Hicks contractions—continue. Women often experience an increase in leukorrhea (a whitish vaginal discharge) and colostrum (pre-milk) leaking from the breasts. Hemorrhoids, pelvic and buttock discomfort, and an itchy abdomen also are common complaints. A woman's interest in sex may decrease.

Fetal Development

The process of development for the fertilized egg is both fascinating and complex. When the cluster of cells reaches the uterus, it is smaller than the head of a pin. Once the cells become embedded into the uterine lining, they are collectively known as an embryo. The embryo soon takes on an elongated shape that is rounded at one end. A sac known as the **amnion** or fetal sac envelops the embryo. As water and other small molecules cross the amniotic membrane, the embryo floats freely. The

amniotic fluid provides protection from shocks and bumps and helps maintain a homeostatic, or constant, environment for the developing embryo. A primitive placenta soon forms. The **placenta** is an organ that supplies the growing fetus with oxygen and nutrients from the maternal bloodstream and serves as a conduit for the return of waste products back to the mother for disposal.

Major changes occur with the developing embryo as it evolves into a fetus (Figure 6.2).

First Month.   The embryo grows to about one-tenth to one-fourth inch in length and one-seventh ounce in weight. Foundations are formed for the nervous system, genito-urinary system, circulatory system, digestive system, skin, bones, and lungs. Arm and leg buds begin to form. Rudiments of the eyes, ears, and nose appear. The head is disproportionately large because of early brain development.

Second Month.   The embryo's length is about 1.2 inches, and it weighs about one-sixth ounce. Fingers and toes are distinct structures. The circulatory system is closed. After eight weeks, the embryo is termed a fetus.

Third Month.   The length of the fetus is about two to three inches, and the weight is nearly half an ounce. The sex of the fetus is defined. The fetal kidneys excrete urine, and the heart beats. The nose and palate take shape, and the ears and earlobes are developed.

Figure 6.2

Fetal development. Top left, human embryo between four and five weeks of development. Top right, human fetus about 11 to 12 weeks of development. Bottom left, human fetus about five months (20 weeks) of development. Bottom right, human fetus nearly full term—eight to nine months.

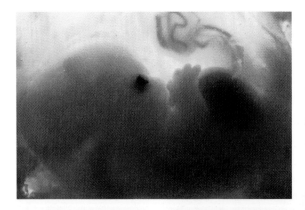
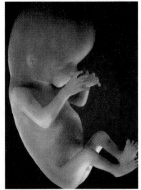
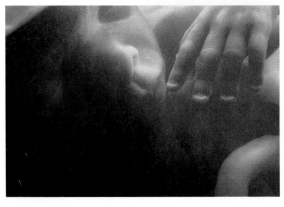
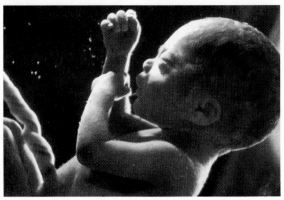

Fourth Month. The fetal length is four to five inches, and the weight is two to four ounces. Fetal movements can be discerned by the mother. Heart sounds can be monitored with external instruments.

Fifth Month. The fetal length is 6.5 to 10 inches, and the weight is 0.75 to 1.4 pounds. The skin is loose and wrinkled. Eyebrows and fingernails develop. Vernix, a white greasy substance, and lanugo, soft fine hair, cover the fetus's skin for protection.

Sixth Month. The length is 10 to 11.5 inches, and the weight is 2.1 pounds. The skin is red. Eyelids remain sealed. The fetus becomes active by kicking, punching, and turning over. The fetus also coughs, hiccups, and responds to sudden noise. If born, the infant will cry and breathe and can survive with intensive neonatal care.

Seventh Month. The fetal length is 14 to 15 inches, and the weight is 2.5 to 3 pounds. The fetus is generally able to survive if born at this time. Eyelids are open. Fingerprints are set.

Eighth Month. The fetal length is 15 to 17 inches, and weight is 4 to 5.5 pounds. The face and body have a loose and wrinkled appearance. Bones harden. Most babies begin to settle in position for birth.

Ninth Month. The fetus gains about an ounce per day. The overall length is 16 to 22 inches, and the weight is six to nine pounds. The skin is filled out and smooth. The skull bones have hardened, and the baby is ready for survival outside the womb. The lanugo hair and most of the vernix have disappeared.

Prenatal Care

A pregnant woman needs to take good care of herself to ensure proper development of her unborn child. Good prenatal care encompasses a spectrum of topics from proper nutrition to regular prenatal health care.

Nutrition

Good nutrition is an integral part of both preconceptional and prenatal care. Throughout pregnancy, a well-balanced diet is critical. Pregnancy increases a woman's need for nutrients and calories, making a balanced diet essential for women of childbearing age (Table 6.2). Sensible eating during pregnancy includes the basic concepts discussed in Chapter 9. Pregnant women should consume approximately an additional 100 calories per day in the first trimester and an additional 300 calories per day during the second and third trimesters. It is important not to diet during pregnancy but rather to eat sensibly. Pregnant women do not need to eat twice as much food or calories, but rather consume the essential nutrients required for healthy development of the fetus.

Although it is recommended that a woman try to meet her vitamin and mineral requirements by eating a balanced diet, many healthcare providers recommend

Table 6.2 Dietary Reference Intakes (DRIs): Recommended Daily Intakes for Pregnant Women*

Vitamins		Mineral/Elements	
A	770 μg	Calcium	1,000 mg
C	85 mg	Chromium	30 μg
D	5 μg	Copper	1,000 μg
E	15 mg	Fluoride	3 mg
K	90 μg	Iodine	220 μg
B₁ (thiamine)	1.4 mg	Iron	27 mg
B₂ (riboflavin)	1.4 mg	Magnesium	350–360 mg
B₃ (niacin)	18 mg	Manganese	2 mg
B₆ (pyridoxine)	1.9 mg	Molybdenum	50 μg
Folate	600 μg	Phosphorus	700 mg
B₁₂ (cobalamin)	2.6 μg	Selenium	60 μg
Pantothenic acid	6 mg	Zinc	11 mg
Biotin	30 μg	Potassium	4.7 g
Choline†	450 mg	Sodium	1.5 g
		Chloride	2.3 g

*These numbers may not be applicable to women age 18 and younger who are pregnant.

†Although adequate intake amounts have been set for choline, there are few data to assess whether a dietary supply of choline is needed at all stages of the life cycle.

Sources: *Dietary Reference Intakes for Calcium, Phosphorous, Magnesium, Vitamin D, and Fluoride* (1997); *Dietary Reference Intakes for Thiamin, Riboflavin, Niacin, Vitamin B₆, Folate, Vitamin B₁₂, Pantothenic Acid, Biotin, and Choline* (1998); *Dietary Reference Intakes for Vitamin C, Vitamin E, Selenium, and Carotenoids* (2000); *Dietary Reference Intakes for Vitamin A, Vitamin K, Arsenic, Boron, Chromium, Copper, Iodine, Iron, Manganese, Molybdenum, Nickel, Silicon, Vanadium, and Zinc* (2001); and *Dietary Reference Intakes for Water, Potassium, Sodium, Chloride, and Sulfate* (2004). Copyright 2004 by the National Academy of Sciences. Reprinted with permission.

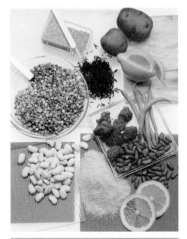

■ Folic acid appears to be a protective factor against neural tube defects, which develop in the first month of pregnancy. It is important for a woman to begin increasing her folic acid intake before she becomes pregnant.

prenatal supplements to ensure adequate intake. **Folate** is a B vitamin that is essential for the healthy development of the fetus. **Folic acid,** the synthetic form of the B vitamin folate found in green leafy vegetables, nuts, beans, citrus fruits, and some fortified cereals, appears to be a protective factor against **neural tube defects** such as spina bifida. Neural tube defects develop in the first month of pregnancy, so it is important for a woman to begin increasing her intake of folic acid or taking supplements before she becomes pregnant. As a result of folic acid's role in preventing neural tube defects, the FDA has required enriched grain products, such as breads, pasta, and bagels, to be fortified with folic acid. Childbearing women should include 400–600 micrograms (0.4–0.6 milligram) of folic acid in their daily diet before and during pregnancy. Since the fortification of cereal grains has become mandatory in the United States, the incidence of neural tube disorders has decreased by 20% to 30%; however, this decrease is lower than was expected. The Centers for Disease Control and Prevention speculates that women at highest risk do not consume as much folic acid–fortified food, do not have easy access to other sources of folic acid, or do not absorb as much folic acid as do women at lower risk.[7]

Calcium and iron are important minerals for all women, including pregnant women. Calcium is essential to the formation of bone and teeth in the fetus, and it prevents the pregnant woman from losing her own bone density while providing for the growing fetus. Iron helps carry oxygen in the blood and reduces the risk of pregnancy-induced hypertension. Women often require iron supplements, because most female iron stores are not adequate to supply both mother and unborn child given the large demand for iron throughout the pregnancy. Iron supplements should be taken with vitamin C to facilitate their absorption.

Women should drink plenty of fluids throughout pregnancy. A woman's blood volume and blood fluids increase significantly during pregnancy, and drinking enough fluids will help to prevent dehydration and constipation. Pregnant women should also avoid certain foods during pregnancy, so as to prevent certain infections that may harm the fetus (see **It's Your Health**).

It's Your Health

Foods to Avoid During Pregnancy

Sushi and other raw fish, especially shellfish (oysters, clams).

Hot dogs or luncheon meats (such as ham, turkey, salami, and bologna) unless they are reheated until steaming hot.

Unpasteurized milk, unpasteurized fruit and vegetable juices, or foods made from unpasteurized milk, including soft cheese (feta, brie, Camembert, Roquefort, queso blanco, queso fresco). Soft cheeses may be eaten if they are made with pasteurized milk.

Refrigerated pates, meat spreads, or smoked seafood. Canned versions of these products are safe to eat.

Raw vegetable sprouts (alfalfa, clover, and radish), which can carry *Salmonella* or *E. coli*.

Raw or undercooked meat, poultry, and eggs, as well as products made with raw or partially cooked eggs (such as eggnog, hollandaise sauce, and some Caesar salad dressings).

Herbal supplements and teas.

Swordfish, shark, king mackerel, and tilefish, which are high in levels of mercury.

- According to the FDA/EPA, women who are pregnant can eat up to 12 ounces (two average-sized fish meals) per week of fish or shellfish that are lower in mercury, such as shrimp, salmon, catfish, and canned light tuna. White (albacore) tuna contains more mercury than canned light tuna, so women should limit their consumption of canned white tuna and tuna steaks to no more than 6 ounces per week.

- Women should check for local advisories about any fish caught in waters by family and friends. If no advice is available, women should limit their consumption to less than 6 ounces per week of this type of fish and not eat any other fish during the week.

Weight gain is another important prenatal nutrition issue. As recently as a generation ago, obstetricians were advising pregnant women not to gain more than 20 pounds during their pregnancies so they would have small, lightweight, easy-to-deliver babies. Today's medical experts advise otherwise. A pregnant woman of average weight should expect to gain 25 to 35 pounds. It is recommended that underweight women gain 28 to 40 pounds and overweight women gain only 15 to 18 pounds.[8] Women who are expecting more than one baby, such as twins or triplets, generally will need to gain more weight, depending on the number of babies. Failure to gain adequate weight increases the risk of problems for the baby. Low infant birthweight is associated with higher infant morbidity, including physical and mental retardation and mortality.

Steady weight gain is important. Erratic weight gains may be symptomatic of an underlying problem such as **toxemia** (also known as **preeclampsia**), in which fluid is retained and toxic substances end up in the blood. Most of a woman's weight gain should occur at the end of the second trimester and the beginning of the third trimester. Women often average a weight gain of four to six pounds in the first trimester and one pound per week in the second and third trimesters.

Exercise

Proper exercise during pregnancy can have many benefits. For a woman who enjoyed regular workouts before becoming pregnant, it can be important psychologically to continue with a regular exercise program. Studies show that women who exercised in the three months before pregnancy felt better during the first trimester than did those who did not exercise; similarly, women who exercised in the first and second trimesters felt better in the third trimester than those who did not exercise. Well-conditioned women often have shorter labor, less need for obstetric intervention during pregnancy and childbirth, and speedier recovery after childbirth. Further studies are needed to determine the effect of exercise or maternal weight gain and infant birthweight.[9]

The exercise program of a pregnant woman must be geared to her current level of fitness, medical history, past pregnancies, stage of fetal development, and maternal complicating factors. Generally, women are advised not to take up a new exercise program during pregnancy. It is better to stay with usual routines. Pregnancy places extra demand on the lungs and heart. In particular, oxygen consumption and heart rate increase during pregnancy. As pregnancy advances, breathing becomes more difficult because of the displacement of the enlarging uterus downward with each inhalation. Walking, swimming, and low-impact aerobics are particularly good exercise choices for pregnant women. Classes or exercise videos made specifically for pregnant women are also good options.

Activities that involve bouncing, jarring, or twisting and any activity that places the abdomen in jeopardy should be avoided during pregnancy. Examples of activities that should be avoided include horseback riding, scuba diving, and downhill skiing. Contact sports are too risky, as is any activity that requires rapid stops and starts or an extreme range of motion. The center of gravity for the body changes dur-

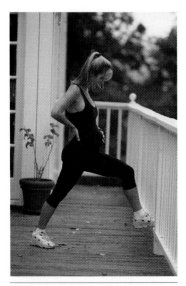

■ Proper exercise during pregnancy can have many benefits. Walking, swimming, and low-impact aerobics are particularly good choices for pregnant women.

ing pregnancy, increasing the risk of loss of balance. A specific exercise position to be avoided during pregnancy is lying on the back, particularly after the fourth month. This position can block the blood supply to the uterus and depress fetal heart rate. A resting position on the side does not compromise fetal blood supply.

The practice of exercising during pregnancy remains controversial, and many questions regarding its safety and benefits remain unanswered. Although women with medical or obstetric complications should avoid rigorous physical activity, healthy women should continue exercising under their healthcare provider's supervision. No firm recommendations have been established and, therefore, women should be advised on an individual basis. Because both pregnancy and exercise require an increase in caloric intake, a woman and her healthcare provider should monitor her weight gain closely throughout the pregnancy.

Another form of exercise, known as pelvic muscle or Kegel exercises, is important during pregnancy. Increasing the strength of the pelvic muscles decreases urine loss during late pregnancy and may speed up the rehabilitation of the pelvic floor after vaginal delivery.

Avoiding Toxic Substances

Maternal exposure to many substances during pregnancy has been shown to have detrimental effects on the developing fetus. Many of these topics are discussed in detail elsewhere in this book. Note, however, that cigarettes, alcohol, and drugs have specific detrimental effects on the fetus.

Cigarette smoking is harmful to both the mother and her developing baby. Despite this fact, a self-reported 12.2% of women in the United States smoked cigarettes during their pregnancy. Overall, maternal smoking declined nearly one-third in the 1990s for all racial and ethnic groups. In 2000, as in previous years, smoking rates in pregnant women were highest among older teenagers (18–19 years), followed by women age 20–24 years. A factor that appears to have a significant relationship with smoking during pregnancy is the education level of the mother: Studies have found that women who had less than 12 years of education were much more likely to smoke than women who had more than a high school education.[10] (See Figure 6.3.)

Maternal smoking has been clearly identified as an important determinant of low birthweight and perinatal death in the United States. Low birthweight (5.5 pounds or less) has been associated with many physical and mental problems in infants. Other complications from maternal smoking that have been reported include the following:

- Infertility
- Spontaneous abortions (miscarriages)
- Ectopic pregnancies
- Placental irregularities
- Intrauterine growth retardation

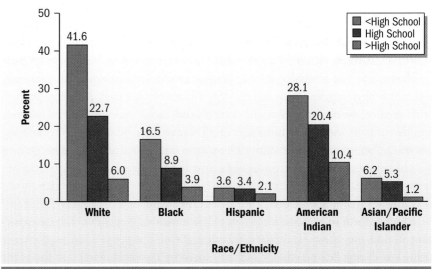

Figure 6.3

Pregnant women who smoke, by education and race/ethnicity,* United States, 2001.

*The white, black, American Indian, and Asian/Pacific Islander categories exclude Hispanics. Percentages are based on only those births for which the mother's smoking status was reported. Data are excluded for California, which did not report the mother's smoking status on birth certificates.

Source: National Center for Health Statistics, CDC. (2001).

- Sudden infant death syndrome (SIDS)
- Other causes of infant mortality
- Long-term effects on the physical, emotional, and intellectual development of the child

Alcohol also is detrimental for both the mother and her developing baby. Alcohol consumption during pregnancy is known to cause alcohol-related defects among infants and **fetal alcohol syndrome (FAS),** which is characterized by growth retardation, facial malformations, and central nervous system dysfunctions, including mental retardation. Alcohol appears to act in concert with several other factors in promoting the development of FAS in infants:

- Differences in the degree of prenatal exposure to alcohol
- Maternal drinking patterns
- Possible genetic susceptibility to FAS
- Differences in maternal metabolism of alcohol
- Time of gestation during heavy alcohol consumption
- Interactions of alcohol use with other drugs and medications
- Maternal nutritional status

The fetus is especially vulnerable during the first trimester of pregnancy, when development of the central nervous system occurs. During this vulnerable period, alcohol-associated effects on the infant may be more closely related to peak blood ethanol levels in the mother than to overall consumption throughout the pregnancy. Because no specific level of alcohol has been identified as causing FAS, women are advised to abstain completely from alcohol consumption throughout pregnancy. Studies have shown that in 2002, 10% of all pregnant women drank alcohol, and approximately 2% of pregnant women were binge or frequent drinkers (five or more drinks per occasion or seven or more drinks per week).[11]

Consumption of other drugs also can adversely affect a developing fetus. No medications or over-the-counter preparations should be taken during pregnancy without first consulting with a clinician. Illicit drug use—most notably the use of cocaine—is associated with fetal distress and impaired fetal growth. The consequences of drug use during pregnancy include severe damage to the baby's brain and nervous system as well as other birth defects. Compared with mothers who did not smoke marijuana, smokers had smaller, sicker babies and a higher risk of stillbirths. Also, babies may be prone to excessive crying and trembling. Drug use may lead to neurochemical birth defects by disrupting normal development of the brain, and, in turn, cause long-term effects on intelligence, mental development, and learning.

In particular, cocaine use increases the risk of premature birth, stillbirths, and malformations. Affected babies are often of lower birthweight, have smaller head circumferences, and are shorter in length. Cocaine use during pregnancy also may cause feeding difficulties, sleep disturbances, unresponsiveness, and inability to concentrate and control moods.

Pregnant women who use heroin are at risk of miscarriage, premature delivery, stillbirth, and poor fetal growth. Babies often suffer from withdrawal symptoms after birth and face an increased risk of sudden infant death syndrome (SIDS). Women who are pregnant and are using heroin should work with a physician to quit using; abruptly stopping the drug can cause miscarriage.[12]

Many over-the-counter prescription medications can prove dangerous during pregnancy as well. The antibiotic streptomycin can cause deafness, and the antibiotic tetracycline can lead to bone abnormalities and discolored teeth. Even aspirin and acetaminophen may affect a developing fetus. Clearly, it is important for pregnant women to consult their physicians before taking any type of medication.

Environmental Risks

Although not all environmental hazards can be avoided, a pregnant woman should take some precautions to protect herself and her baby. Although data are scarce, it is believed that the rapidly developing fetus is especially vulnerable to pollutants, toxic wastes, heavy metals, pesticides, gasses, and other hazardous compounds. For example, the element lead can cross the placenta and has been associated with intrauterine death, prematurity, and low birthweight.[13] Air pollution,

■ Performed at various times during pregnancy, ultrasound uses sound waves to show a picture of the baby. Ultrasound can check the age, growth, and size of a baby; identify multiple pregnancies; and diagnose complications or birth defects.

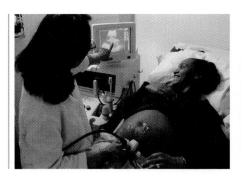
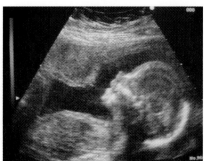

such as secondhand smoke, can be detrimental to both a woman's health and the developing fetus.

In addition, high levels of radiation of the type used for cancer therapy have been associated with birth defects. Diagnostic X rays should be avoided if possible throughout the pregnancy or if there is the possibility of pregnancy. X-ray exposure is associated with respiratory diseases and blood disorders in the fetus, as well as miscarriage.

Another environmental risk to be considered during pregnancy is heat exposure. Women who use hot tubs and saunas or who have high fevers early in pregnancy have been found to be at greater risk of having children with neural tube defects such as spina bifida. Although more research is needed on this subject, it appears that the greatest risk arises early in the pregnancy when the fetal central nervous system is developing.

Prenatal Testing

Prospective parents often worry about whether their unborn baby is normal and healthy. Blood and urine tests are used routinely for checking pregnant women for sexually transmitted diseases, antibodies for rubella and chickenpox, anemia, urinary tract infections, and signs of diabetes. The American College of Obstetrcians and Gynecologists (ACOG) also recommends that a screening test for cystic fibrosis be offered to all couples who are planning a pregnancy or are pregnant. Sophisticated testing has evolved so that some questions can be answered about specific diseases and birth defects. These procedures include ultrasound, alpha-fetoprotein screening, chorionic villus sampling (CVS), and amniocentesis (Figure 6.4).

Ultrasound is a noninvasive procedure that uses high-frequency sound waves to project an image or sonogram of the fetus. This procedure is valuable for ascertaining fetal age, determining the fetal size or location, and detecting certain birth defects. Although ultrasound may be performed at any time in the pregnancy, first-trimester procedures may not be effective in detecting fetal abnormalities. Ultrasound is most accurate between the sixth and twentieth weeks of pregnancy.

Maternal serum alpha-fetoprotein screening (MSAFP) is a blood test that measures alpha-fetoprotein (AFP), a substance produced by the fetal kidneys be-

Prenatal Testing

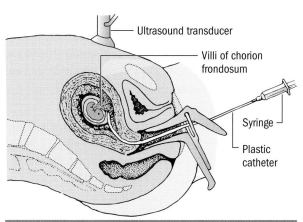

Figure 6.4A

In chorionic villus sampling, fetal cells from the chorionic villi (fingerlike projections on the developing placenta) are suctioned out through the cervix.

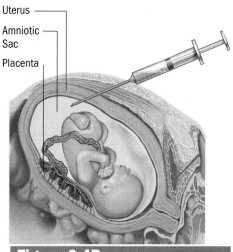

Figure 6.4B

Amniocentesis is a test for fetal abnormalities that involves withdrawing amniotic fluid and inspecting the cells contained within it.

tween the thirteenth and twentieth weeks of pregnancy. A small amount of AFP crosses the placenta into the mother's blood in a healthy pregnancy, so levels of AFP are measured in the maternal blood. High levels may indicate a neural tube defect, and abnormally low levels may indicate Down syndrome.

A triple test is a type of maternal blood test that includes the MSAFP plus tests for hCG and estriol. Low levels of AFP and estriol, combined with elevated levels of hCG, can indicate Down syndrome. Triple screen testing of maternal blood has aided in prenatal diagnosis of 95% of cases of anencephaly, 80% of cases of serious spina bifida, and 60% of cases of Down syndrome.

Chorionic villus sampling (CVS), another prenatal screening procedure, can be done as early as six weeks after conception. It is generally performed in the tenth to twelfth weeks of pregnancy and involves suctioning a small sample of the chorionic villi, the tissue surrounding the fetus, for laboratory analysis. The villi are retrieved through a catheter placed into the vagina through the cervix. CVS has been associated with several concerns. The chromosome results may be inconclusive and require a follow-up amniocentesis procedure. Although the risk appears low, concern exists regarding the association of the procedure with infant limb abnormalities, uterine infection, and fetal loss.[14] The advantage of the procedure is that it is performed during the first trimester, permitting a greater range of decision-making options for the pregnancy.

Amniocentesis is a procedure performed between the fifteenth and eighteenth weeks of pregnancy. It involves the removal of a small amount of amniotic fluid surrounding the fetus. A long, thin needle is inserted through the abdomen into the amniotic sac to remove this fluid. The fluid contains cells shed by the fetus, which are grown in tissue culture and then checked for any chromosomal, biochemical, or genetic defects, such as Down syndrome. A slight risk of fetal loss is associated with the procedure.

It is difficult to calculate risks associated with these procedures. Risks for ultrasound and AFP are considered to be very low. Both CVS and amniocentesis are associated with a 1% to 3% chance of miscarriage.[14,15] For this reason, these tests are generally recommended only if the mother is older than age 35 or if the couple has a personal or family history of genetic disorders.

Women also should be tested for **Rh incompatibility** through a simple blood test. Most people produce Rh factor, a protein located on the surface of a red blood cell. A person who does not produce Rh factor has Rh-negative blood. Rh incompatibility occurs when an Rh-negative mother and an Rh-positive father conceive a baby who inherits the father's Rh-positive blood type. This situation may present problems during pregnancy and in labor and delivery if the fetal Rh-positive blood cells enter the mother's bloodstream. The mother forms antibodies against the fetal blood cells in a process called maternal sensitization. This situation often occurs in a first pregnancy with an Rh-positive fetus, but because of the small amount of antibodies produced, it does not cause problems with the fetus. Future pregnancies, however, are at greater risk of antibodies crossing the placenta and causing Rh disease in the fetus. Rh-negative mothers should receive an injection of Rh immune globulin after delivery, during pregnancy, after a miscarriage, and after certain procedures such as amniocentesis. Without treatment, the most severely affected fetuses will be stillborn. In the newborn, Rh disease can result in jaundice, anemia, brain damage, heart failure, and death. Rh disease does not affect the mother's health.

Complications of Pregnancy

Several complications can arise during pregnancy. Perinatology is the medical specialty concerned with the diagnosis and treatment of pregnant women with high-risk conditions and their unborn babies.

Miscarriage

I had some rather severe abdominal pain and some bleeding. I knew my period was late, but I was shocked to learn from my doctor that I had had a miscarriage. I didn't even know that I was pregnant.

24-year-old woman

A **miscarriage,** or spontaneous abortion, is defined as a pregnancy that ends before the twentieth week of gestation. Of the more than 6 million pregnancies in the United States per year, 16% end in a miscarriage or stillbirth.[16] A miscarriage can occur early in the pregnancy, and many women who miscarry are not even aware of their pregnancy.

A miscarriage may be characterized by bleeding and cramping. Generally, when a woman experiences bleeding or cramping early in the pregnancy, bed rest is recommended. In some cases, these symptoms stop, and the pregnancy proceeds normally. In other cases, the bleeding becomes intense, the cervix dilates, and the embryo is released from the body. If the miscarriage is complete, the bleeding stops and the uterus returns to its normal shape and size. If the miscarriage is incomplete, any remaining fragments must be removed in a procedure known as a dilation and curettage (D&C). The risk for miscarriage decreases after the first trimester of pregnancy.

The causes of miscarriage vary and are not always definable. This uncertainty is a source of frustration for many couples who feel the need to understand why the miscarriage happened. Grief associated with miscarriage is often underestimated, so many affected women find themselves with inadequate support from their partners, friends, family, and healthcare providers. Most women experience grief immediately following their loss, as well as feelings of guilt, self-blame, and abandonment. The intensity of a woman's emotional distress may be related to certain other factors, such as the desirability of the pregnancy, late gestational age of the fetus, lack of social support, a lengthy period trying to get pregnant, and use of infertility treatments. Women also may feel that they have disappointed their partners or families.[17]

Ectopic Pregnancy

Ectopic pregnancy, in which a fertilized egg becomes implanted and begins to grow outside the uterine cavity, is a hazard for women in the early months of a pregnancy. This problem occurs in one in every 40–100 pregnancies and can be a life-threatening condition. Complications of ectopic pregnancies have emerged as one of the leading causes of maternal death during the first trimester, although this death rate has decreased in the last 30 years to less than 0.1% in the United States.[18]

Most ectopic pregnancies occur inside a fallopian tube. As the tubal pregnancy advances, the tube stretches and can tear or rupture. Symptoms of ectopic pregnancy usually begin at about the seventh or eighth week of gestation. The most common complaints are abdominal pain and tenderness, and an overdue menstrual period. The abdominal pain can be quite subtle initially and progress in severity if tearing of the fallopian tube causes internal bleeding. Tubal rupture is a serious condition that is a leading cause of pregnancy-related death. Abnormal vaginal bleeding or spotting also occurs in a majority of cases of ectopic pregnancy. In some cases, an ectopic pregnancy may degenerate on its own and require no intervention. In most cases, however, surgery is indicated to remove the fertilized egg.

Pelvic inflammatory disease is the major risk factor for ectopic pregnancy. Other risk factors, such as past use of an intrauterine device, infection of the lower genital tract, tubal infertility, pelvic surgery, and postabortion infection, are probably associated with ectopic pregnancy through their relationship to pelvic infection. Protective factors for ectopic pregnancy include the use of barrier methods of contraception and oral contraceptives. Ectopic pregnancies occur more often in women of color and women age 35 to 44 years.[18]

Premature Labor

Pregnancy usually lasts from 38 to 42 weeks. Labor that starts before week 37 of a pregnancy is called **premature labor.** Babies born prematurely may have problems with breathing, eating, and temperature control and are more likely to die in the first month of life.

Approximately 12% of babies in the United States are born preterm, an increase of 3% over the last 20 years.[19] Women are at higher risk of preterm birth if they have had a previous preterm birth, are pregnant with twins or more, have certain uterine or cervical abnormalities, or have certain medical conditions. In addition, women who seek late prenatal care or no care at all, as well as women who may smoke, drink alcohol, use drugs, or experience stress, are at greater risk. The March of Dimes Prematurity Campaign, launched in 2003, is working to increase awareness about prematurity, thereby reducing the rate of premature births. Women can decrease their risk of premature birth by recognizing the warning signs of preterm labor (see **It's Your Health**).

Genetic Disorders and Congenital Abnormalities

Genetic disorders are responsible for a significant number of miscarriages. In fact, an estimated 3% of all newborns have some sort of genetic abnormality, which vary widely in terms of their seriousness. Certain genetic disorders are more prevalent among specific populations—for example, the most common genetic disorder among American whites is **cystic fibrosis**, an abnormality of the respiratory system and the sweat and mucous glands. Babies also may be born with abnormalities that are caused by infection, chemical imbalance, or environmental hazards. These problems may range from defects of internal systems to abnormalities in the skeletal development.

Examples of Birth Disorders

Down syndrome is caused by the presence of an extra chromosome, usually number 21 or 22. This abnormality, which occurs about once in every 900 births, is characterized by varying degrees of physical and mental retardation. A woman's risk of having a baby with Down syndrome increases as she gets older. Amniocentesis and alpha-fetoprotein screening may indicate the presence of Down syndrome.

Sickle cell anemia is a blood disorder that primarily affects people of African descent; it is also common in people from South America, Central America, Saudi Arabia, India, and the Mediterranean countries. In this condition, hemoglobin, the oxygen-carrying protein of red blood cells, is abnormal and causes red blood cells to assume a crescent or sickle shape. The sickled cells are unable to provide adequate oxygen to vital organs of the body. As a result, the affected person becomes tired and lethargic and often experiences pain and a loss of appetite. Blood transfusions provide some relief but do not cure the condition. Worldwide, some 120,000 to 250,000 infants are born with sickle cell disease each year.[20] In the United States, about 2 million people carry the sickle cell trait. One in every 600 African Americans, and one in every 1,000–1,400 Hispanic Americans are born with the disease.[21]

Phenylketonuria (PKU) is a genetic disorder in which a crucial liver enzyme needed by the body for the metabolism of the amino acid phenylalanine is absent, resulting in severe mental retardation if left untreated. All states routinely screen newborns for PKU; the test should be performed at least 24 hours after birth but before the baby is seven days old. Treatment for the condition is a long-term therapeutic diet, which reduces the effect of the disorder.

Tay-Sachs disease is a genetic disorder that results in death by age five or six years. It presents almost exclusively among Jews of Eastern European ancestry. Tay-Sachs victims appear normal at birth but experience gradual physical and mental deterioration. Carriers of the condition may be identified by a blood test.

Spina bifida involves a neural tube defect in which the spine does not close and exposed nerves are thereby damaged. Many babies with spina bifida experience a variety of symptoms, ranging from muscle weakness to paralysis to fecal and urinary incontinence. Maternal intake of folic acid greatly reduces the risk of spina bifida. The condition may be identified through alpha-fetoprotein screening, although the test is not always accurate.

Infections

Any infection in the mother can potentially cause harm to an unborn fetus. Sexually transmitted diseases, including HIV infection (see Chapter 7), are particularly dangerous during a pregnancy.

- Gonorrhea, chlamydia, and syphilis can cause preterm delivery and miscarriages.

- Bacterial vaginosis (BV), an infection of the vaginal area that is usually benign and asymptomatic, can lead to preterm delivery as well as low-birthweight babies. In addition, the presence of BV has been associated with an increased risk of HIV infection, which can further complicate a pregnancy.

- Perinatal transmission of AIDS is a special concern for women because the majority of HIV-infected women are of reproductive age. The use of anti-HIV drugs by pregnant women has reduced the rate of HIV transmission from mother to baby by more than 70%. Recent studies, however, have led to concerns regarding resistance to common HIV drugs used during pregnancy, which ultimately could result in an increase in the number of babies born with resistant HIV infection.[22]

The 2002 CDC STD Treatment Guidelines recommend that pregnant women be screened for chlamydia, gonorrhea, hepatitis B, HIV infection, and syphilis. Women should also be tested for bacterial vaginosis.[23] Pregnant women should request these tests specifically because some doctors do not routinely perform them.

The most common prenatal infection today is **cytomegalovirus (CMV),** a viral infection that causes mild flulike symptoms in adults but that can cause small birth

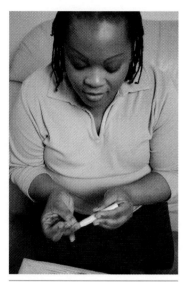

■ Women with diabetes are at an increased risk for complications with pregnancy.

size, brain damage, developmental problems, enlarged liver, hearing and vision impairment, and other malformations in newborns.[24] Babies with CMV are infected in utero and only 10% of those infected have symptoms. Pregnant women often acquire CMV from young infected children who show few or no symptoms.

The infectious disease most clearly linked to birth defects is **rubella,** also known as German measles. All women of reproductive age should be vaccinated against rubella if they have not had this formerly common childhood illness.

Group B streptococcus (GBS) is a type of bacterium that can cause illness in newborn babies and pregnant women. Although the rate of GBS infection has declined in the United States, 1,600 cases and 80 deaths from GBS still occur every year, making GBS one of the leading causes of newborn morbidity and mortality. Pregnant women with GBS do not necessarily infect their babies; however, babies who develop signs and symptoms are at risk of sepsis, pneumonia, meningitis, long-term disabilities such as hearing or vision loss, and death. Obstetricians should screen all women for GBS at 35 to 37 weeks of gestation and can prevent disease by administering antibiotics intravenously during labor. A consequence of antibiotic treatment for women with GBS has been the emergence of antibiotic-resistant strains of GBS in recent years.[25]

Other Complications

Pregnancy-induced conditions, such as gestational diabetes or hypertension, may arise in women who have shown no previous signs of high blood sugar or high blood pressure. Gestational diabetes is one of the more common conditions in older women. It can usually be controlled with dietary changes, but may require insulin in severe cases. Babies born to mothers with gestational diabetes are often large in size, and a cesarean section may be recommended. Gestational hypertension also is more common in older women. It usually develops late in the second trimester and can be controlled by diet and medication. One form of pregnancy-induced hypertension known as preeclampsia is characterized by very high blood pressure, protein in the urine, and excessive water retention. Bed rest, medication, and possible hospitalization are necessary to prevent the occurrence of **eclampsia,** seizure activity or coma unrelated to other cerebral conditions in a pregnant woman with preeclampsia.

Women also should be aware of postpartum issues, such as depression. Many women will experience postpartum "blues," mood swings, and slight depression for several days after a baby's birth. These feelings are normal and will go away in the first few weeks. Some women experience more severe symptoms, however, which will warrant treatment. Women who are more susceptible to postpartum depression include those women who suffer from depression, have experienced postpartum depression in a previous pregnancy, have severe PMS or PMDD, and/or are experiencing other stressors in their family, marriage, or life at the time of the birth. (See Chapter 12 on mental health.)

Women with disabilities and chronic conditions who want to become pregnant may have special considerations to discuss with their healthcare providers. Certain conditions that are common in pregnant women, such as vaginal and urinary tract infections, fluid retention, and decreased mobility, may create even more significant problems for women with preexisting conditions or disorders. Other difficulties may also affect women with physical disabilities that impair their mobility. As her body changes with pregnancy, a woman with impaired mobility may experience balance problems and new pressure points if she is in a wheelchair. Each disability or condition may present with different issues, just as each pregnant woman may present with different complications and issues. Throughout the pregnancy, from preconception to postpartum, women with disabilities or chronic conditions should work with a team of healthcare providers to ensure favorable pregnancy and post-pregnancy outcomes.

Childbirth

Many women have special concerns about the childbirth experience. It is important to discuss these concerns with the clinician early in the pregnancy. Self-Assessment 6.1 provides a checklist for childbirth considerations. This list can serve as a basis for further questions and decision making.

Preparation for Childbirth

Preparation for childbirth is a concept that has been popular in the United States for the last 40 years. "Preparation" usually entails attending organized classes to prepare a woman and her partner for labor and delivery. Some individuals anticipate or desire having a "natural childbirth" experience (meaning childbirth without use of medications for pain relief and with minimal mechanical monitoring), and others wish to learn more about the birthing events. Regardless of the plans for the childbirth experience, organized classes provide an opportunity to learn about local birthing options and a chance to discuss personal issues and concerns. They also provide an opportunity to gain knowledge about pregnancy and childbirth and to develop pain management skills. Strategies that are taught may include breathing techniques, such as **Lamaze,** relaxation techniques, muscle-strengthening exercises, and different positions that facilitate labor, thereby promoting an uncomplicated birth. Perhaps the greatest advantage of childbirth education is the opportunity to prepare for a more satisfying birth experience.

Labor and Delivery

Labor and delivery can be a rewarding and satisfying experience when a woman anticipates the sequence of events and is prepared for the process. Long before actual labor begins, the uterus changes so as to prepare itself to function efficiently during labor and delivery. By the end of the pregnancy, the uterus measures about 10 to 14 inches. Its capacity has increased nearly 500 times during the pregnancy, and it increases in weight from 1.5 ounces to 30 ounces. The uterine muscle fibers grow to 10 times their original thickness. The uterus is one of the strongest muscles in a woman's body, and it contracts powerfully during labor. Throughout pregnancy,

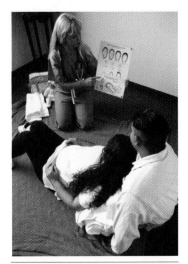

Childbirth education classes help a couple prepare for delivery by teaching relaxation and pain management techniques. The classes also provide the opportunity for the couples to discuss their concerns and excitement.

Self-Assessment 6.1

Childbirth Considerations

Birthing Issues	Very Important	Not Important	Don't Want
Hospital delivery room	_____	_____	_____
Hospital birthing room	_____	_____	_____
Birthing center	_____	_____	_____
Home	_____	_____	_____
Obstetrician	_____	_____	_____
Family practitioner	_____	_____	_____
Certified nurse-midwife	_____	_____	_____
Partner/coach			
Present during labor	_____	_____	_____
Present during delivery	_____	_____	_____
Present for all procedures	_____	_____	_____
Present during cesarean	_____	_____	_____
Present during recovery	_____	_____	_____
Early labor			
Stay home as long as possible	_____	_____	_____
Arrive early and settle in	_____	_____	_____
Wear own clothes	_____	_____	_____
Perineal shave	_____	_____	_____
Enema	_____	_____	_____
Intravenous tube	_____	_____	_____
First-stage labor			
Labor room	_____	_____	_____
Birthing room	_____	_____	_____
External fetal monitor	_____	_____	_____
Internal fetal monitor	_____	_____	_____
Second-stage labor			
Labor room	_____	_____	_____
Delivery room	_____	_____	_____
Birthing room	_____	_____	_____
Family present	_____	_____	_____
Delivery position flexibility	_____	_____	_____
Episiotomy	_____	_____	_____
After delivery			
Prolonged holding of baby	_____	_____	_____
Warm-water bath for baby	_____	_____	_____
Breastfeeding in birthing area	_____	_____	_____
Postpartum			
Private room	_____	_____	_____
Baby rooming in with mother	_____	_____	_____
Breastfeeding	_____	_____	_____
Bottle-feeding	_____	_____	_____
Length of stay in facility	_____	_____	_____
Sibling/family visitation	_____	_____	_____
Postpartum depression concerns	_____	_____	_____

Decisions on places of birth, birthing positions, pain relief, and breastfeeding can be made based on this checklist. After completing the assessment, women should discuss their issues of concern with their partner and their healthcare provider.

the uterus contracts at slightly irregular intervals. These irregular contractions, known as Braxton-Hicks contractions, differ from "real" labor contractions in that they do not gradually increase in frequency, intensity, or duration. Instead, they serve to increase the blood circulation and help the uterus to accommodate the growing baby.

Three distinctive signs indicate that labor is beginning:

- Regular, progressive uterine contractions that occur every five minutes or so and last from 45 seconds to a minute. The contractions gradually become longer, stronger, and closer together.
- Rupture of the membranes, or "bag of waters." This rupture may be a "slow leak" or a gush. The fluid is usually clear.
- The "bloody show." It involves the passage of a small amount of bloodstained mucus, which served as a plug in the cervix to protect the fetus from infection. As the cervix begins to dilate, this plug is released.

Other less distinctive signs of approaching labor include diarrhea, backache, and an increase in Braxton-Hicks contractions. The only confirmation that labor has begun is a pelvic examination that reveals a softening, thinned-out, and dilating cervix.

Many factors affect the progress of labor, including the position of the baby and the shape of the mother's pelvis. Although all experiences are different, each labor progresses through three distinct stages (Figure 6.5).

Stage I is from the onset of labor to full dilation of the cervix. Before labor begins, the wall of the uterus is thin, the cervix is long and thick, the birth canal is narrow, and the membranes may still be intact. As labor begins, the bands of longitudinal muscle fiber in the upper part of the uterus contract and thus gradually draw up, thin, and open the mouth of the cervix. The cervical canal shortens until the cervix is of the same thickness as the uterine wall. This process, in which the cervix is "taken up" into the uterus, is known as **effacement.** Once the cervix is effaced, the force of the uterine contractions begins to dilate the cervix, although effacement and dilation may occur simultaneously. Dilation refers to the size of the round opening of the cervix. It is measured in centimeters or finger widths. Full dilation is 10 centimeters or five finger widths (Figure 6.6).

Stage II of labor begins when the cervix is completely dilated and ends with the birth of the baby. The presentation of the baby—the part of the body positioned to emerge first—is usually by the top of the head, known as a vertex presentation. When the feet or buttocks present first, it is known as a **breech** presentation. The breech position occurs in about 3% of deliveries. A breech presentation usually results in a longer labor. Because a breech delivery presents greater risks to the mother and baby, a cesarean delivery is often performed.

As the baby's head appears, or crowns, an episiotomy may be performed. An episiotomy is an incision in the perineum that enlarges the vaginal opening for birth. The traditional argument for performing this procedure is that a surgical incision heals better and faster than a jagged tear. Once routine with vaginal deliveries,

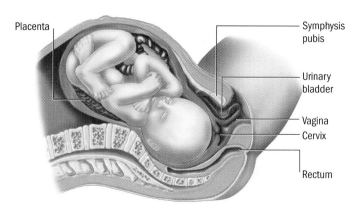

(a) Early first-stage labor

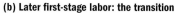

(b) Later first-stage labor: the transition

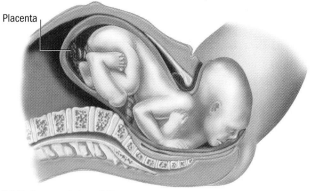

(c) Early second-stage labor

(d) Third-stage labor: delivery of afterbirth

Figure 6.5

Labor and delivery. Stage I: the cervix becomes fully dilated; stage II: the infant is born; stage III: the afterbirth is delivered.

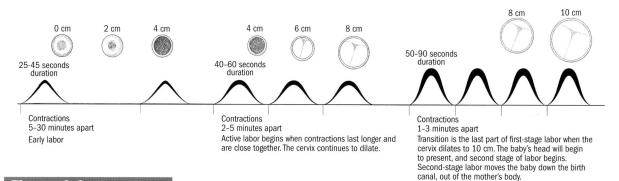

Figure 6.6

Dilation through stages of labor.

the practice of episiotomies has been seriously questioned as to its necessity and benefits for all pregnancies. A recent study showed that episiotomies were linked with more pain, more difficulty healing, and a longer wait for resuming sex after childbirth, with no obvious benefits for most women. Only women requiring a quick delivery for babies in distress should receive an episiotomy. The study noted that an estimated 1 million women had unnecessary episiotomies every year.[26]

Some mothers find that a sitting or squatting position facilitates the second stage of labor. Such positions permit gravity to help with the birth. Squatting specifically enlarges the pelvic opening. Under usual circumstances, the birth of the baby is a gradual process with head first, then shoulders, and then the body.

Stage III lasts from the completion of delivery of the baby to completion of delivery of the **afterbirth,** or placenta. In this final stage of labor, the uterus contracts firmly after the delivery of the baby. The placenta separates from the uterine wall and is expelled. If an episiotomy has been performed, it is sutured at this time.

Pain Relief in Childbirth

Different women experience different levels of pain during childbirth. The reality of childbirth is that it usually involves some physical hurt. The physical and psychological techniques promoted in childbirth preparation classes can dramatically influence the perception of pain and the confidence in dealing with labor difficulties. These pain relief measures have the inherent advantage of not producing any chemical disruption in the mother's body, which could then affect the baby or the birthing process.

A variety of pain-relieving medications also are available for childbirth. Most decisions about medications are actually personal choices, not medical decisions. For this reason, it is important for a pregnant woman to learn about possible medications before she goes into labor. Tranquilizers and analgesics are often used together for general relaxation and to take the edge off contractions. Anesthetics used during labor and delivery may be given in different forms, including epidural, spinal, and pudendal.

- **Epidural anesthesia,** the most popular choice among pregnant women, allows the mother to be awake for the birth. The anesthetic is injected through a catheter placed in a space beside the spinal cord.
- Spinal anesthesia is injected directly into the spinal canal. Like epidural anesthesia, spinal anesthesia prevents a woman from being able to move around in labor and often inhibits a woman from pushing.
- Pudendal anesthesia is injected into the area around the vagina and perineum. This method is least likely to affect the baby.

Cesarean Delivery

A **cesarean delivery** (also known as a cesarean section) is the birth of a baby through surgical incisions made in both the wall of the mother's abdomen and her uterus. Anesthesia is required for the procedure. Considerable controversy exists today over whether this type of delivery is being performed too often. The rate of cesarean sections had increased dramatically between 1970 and 1988, rising from 5.5% of all births in 1970 to a high of 24.7% in 1988. Between 1991 and 1996, however, the U.S. cesarean rate dropped by 8%, but then increased again between 1996 and 2003 to the highest percentage ever recorded in the United States.[27] Clearly, a cesarean birth is sometimes necessary for the safety of the mother or the baby—for example, when there are problems with the baby, problems with the woman's passage area, or problems with the delivery process.

One cause for cesarean section is **fetal distress,** a condition in which some aspect of labor or the baby's environment places the baby at risk. For example, the baby's oxygen supply might be cut off owing to **abruptio placentae,** in which the placenta separates prematurely from the wall of the uterus. This event threatens not only the baby, but also the mother with a risk of hemorrhage. A **prolapsed cord** is another risky situation in which the umbilical cord comes through the pelvis before the baby and can disrupt the flow of oxygen to the baby due to a compressed cord.

Problems with the birth passage also influence the decision for a cesarean delivery. **Cephalopelvic disproportion,** in which the baby is too large for the pelvis, is a common reason for choosing this type of delivery. Often a fetus indicates that

It's Your Health

Cesarean Birth in America

- There are over 1.1 million cesarean surgeries performed in the United States every year, making it the most common major surgery in the country.

- Birth via cesarean section in the United States and abroad has been rising rapidly since the mid-1990s. There is wide divergence in rates; in Italy and South Korea almost 40% of births are cesarean, while in other countries, such as the Netherlands, Sweden, and Czech Republic, the rates are less than 20%.

- The leading causes of cesareans in the United States are malpresentation of the baby (for example, feet first); apparent problems with the infant's health during labor as identified by fetal monitoring; prolonged labor; and concerns about the baby's weight.

- Vaginal births after cesareans in the United States are now largely limited to selected large hospitals. Because of this, more than 90% of mothers with prior cesareans will have a repeat cesarean.

- Demographically, the mothers most likely to experience a cesarean are black, non-Hispanic, 35 or older, overweight, or obese when they become pregnant.

- There has been a lot of attention on cesarean deliveries based on maternal request, but a 2006 national survey, entitled *Listening to Mothers* (available at http://www.childbirth connection.org), found far less than 1% of mothers having a cesarean based on their own request. General shifts in obstetrical practices—primarily a lowering of threshold for performing a cesarean—largely accounts for the rise in the cesarean rate.

Source: DeClercq, Eugene. Boston University School of Public Health. Reprinted with permission.

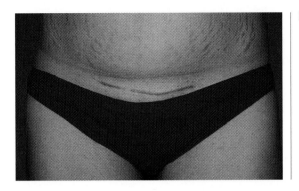

■ Many women with a prior history of cesarean birth are able to deliver their subsequent pregnancies vaginally.

the pelvis may not be a comfortable "fit" by assuming a position other than the normal head-first position for birth. A woman in labor whose baby is in a transverse lie, a crosswise position in the uterus, will need a cesarean delivery because neither the head nor the buttocks are in the pelvis. When a baby is in a breech position, the buttocks emerge before the head. The head has a larger diameter than the buttocks, and the risk is that it will not fit well through the passage because it has not had the opportunity to mold and nestle into the pelvis throughout the labor process. Multiple births are also more likely to require cesarean delivery. A relatively rare complication of the passageway is obstruction by a fibroid, a benign tumor, or even the placenta **(placenta previa)**. Usually these obstructions or other problems with fetal passage can be diagnosed before labor and delivery, which permits time to discuss various options with the healthcare provider.

Other conditions may also be an indication for cesarean delivery. For example, "failure to progress" is a term that describes cervical failure to dilate adequately despite regular uterine contractions. To avoid prolonged distress to mother and baby in this situation, a cesarean delivery may be performed. Herpes is another reason for a cesarean delivery. If a woman has active lesions in the birth canal, a cesarean delivery is indicated to avoid infecting the baby.

Vaginal Birth After Cesarean Delivery

For many years, a widely held philosophy about childbirth was "once a cesarean, always a cesarean." This philosophy may be partially responsible for the overall increase in cesarean birth rates in the United States during recent years. National data indicate a steady decline in cesarean sections through 1996, owing in part to the movement encouraging vaginal birth after cesarean delivery (VBAC). By the late 1990s, however, studies revealed that some women should not attempt VBAC for fear of uterine rupture or the need for an emergency cesarean section. Many smaller hospitals stopped offering VBAC out of medical liability concerns.[28]

The American College of Obstetricians and Gynecologists (ACOG), as well as many hospital boards, has taken a strong position on VBAC to help control the morbidity associated with major abdominal surgical procedures and to help reduce the spiraling costs of health care. A trial of labor is recommended for most women who underwent a previous cesarean section and have no unusual circumstances or conditions. ACOG has found that the mother usually experiences fewer complications with VBAC than with cesarean birth in terms of infection, bleeding, and anesthesia. Other advantages of VBAC include a shorter hospital stay and recovery period as well as significant cost savings. Women giving birth in hospitals that are not equipped for emergency cesarean sections and women with certain medical contraindications should not undergo VBAC.[28]

Breastfeeding

The practice of breastfeeding varied greatly throughout the second half of the twentieth century. As formula became popular in the 1950s and 1960s, many women who had the money to purchase formula, bottles, and nipples as well as the time to sterilize the bottles and nipples stopped breastfeeding. Reports in the 1970s on the benefits of breastfeeding resulted in a return to breastfeeding, especially for educated women and women of higher socioeconomic status. This trend continued until the 1980s, when many women again returned to formula feeding. Since 1991, the popularity of breastfeeding has increased again, with nearly 70% of mothers initiating breastfeeding.

Physiological Changes of the Breast

Hormones during pregnancy cause changes in the breasts so as to prepare them for **lactation** (milk production). The breasts enlarge as the cells that produce milk increase in number and the ducts that carry milk develop (Figure 6.7). The nipple and areola become more elastic and are protected by a natural lubricant secreted from tiny glands under the skin. After delivery, levels of estrogen and progesterone in the body rapidly decrease, triggering the production of milk. Two hormones are released in response to a baby's suckling:

- *Prolactin* stimulates lactation.
- *Oxytocin* is responsible for the transportation of milk from the producing cells to the milk ducts to the nipple.

The composition of breast milk varies depending on the stage of lactation, the stage of feeding, and the mother's diet. Early milk, or milk produced during the pregnancy and for 3 to 5 days after birth, is called **colostrum.** Colostrum is yellowish in color, thicker than milk, and rich with protective antibodies and protein. Transitional milk leads to regular mature milk after about 10 days. During feedings, low-fat, thirst-quenching milk is released first, followed by higher-fat, more nourishing milk. The milk's vitamin content is representative of the mother's vitamin intake.

Benefits of Breastfeeding

The benefits of breastfeeding are numerous, providing protective features against many acute and chronic diseases as well as advantages for general health, growth, and development (see **It's Your Health**). Breast milk is highly nutritious, providing

It's Your Health ▪▪

Benefits of Breastfeeding

Infant's Benefits

- Fewer episodes and decreased severity of diarrhea and gastrointestinal difficulties
- Decreased incidence of ear infections, urinary tract infections, and upper respiratory infections
- Fewer hospitalizations and visits to the doctor's office
- Fewer food allergies
- Possible protection against diabetes, Crohn's disease, SIDS, chronic digestive disease, and childhood cancers
- Possible benefits of cognitive development

Mother's Benefits

- Less postpartum bleeding
- Faster return to pre-pregnancy weight
- Possible decreased incidence of ovarian cancer, breast cancer, and osteoporosis

Benefits for Both

- Special bond between mother and infant

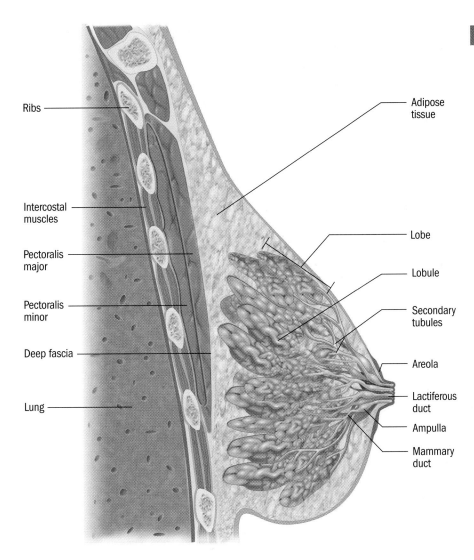

Figure 6.7

The female breast.

Ribs

Intercostal muscles

Pectoralis major

Pectoralis minor

Deep fascia

Lung

Adipose tissue

Lobe

Lobule

Secondary tubules

Areola

Lactiferous duct

Ampulla

Mammary duct

all of the nutrients that a growing baby needs. It is ideal as a baby's sole source of nutrients for the first six months of life. In addition, breast milk contains enzymes to aid in the infant's digestion as well as antibodies to protect against infection. Evidence has shown that breastfed infants have less frequency and severity of diarrhea; fewer cases of upper respiratory, ear, and even urinary infections; and fewer hospitalizations and doctor's visits. Many studies show the possibilities of breast milk protecting against type 1 diabetes mellitus (childhood-onset diabetes), Crohn's disease, SIDS, chronic digestive disease, and childhood cancers, such as lymphoma and leukemia. Breastfeeding is also believed to bestow cognitive benefits.[29]

New mothers may also reap benefits from breastfeeding. Due to the increased levels of oxytocin from breastfeeding, the uterus returns to its normal size more quickly and the woman experiences less postpartum bleeding. Breastfeeding also helps a woman to return to her pre-pregnancy weight more quickly, although she is less likely to lose her last five pounds of weight. Women who breastfeed may have a lower incidence of ovarian and premenopausal breast cancer, as well as improved bone mass leading to reduced fractures and risk of osteoporosis in the post-menopausal years.[29] Besides all of the physical health benefits, breastfeeding can create a special bond between mother and infant.

While any length of breastfeeding is better than no breastfeeding, research indicates that exclusive and prolonged breastfeeding has a greater protective effect than short-term nursing or nursing along with supplemental formula feeding. Experts recommend that mothers breastfeed their babies exclusively for six months, and that they continue to breastfeed while supplementing with solid foods until the baby's first birthday.

Complications of Breastfeeding

Breastfeeding is not always the best option for some infants. Women who are infected with HIV; have untreated active tuberculosis; are users of alcohol, tobacco, or other recreational drugs; are undergoing cancer chemotherapy or radiation treatment; or are using certain necessary medications that may not be healthy for the developing infant should not breastfeed. Infants with **galactosemia** (an inherited disease caused by a lack of enzyme for processing galactose that can lead to organ enlargement, cataracts, and mental retardation) should not be breastfed.

Women may experience difficulties with feeding, including the following problems:

- Inverted or flat nipples
- Raw or cracked nipples
- Severely swollen breasts
- Problems with the infant latching on
- Pain during latch-on

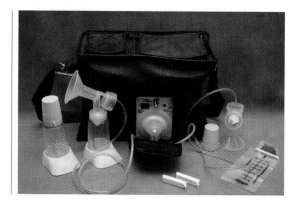

■ Breast pumps are useful to mothers who work or who have difficulty breastfeeding.

These problems often can be resolved by changing positions, massaging the breasts, or using a nipple shield to protect the breast. Other complications may require medical attention, such as **mastitis** (bacterial infection of the breast) or **thrush** (yeast infection that affects the mouth of the baby). Women should talk to their healthcare provider or a nursing specialist if they experience problems with feeding.

Diet, Drugs, and Alcohol During Breastfeeding

Women who choose to breastfeed should consume a healthy diet to ensure adequate intake of the necessary vitamins and minerals (Table 6.3). Caloric intake

Table 6.3 Dietary Reference Intakes (DRIs): Recommended Daily Intakes for Lactating Women*

Vitamins		Mineral/Elements	
A	1,300 μg	Calcium	1,000 mg
C	120 mg	Chromium	45 μg
D	5 μg	Copper	1,300 μg
E	19 mg	Fluoride	3 mg
K	90 μg	Iodine	290 μg
B_1 (thiamine)	1.4 mg	Iron	9 mg
B_2 (riboflavin)	1.6 mg	Magnesium	310–320 mg
B_3 (niacin)	17 mg	Manganese	2.6 mg
B_6 (pyridoxine)	2.0 mg	Molybdenum	50 μg
Folate	500 μg	Phosphorus	700 mg
B_{12} (cobalamin)	2.8 μg	Selenium	70 μg
Pantothenic acid	7 mg	Zinc	12 mg
Biotin	35 μg	Potassium	5.1 g
Choline[†]	550 mg	Sodium	1.5 g
		Chloride	2.3 g

*These numbers may not be applicable to women age 18 and younger who are pregnant.

[†]Although adequate intake amounts have been set for choline, there are few data to assess whether a dietary supply of choline is needed at all stages of the life cycle.

Sources: *Dietary Reference Intakes for Calcium, Phosphorous, Magnesium, Vitamin D, and Fluoride* (1997); *Dietary Reference Intakes for Thiamin, Riboflavin, Niacin, Vitamin B_6, Folate, Vitamin B_{12}, Pantothenic Acid, Biotin, and Choline* (1998); *Dietary Reference Intakes for Vitamin C, Vitamin E, Selenium, and Carotenoids* (2000); *Dietary Reference Intakes for Vitamin A, Vitamin K, Arsenic, Boron, Chromium, Copper, Iodine, Iron, Manganese, Molybdenum, Nickel, Silicon, Vanadium, and Zinc* (2001); and *Dietary Reference Intakes for Water, Potassium, Sodium, Chloride, and Sulfate* (2004). Copyright 2004 by the National Academy of Sciences. Reprinted with permission.

should be increased by 500 calories per day relative to a woman's pre-pregnancy diet. Women should maintain a sufficient amount of calcium (1,000 mg per day) to rule out any possibility of long-term effects of breastfeeding on the mother's bone density. Note that any substance taken in by the mother can be passed to the infant through the breast milk, including harmful substances such as caffeine, alcohol, and certain drugs. For this reason, breastfeeding women should consult their healthcare providers before taking any medications.

Infertility

Fecundity refers to the physical ability of a woman to have a child. Women with impaired fecundity include those who find it physically difficult or medically inadvisable to conceive or deliver a child. The term *impaired fecundity* is also used to describe women who, although having sexual intercourse on a regular basis without contraception for 36 months or more, fail to become pregnant. This definition of reduced ability to bear children differs from the medical definition of infertility, which is the inability of couples who are not surgically sterile to conceive after 12 months of regular intercourse without contraception.[30]

Causes

Fertility-related difficulties can arise at many points, including the process of ovulation in women, sperm production in men, or the maintenance of the embryo once the egg has been fertilized by the sperm.

- In 25% to 35% of couples, the fertility problem is in the male.
- In 25% to 35% of couples, the fertility problem is in the female.
- For the remaining couples, infertility is a result of both a male and a female factor or unknown causes.

Although many causes of infertility are possible, many couples cannot find a reason for their infertility. A woman may have scarring or an obstruction in her fallopian tubes, a structural problem in the uterus causing difficulties with implantation, or endometriosis. Men may have weak or immobile sperm, or the sperm may not be able to survive in the vaginal environment. The most common female infertility factor is an ovulation disorder. The most common male infertility factors include **azoospermia** (no sperm cells are produced) and **oligospermia** (few sperm cells are produced). Certain substances or environmental conditions, such as chemotherapy or radiation treatment, alcohol and drugs, anabolic steroids, or excessive heat, are harmful to sperm and can decrease sperm count or affect the viability of the sperm. An important cause of infertility in both men and women is sexually transmitted disease. In women, for example, untreated chlamydia or gonorrhea can lead to pelvic inflammatory disease (PID), an infection of the uterus and fallopian tubes that often causes infertility.

Diagnosis

To determine the cause of infertility and thus the appropriate treatment method, various tests can be performed. A simple method of determining whether ovulation is occurring, for example, is to monitor a woman's basal body temperature to see whether a slight increase in her temperature occurs midway through her menstrual cycle.

Cervical mucus tests also can be performed to test the quality of the mucus. The ferning test involves collecting mucus near the time of ovulation to see if, when smeared, it resembles the fronds of a fern. If so, the woman's estrogen levels are normal, and the mucus is creating a desirable environment for the sperm to travel.

A postcoital test may also be performed before ovulation. Mucus is collected within six hours after intercourse and is viewed under a microscope to see whether it contains multiple, active sperm.

Other tests used to diagnose infertility include the following:

- Blood tests for measuring hormone levels
- Radiograph studies such as a hysterosalpingogram, which outlines obstructions or abnormal growths in the uterus or fallopian tubes
- Laparoscopic surgery to view the uterus, fallopian tubes, and ovaries

A common test used to diagnose male infertility is semen analysis. Semen is evaluated for the number of sperm present, the volume of ejaculate, the motility of the sperm, and the size and shape of the sperm. If a man has a low sperm count, blood tests may be performed to measure various hormones and proteins. A physical examination and an ultrasound of the scrotum also may be performed to detect varicose veins that may need repair.

Even if no diagnosis is made, couples may still be able to conceive using various measures.

Treatment

A variety of treatment approaches can be employed depending on the cause of the infertility. The most basic form of treatment relies on a change in sexual activity. By using a basal body temperature chart, for example, women can monitor their temperature changes and better determine their exact time of ovulation. About 85% to 90% of infertility cases are treated with drug therapy or surgical repair of reproductive organs. Medical approaches to infertility may involve hormones to treat cervical mucus problems or difficulties in ovulation, while ultrasound is used to monitor the response of the ovaries during treatment.

- Estrogen and prednisone may be given to improve the quality of cervical mucus, thereby allowing sperm to penetrate the mucus.
- To stimulate ovulation, a medication called clomiphene citrate (trade name Clomid) is often prescribed. It stimulates the release of luteinizing hormone and causes an increase in estradiol, thereby triggering ovulation.

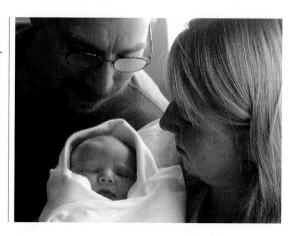

▪ Many couples who have had trouble conceiving use assisted reproductive technologies to assist them in getting pregnant.

- Gonadotropin-releasing hormone (GnRH) may be administered to improve a woman's response to ovulation stimulants.

Microsurgery is a useful technique for male and female problems that require surgical intervention. Using a laparoscope, doctors can open blockages in a woman's fallopian tubes or correct structural abnormalities of the uterus or ovary. Surgery may also be used in males to open blocked sperm ducts or to repair a **varicocele** (a mesh of varicose veins in and around the testicle), which is often associated with infertility.

Other techniques that have shown success to date include **artificial insemination** and **assisted reproductive technologies (ART).** Artificial insemination is the process of implanting sperm from a donor into a woman near the time of her ovulation. Sperm donors are screened for HIV infection and various genetic disorders, as well as categorized by certain features to create as optimal a match as possible between the woman and the donor. Artificial insemination is often used when the infertility problem is based on a male factor.

Any treatment or procedure that involves the handling of human eggs and sperm for the purpose of helping a woman become pregnant qualifies as a type of ART. All ART procedures involve stimulating the ovary to produce eggs, harvesting the eggs with a microscopic needle, and then removing the eggs from the woman's body. ART methods are listed below.

- **In vitro fertilization (IVF)** involves removing the ova from a woman's ovary just before normal ovulation would occur. The woman's egg and her partner's sperm are placed in a special fertilization medium for a specific period of time and are then transferred to another medium for continued development. If the fertilized egg cell shows signs of development, it is returned to the woman's uterus within several days by means of a hollow tube placed through the vagina and cervix. The egg cell implants itself in the lining of the uterus, and the pregnancy continues as normal. Data indicate that 15% to 20% of these procedures are successful.[31]

- **Gamete intrafallopian transfer (GIFT)** involves placing sperm and eggs into the fallopian tubes. This procedure is less time-consuming and less expensive than IVF. GIFT mimics nature by permitting fertilized eggs to divide in the fallopian tubes. It has a success rate similar to that seen with IVF, but is more invasive than IVF.

- **Zygote intrafallopian transfer (ZIFT)** involves placing the egg and the sperm in a test tube for fertilization, just as in IVF. The fertilized egg is removed from the tube at an earlier stage than in IVF, however, and placed in the fallopian tube in the woman's body. The zygote can then continue its cell division during its trip down the fallopian tube and become implanted in the uterus naturally.

- **Intracytoplasmic sperm injection (ICSI)** involves injecting sperm directly into the egg with a microscopic needle.

- **Egg donation** is used when a woman is unable to produce eggs or she has a genetic disorder that will be passed on to the child. Egg donors must be willing to dedicate an enormous amount of time to this process because of the amount of drug treatment and monitoring that they must undergo. It is not a simple procedure for either the donor or the recipient of the egg.

- **Embryo transfer** is a procedure in which the sperm of the infertile woman's partner is placed in another woman's uterus during ovulation. Approximately five days later, the fertilized egg is transferred to the uterus of the infertile woman, who then carries the developing embryo.

- **Host uterus** is a procedure in which the sperm from a man and the egg from a woman are combined in a laboratory. The fertilized egg is then implanted into the uterus of a second woman who agrees to bear the child, which is not genetically related to her.

- **Surrogacy** occurs when a woman is artificially inseminated with the sperm of an infertile woman's partner. She carries the baby to term, usually for an established fee and the provision of her health care. After delivery, the baby is turned over to the couple.

Each of these procedures, while offering hope to infertile couples, can raise ethical and legal questions.

Emotional Effects of Infertility

Infertility and the procedures used to treat it are extremely stressful for most couples. In some cases, women who undergo the often arduous tests experience anger and resentment toward their partners, especially if their partners do not provide adequate support and share in their experiences. If the cause of infertility is determined, the man or woman who is experiencing the medical problem may feel guilty and blame himself or herself for failing to become pregnant. The experience of becoming pregnant and miscarrying can also lead to excitement and anticipation

We had been trying to have a baby for several years. It was so frustrating because all of our friends were having babies. We felt so many things—guilt, embarrassment, fear, and anger. Finally, after a lot of testing, we tried IVF and it worked! We have a little girl. It was a long and difficult journey to have her, but we are so pleased.

35-year-old woman

followed by depression and frustration. Once involved in testing, couples may become hopeful again but hesitant. The mix of emotions often leads to confusion and miscommunication between the couple.

As a couple prepares to undergo an ART procedure such as IVF, more grief may be experienced. In addition to fearing that it is the last option available, couples must shoulder the exorbitant costs of infertility treatment and face the possibility that it may be unsuccessful.[32] Women who fail to become pregnant following any type of fertility therapy experience grief and depression before, during, and after treatment. Women have reported feeling despair, anger, and a loss of control as their hopes of becoming pregnant faded. Effective coping behaviors and a strong network of family and friends appear to reduce a couple's emotional stress. If treatment fails, some couples accept happiness without their own children in their lives, whereas other couples may opt for adoption.

Epidemiology

Traditional epidemiological data on pregnancy and childbirth have focused on issues of maternal and child morbidity and mortality. In recent years, an expanded focus has provided insight into other important epidemiological considerations of pregnancy, childbirth, breastfeeding, and infertility.

Pregnancy

In 2004, the U.S. birth rate was 14 per 1,000 persons. Teenage birth rates fell to a new record low, continuing a decline that began in 1991. The birth rate fell to 41.2 births per 1,000 females 15–19 years of age in 2004. Significant variations exist in the birth rates for teenagers among racial groups; Figure 6.8 provides a comparison of 1991 and 2004 birth rates for white, black, Hispanic, American Indian and Asian/Pacific Islander teenagers, age 15–19. Birth rates for women in their twenties were generally down, while births to older mothers (30–49) were still on the rise.[33]

Figure 6.8

Birth rates for teenagers 15–19 years of age by race and Hispanic origin.

Source: Hamilton, B. E., Martin, J. A., Ventura S. J., Sutton, P. D., and Menacker, F. (2005). Births: preliminary data for 2004. *National Vital Statistics Reports* 54(8). Hyattsville, MD: National Center for Health Statistics.

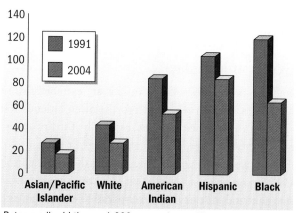

Rates are live births per 1,000 women in specific group.

Pregnancy and childbirth are safe experiences for many women; however, any medical or obstetric complication is one too many. In the early 1900s, 1 in 150 women died from causes related to pregnancy, with the death rate among women of color being nearly double that of white women.[34] These deaths were typically caused by infection, toxemia, abortion, and hemorrhage. Today, the leading causes of pregnancy-related deaths are embolism, hemorrhage, and pregnancy-related hypertension. In 1900, there were approximately 850 maternal deaths per 100,000 live births in the United States; since 1982, the rate of maternal deaths has not changed much and hovers around 7 to 8 maternal deaths per 100,000 live births. Although this reduction in maternal mortality is impressive, data indicate that women of color are still three to four times more likely than white women to die of pregnancy-related causes, and the risk for black women is the highest among all racial groups (Figure 6.9). Women 35 years of age and older also are at increased risk for maternal mortality.[35]

Infant mortality is another complication of pregnancy. The three leading causes of infant death are congenital malformations, disorders relating to short gestation and low birthweight, and **sudden infant death syndrome (SIDS).** Together, these causes accounted for nearly one-half of all infant deaths in the United States in 1999.[36] The infant mortality rate was 6.9 infant deaths per 1,000 live births in the United States in 2000, down from 8.9 deaths per 1,000 live births in the early 1990s. The decline in infant mortality since the 1970s is largely attributable to advances in neonatal intensive care and the dissemination of these advances across the country. The neonatal period consists of the first month of life, and about two-thirds of infant deaths occur in this time frame. Data analyses, however, indicate that black infants die at more than twice the rate of white, Hispanic, Asian, or Pacific Islander infants.

Low birthweight is defined as a birthweight of less than 2,500 grams (5.5 pounds) and is the single most important predictor of infant survival. This condition may result from preterm birth (before 37 weeks gestation), poor fetal growth for a given

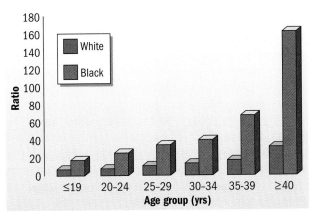

Deaths per 100,000 live births.

Figure 6.9

Pregnancy-mortality ratios, by age and race, United States, 1991–1999.

Source: Chang, J., et al. (2003). Pregnancy-related mortality surveillance—United States, 1991–1999. *Morbidity and Mortality Weekly Report* 52(SS02): 1–8.

duration of pregnancy (known as **intrauterine growth retardation**), or both. Black infants are twice as likely as white or Hispanic infants to have low birthweight. In the United States, the rate of low birthweight increased from 7.0% of all births in the 1990s to 8.1% of total births in 2004, in part due to the increase in multiple births resulting from expanded use of fertility treatments.[33] (See Figure 6.10.)

Breastfeeding

Rates for breastfeeding have increased every year since 1991; however, the rate of breastfed babies is still lower than desired. Between 1993 and 1994, 58.1% of mothers breastfed their babies. This was almost double the percentage of women breastfeeding between 1972 and 1974. In 1998, 64% of all mothers breastfed their babies in the early postpartum period. The percentage of African American women breastfeeding, however, is still significantly lower than it is for other races (whites: 68%; Hispanics: 66%; blacks: 45%). The rate increases as the educational level and age of the mother increase.[37] According to findings from the 2003 CDC National Immunization Survey,[38] a nationally representative sample of the U.S. population:

- 70.9% of all U.S. infants were ever breastfed.
- 36.2% of infants were breastfeeding at 6 months of age.
- 17.2% of infants were still breastfeeding at 1 year of age.

Infertility

Approximately 15% of U.S. women of childbearing age have sought some type of treatment for infertility. In 2000, a total of 35,025 babies were born using ART. In vitro fertilization was the most common procedure used (Figure 6.11). The majority of women using ART are between the ages of 30 and 39. A woman's age is the most important factor when determining the chance of a live birth using her

Figure 6.10

Percentage of infants born preterm and born low birthweight, United States, 1990, 1995, 2000, and 2004.

Source: Martin, J. A., Hamilton, B. E., Menacker, F., Sutton, P. D., and Mathews, T. J. (November 15, 2005). Preliminary births for 2004: infant and maternal health. Health E-stats.

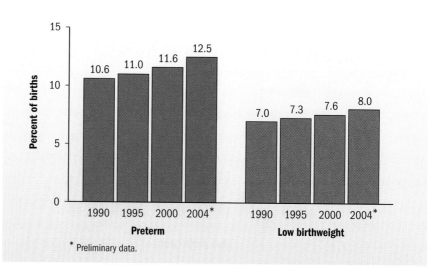

* Preliminary data.

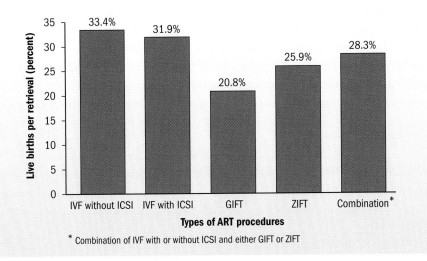

Figure 6.11

Live births per retrieval for different types of ART procedures using fresh nondonor eggs or embryos, 2003.

Source: National Center for Chronic Disease and Prevention and Health Promotion of the CDC in consultation with the American Society for Reproductive Medicine and the Society for Assisted Reproductive Technology. (2003). *2003 Assisted Reproductive Technology (ART) Report.*

own eggs. Both rate of pregnancy and rate of live births drop for women in their early thirties and decline sharply for women in their mid-thirties. Women in their twenties have the best success rates.[39]

Informed Decision Making

Informed decision making about pregnancy should begin before conception. The newly conceived offspring depends on its mother for nutrition and well-being weeks before the mother may know that she is pregnant. If the mother is a smoker or is abusing alcohol or drugs during this critical early period of development, her child is at a decided disadvantage.

Pregnancy

A pregnant woman has to take good care of herself to provide the best care for her unborn child. Regular prenatal care that begins early in the pregnancy is essential and is associated with reduced infant morbidity and mortality. Most women see their clinician once a month during the pregnancy until week 28. In the last trimester, this frequency increases to every other week until week 36, when weekly visits until delivery are indicated. Proper nutrition, adequate and appropriate exercise, and avoidance of alcohol, tobacco, caffeine, and illegal drugs are all essential components of good prenatal care.

Childbirth

Childbirth is a personal, special, one-time-only event. Preparation for birthing ensures the best possible experience. Childbirth education classes provide many

I cannot remember much about the birth of my first baby. I was young and scared, and I only wanted to be "knocked out." Afterwards, I realized that I had missed one of the most important events of my life. With my second baby, we went to classes and I read everything I could. I really was prepared. I felt so much more in control of what was happening to me. Birth is something too wonderful to miss.

30-year-old woman

valuable opportunities for learning, practical preparation, and building skills for a rewarding and facilitated childbirth experience. They also provide an opportunity to share concerns and discuss plans. Local resources for childbirth options, such as birthing centers or home deliveries, can be evaluated. Classes provide motivation to learn relaxation and pain management techniques.

Resources in childbirth preparation vary. Some communities offer many resources; in other communities, resources are rather few and far between. To maximize the benefits from a childbirth education class, the qualifications of the instructor, class size, and class focus should be carefully evaluated.

Instructors in childbirth education should be certified. The most prestigious certification program for childbirth educators is conducted by Lamaze International. Educators with this certification use the credential LCCE (Lamaze Certified Childbirth Educator). Those who have made significant contributions to the field may use the credential FLCCE (Fellows of the College).

The most appropriate class size is eight to twelve couples. This number allows for individual attention, time for discussion, and adequate floor space for practice. In addition to providing the basic information on pregnancy and childbirth, classes should discuss birthing options and developing personal plans for birth based on personal medical requirements and resources.

Breastfeeding

Breastfeeding can be a very rewarding experience. Women who have difficulty beginning the process are encouraged to "stick with it" as both the mother and the infant learn how to work with each other. Although suckling is instinctual for the infant, feeding from the breast is a learned behavior for the mother. Adjusting positions, anticipating the infant's hunger, and relaxing during the feeding are ways to make breastfeeding more pleasurable for both mother and infant. Breastfeeding assistance is usually offered postpartum at the hospital, and lactation specialists also are available for women when they return home with the baby. Aside from the bond created between mother and child, breastfeeding offers significant health benefits to both parties.

■ Hospitals and birthing centers often have lactation specialists on staff to help new mothers learn the ropes of breastfeeding.

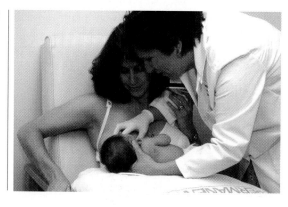

Profiles of Remarkable Women

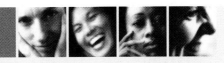

Martha May Eliot, M.D. (1891–1978)

Martha May Eliot, a pioneer in maternal and child health, graduated from Radcliffe College and the medical school at Johns Hopkins University. She taught at Yale University's Department of Pediatrics until 1935, while also directing the National Children's Bureau Division of Child and Maternal Health. In 1951, Eliot became Bureau Chief. She conducted community studies, exploring issues of social medicine and ways that public health measures could prevent disease. She also drafted most of the Social Security Act's language dealing with maternal and child health in 1934. During World War II, Eliot provided care for more than 1 million servicemen's wives through the Emergency Maternity and Infant Care program. She continued her involvement with women's and children's health after the war by working with the World Health Organization (WHO) and the United Nations Children's Fund (UNICEF) in significant capacities.

After leaving her position as Bureau Chief of the National Children's Bureau Division of Maternal and Child Health, Eliot became Department Chair of Child and Maternal Health at Harvard University's School of Public Health. She received many honors throughout her lifetime that recognized her work as a leading pediatrician and the force behind many maternal and child health programs. She was one of the first women admitted into the American Pediatric Society, the first woman elected president of the American Public Health Association (APHA), and the first woman to receive APHA's Sedgwick Memorial Medal. APHA now awards the Martha May Eliot Award to recognize others' achievements in maternal and child health.

Infertility

Infertility should be recognized as a problem of a couple, not the woman or her partner. Because the factors that reduce fertility are shared, both partners must be evaluated when initiating an infertility workup. Infertility services are widely available today, and evolving technologies have enabled many couples to have a child. Infertility clinics can offer couples information, support, and procedures to address their specific needs. Identification of infertility services is often facilitated through referral from a gynecologist.

Summary

Pregnancy, childbirth, and breastfeeding are exciting, yet complex, dimensions of women's health. In addition to the biological aspects, pregnancy, childbirth, and breastfeeding are greatly influenced by social, cultural, historical, legal, and ethical dimensions. Understanding the physiological causes for the physical and emotional changes that occur in a pregnant woman can often help make the pregnancy process more manageable. Prenatal care is a vital component of a healthy pregnancy, and usually includes nutritional counseling, genetic testing, ultrasounds, and ongoing monitoring of the mother and baby. Many women experience the changes of pregnancy and the birth of their child without complications. Others learn firsthand the emotional hardships of infertility, miscarriage, diagnosis of abnormalities in the fetus, premature delivery, or complications during the delivery. For couples who have difficulty conceiving, a host of medical and surgical options exist to achieve a pregnancy. As with other areas of women's health, informed decision making is a critical determinant throughout the prenatal to postnatal periods.

■ ■ ■ ■

Topics for Discussion

1. Should childbirth retain its "medicalized" focus? Why or why not?
2. Should pregnant women be restricted in their access to tobacco, alcohol, or drugs?
3. Should prenatal testing be routine for all pregnant women?
4. Should preparation for childbirth be required for all women?
5. Discuss the rights of pregnant teenagers as parents. What rights do a teen's parents have in regard to her pregnancy? Does the father of the child have any say in the pregnancy?
6. What are possible ethical and legal dilemmas associated with infertility techniques and treatment?

■ ■ ■ ■

Web Sites

American Academy of Pediatrics: http://www.aap.org

Centers for Disease Control and Prevention—Breastfeeding: http://www.cdc.gov/breastfeeding

Centers for Disease Control and Prevention—Reproductive Health Information Source: http://www.cdc.gov/reproductivehealth

La Leche League International: http://www.lalecheleague.org

March of Dimes: http://www.marchofdimes.com

National Campaign to Prevent Teen Pregnancy: http://www.teenpregnancy.org

Resolve, The National Infertility Association: http://www.resolve.org

■ ■ ■ ■

References

1. Bogdan, J. C. (1990). Childbirth in America, 1650 to 1990. In R. D. Apple (ed.), *Women, Health and Medicine and America*. New York: Garland Publishers.
2. Wertz, R. W., and Wertz, D. C. (1977). *Lying-In: A History of Childbirth in America*. New York: Free Press.

3. Leavitt, J. W. (1986). *Brought to Bed: Childbirthing in America, 1750–1950.* New York: Oxford University Press.

4. Barness, L. A. (1991). Brief history of infant nutrition and view to the future. *Pediatrics* 88: 1054–1056.

5. Ansley, D. (1992). Spermtales. *Discover* 13(6): 66–69.

6. De Jonge, C. J. (1998). An update on human fertilization. *Seminars in Reproductive Endocrinology* 16(3): 209–217.

7. Mathews, T. J., Honein, M. A., and Erickson, J. D. (2002). Spina bifida and anencephaly prevalence—United States, 1991–2001. *Morbidity and Mortality Weekly Report* 51(RR13): 9–11.

8. Kolasa, K. M., and Weismiller, D. G. (1997). Nutrition during pregnancy. *American Family Physician* 56(1): 205–212.

9. Morris, S. N., and Johnson, N. R. (2005). Exercise during pregnancy: a critical appraisal of the literature. *Journal of Reproductive Medicine* 50(3): 181–188.

10. Mathews, T. J. (2001). Smoking during pregnancy in the 1990s. *National Vital Statistics Reports,* 49(7). Hyattsville, MD: Centers for Disease Control and Prevention, National Center for Health Statistics.

11. Centers for Disease Control and Prevention. (2004). Alcohol consumption among women who are pregnant or who might become pregnant—United States, 2002. *Morbidity and Mortality Weekly Report* 53(50): 1178–1181.

12. March of Dimes. (2004). *Illicit Drug Use During Pregnancy. Quick Reference Fact Sheets for Professionals and Reseachers.*

13. Papanikolaou, N. C., et al. (2005). Lead toxicity update. A brief review. *Medical Science Monitor* 11(10): RA329–336.

14. Wapner, R. (1997). Chorionic villus sampling. *Obstetric and Gynecologic Clinics of North America* 24(1): 83–110.

15. Tongsong, T., et al. (1999). Amniocentesis-related fetal loss: a cohort study. *Obstetrics and Gynecology* 92: 64–67.

16. Ventura, S. J., Abma, J. C., Mosher, W. D., and Henshaw, S. (2003). Revised pregnancy rates, 1990–97 and new rates for 1998–99, United States. *National Vital Statistics Report* 52(7). Hyattsville, MD: National Center for Health Statistics.

17. Brier, N. (1999). Understanding and managing the emotional reactions to a miscarriage. *Obstetrics and Gynecology* 93(1): 151–155.

18. Goldner, T. E., Lawson, H. W., Xia, Z., and Atrash, H. K. (1993). Surveillance for ectopic pregnancy—1970 to 1989. *Morbidity and Mortality Surveillance Summaries* 42(SS-6): 73–85.

19. Martin, J. A., Hamilton, B. E., Sutton, P. D., Ventura, S. J., Menacker, F., and Munson, M. L. (2005). Births: final data for 2003. *National Vital Statistics Reports* 54(2). Hyattsville, MD: National Center for Health Statistics.

20. Olney, R. S. (1999). Preventing morbidity and mortality from sickle cell disease: a public health perspective. *American Journal of Preventive Medicine* 16(2): 116–121.

21. National Heart, Lung, and Blood Institute. (2003). Sickle Cell Anemia. Accessed online: http://www.nhlbi.nih.gov/health/dci/Diseases/Sca/SCA_WhatIs.html.

22. Fowler, M. G., Mofenson, L., and McConnell, M. (2003). The interface of perinatal HIV prevention, antiretroviral drug resistance, and antiretroviral treatment: what do we really know? *Journal of Acquired Immune Deficiency Syndrome* 34(3): 308–311.

23. Centers for Disease Control and Prevention. (2002). Sexually transmitted diseases treatment guidelines: 2002. *Morbidity and Mortality Weekly Report* 51(RR-6): 2.

24. Bodeus, M., Hubinont, C., and Goubau, P. (1999). Increased risk of cytomegalovirus transmission in utero during late gestation. *Obstetrics and Gynecology* (93)5: 658–660.

25. Schrag, S, Gorwitz, R., Fultz-Butts, K., and Schuchat, A. (2002). Prevention of perinatal Group B streptoccocal disease: revised guidelines from CDC. *Morbidity and Mortality Weekly Report* 51(RR11): 1–22.

26. Hartmann, K., et al. (2005). Outcomes of routine episiotomy: a systematic review. *Journal of the American Medical Association* 293: 2141–2148.

27. Centers for Disease Control and Prevention. (2005). Quickstats: total and primary cesarean rate and vaginal birth after previous cesarean (VBAC) rate—United States, 1989–2003. *National Vital Statistics Reports* 54(02). Hyattsville, MD: National Center for Health Statistics.

28. American College of Obstetricians and Gynecologist. (2004). Vaginal birth after previous cesarean delivery. ACOG Practice Bulletin No. 54. *Obstetrics and Gynecology* 104(1): 203–212.

29. American Academy of Pediatrics: Work Group on Breastfeeding. (1997). Breastfeeding and the use of human milk. *Pediatrics* 100(6): 1035–1039.

30. Stephen, E. H., and Chandra, A. (2000). Use of infertility services in the United States: 1995. *Family Planning Perspectives* 32(3): 132–137.

31. Carson, S. A., and Casson, P. R. (1999). *The American Society for Reproductive Medicine Complete Guide to Fertility.* Chicago, IL: Contemporary Books.

32. Lukse, M. P., and Vacc, N. A. (1999). Grief, depression, and coping in women undergoing fertility treatment. *Obstetrics and Gynecology* 93(2): 245–251.

33. Hamilton, B. E., Martin, J. A., Ventura, S. J., Sutton, P. D., and Menacker, F. (2005). Births: preliminary data for 2004. *National Vital Statistics Reports,* 54(8). Hyattsville, MD: National Center for Health Statistics.

34. Rochat, R. W., Koonin, L. M., Atrash, H. K., and Jewett, J. F. (1988). Maternal mortality in the United States: report from the Maternal Mortality Collaborative. *Obstetrics and Gynecology* 72: 91–97.

35. Centers for Disease Control and Prevention. (2003). Pregnancy-related mortality surveillance—United States, 1991–1999. *Morbidity and Mortality Weekly Report* 52(SS02): 1–8.

36. Anderson, R. N. (2002). Deaths: leading causes for 2000. *National Vital Statistics Reports* 50(16). Hyattsville, MD: National Center for Health Statistics.

37. U.S. Department of Health and Human Services. (2000). *Healthy People 2010,* 2nd ed. With *Understanding and Improving Health and Objectives for Improving Health.* 2 vols. Washington, DC: U.S. Government Printing Office.

38. Centers for Disease Control and Prevention. (2003). *National Immunization Survey.*

39. Centers for Disease Control and Prevention, American Society for Reproductive Medicine, and Resolve. (2000). *2000 Assisted Reproductive Technology Success Rates: National Summary and Fertility Clinic Reports.*

Chapter Seven

Reproductive Tract Infections

Chapter Objectives

On completion of this chapter, the student should be able to discuss:

1. Basic information about sexually transmitted diseases (STDs) and how they differ from other reproductive tract infections.

2. Relative prevalence and infection rates of STDs in women, the United States as a whole, and different ethnic groups.

3. Biological and cultural reasons why STDs disproportionately affect and infect women.

4. The diagnosis process, transmission, symptoms, and course of infection of each of the major reproductive tract infections in the United States.

5. The stigma associated with many STDs and how it both hurts people who are infected and slows prevention and treatment efforts.

6. The role of open communication, both with clinicians and with partners, in regard to STDs.

7. The importance of personal responsibility and risk reduction in making decisions about one's sexual life.

8. The course of HIV/AIDS infection and how treatment works.

9. National and global trends related to the AIDS epidemic.

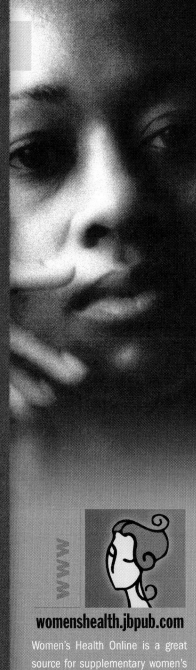

womenshealth.jbpub.com

Women's Health Online is a great source for supplementary women's health information for both students and instructors. Visit

http://womenshealth.jbpub.com

to find a variety of useful tools for learning, thinking, and teaching.

Introduction

Reproductive tract infections (RTIs) are infections caused by a variety of organisms that affect the upper reproductive tract, the lower reproductive tract, or both. Most women experience at least one—and often several—reproductive tract infections in their lifetimes. Reproductive tract infections pose a significant health risk for women. Women are not only at higher risk for acquiring RTIs than men, but also suffer more significant sequelae from these conditions. Most infections are transmitted by sexual intimacy and, therefore, are referred to as **sexually transmitted diseases (STDs).** STDs include chlamydia, gonorrhea, syphilis, herpes, genital warts, hepatitis, and human immunodeficiency virus (HIV) infections. Sexually associated infections include vaginitis, trichomoniasis, yeast infections, and bacterial vaginosis.

The consequences of an STD depend on the organism causing the infection. Gonorrhea and chlamydia can cause permanent damage to the reproductive system, even in the absence of symptoms. Herpes is an incurable disease with painful and often emotionally devastating symptoms, but the disease generally does not pose a long-term health risk. AIDS, and in some cases syphilis and hepatitis, can threaten life itself. Although some infections attack a single structure, such as the labia or cervix, others ascend upward from the vagina, through the cervical canal, and into the uterus, where further invasion into the fallopian tubes, ovaries, and entire pelvis can occur. Having one STD increases a person's risk of acquiring another STD and may make that individual up to seven times more likely than an uninfected person to acquire HIV through sexual contact.[1] STDs also increase a person's infectiousness, making an HIV-positive individual who is infected with another STD more likely to transmit HIV through sexual contact.[2] Some bacteria and viruses may enter the bloodstream and result in systemic effects. Other infections, such as bacterial vaginosis or yeast infections, may be major annoyances, but they do not have serious life-threatening sequelae.

STD organisms know no class, racial, ethnic, or social barriers—all individuals are vulnerable if exposed to the infectious organism. Society, however, has a tendency to look on STDs as punishment for immoral activity. In addition, women have been viewed as the source of disease. Thus, when a woman learns that she has an STD, her reaction may include disbelief, hurt, a feeling of victimization, guilt, embarrassment, anger, fear, shame, and a feeling of loss of control over her sexuality and health. With viral diseases, there is often the added pressure of worry over how the lingering virus will affect present and future relationships. The emotional effects for women are often as serious or worse than the physical effects of reproductive tract infections. Clearly, knowledge and prevention are the best defenses against STDs, followed by early diagnosis and treatment to reduce or eliminate the consequences of infection.

Perspectives on STDs

Historical Overview

Although STDs are a modern epidemic, they are not modern diseases. STDs have been referenced in medical literature for hundreds and, in some cases, thou-

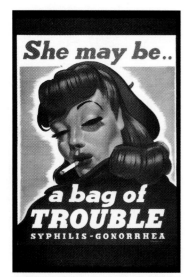

■ Historically, society has looked on STDs as punishment for immoral activity. In addition, women have been viewed as the source of disease.

sands of years. The oldest books in the Bible describe diseases that probably were gonorrhea and syphilis. Early Biblical descriptions of leprosy more accurately fit the conditions of diseases now called syphilis or scabies. Ancient Greek and Roman physicians identified genital warts and syphilis chancres in their writings. Even the term *condyloma*, once defined as meaning "fig" and now solely used to refer to genital warts, is of Greek origin. Hippocrates described the mechanism for gonorrhea transmission as "excesses of the pleasures of the Venus." Susruta, an ancient Hindu, also described gonorrhea. In ancient Rome, Tiberius issued a decree outlawing public kissing to curb a herpes epidemic. Spanish explorers may have brought syphilis to Europe from the New World; even the character of Falstaff from Shakespeare's *Henry IV* appears to be suffering from the disease. Between 1495 and 1500, syphilis ravaged Europe, killing hundreds of thousands of people. The HIV/AIDS epidemic today has been likened to these historical STD ravages.

Epidemiological Data and Trends

STDs, previously called "venereal diseases," are a major health problem and have been identified as a national health priority.[3] They are at epidemic proportions among reproductive-age Americans and present serious threats, especially to young women. In 2000, there were 9.1 million new cases of STDs among U.S. youth from the ages of 15 to 24 alone.[4] Adolescents have a greater biological risk of infection, and their risk of exposure is higher because of difficulties accessing appropriate health care, the increased risk of multiple short-term sexual relationships, and inconsistent use of barrier contraception.[2] The United States has the highest rate of STD infection in the industrialized world. By age 24, at least one out of every four Americans is believed to have contracted an STD, and an estimated 65 million Americans are now living with an incurable STD.[5]

Despite the availability of antibiotics that work effectively against several of the pathogens, STD rates continue to climb. More than 20 organisms and numerous syndromes are currently recognized as being transmitted sexually.

Measuring the scope of the STD epidemic is a difficult task. Some STDs are reportable conditions (diseases required by federal law to be reported to prevent and control their spread), and national data on them are available. Healthcare providers are required to report cases of chlamydia, gonorrhea, and syphilis, but healthcare facilities vary widely in the manner that they report these diseases. Chlamydia, the reportable disease with the highest incidence, is spreading at a rate of 3 million new cases each year in the United States (Figure 7.1).[6] Many STDs are asymptomatic, so many infected individuals are not diagnosed. Other STDs are not reportable, and actual incidence rates can only be estimated.

Prevalence rates provide an even more startling picture of the STD epidemic. For example, an estimated 45 million Americans harbor the herpes virus, and human papillomavirus (HPV) may afflict as many as 20 million people in the United States (Figure 7.2).[4] In 2004, infections of chlamydia were more than seven times higher among African American females than among white females. In the same year, the rates of gonorrhea infections in African Americans,

Figure 7.1

Estimated incidence (new cases) of major STDs in the United States among American youth (ages 15–24) in 2000.

Source: Weinstock, H., Berman, S., and Cates, W. Jr. (2004). Sexually transmitted diseases among American youth: incidence and prevalence estimates, 2000. *Perspectives on Sexual and Reproductive Health* 36(1): Table 2. Reprinted with permission from The Guttmacher Institute.

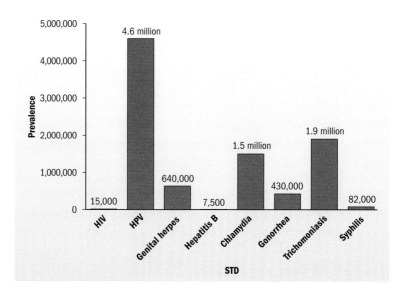

Native Americans, and non-white Hispanics were 19, 4, and 2 times higher than among whites.[7] STDs also affect Hispanics at higher rates than non-Hispanic whites (Figure 7.3). Native American/Alaska Native and Asian/Pacific Islander women have rates of chlamydia consistently higher than whites.[7] Although rates appear to be consistently higher among minorities, some reporting bias may affect the data collected. Minorities are more likely than Caucasians to visit public clinics, which are often the main source of STD estimates, possibly accounting for increased reporting of disease among these groups.

Figure 7.2

Estimated prevalence (existing cases) of selected common STDs in the United States among American youth (ages 15–24) in 2000.

Source: Weinstock, H., Berman, S., and Cates, W. Jr. (2004). Sexually transmitted diseases among American youth: incidence and prevalence estimates, 2000. *Perspectives on Sexual and Reproductive Health* 36(1): Table 2. Reprinted with permission from The Guttmacher Institute.

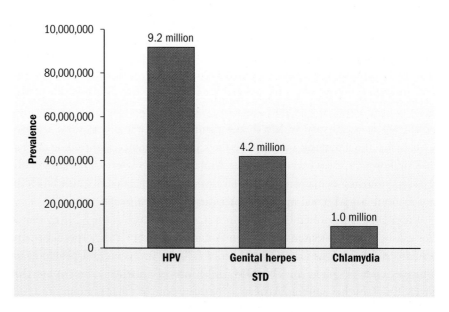

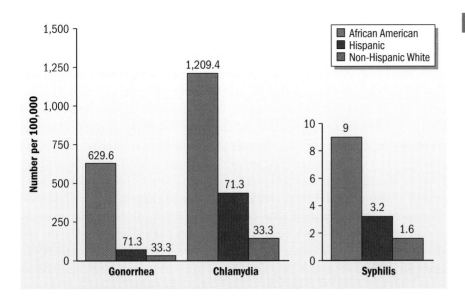

Figure 7.3

Race/ethnicity differences in rates of gonorrhea, syphilis, and chlamydia, 2004.

Source: U.S. Department of Health and Human Services, Centers for Disease Control and Prevention. (2005). Sexually Transmitted Disease Surveillance 2004. Atlanta, GA. Retrieved January 4, 2006, from http://www.cdc.gov/std/stats/natoverview.htm.

Social Issues and Dimensions

STDs are biologically sexist, presenting greater risk and causing more complications for women than for men. Women experience most of the STD burden and complications, including infertility, perinatal infections, genital tract neoplasia, and death. In women, these diseases are often silent, presenting as asymptomatic but remaining damaging and infectious. STDs in pregnant women frequently place unborn babies and children at risk of illness, congenital anomalies, developmental disabilities, and death. Because STDs are most prevalent among women 15 to 24 years of age,[2] these women experience the greatest burden of chronic pelvic pain, pelvic inflammatory disease (PID), ectopic pregnancy, and infertility. Women constitute the majority of individuals living at or below the poverty line in the United States, and the poor bear the added burden of limited access to comprehensive STD diagnostic, treatment, and follow-up services.

Considerable stigma accompanies an STD diagnosis, regardless of the culprit organism. This stigma arises because people often mistakenly assume that "deviant" sexual behavior or decisions make people more prone to infection. In reality, all sexually active people are at risk for acquiring an STD, especially if they have unprotected sex. Reproductive tract infections may be perceived as dirty or shameful, and an infected woman may fear that healthcare providers will not care for her or will be offended by doing so. Women are more vulnerable than men to the STD stigma owing to society's double standard that requires women to be "pure" or virginal, while men are often expected to "sow their wild oats," or engage in sexual activity with multiple partners. Some women may view an STD as punishment for previous behavior. Many people still equate STDs with immorality, promiscuous behavior, and low social status. Public health education efforts need to focus on countering these false perceptions.

Cultural dimensions often complicate public health and education efforts. Although STD educational and behavioral issues cut across all racial and ethnic groups, the situation is far worse in poor African American communities due to other social problems complicating the STD epidemic. Men in cultures or regions that are intolerant of homosexuality may have high-risk encounters with other men while keeping these behaviors secret, identifying themselves as "straight," and ultimately infecting their girlfriends or wives. Many women are not in charge of contraceptive decision making and may put themselves at risk by engaging in sexual activities with philandering or infected partners. Crack-related sexual behaviors ("selling" sex for crack), as well as risky sexual activity while under the influence of various drugs including alcohol, compound STD transmission.[8] Emotional dimensions often dominate logical behavior and rational thinking—for example, among prostitutes who wear condoms with clients but not with boyfriends, and among teenage girls who believe that condoms are unnecessary when a boyfriend declares his love.

In addition, healthcare providers may neglect certain populations of women when it comes to screening for these diseases. Women whose sexual partners are exclusively women appear to have a lower prevalence of some STDs, but they are still at risk for infection and therefore should be advised on prevention guidelines. Various types of latex barriers can be used for oral-genital or oral-anal contact, as well as for direct skin-to-skin contact, so as to prevent STD transmission among people of all sexual orientations. Healthcare providers also may not screen women with disabilities for STDs. To complicate matters, a woman with a disabling condition may have sensory impairments that limit self-diagnosis or may manifest altered symptoms of common STDs. It is important that women's healthcare providers always test for STDs on any sexually active woman.

Economic Dimensions

In 2000, STDs among youth (ages 15–24 years) in the United States had a direct economic burden of $6.5 billion. The entire economic burden of STDs on all age groups would undoubtedly be significantly higher.[9] This estimate does not include costs like lost wages, loss of productivity due to STD-related illness, out-of-pocket costs, or costs incurred by the transmission of STDs to infants, which can result in significant lifelong expenditures.

By far, the greatest costs associated with bacterial STDs result from complications of untreated chlamydia and gonorrhea. Without medical attention, these STDs can lead to PID and future fertility problems, leading to even more significant costs.

Because viral STDs cannot be cured and may require treatment over a period of years, they tend to cost more than bacterial STDs. The greatest costs associated with viral STDs result from treatment of precancerous cervical lesions caused by HPV infection and treatment of sexually transmitted HIV infection (Figure 7.4). In addition to their economic dimensions, STDs carry a high human cost of pain, suffering, and grief. Chlamydia and gonorrhea complications can lead to chronic

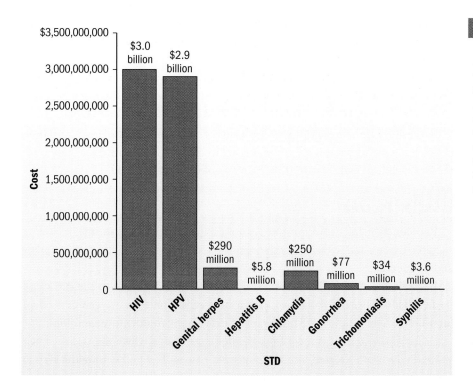

Figure 7.4

Estimated cost of major STDs among U.S. youth, 2000.

Source: Chesson, H. W., Blandford, J. M., Gift, T. L., Tao, G., and Irwin, K. L. (2004). The estimated direct medical cost of sexually transmitted disease among youth, 2000. *Perspectives on Sexual and Reproductive Health* 36(1): Table 1. Reprinted with permission from The Guttmacher Institute.

pain, infertility, and tubal pregnancies, which can affect a woman's health and well-being throughout her lifetime.

HIV/AIDS creates enormous costs at both the societal and individual levels. The devastating effects of the disease on entire communities in some parts of the world—for example, in sub-Saharan Africa—have brought catastrophic economic consequences. In the United States, many families' primary wage earners are sick with the disease, leading to significant economic hardship. In addition, the cost of the drugs required to keep HIV infection in check can approach $15,000 per year. People living with HIV/AIDS in the United States are thus a special population to consider in terms of their needs for health insurance and prescription drug coverage, as the costs of the disease far exceed the ability of most individuals to pay for necessary services and treatments. Globally, governments and non-governmental organizations alike are working together to help fund programs that provide access to diagnostic and treatment services for people living with HIV/AIDS.

In 2004, senior researchers from UNAIDS, the department within the United Nations that addresses AIDS-related issues, estimated that the annual cost of battling HIV/AIDS would reach $9.2 billion in 2005 and could reach $20 billion in 2007, compared with about $1.8 billion in 1998. The 2005 estimate included $4.8 billion to prevent the spread of HIV infection through education, the provision of condoms, and the use of the relatively cheap and effective drugs that can stop infection from passing from mothers to their newborns. The other $4.4 billion will be spent on treatment, including the expensive antiretroviral drugs that keep HIV-carriers alive and well in rich countries, and on supporting orphans.[10]

Clinical Dimensions and Treatment Issues of Sexually Transmitted Diseases

Because STDs are caused by a spectrum of organisms, considerable variation exists in the manifestation of symptoms and in treatment options. This section reviews the clinical and treatment perspectives of each major STD.

Infection Process

Reproductive tract infections are caused by a variety of organisms, including bacteria, viruses, and parasites. Each organism requires a unique diagnostic strategy and treatment.

Bacteria behave in different ways. For example, some attach to the surface of normal body cells, and some live within host cells. Some are oxygen dependent (**aerobic**), whereas others are intolerant of oxygen environments (**anaerobic**).

Bacteria receive nourishment from the fluid or tissue in which they reside. Their waste products are released into these invaded tissues. The body's **immune system** senses the presence of the foreign bacteria, and mobilizes white blood cells to attack them. The infected area becomes warm, red, and swollen owing to the increased circulation and the accumulation of **pus**. The local host cells may be destroyed directly from the bacteria, indirectly from the excessive swelling and waste products, or even by the body's own overzealous immune response. In many cases, bacterial waste products are toxic beyond the localized area and may result in systemic conditions of aches, fever, chills, and malaise. An example of a systemic illness produced by bacterial waste products is **toxic shock syndrome**, which is caused by certain strains of *Staphylococcus aureus* bacteria.

Although normal infection defenses routinely fight off invading organisms throughout the body, reproductive tract infections are particularly challenging. The pelvis contains ideal media for bacterial growth and proliferation, especially during menstruation and after a miscarriage or abortion. Bleeding seems to facilitate bacterial invasion, and blood enhances bacterial growth. In addition, many kinds of bacteria normally live in the intestine and vaginal area. Thus the normal ecosystem of these areas involves a delicate balance of organisms. Harmful bacteria that upset this balance can be killed by antibiotics, but taking such drugs to kill one organism often results in the "killing off" of the normal bacteria and may produce a domino effect. When bacteria levels are reduced, yeast colonies may proliferate, and additional treatment may be necessary.

Viruses follow unique invasion patterns. These tiny organisms are made of DNA or RNA and are hundreds to thousands of times smaller than bacteria. Their attack mechanism also differs from that of bacteria. Viruses invade normal cells and take over the metabolic functions, fueling themselves on the cells' resources. In the

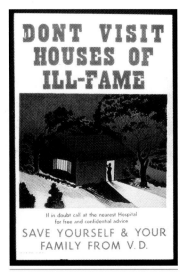

DONT VISIT HOUSES OF ILL-FAME

If in doubt call at the nearest Hospital for free and confidential advice

SAVE YOURSELF & YOUR FAMILY FROM V.D.

■ Although this public service announcement is many decades old, people still equate STDs with immorality, promiscuous behavior, and low social status.

process, the viruses often destroy their host cells. The body's immune system is able to recognize invading viruses and mobilize responses to them, creating an immune response manifested by symptoms of pain, swelling, heat, redness, and/or fever. Unfortunately, a compromised immune system is ineffective against viral invaders. Viral STDs, especially HIV, present difficult challenges to medical researchers. HIV weakens and even subverts the host immune system, allowing **opportunistic infections** that the body normally fights off easily, to invade and proliferate. Because antibiotics are ineffective against viral organisms, researchers are constantly looking to develop effective antiviral drugs that are not too toxic to use. Herpes, genital warts, hepatitis, and AIDS are all reproductive tract infections caused by viruses.

Ectoparasitic infections are caused by tiny parasites that reside on the skin and survive on human blood and tissue. Infections include scabies and pubic lice ("crabs"). Parasites cause itching and may cause bumps or a rash, but are easily treated with a topical cream. Parasitic infections are not considered major STDs; although they affect many people, they are more an annoyance than a serious health threat.

Gonorrhea

Despite a national public health effort, gonorrhea remains prevalent in the United States. Gonococcal infections have the same sequelae as chlamydia. Many women do not experience any symptoms with gonorrhea, especially in the early stages. Instead, gonorrhea in women is often detected at routine gynecological screenings or when their male partners develop symptoms that lead to clinical treatment. When symptoms do present in women, they may include unusual vaginal discharge or bleeding, painful urination, painful intercourse or bleeding after intercourse, pelvic pain or tenderness, or fever. The gonococcus bacterium thrives

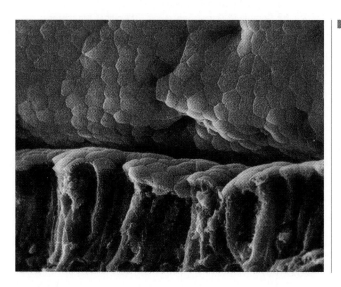

Magnified view of virus. Viral infections such as herpes simplex or human papillomavirus are lifelong conditions.

in moist warm cavities, such as the mouth, throat, rectum, cervix, and urinary tract. As a consequence, gonococcal infections may present in the reproductive tract, throat, eyes, and rectum. Accurate diagnosis of gonorrhea requires a culture taken from the cervix and urethra, and from the throat and anal area if those areas may have been exposed.

There are several treatment options for gonorrhea (Table 7.1). Gonorrhea treatment is complicated by the frequent coexistence of unrecognized chlamydial infection and the increasing incidence of gonorrheal antibiotic-resistant strains. Because neither gonorrhea nor chlamydia may be apparent upon physical examination, gonorrhea treatment usually includes screening for resistant strains of gonorrhea and prescribing additional antibiotics to treat chlamydia effectively. The sequelae of gonorrhea are so severe and threatening to general health and reproductive capability that any woman exposed to a partner with gonorrhea, even in the absence of symptoms, should be treated. If a woman has symptoms that would indicate gonorrhea has spread, longer and more intensive antibiotic treatment is indicated. This often means hospital admission for intravenous antibiotic therapy. About a week after antibiotic treatment for gonorrhea, reculture is necessary for a woman and her partner(s). This follow-up is especially important because, as noted previously, some strains of gonorrhea are resistant to certain antibiotics, and further treatment may be necessary to eliminate the disease.

Reinfection with gonorrhea is common, so sexual intercourse should be avoided until cultures on both partners confirm that treatment was successful. Untreated or unsuccessful treatment of gonorrhea may result in PID or a syndrome caused by disseminated gonococcal infection, which can include septicemia (blood poisoning), joint infection, skin problems, and heart and brain infections.

Table 7.1 Gonorrhea Treatment

Antibiotic Treatment Options for Gonorrhea	Antibiotic Treatment Options for Combined Gonorrhea and Chlamydia Infections	Personal Measures with Treatment
Penicillin was once the most useful treatment, but with resistant strains, other antibiotics must be used: ■ Sulfonamides ■ Tetracyclines ■ Ceftriaxone ■ Cefixime ■ Ciprofloxacin ■ Ofloxacin	Ceftriaxone Doxycycline Azithromycin	Avoid sexual activity. Use careful hygiene to avoid contagion. Avoid rubbing eye.

Source: Centers for Disease and Prevention. (2002). Sexually transmitted disease treatment guidelines. *Morbidity and Mortality Weekly Report* 51: 1–80.

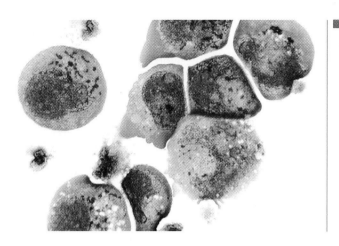

■ Magnified view of bacteria. Bacterial sexually transmitted diseases can be treated with antibiotics.

Chlamydia

Chlamydia is ranked as the most commonly reported infectious disease in the United States (Figure 7.5). Young women are most likely to be infected. Almost one in 35 women between 15 and 24 years old in the United States is infected.[11] Chlamydia is also becoming even more common: the percentage of Americans infected with chlamydia in 2002 was six times the percentage of Americans infected in 1987.[12] Chlamydia infections, which are caused by a bacterium that is transmitted sexually, are the leading cause of preventable infertility and ectopic pregnancy. Most women and about half of men with this STD do not have any symptoms. If symptoms are present, women usually experience a yellowish vaginal discharge,

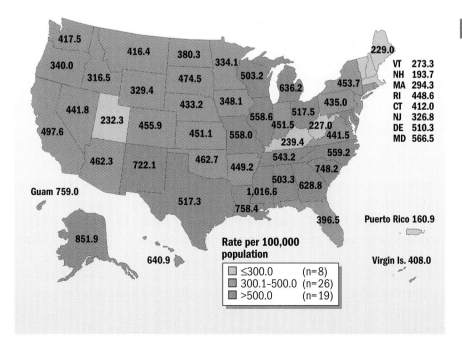

Figure 7.5

Rates of chlamydia among women by state; United States and outlying areas, 2004. Chlamydia rates among women are not consistent across all U.S. States.

The total chlamydia infection rate among women in the United States and outlying areas (Guam, Puerto Rico, and Virgin Islands) in 2004 was 480.7 per 100,000 female population

Source: http://www.cdc.gov/std/stats/slides.htm.

burning with urination, or general pain in the lower abdomen. Chlamydia can invade the uterus, fallopian tubes, cervix, urethra, and even liver, without symptoms ever manifesting themselves. When the chlamydia infection moves into the upper reproductive tract, the condition is known as pelvic inflammatory disease.

Chlamydia screening remains one of the most important national efforts to maintain and improve fertility. It is estimated that routine chlamydia screening could prevent half of the new cases of pelvic inflammatory disease (PID) in the United States.[11] To screen for chlamydia, a culture may be obtained, although this bacterium is difficult to grow in solution and inaccurate results are not uncommon. Newer, more accurate urine-based tests that identify the genetic makeup of the chlamydia bacteria are now being used more often. Clinician suspicion of chlamydia is heightened in a woman with a reddened, swollen cervix and a yellowish cervical discharge. Because gonorrhea and chlamydia often coexist, culture for gonorrhea is a standard procedure when chlamydia is suspected.

A woman may be treated for chlamydia, even without a confirmed diagnosis, based on symptoms and physical examination. A seven-day regimen of doxycycline or a single dose of azithromycin is the preferred treatment for uncomplicated cases. The affected woman's partner(s) should be treated at the same time, and a follow-up examination is usually performed about four weeks after treatment to ensure that the therapy was successful. Sexual intercourse should be avoided until after treatment is successful.

Aggressive treatment is necessary with chlamydia because uterine invasion occurs fairly rapidly, and the invasion process may be asymptomatic. Full PID treatment is undertaken if any evidence indicates that the organism has invaded the uterus. Treatment delay may result in the organism reaching the fallopian tubes with resultant scarring, tubal obstruction, infertility, and ectopic pregnancy. Pregnant women infected with chlamydia may be at increased risk for spontaneous abortions, stillbirth, preterm delivery, and delivery of low-birthweight infants. Transmission of the organism to the baby may result in eye infections and pneumonia in the infant.

Pelvic Inflammatory Disease

Pelvic inflammatory disease (PID) is the most frequent serious complication of bacterial infections, particularly chlamydia and gonorrhea. Each year more than 1 million women experience an episode of PID, causing more than 100,000 cases of infertility and 150 deaths in women.[13] PID from chlamydia is a leading cause of ectopic pregnancies. In 2002, 40,000 women were hospitalized in the United States for ectopic pregnancy.[14] PID also may result in infertility. The Centers for Disease Control and Prevention (CDC) has estimated that 12% of those affected become infertile after the first episode of PID.[15] PID costs to society remain high. Estimates (in 2000 dollars) were as high as $10 billion annually.[16] Recent emphasis on national screening seems to be producing a downward trend of overall PID, with documented decreases in hospital and ambulatory settings from 1985 through 2001.[17]

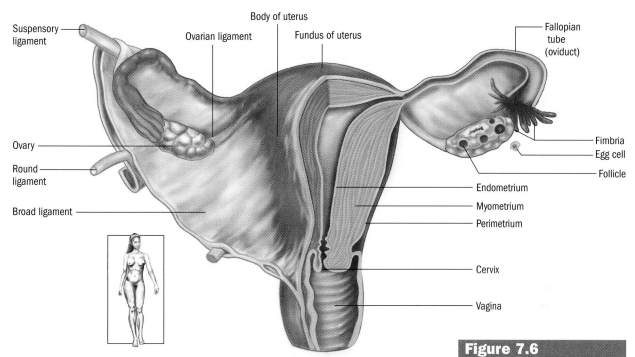

Suspensory ligament

Ovarian ligament

Body of uterus

Fundus of uterus

Fallopian tube (oviduct)

Ovary

Round ligament

Broad ligament

Fimbria

Egg cell

Follicle

Endometrium

Myometrium

Perimetrium

Cervix

Vagina

Figure 7.6

Pelvic inflammatory disease can affect any or all of a woman's reproductive organs.

Chlamydia and gonorrhea are responsible for the majority of cases of PID. *Pelvic infection* and *PID* are both general terms for an infectious process that occurs anywhere in a woman's pelvic organs (Figure 7.6). The infection process may be diffuse—that is, spread out throughout the pelvic cavity—or it may be localized in specific areas. Terms for localized infections include the following:

- Endometritis—infection of the lining of the uterus
- Myometritis—infection of the muscular layers of the uterus
- Salpingitis—infection of the fallopian tubes
- Oophoritis—infection of the ovaries
- Peritonitis—infection of the lining of the abdominal cavity

There is considerable variability with PID symptoms. Some women experience very insidious symptoms, including vaginal discharge, mild but persistent abdominal or back pain, or pain during intercourse. Other women experience sudden and severe pelvic pain, fever, shaking chills, or heavy vaginal discharge or bleeding. Chlamydial PID is more likely to present with the former, more subtle symptoms, and gonorrheal PID is more likely to present with the latter, more severe set of symptoms.

Clinical evaluation is necessary for PID diagnosis. The first step in confirming the presence of PID is eliminating the possibility of other serious conditions that may manifest themselves in a similar manner. Although uterine tenderness and discharge are indications of possible infection, bacterial culture is necessary to identify the causative bacterium and to determine the most appropriate treatment course.

If PID is limited to the uterus, antibiotic treatment usually is sufficient to resolve the problem with little likelihood of permanent damage or future complications. In contrast, infection in the fallopian tubes, ovaries, or abdominal cavity is a cause for significant concern. Permanent damage from PID is more likely if the infection has invaded the fallopian tubes, because the tubes are fragile and easily damaged by an infectious process. Infection causes swelling and scarring of the tubes, which can lead to blockage and distortion, impairing future fertility.

Pelvic abscess is another serious PID complication. Pus and live bacteria may leak from the open end of a fallopian tube and result in peritonitis and an abdominal abscess. A sonogram may be performed if an abscess is suspected; if one is present, the sonogram can help determine whether laparoscopy is indicated to drain the abscess.

Women who have had PID must take elaborate precautions to avoid reinfection. Present and previous sexual partner(s) must be treated with the same antimicrobial regimen as the infected woman, whether or not the partners have symptoms.

Human Papillomavirus

Many types of **human papillomavirus (HPV)** exist—some causing genital warts and others associated with vaginal, anal, and cervical dysplasia.[18] Because of the symptoms that it can cause, HPV often is referred to as genital warts, venereal warts, condylomata, or condyloma acuminatum. From a physiological perspective, HPV is usually not a serious disease. HPV is a local virus; it stays within the anogenital area and cannot spread or do harm to other parts of the body. The HPV strains that cause genital warts can be easily transmitted through sexual contact, and the warts themselves may require treatment, but this is normally the limit of infection. The strains of HPV that can cause cervical dysplasia can produce serious harm and even death in the cases that do progress, but they do so only in a small minority of cases. Most infections with these strains of HPV are asymptomatic and are efficiently cleared by the body's immune system. However, the sheer number of HPV infections in the United States makes HPV a major STD, even if most people with the virus do not develop serious consequences. An accurate determination of HPV prevalence is difficult because genital HPV infections are not reportable conditions, and many infections have no symptoms. While estimates vary, cumulative prevalence rates of HPV are as high as 82% among adolescent women in select populations.[19]

HPV is spread by direct genital skin-to-skin contact. This infection affects both males and females of all ages.

HPV infection with the strains of HPV that cause genital warts is usually characterized by single or multiple lesions or warts, which may first appear as small wens (round elevations in the skin) but may grow in size and number and blend together in a cauliflower-like growth. Genital warts vary in size, may exist in single or multiple units, and may be raised or flat. In women, these painless lesions may occur on the buttocks, anus, inner thighs, vulva, vagina, and cervix. In women, symptoms may appear on the walls of their vagina or cervix and, therefore, they may not realize they have HPV infection. The lesions may increase in size during pregnancy and regress—that is, spontaneously disappear after delivery. In some cases, a doctor may treat warts before childbirth to prevent them from possibly interfering with delivery.

When warts regress, HPV is still present, just not readily apparent. Once contracted, the virus has a variable incubation period during which no symptoms are visible and the person is not yet infectious. Warts usually appear one to eight months after exposure, may not manifest themselves for years, or may not appear at all. A **prodrome** period follows the incubation period, during which there are still no symptoms but the disease is contagious. This is the most dangerous period because the infected person does not know that she or he is capable of transmitting the virus to others. HPV lesions develop in more than 50% of the sexual partners of infected individuals.

Diagnosis of these strains of HPV is usually based on visual detection during clinical examination. A clinician may biopsy a suspicious area if there is an increased risk of malignancy, if the patient is immunocompromised, or if warts persist or enlarge despite therapy. Because warts are dry and painless and usually present on the vulva, cervix, inside the vagina, or around the rectum, women may be unaware that they are infected. Diagnosis may be difficult because many HPV infections are not macroscopically visible. Women with the strains of HPV that cause cervical cell changes usually have no symptoms. Often the first indication of an abnormal condition is a routine Pap smear that identifies cervical cellular changes consistent with HPV infection. For a woman with an inconclusive Pap test, HPV DNA testing conducted on the residual material collected from a Pap can help identify the presence of HPV to determine if she is at risk of cervical dysplasia. Women who are 30 and older can get an HPV test along with their Pap tests. Women who are negative on both tests can be reassured that they do not have HPV and they are not at risk of developing cervical cancer in the near future. If the HPV DNA test is positive, a **colposcope** may be used to look for evidence of warts in the cervix or vagina.

While warts may regress spontaneously, they are frequently symptomatic or psychologically distressing, so treatment is often indicated. The goal of treatment is to get rid of visible warts, although the virus itself cannot be cured. HPV infections can be quite persistent and have a tendency to recur regardless of which treatment method is selected. Treatment is easier and less painful in earlier stages. While no treatment can "cure" HPV, evidence suggests that most individuals' immune systems will eventually clear the virus even without treatment. The particular treatment modality depends on the extent of HPV infection and its location. Treatment options include the following choices:

- Topical agents applied by the patient (such as imiquimod and podofilox)
- Cryotherapy (freezing of warts)
- Podophyllin or trichloroacetic acid (TCA)
- Laser surgery (vaporization of warts)

- Electrosurgery (surgery with electrified blade)
- Surgical excision

Patient-applied therapies are usually more acceptable to patients, more cost-effective, and less harmful to cervical tissue. There is risk of recurrence after any therapy for external genital warts; however, recurrence rates may be the lowest with patient-applied topical therapies. Sexual partners may also be treated, and use of condoms is often recommended to prevent reinfection.

HPV can present problems in pregnancy, though this is relatively rare. Occasionally genital warts may become large enough to interfere with labor, requiring a cesarean delivery. A pregnant woman with HPV has a rare chance of passing the virus to her child during vaginal delivery.

Relationship with Cervical Cancer

Of all the STDs, HPV may be the most biologically sexist. Both men and women can get gentital warts, but the kind of HPV that can cause cervical cancer appears to affect almost exclusively women (some HPV strains have been associated with penile or anal cancer in men, but these cancers are extremely rare). Several of the more than 100 identified strains of HPV have been shown to be causal factors in the development of cervical cancer. The HPV types that are linked to cervical cancer are different than the types that cause genital warts. The cancer-causing strains usually have no initial symptoms, but persistent infection can lead to cervical lesions that a physician can detect using colposcopy. Research suggests that these warts may work with other factors to cause a DNA mutation in immature cervical cells, leading to the development of cervical cancer. Strains 16, 18, 45, and 56 have been specifically implicated in cervical cancer development.[18]

The percentage of women with HPV infection who actually develop cervical cancer, however, is very small. Instead, most women will clear the infection based on their bodies' own immune response. The strength of the immune system appears to affect the course of infection: conditions that alter or slow the immune response may encourage dysplasia. Men infected with these strains of HPV are still capable of transmitting the virus, even if the virus never affects them or causes symptoms. HPV DNA testing is more sensitive and the results more easily reproducible than Pap testing and colposcopy for the detection of existent and incipient cervical precancerous conditions and cancer. A negative HPV test provides a degree and duration of reassurance not achievable by any other diagnostic method[20] (Table 7.2).

Special Precautions

Women who have cervical dysplasia may need to seek aggressive treatment to prevent possible cancer development. Colposcopic examination and biopsy of suspicious areas are indicated. It also is important to be diligent about personal care, medical follow-up care, and annual Pap smears and pelvic examinations.

While latex condoms may reduce the likelihood of HPV transmission, they probably do not provide as reliable protection from HPV as they do against some other

Table 7.2 Understanding Cervical Cancer Screening: The Pap and HPV Tests

Normal and Abnormal Pap Test Result	What It Means
Normal Pap smear (Pap test)	Your cervical cells appear to be healthy.
Abnormal Pap smear (Pap test)	These appear to be changes in your cervical cells that need to be evaluated further.
Borderline, or inconclusive Pap test result (officially called "ASC-US," which stands for atypical squamous cells of undetermined significance)	Your cervical cells are not obviously normal, but they are not clearly abnormal either. Having an HPV test can help determine whether you need further evaluation.

	Looks for	How It Works
Pap test	Signs of abnormal cell changes	A lab professional looks at a sample of cervical cells through a microscope
HPV test	The virus that *causes* the abnormal cell changes that can lead to cervical cancer	A molecular test is done on the sample of cervical cells by an automated system

STDs, such as HIV. HPV is spread by genital skin-to-skin contact, not by bodily fluids. Because a latex condom does not cover all of the genital skin, it cannot guarantee prevention of transmission, even if no visible symptoms are present. A female condom may provide more protection than a traditional condom that covers the penis, but there are no guarantees with either type of condom usage.

Herpes Simplex Virus

Herpes genital infections are recurrent and incurable STDs. There are two types of **herpes simplex virus (HSV)** that are transmitted sexually: HSV-1 and HSV-2. The viruses that cause chickenpox and mononucleosis are also part of the herpes family. At one time, it was believed that HSV-1 was geographically localized above the waist, and HSV-2 was localized below the waist. It is now known that HSV-1 and HSV-2 are capable of invading each other's territory. HSV-1 causes infections of the mouth area, which are commonly known as cold sores or fever blisters. HSV-2 has traditionally been known as genital herpes. While as many as 30% of first episodes are due to HSV-1 infection, HSV-2 causes the majority of recurrent genital infections. An estimated 45 million Americans are infected with HSV, although most of these infections are asymptomatic.[21] Most cases of herpes are spread by people who do not know they have it.[22]

Symptoms of HSV are usually most severe just after acquiring the infection. Symptoms may appear as soon as one day or as long as three to four weeks after exposure. Lasting about 12 days, herpes generally presents as single or multiple small, painful blisters that appear in the vulva or buttocks of women. If they are present on the cervix, they usually go unnoticed. The blisters evolve into painful ulcers in a couple of days. These symptoms may be accompanied by vulvar swelling, fever, and enlarged and tender lymph nodes. Sores usually heal in one to four weeks with little or no scarring. The time between outbreaks is referred to as the latent or inactive phase. During this time, genital sores have healed but the infection remains. A prodrome or warning phase often precedes a herpes outbreak. The warnings may consist of tingling or itching sensations in the area where sores later appear. It is not known what causes repeat outbreaks of herpes. Some people find that irritating stimuli to the infected area, such as tight clothing, menstrual changes, or exposure to sunlight or extreme heat or cold, can trigger an outbreak while others do not notice any such effects.

The human body can never rid itself of the herpes virus. Between outbreaks, the virus evades the immune system by lying dormant within host nerve cells, where the immune system cannot reach it. In most cases, however, the immune system does get better at fighting the virus during outbreaks, so that recurrent outbreaks are usually milder in severity and shorter in duration than the original outbreaks, lasting, on average, five days. People with herpes generally have fewer outbreaks as time goes by. While there is no surefire way to prevent all outbreaks, maintaining a healthy lifestyle helps the immune system keep the virus in check. Any stress on the body can also stress the immune system; indeed, many people report that outbreaks begin when they are already sick with a cold or flu, have gone a long time without getting enough sleep, or are experiencing stressful times in their lives—all things that can burden the immune system. Ironically, refraining from obsessing or worrying excessively about a herpes infection, while still remaining knowledgeable about the disease, may help prevent outbreaks.

Herpes outbreaks show considerable variability from person to person. Some herpes outbreaks last as long as three weeks; others are as short as a few days. Some outbreaks are characterized by multiple blisters; others involve only a single blister. Some individuals experience outbreaks every few months; others have one or more each month. Although uncommon, some individuals never experience recurrent outbreak symptoms after the initial event. Infectiousness remains an important concern, even for individuals who are unaware of their herpes symptoms.

Active herpes sores are very contagious during both the initial attack and the recurrences. Both HSV-1 and HSV-2 can be spread from sores to the eye, where serious infection is possible. An oral infection be spread to infants and children via kissing or casual contact. People infected with herpes undergo periods of **asymptomatic viral shedding.** During these periods, active herpes virus is present on a person's infected area and may be infectious, whether or not symptoms are present. Viral shedding typically lasts for two to 20 days during an initial outbreak and for two to five days during recurrent outbreaks. Researchers have not been able to determine exactly how infectious an individual is when asymptomatic shedding occurs. However, the risk of transmission is highest when active sores are present. Active sores contain hundreds of times more virus than viral sheddings from genital secretions.

I don't sleep around a lot. I have been with only three guys. But I have herpes. I can't tell where I got it . . . I mean, it's like I have slept with not only those guys, but everyone else they have had sex with. How can a person really trust someone not to have an STD these days?

21-year-old woman

Diagnosing herpes may be based on the person's history or a recurrent pattern of illness. Because clinical diagnosis is often inaccurate, viral culture and type-specific serology are used to confirm a diagnosis.

There is not yet a cure for herpes. Prescribed antiviral medications may reduce or suppress symptoms, and antibiotic ointment may help prevent a secondary bacterial infection of the sores. Taking herpes medication may also reduce, but not eliminate, the chance of transmission between outbreaks.[22] Acyclovir, valacyclovir, and famciclovir are the current treatments of choice for herpes; while they do not cure the condition, they can relieve symptoms and shorten healing time. All three medications work by inhibiting the ability of the virus to use proteins, thereby interfering with its ability to replicate. Clinicians may prescribe acyclovir to women who acquire herpes during pregnancy or who have severe outbreaks around the time of delivery.[23] The FDA has approved three different treatment regimes for herpes: (1) therapy for an initial outbreak, (2) episodic therapy to speed healing and relieve discomfort during recurrences, and (3) suppressive therapy on a daily basis to attempt to prevent outbreaks. Because the effects of a herpes transmission are usually limited to symptoms and transmission, a woman with herpes should take an active role in deciding the treatment regimen, if any, that is right for her. Women with severe symptoms may wish to take suppressive therapy, whereas women who have outbreaks that are mild or not noticeable may opt for episodic therapy or seek to manage the virus without medication.

Special Precautions

Good personal hygiene is essential during a herpes outbreak. The infected individual must wash his or her hands thoroughly after touching a herpes sore to avoid possible transmission to another mucous membrane, such as the eyes or mouth. Care should be taken to avoid spreading the virus to others, including infants and children. If active herpes is present in or near the mouth, kissing should be avoided. As a precautionary measure, personal objects such as washcloths, toothbrushes, drinking cups, and towels should not be shared. Although clinical studies have not demonstrated effective indirect transmission, the virus can remain alive outside the body for several hours in a moist environment.

There are no guarantees of "safe sex" with herpes. At a minimum, sexual intercourse, including oral sex, must be avoided when active herpes sores are present. Because viral populations are so high in sores, individuals should wait until the sores are completely healed before resuming sexual activity. Because it is difficult to tell when a herpes outbreak is beginning, open communication about risks and feelings is essential. Condoms appear to provide some protection, with female condoms providing better coverage than male condoms.[24] Because herpes sores can be present in areas not covered by either condom, however, there are no guarantees against transmission. Condoms are especially important in a situation in which the male partner has herpes and the female partner does not and is pregnant. An initial attack of herpes during pregnancy presents serious risks to the developing fetus, including possible pregnancy loss or preterm delivery.

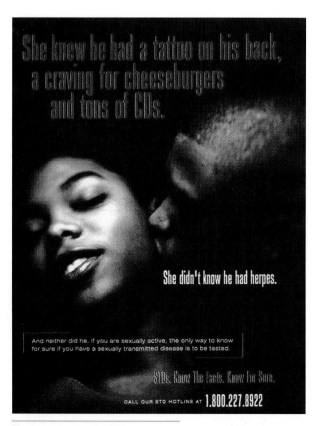

She knew he had a tattoo on his back, a craving for cheeseburgers and tons of CDs.

She didn't know he had herpes.

And neither did he. If you are sexually active, the only way to know for sure if you have a sexually transmitted disease is to be tested.

STDs. Know The Facts. Know For Sure.

CALL OUR STD HOTLINE AT 1.800.227.8922

■ Many people with HSV are asymptomatic but can still transmit the herpes virus. The only way to be definitively diagnosed with an STD is to be tested. Reprinted with permission from the American Social Health Association.

Women with herpes should be especially diligent about protecting themselves from further infection by other STDs. Such women are at increased risk for acquiring HIV and HPV because of the open sores associated with the herpes virus.

Pregnant women with herpes should begin prenatal care early. The risk is greatest for women who contract herpes during their pregnancy. If active lesions are present in the vaginal canal at the time of birth, a cesarean delivery may be undertaken to avoid exposing the infant to the virus. Infant exposure to the virus may cause infections of the eyes, skin, mucous membranes, and central nervous system, and even death. However, most pregnant women with herpes deliver vaginally and give birth to healthy babies.[22]

Although no one wants to get genital herpes, in most cases the stigma of the disease vastly outweights its physiological effects. Herpes is closely related to the viruses that cause chickenpox and mononucleosis (mono), yet because herpes is sexually transmitted, people with herpes may describe themselves as "dirty" or "tainted" or feel that they will never be lovable or able to enter a sexual relationship again. The truth is that many people with herpes have strong relationships and healthy sex lives. Although there is no way to guarantee prevention of sexual transmission, there are many ways to reduce risk, from avoiding sex or wearing condoms between outbreaks, to taking suppressive therapy to reduce outbreaks and asymptomatic shedding. Some people decide to enter relationships with other people who have herpes, although other STDs would still be a potential concern. Because the symptoms of herpes infections are transient and often ultimately quite mild, some couples with one infected partner decide that the benefits of a healthy, unique loving relationship outweigh the drawbacks of possible herpes transmission.

Comfort Measures

Keeping the genital area clean and dry minimizes discomfort during a herpes flare-up. A hair dryer on a cool setting may be used to dry the area thoroughly without irritation or discomfort. Genital cleansing must be gentle because rubbing can cause lesions to break and bleed. Many women find **sitz baths** comforting during outbreaks of herpes. Domeboro solution or baking soda may be added to the sitz bath. Cold, wet compresses or individually wrapped cleansing pads containing glycerol and witch hazel applied to the sores may also provide temporary relief of discomfort, especially during oozing. In addition, some women find icepacks helpful in reducing discomfort during outbreaks.

Syphilis

In 2000, the rate of **syphilis** cases in the United States reached its lowest level since data began being recorded in 1941, although rates remain high in the South, particularly among African Americans. Public health officials had hopes of completely eliminating syphilis in the United States. However, the incidence of syphilis cases has increased every year since 2001, mostly among men. While minorities are still more likely than their white counterparts to be infected with syphilis, there has been considerable reduction in these differences over the past five years.[7]

Syphilis is caused by infection with the bacterial organism *Treponema pallidum.* Dubbed the "Great Pox," syphilis is highly infectious and has a long, varied clinical course. If untreated, it may result in serious consequences, including cardiac and neurological damage and ultimately death. Although syphilis is curable—the syphilis bacterium can be killed with antibiotics—the damage caused by long-term infection is permanent.

There are three major stages of syphilis, which present with unique symptoms: primary, secondary, and tertiary.

Primary syphilis, the first disease stage, usually occurs in about three weeks but can occur as long as 12 weeks after sexual contact with an infected individual. Usually the first symptom is an open sore, called a chancre, at the site of sexual contact. Only a small number of women who develop a chancre know it because this sore is often located deep inside the vagina. The chancre is usually painless regardless of its location, despite its appearance. The chancre heals and disappears without scarring within two to six weeks, whether or not the individual receives treatment. A few people may experience dormancy of the bacterial infection at this point and never be affected by it again.

The course of *secondary syphilis* is also variable and occurs within one week to six months after primary syphilis. There are a variety of secondary-stage symptoms, most notably a rash on the palms of the hands and soles of the feet. This rash often appears on the external genitals as well and may develop into open sores. Other symptoms during the secondary stage include a fever; flulike symptoms; sore mouth and throat; joint pain; loss of appetite; nausea; headache; and inflamed, sensitive eyes. Some individuals lose hair from their scalp in patches. Condylomata (broad-based moist sores) may appear around the genital and anal areas. Individuals are highly infectious in the secondary stage of syphilis. Symptoms usually last three to six months but may reappear and then disappear again for several years. This latent phase of syphilis may be temporary or permanent.

A few people progress to the most dangerous phase, *tertiary syphilis.* Tertiary syphilis may produce gummas (a kind of soft tumor), in addition to vascular, ophthalmologic, and neurologic sequelae. Tertiary syphilis symptoms appear 10 to 20 years after initial exposure if the individual has not received treatment. They may include heart disease, nerve and brain damage, spinal cord damage, blindness, and death.

Syphilis can pass from an infected woman to her developing fetus. Early screening and treatment of pregnant women are essential to reduce the incidence of congenital syphilis. Untreated syphilis infection during pregnancy often results in miscarriage, stillbirth, or severe birth defects. Babies born with syphilis who survive may suffer from skin sores, rashes, swollen liver and spleen, jaundice, and anemia, and if they are untreated after birth, damage to the heart, brain, and eyes.

A diagnosis of syphilis is confirmed by identification of antibodies in a blood test, although the antibodies do not appear until six to seven weeks after exposure. Syphilis sores may be recognized during a physical examination and may help in identifying the stage of the disease. The syphilis organism sometimes may be visualized with dark-field microscopy from sore secretions.

High doses of antibiotics are prescribed for early-stage syphilis. More prolonged, intensive treatment is indicated if the individual has been infected for a year or longer. Although antibiotics can stop the course of syphilis progression, they cannot undo its damage. For all stages of syphilis, sexual partner(s) must be concurrently treated.

Special Precautions

Syphilis is a highly infectious, destructive disease. Preventive measures for this STD are similar to those for other STDs (see "Informed Decision Making: Reproductive Tract Infections"). As noted earlier, a woman infected with syphilis and her sexual partner(s) should be treated at the same time. Both should avoid intercourse and all sexual intimacy for at least a month until repeat blood tests indicate that the treatments have been effective. Effective treatment and follow-up in the primary and secondary stages of the disease can prevent further serious, permanent damage.

Hepatitis

Hepatitis, an inflammation of the liver, is caused by infection with one of several viruses—type A, B, C, D, E, F, or G. Although hepatitis A, B, and C may be transmitted via sexual intimacy, hepatitis B is the only infection transmitted primarily through sexual contact.

Hepatitis A is usually a mild illness that resolves within a few weeks. It primarily affects young adults and children and usually spreads through consumption of contaminated food or water. It also may be spread through exposure to fecal matter of an infected person. A common source of hepatitis A is uncooked shellfish from contaminated waters. Sexual oral–anal contact is another mode of transmission. A two-shot vaccine can provide lifetime immunity to hepatitis A.

Hepatitis B is spread mainly by sexual contact, although it is also transmitted via needle sharing among intravenous drug users and accidental needle-sticks or contaminated surgical instruments among healthcare workers. Hepatitis B has the distinction of being the one STD that is entirely preventable; a three-shot series can provide lifetime immunity to heptatis B.[25] In the past, hepatitis B was often transmitted via contaminated blood. Thanks to today's more sensitive laboratory tests, transmission via this route is now rare.

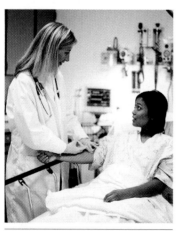

▪ Both hepatitis A and B can be prevented with immunization.

Hepatitis B symptoms range from nonexistent to severe incapacitation. Those who do have symptoms often experience low-grade fever, fatigue, headache, generalized aches, loss of appetite, nausea and vomiting, abdominal pain, and **jaundice**. Liver failure is a severe complication of hepatitis B. Another serious complication is persistent infection, which can occur with no apparent symptoms (called a carrier state) and can lead to chronic liver disease, resulting in permanent liver scarring and liver failure. Hepatitis B infected approximately 73,000 individuals in the United States in 2003.[25] It is also a common infection in Africa and Southeast Asia.

Hepatitis C is the most common cause of chronic liver disease in the United States.[26] It is mostly transmitted through contact with infected blood, intravenous drug use, or contaminated blood transfusion. Sexual transmission accounts for 10% to 15% of hepatitis C infections, but this route is most likely to occur when there is possible exposure to blood in addition to sexual fluids.[26] Transmission rates from mother to child during pregnancy are about 4%.[27] Most people with hepatitis C will go on to have chronic infections, and some may die from severe liver complications.

Diagnosis of hepatitis is based on clinical symptoms and laboratory blood tests, which confirm the type of virus involved. Diagnosis is often difficult because any form of hepatitis can be present without symptoms. There is no cure for hepatitis. Symptoms are treated, and rest and supportive care are recommended. A healthy diet is important, and alcohol should be avoided until liver function tests indicate that the liver is functioning normally. Women on estrogen therapy, either birth control pills or replacement therapy, should discontinue these medications until normal liver function returns.

Although most individuals with hepatitis recover within a few weeks, 10% to 30% of infected individuals develop a persistent hepatitis infection, either with or without symptoms. Chronic hepatitis may lead to severe liver impairment and is associated with the later development of liver cancer. Chronic infections may be treated with alpha-interferon to relieve symptoms and improve liver function; unfortunately, this treatment regime is expensive, may cause severe side effects, and in the majority of cases is not effective in eliminating infection.

Special Precautions

Under most circumstances, B is the only type of hepatitis that is transmitted sexually. Individuals need to take the same precautions against infection with hepatitis as other viral STDs.

A unique feature of hepatitis is that both hepatitis A and B may be prevented by vaccination or treatment with immune globulin within two weeks of exposure. The vaccine actually prevents infection with three forms of hepatitis, since hepatitis D is a defective virus that requires co-infection of heptatitis B to survive. Immune globulin is made from pooled antibodies taken from blood donations, and it provides a temporary passive immune effect. The vaccination consists of a three-injection series that must be given in a six-month period and provides long-term

It's Your Health

Individuals Who Should Be Vaccinated for Hepatitis A

People traveling to certain countries where hepatitis A is common (e.g., Africa, Asia)

People engaging in anal-oral sex

Intravenous drug users

Daycare and institutional workers

People with chronic liver problems

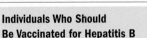

It's Your Health

Individuals Who Should Be Vaccinated for Hepatitis B

Healthcare workers who come in contact with blood or other bodily fluids

Household contacts of a person infected with hepatitis B

Sexual partner(s) of a person infected with hepatitis B

Individuals with multiple sexual partners

Staff and clients of residential institutions, including prisons

Individuals receiving hemodialysis or blood products

Intravenous drug users

Individuals with recent sexually transmitted diseases

Infants born in the United States

immunity. Vaccination is expensive but is recommended for groups who are at higher risk for exposure to the virus.

Sexual partners of infected individuals, pregnant women with hepatitis B (to prevent transmission to the fetus), a newborn baby of an infected mother, and household contacts of an individual with hepatitis A or B should receive immune globulin for hepatitis A and B. If the infected person is a member of an institutional facility, such as a daycare center, prison, or nursing home, staff and fellow clients should also receive immune globulin.

Vaginitis

Several kinds of vaginal infections can be transmitted through sexual interaction. Because they may be frequently transmitted through nonsexual means, however, they are not generally referred to as STDs. *Trichomonas* infection, yeast infections, and bacterial vaginosis are fairly common reproductive tract infections. Although they are responsible for physical and emotional discomfort, they do not pose long-term health problems among otherwise healthy women.

Trichomoniasis

Trichomonas infection is caused by a one-celled protozoan and is usually transmitted between individuals via sexual contact. The infectious organism is, however, capable of surviving outside a human host in a wet environment, such as on a swimsuit or wet towel, and transmission between individuals can occur via these objects.

Some women do not experience any symptoms with **trichomoniasis**. When symptoms do occur, they typically include a frothy, thin, grayish or greenish vaginal discharge; intense vaginal itching; an objectionable odor; pain during urination and intercourse; and urinary frequency. Diagnosis of *Trichomonas* infection is confirmed with a wet smear of vaginal secretions.

Metronidazole (Flagyl, Metryl, Protostat, Satric) is the most effective antibiotic treatment for *Trichomonas* infection and is available in either a single-dose or multiple-dose format. Because many women and most men infected with *Trichomonas* do not experience symptoms, sexual partners should be treated at the same time, and condoms should be used for the first four to six weeks after treatment to avoid reinfection. Recurrent infections are common with trichomoniasis in pregnant women. This disease may result in premature rupture of membranes, preterm delivery, low birthweight, or a genital or lung infection in the newborn.

Yeast Infections

Yeast organisms (also known as *Candida albicans,* fungus infection, monilia, and candidiasis) normally exist in the microscopic ecosystem of a woman's body. Yeast is usually not sexually transmitted. When yeast overgrows, however, the symptoms are quite annoying. A thick, white, cottage cheese-type vaginal discharge, redness, swelling, and itching are common symptoms. Diagnosis is gen-

---

It's Your Health

Tips for Avoiding Vaginal Infections

Wipe from front to back to avoid bacteria from the rectum entering the vagina.

Avoid sexual contact with someone who has a sexually transmitted disease.

Wear cotton underwear; avoid tight or wet garments for extended periods of time.

Avoid irritating substances, such as bubble baths, harsh soaps, feminine hygiene sprays, douches, and deodorant tampons.

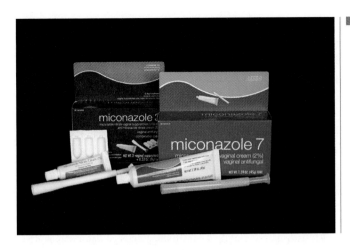

■ Yeast infections can be treated with many products that are available over the counter.

erally made by microscopic examination of a sample of the vaginal discharge. If yeast is not apparent but symptoms point to a yeast infection, a culture may be performed.

Yeast infections are usually treated with antibiotic vaginal cream (Monistat, Gyne-Lotrimin, Vagistat, Femstat) with dosage regimens of one, three, or seven days, depending on the medication. Treatment of partners is usually unnecessary. FDA approval has made these medications available in over-the-counter forms. For women with chronic and recurrent infections, this has facilitated treatment by reducing the waiting time for a prescription and the expense of a clinical visit. For women who are not sure what type or kind of vaginal infection they may have, self-treatment is not a good idea. Although some groups advocate treatments such as yogurt douches, commercial douches, *Lactobacillus* capsules, and cranberry juice, these regimens have not been subjected to clinical trials, and their efficacy is unknown.

Although yeast infections do not usually invade the pelvis and affect fertility, reinfection is common and annoying. Recurrent attacks may occur shortly after treatment or be delayed for a considerable period of time. What causes yeast to grow out of control is unknown. Yeast is a ubiquitous inhabitant of intestinal and vaginal tracts. Persistent yeast problems often present during pregnancy and in women who take oral contraceptives. Women with diabetes and women who are overweight also report higher frequencies of such infections. For women with recurrent infections, prolonged or intermittent treatment is often recommended to keep yeast growth under control. Concurrent treatment for yeast whenever antibiotics are prescribed may also help women with chronic yeast infections.

Bacterial Vaginosis

Bacterial vaginosis (BV) is known by many terms, including nonspecific vaginitis, *Gardnerella vaginalis*, bacterial vaginitis, *Haemophilus vaginalis*, *Corynebacterium vaginalis*, and anaerobic vaginosis. This condition is caused by an overgrowth of several species of vaginal organisms, which may be transmitted by sexual activity.[28] Bacterial vaginosis is considered a sexually associated condition but not necessarily a sexually transmitted disease. Although BV does not usually cause complications on its own, it is considered to be a co-factor in the acquisition of other sexually transmitted diseases, including HIV.[29] BV is more prevalent among women with more than one sexual partner, intrauterine device (IUD) users, and women who have cervicitis.

The most common cause of abnormal vaginal discharge, BV is very common, usually detected in 10% to 40% of women worldwide.[30] Symptoms include a gray or white frothy discharge that may be thick or watery and that may have an objectionable odor. Painful urination, vaginal pain or burning during intercourse, redness, and itching may also be present.

While many women complain of vaginal odor, discharge, or irritation, as many as 50% of women with BV may be asymptomatic; thus, routine screening is recommended whenever STD testing is indicated.[2] Identifying bacterial vaginosis is relatively straightforward. Diagnosis may be made with microscopic examination of a discharge sample or a wet mount of vaginal cells. Recent studies have shown that pregnant women with bacterial vaginosis have an increased risk of delivering preterm, low-birthweight infants. Bacterial vaginosis may coexist with other STDs and has been identified as a possible factor in HIV transmission. Because BV also may be associated with PID, definitive diagnosis is important to ensure adequate treatment.

Recommended treatment regimens include both oral and vaginal metronidazole and vaginal clindamycin. The vaginal treatment regimen is associated with fewer gastrointestinal side effects than the oral regimen.[2] Treatment of sexual partners is not standard procedure, although it may be indicated if reinfection occurs after treatment or if sexual transmission is suspected as the mode of acquisition. Topical treatments such as metronidazole gel and clindamycin cream may be effective for relieving symptoms.

One activity that can increase a woman's risk of bacterial vaginosis is regular douching. Douching may harm the vaginal flora and can increase the risk for bacterial vaginosis as well as other infections.[31]

Informed Decision Making: Reproductive Tract Infections

Joe had a long-term relationship with this girl, and they broke up last year. I used to worry about that relationship, but now I am more worried about the insignificant encounters he had after they broke up. He doesn't know anything about them, and neither do I. How do I evaluate my risk?

23-year-old woman

When a woman elects to become sexually active, she assumes responsibility for her decision. This responsibility extends beyond the pregnancy protection arena to include STD protection. A strong knowledge base is the first step in STD protection. Every woman should have a thorough understanding of STD risk, symptoms to watch for, and prevention strategies. An ounce of prevention is worth far more than a pound of cure in this case, because many STDs are incurable.

Apart from abstinence, the most reliable prevention strategy for reproductive tract infections is long-term mutual monogamy with a single partner. The most significant risk factor for any STD is the woman's partner(s). The risk of contracting an STD increases when a woman has more than one sex partner and when her partner has more than one sex partner. STDs should be considered a possibility whenever a woman is not in a strictly exclusive monogamous long-term relationship.

STDs are transmitted by sexual intimacy. Intimacy includes "traditional" sex (penis in vagina) and other forms of intimate skin-to-skin and mucous membrane-to-mucous membrane contact. These diseases can, therefore, be transmitted with oral or anal sex. STDs can be transmitted in both homosexual and heterosexual encounters, although many STDs are less common among lesbian women. Although the notion of safe sex is misleading, safer sex practices do exist that reduce the overall risk of acquiring an STD. Table 7.3 provides a comparison of safer, risky, and dangerous sex practices.

Birth control choice influences STD risk. Consistent and correct use of latex condoms can reduce the risk of STD transmission.[32]

HIV and many other STDs are spread when blood or sexual fluids from one person get into the mucous membranes (areas of the body not covered by skin, such as the interior of the vagina, the tip of the penis, or even cuts or nicks in the skin) of another person. While latex condoms are effective at preventing fluid exchange, they probably provide less protection for STDs that have other modes of transmission. Herpes and HPV, for example, are spread by contact with symptoms or infected genital skin. Because a condom covers some but not all of the potentially infectious area, it is not a reliable means of protection against these STDs. Some practices are more risky for contracting some STDs than for others. A person is extremely unlikely to get HIV from receiving oral sex even without a condom, for

I felt weird when Karen insisted that we go to the doctor together before we had sex. I guess I was afraid that one of us would have something. But we didn't and, you know, I think that our relationship is stronger because she insisted. I respect her for having the courage it took to do that. I wish that it had been my idea.

22-year-old man

Table 7.3   Some Sexual Activities and Their Relative Risk Levels

Activity	Level of Risk	Ways to Reduce Risk
Anal intercourse without a condom	High	Use a latex condom; only have sex with a mutually monogamous, tested partner
Vaginal intercourse without a condom	High	Use a latex condom; only have sex with a mutually monogamous, tested partner
Oral sex	High, though less risky than vaginal or anal intercourse for several STDs, including HIV	Use a latex condom for oral sex with a man or a dental dam or other moisture barrier for oral sex with a woman; only have sex with a mutually monogamous, tested partner
Mutual masturbation (hand-to-genital contact)	Very low, assuming no visible symptoms or cuts in the skin are present	Refrain from activity when there are symptoms or cuts in the skin
Kissing, no sores or broken skin	Very low; slight risk of oral herpes or syphilis infection	Refrain from kissing when possible symptoms are present
All sexual activities with a mutually monogamous partner who is free from infection	None, assuming partner is truly negative	Make sure partner has been tested for *all* STDs and is trustworthy
Abstaining from all sexual contact	None	

Source: Alexander, W. (2006). Summarized from several Centers for Disease Control and national STD and AIDS hotline sources.

example, but could easily get syphillis, an oral gonorrhea infection, or herpes in this way.

Spermicides may provide some additional protection from the viruses that cause herpes, genital warts, and AIDS. There are no guarantees, however; viruses located at sites other than the penis, such as the scrotum, anal region, vulva, or inner thighs, are not affected by spermicides or covered by condoms, and transmission from these sites can still occur.

Frank, honest communication before sexual intimacy is essential. Although it may be difficult to have an honest discussion about infections and previous risk behaviors, the price of not communicating can be high. Honest communication is a mark of personal maturity. If a potential partner is unable or unwilling to discuss infections and intimacy concerns, it may be an indication of other issues that merit evaluation before proceeding with sexual closeness. Sexual closeness should be avoided if either partner has any symptoms of infection or if there are any suspicions of infection. Delaying activity for a few days and having symptoms evaluated may prevent lifelong consequences. Because many people with STDs honestly do not know they are infected, many couples now see a clinician together for examination and STD testing before initiating a sexual relationship.

Communicating about incurable STDs such as herpes and HPV is especially difficult. The timing of communication is important—waiting until after sex to tell someone about a herpes infection may understandably upset a partner. But because of the stigma of the disease, a person with herpes may want to wait until some level of trust has been established before informing a potential sex partner. Being calm and knowledgeable about an infection also aids in communication. Many people are ignorant about the course of infection of STDs or the means by which they are spread. Open and frank discussion benefits both partners; studies have found that sharing a herpes diagnosis with a supportive spouse or lover and avoiding denial as a coping mechanism help people with herpes come to better and healthier terms with their infections.

When to See a Clinician

STDs present special clinical challenges for women. As noted earlier, symptoms may be present, absent, or mistaken for other conditions. There are several critical times when a woman should seek assistance in evaluating a possible reproductive tract infection. If a woman suspects that she *may* have an infection, she should be evaluated. STDs can be accompanied by a spectrum of symptoms or no symptoms. Waiting for symptoms to go away is an exercise in futility, because although some symptoms may temporarily disappear, the disease may still be present, transmissible, and damaging.

If a partner has an infection or is suspicious of an infection, it is important to curtail sexual activity, and both individuals should seek clinical evaluation. Treating one partner and not the other often results in a "ping-pong" reinfection process. In addition, sharing one antibiotic prescription between two people usually means that neither partner receives adequate treatment. Using leftover antibiotics from previous infections is equally foolhardy because supplies are usually inappropriate and inadequate, and may serve merely to mask the symptoms, complicating an accurate diagnosis later. Sexual activity should be curtailed or condoms diligently used until both partners are certain of an STD cure.

Women are often embarrassed to mention their fears about STDs to a clinician. If there is a risk of infection, it is important to mention this possibility. Although no woman wants to find out that she has an STD, it is always better to know than not to know: STDs can be spread and do serious biological damage even in the absence of symptoms, and all STDs are treatable, if not curable. Clinicians may not routinely test for STDs or look for them in a routine gynecological examination. If a woman knows she has an infectious condition such as HSV or HPV, she should advise her clinician to reduce the likelihood of accidental transmission to the clinician. If oral or anal sex has been part of a woman's sexual experience, the clinician should be advised so that a comprehensive examination may be conducted for an accurate diagnosis. A clean bill of health from a gynecologist is not of much value if an undiagnosed gonococcal throat infection is present. Finally, it helps to be prepared. Writing down a list of questions to ask a clinician and practicing questions to ask with a friend beforehand are two strategies women can use to make sure they get all the information they need without making additional visits.

A physical examination for STDs is often like a routine gynecological examination, but it is not limited to the genital area. An examination of the mouth, throat, and lymph nodes usually precedes the genital examination. The genital examination is conducted in a lithotomy position, which requires that the woman lie on her back with her legs spread and positioned in stirrups. This position enables the healthcare provider to examine the perineal area. The examination begins with a careful visual inspection by the clinician. A speculum is inserted into the vagina for an internal examination. The clinician then examines the vagina for discharge, odor, ulcerations, or inflammation. If a woman has douched before the visit, the clinician may not be able to diagnose the condition accurately. A bimanual examination follows the

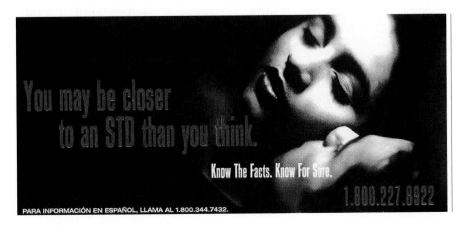

Honest communication before sexual intimacy is essential for assessing risk behaviors and avoiding transmission of disease. Reprinted with permission from the American Social Health Association.

internal examination (see Chapter 4 for details of the gynecological examination). Any suspicious lesion in the perineal area is cultured, and a rectal culture is obtained if the woman has had anal intercourse.

Treatment Concerns

Treatment regimens for STDs vary according to the specific pathogen involved, severity of infection, location of infection, previous infections, and personal medical history. A woman should inform her clinician if she is taking any prescriptions or over-the-counter medications. Previous drug reactions also constitute important information, because any previous reaction to a drug ending in "cillin" is a contraindication to any other "cillin" drug. If a woman suspects that she may be pregnant, it is important to advise the clinician of that possibility as well. Tetracycline should not be taken by pregnant women because it produces severe staining of the permanent teeth of the developing fetus. Sulfa drugs, acyclovir, lindane, and Flagyl (metronidazole) also should be avoided by pregnant women.

It is of paramount importance that prescribed medications be taken as recommended. If antibiotics are prescribed for 10 days, then they need to be taken for 10 days, even if symptoms dissipate earlier.

Several STDs require follow-up examinations to ensure that the treatment regimen was successful. Failure to comply with follow-up guidelines may result in unsuccessful treatment and continued disease transmission and damage. Because reproductive tract infections may cause abnormal Pap test findings, after an infection has cleared up, it is a good idea to have a Pap test repeated in six to 12 weeks. A reading at that time will give a more accurate report of the cervical status than one conducted during a period of inflammation.

AIDS

AIDS (acquired immunodeficiency syndrome), a progressive disease caused by **HIV (human immunodeficiency virus),** is characterized by the destruction of the immune system. There are no constant, specific symptoms associated with this condition, and no effective cure or vaccine is available. The best way to stop HIV is to prevent infection. HIV is no longer an automatic death sentence, however, as recent therapeutic advances have enabled people infected with HIV to live longer, fuller lives.

HIV is a **retrovirus**, a virus that incorporates its genetic material into the genome of the cell it attacks. When HIV, also known as the AIDS virus, enters the bloodstream, it attacks specific white blood cells called CD4 or T lymphocytes. The virus also replicates. The CD4 cells are no longer able to stimulate a cellular defense response, and the body's systemic immune system is compromised. The number of CD4 cells in an infected person's body decreases as the number of HIV-infected cells increases. AIDS is the final stage of HIV; it is diagnosed when the person has a positive test for antibodies to HIV and a low T lymphocyte count. An

HIV-positive person also may be diagnosed with AIDS when one of 26 known infections, called opportunistic infections, is present. Opportunistic infections present a potentially fatal risk to individuals with AIDS.

HIV is transmitted from one person to another through sexual intercourse, shared intravenous needle use, or contaminated blood or blood products. HIV is not spread by casual, social, or family contact. Although HIV is a sophisticated and elusive killer within the body, the virus quickly dies when exposed to the open air; unbroken human skin actually provides excellent protection from HIV. One cannot acquire the virus by touching or being near a person with AIDS. An individual with HIV may have no physical symptoms, so it is impossible to tell whether a person is infected just by looking at him or her. HIV-infected individuals are capable of transmitting the virus to others, however, even in the absence of symptoms. The HIV incubation period ranges from a few months to several years or more. As evidenced by revelations from Hollywood and the national sports scene, no individual or groups of individuals are immune to HIV/AIDS.

Perspectives on AIDS

Historical Overview

Although the history of AIDS is relatively short, the human toll exacted by the disease cannot be calculated. It is not known for sure when or where AIDS started, although some experts have speculated that the disease originated in Africa in the 1970s. AIDS was first diagnosed in the United States in 1981.

One myth associated with this disease is that AIDS is a homosexual disease. In reality, anyone who engages in risky sexual behavior or intravenous drug use behaviors—whether homosexual, bisexual, or heterosexual—is susceptible to HIV.

Men who have sex with men still constitute a disproportionate percentage of people infected with HIV, accounting for 63% of all the new cases diagnosed in 2003.[33] However, this does not mean that homosexual men are doomed to get HIV or that other population groups are safe. HIV epidemics in other countries have been spread primarily by intravenous drug users or heterosexual sex. An even further complicating factor is that, like many intravenous drug users, many men who have sex with men hide or deny their risky behaviors and pose as non-injecting, straight men.[33]

The CDC estimates that HIV infects about 40,000 people in the United States per year.[34] Three-quarters of American women with HIV acquire their infections through heterosexual sex; almost all of the rest acquire it through intravenous drug use. Minority women, especially African American women, bear a heavy HIV disease burden: African American women are more than 12 times as likely to have HIV as their white counterparts.[33]

The number of people living with HIV in the United States reached 1 million for the first time in 2003.[34] This milestone reflects the successes and the failures of the fight against AIDS in the United States. On the one hand, advances in antiretroviral treatment mean that people are living longer with HIV and therefore

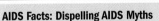

It's Your Health

AIDS Facts: Dispelling AIDS Myths

AIDS is not a disease of homosexual men.

Women are susceptible to AIDS.

AIDS may not be spread by casual contact.

AIDS cannot be transmitted to humans from insects.

There is no risk of acquiring AIDS by donating blood.

Information and education are the best weapons against AIDS.

Confidential, anonymous testing for AIDS is available.

dying less rapidly. On the other hand, stagnating prevention efforts have not been nearly as effective as they were in the 1980s and early 1990s. The number of people newly infected with HIV has remained stable for more than a decade.

Global Perspective

The joint United Nations Programme on HIV/AIDS estimates that more than 40 million people—95% of whom live in developing countries—are living with HIV. Globally, 46% of all people living with HIV in 2005 were women. More than 3 million people died of AIDS in 2005; nearly 600,000 of these deaths were children.

This global epidemic has hit sub-Saharan Africa the hardest. Even though sub-Saharan Africa contains only 10% of the world's population, it is home to 60% of the total number of people living with HIV. One out of every 14 people living in the area has HIV. The main factor preventing this number from growing even higher is the spiraling number of deaths from AIDS. Estimates of deaths and people infected reveal only a small part of this grim picture, however. More than 30 million children have lost their parents to AIDS, and sickness and death among the generation of young adults may cripple many economies for decades.[33]

Sub-Saharan Africa is not the only region affected by AIDS. Many countries in Southeast Asia are on the cusp of potentially explosive AIDS epidemics. Despite these bleak statistics, no country is entirely without hope. Studies have shown that HIV transmission can be dramatically reduced with intensive and long-term prevention efforts. Establishing and maintaining effective programs to manage AIDS in developing countries, however, will undoubtedly be one of the most difficult challenges of the twenty-first century.

Epidemiological Data and Trends

AIDS in women presents a different epidemiological pattern than that found among men. Women did not constitute a sizable proportion of the total number of HIV cases in the United States until several years into the AIDS epidemic, but this number has since grown. In 1992, women accounted for 13.8% of people infected with HIV; by 1998, they represented 20% of this total. Recently this proportion appears to have stabilized at 25%.[35] Women infected with AIDS are more likely to be living in the Northeast or the South.[35] Figure 7.7 shows AIDS cases by region and race/ethnicity in the United States. Most HIV-infected women acquire the virus through heterosexual transmission, as shown in Figure 7.8. Nearly 20% of newly reported women's HIV cases are the result of injection drug use.

Despite these alarming numbers, the epidemiological data on HIV/AIDS among women probably underrepresent the true magnitude of the disease. The CDC had initially identified criteria for AIDS diagnosis based on symptoms in male populations who contracted AIDS via homosexual contact or intravenous drug use. HIV-infected women often develop serious gynecological problems that are HIV-related, but because their problems did not meet the original CDC criteria, these individuals were not diagnosed with AIDS. Later, the diagnostic criteria were modified to address the gynecological symptoms consistent with the clinical picture of AIDS in

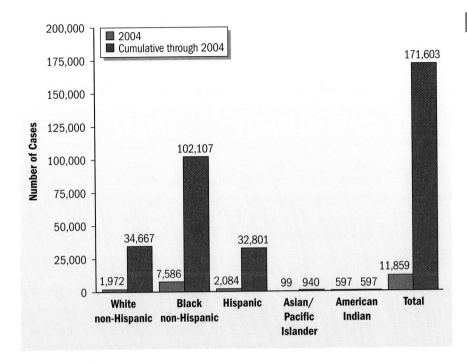

Figure 7.7

Reported AIDS cases in female adults and adolescents, United States.

Source: Centers for Disease Control and Prevention. (2005). *HIV/AIDS Surveillance Report, 2004. Vol. 16.* Atlanta: U.S. Department of Health and Human Services, Centers for Disease Control and Prevention. Retrieved January 4, 2006, from http://www.cdc.gov/hiv/stats/hasrlink.htm.

women. Today information on the HIV disease process in women and appropriate treatment regimens remains scarce. Women have more recently been included in HIV/AIDS clinical trials, but they still lack equal representation.

Special Concerns for Women

Today women are finally being recognized as an at-risk, HIV-susceptible population. The initial focus on male homosexuality as a risk factor is one reason for the delay in acknowledging their vulnerability. In North America and Western Europe,

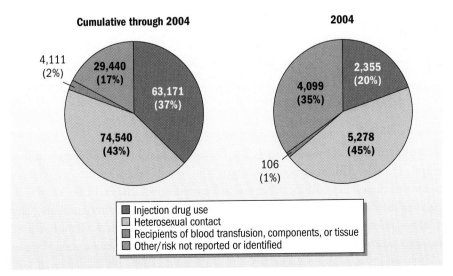

Figure 7.8

Reported AIDS cases in women by exposure category, United States. Because people typically develop AIDS years after infection, current AIDS diagnoses actually represent trends in HIV infection from several years ago.

Source: Centers for Disease Control and Prevention. (2005). *HIV/AIDS Surveillance Report, 2004. Vol. 16.* Atlanta: U.S. Department of Health and Human Services, Centers for Disease Control and Prevention. Retrieved January 4, 2006, from http://www.cdc.gov/hiv/stats/hasrlink.htm.

where the primary modes of HIV transmission had traditionally been homosexual and bisexual contact and intravenous drug use, the threat posed by heterosexual contact had been largely disregarded. In addition, women are more likely to develop AIDS and die at higher CD4 cell counts than men, which may explain why women experience a delay in receiving treatment relative to men. Also, women experience more rapid declines in CD4 cell counts over time than do men.

The frequency of HIV/AIDS transmission continues to increase in women. Heterosexual women are far more likely to contract HIV from a man than a man is to contract the infection from a woman. This difference in part reflects a woman's exposure to a greater quantity of secretions that are possibly carrying the virus (i.e., semen) and the greater mucosal surface area of the vagina and cervix in which infection can occur. In addition, women are likely to experience small tears in the vaginal lining during intercourse, increasing their susceptibility to infection by HIV-positive semen.

Women who partner with women are not free from risk, however. Many women who consider themselves lesbians have had heterosexual intercourse and may have received HIV through that avenue without knowing it. And while woman-to-woman sexual contact does appear to be less risky for transmission of HIV, many other STDs, such as herpes, chlamydia, or syphilis, may be easily spread that way.

Failure to focus on women as unique high-risk group for HIV has created significant obstacles in diagnosis, prevention, and treatment. As a consequence, women may be subject to delayed recognition of symptoms, diagnosis, and treatment. In the United States, women are more likely to die from AIDS than men; however, when both groups have equal access to health care, no differences in rates of survival are expected.

Since 1985, the proportion of all AIDS cases involving adult and adolescent women has more than tripled, from 7% in 1985 to 23% in 2004. The epidemic has increased most dramatically among women of color. African American women are 12 times more likely than white women to be infected with HIV. Hispanic women are also disproportionately more likely to be infected, albeit not as dramatically.[36] In 2001, HIV infection was the leading cause of death for African American women aged 25–34 years and was among the four leading causes of death for African American women aged 20–24 and 35–44 years, as well as Hispanic women aged 35–44 years.[37]

Social Issues

African American women with HIV face the dual burden of being neither white nor male. African American women who have HIV are less likely to recieve treatment than other ethnic groups and are more likely to die early. Half the people who died of AIDS in 2003 were African American.[36] Class undoubtedly plays a large role in this disparity. Women who are economically deprived often have inadequate access to heatlhcare facilities and are more likely to be unhealthy in

Table 7.4   Basic Information about the Major Sexually Transmitted Diseases *(continued)*

Treatment:	Antibiotics will stop infection but may not be able to repair damage from long-term infection
Special Concerns for Women:	Pelvic inflammatory disease *(see PID)*, possible co-infection with gonorrhea, re-infection with an untreated partner, perinatal (mother to child) transmission
Potential Long-Term Consequences:	Infertility, ectopic pregnancy, chronic pelvic pain, possibility of systemic infection

HPV (Human Papillomavirus)

Organism:	Virus—human papillomavirus (almost 100 strains, about a dozen of which are sexually transmitted)
Transmission:	Genital skin-to-genital skin contact
Symptoms:	Some kinds of HPV can cause warts to appear on the external genital or anal areas; others may cause abnormal cell growth in the cervix
Diagnosis:	Warts may be diagnosed by physical examination; cervical dysplasia may be diagnosed with biopsy; DNA testing of the virus can identify the presence of HPV
Treatment:	Treatment for genital warts revolves around removing symptoms, not eliminating virus, and consists of topical caustic agents, electrocautery, cryotherapy, and laser surgery; abnormal cell changes in the cervic may be treated by cryotherapy, loop electrosurgical excision (LEEP), cone biopsy, or laser surgery.
Special Concerns for Women:	Cervical changes, if untreated, may develop into cervical cancer; warts may interfere with pregnancy in rare cases
Possible Long-Term Consequences:	Cervical growths can lead to cervical cancer if undiagnosed or untreated; most cases of HPV go away on their own eventually

Herpes Simplex Virus (HSV)

Organism:	Virus—herpes simplex (two types—1 and 2)
Transmission:	Direct contact with symptoms; contact with the infected area carries a low but real risk even without symptoms
Symptoms:	Possibly painful sores, blisters, or rashes on the genital area, rectum, or mouth that appear and disappear periodically; women are often asymptomatic or have symptoms in the cervical area that go unnoticed
Diagnosis:	Examination or culture of symptoms; blood tests can identify herpes antibodies
Treatment:	No cure or vaccine available; three antiviral medications (acyclovir, famvir, and valacyclovir) can reduce duration or number of outbreaks
Special Concerns for Women:	Possible perinatal transmission, especially if herpes infection takes place during pregnancy; herpes sores may increase likelihood of receiving HIV if exposed
Possible Long-Term Consequences:	Rare in otherwise healthy adults; severity, duration, and frequency of symptoms usually diminish over time

Hepatitis B (HBV)

Organism:	Virus—hepatitis B virus
Transmission:	Entrance of blood or sexual fluids into the body; most cases occur through unprotected sexual contact or shared needles
Symptoms:	Often asymptomatic; symptoms include nausea, fever, dark urine, jaundice (yellowing of the skin and eyes), and abdominal discomfort
Diagnosis:	Blood tests to identify virus or antibodies; liver tests and symptoms may also be used in diagnosis
Treatment:	No cure for hepatitis B exists, but antiviral medications may help in some chronic cases; a three-shot vaccine will prevent hepatitis B infection

Table 7.4 Basic Information about the Major Sexually Transmitted Diseases (continued)

Hepatitis B (HBV) (Continued)

Special Concerns for Women:	Perinatal transmission
Possible Long-Term Consequences:	Possible liver disease or liver cancer in chronic cases; most infections eventually resolve on their own

Trichomoniasis

Organism:	Single-celled protozoan—*Trichomonas vaginalis*
Transmission:	Direct sexual contact, less likely through contaminated wet objects (towels, swimming suits)
Symptoms:	Many women and most men are asymptomatic; symptoms may include white or greenish yellow discharge, vaginal itching, or painful urination
Diagnosis:	Examination of symptoms or culture of infected area
Treatment:	Oral antibiotics
Special Concerns for Women:	Re-infection from untreated or undertreated partners
Possible Long-Term Consequences:	Rare for otherwise healthy women

Pelvic Inflammatory Disease (PID)

Organism:	Bacteria—usually *Chlamydia trachomatis* (chlamydia) or *Neisseria gonorrhoeae* (gonorrhea)
Transmission:	PID itself is not transmitted but usually develops as a complication of gonorrhea or chlamydia
Symptoms:	Cases may be asymptomatic; abdominal pain or pain during intercourse, unusual vaginal discharge or bleeding, fever, and nausea
Diagnosis:	Clinical evaluation based on symptoms and possible presence of a causative bacterial agent
Treatment:	Antibiotics; surgery may be necessary in advanced cases
Special Concerns for Women:	Re-infection of bacterial infection from untreated or undertreated partners; possible perinatal transmission of bacterial agent
Possible Long-Term Consequences:	Infertility, ectopic pregnancy, recurrent infection, chronic pelvic pain

■ ■ ■ ■ ■

Web Sites

AIDS Education Global Information System: http://www.aegis.com

American Social Health Association: http://www.ashastd.org

Centers for Disease Control, Division of STDs: http://www.cdc.gov/STD

EngenderHealth: http://www.engenderhealth.org

Hepatitis Foundation International: http://www.hepfi.org

HIVandHepatitis.com: http://www.hepatitisandhiv.com

International Herpes Alliance: http://www.herpesalliance.org

Planned Parenthood: http://www.plannedparenthood.org

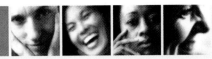

Profiles of Remarkable Women

Felicia Hance Stewart, M.D. (1943–2006)

Felicia Hance Stewart was an obstetrician/gynecologist who was also a distinguished clinician and researcher. She received her Bachelor of Arts degree at the University of California, Berkeley, her medical degree from Harvard Medical School, and postgraduate training at Cambridge City Hospital in Massachusetts and at the University of California San Francisco Medical Center. From 1973 to 1994, Stewart practiced at the Sutter Medical Group/Sutter Medical Foundation in Sacramento, California. She served as Director of Medical Research for the Sutter Medical Foundation and carried out numerous clinical studies focusing on contraceptive development. During this time, Stewart also worked as staff physician and Associate Medical Director at Planned Parenthood of the Sacramento Valley. In addition, she served as a member of the Technical Advisory Committee for the CONRAD (Contraceptive Research and Development Program) that oversees research funding in this field for the U.S. Agency for International Development.

Following her time as practicing physician, Stewart served as Deputy Assistant Secretary for Population Affairs in the Department of Health and Human Services, making her the most senior official in the United States responsible for domestic and international policies on family planning and population issues. In this position, she had direct responsibility for management of the National Family Planning Program (Title X) and the Adolescent Family Life Program (Title XX).

In 1996, Stewart was appointed the Director of Reproductive Health Programs for the Henry J. Kaiser Family Foundation, where she focused on improving services for low-income women and preventing unintended pregnancy. In 1999, she joined the Center for Reproductive Health Research and Policy at the University of California, San Francisco. As a Co-Director of the Center, Stewart conducted a wide range of U.S. and international projects that span the disciplines of contraception, abortion, and sexually transmitted diseases.

Stewart served as the principal investigator on many research projects and published numerous articles and textbooks on contraception and family planning. She contributed greatly to issues concerning reproductive health and, consequently, served on many national scientific and professional advisory and review committees. Stewart authored *Understanding Your Body: The Concerned Woman's Guide to Gynecology and Health,* a nontechnical reference book, and co-author of *Contraceptive Technology,* a professional reference for family planning. Stewart may be most remembered for her leading role in the research establishing that the emergency contraceptive known as "Plan B" is both safe and effective when sold without a physician's prescription. Her published research led to the availability of over-the-counter "Plan B" in a number of states, including California.

Sexuality Information and Education Council of the U.S.: http://www.siecus.org

The Body: An AIDS and HIV Information Resource: http://www.thebody.com

UNAIDS: http://www.unaids.org

References

1. Hanson, J., Posner, S., Hassig, S., and Farley, T. (2005) Assessment of sexually transmitted diseases as risk factors for HIV seroconversion in a New Orleans sexually transmitted disease clinic, 1990–1998. *Annals of Epidemiology* 15(1): 13–20.

2. U.S. Centers for Disease Control and Prevention. (2002). Sexually transmitted disease treatment guidelines. *Morbidity and Mortality Weekly Report* 51: 1–80.

3. U.S. Department of Health and Human Services. (2000). *Healthy People 2010* (second edition). With *Understanding and Improving Health and Objectives for Improving Health.* 2 vols. Washington, DC: U.S. Government Printing Office.

4. Weinstock, H., Berman, S., and Cates, W. (2004). Sexually transmitted diseases among American youth: incidence and prevalence estimates. *Perspectives on Sexual and Reproductive Health* 36(1): 6–10.

5. Rietmeijer, C. A., Van Bemmelen, R., Judson, F. N., and Douglas, J. M. (2002). Incidence and repeat infection rates of *Chlamydia trachomatis* infections among male and female patients in an STD clinic: implications for screening and rescreening. *Sexually Transmitted Diseases* 29: 65–72.

6. U.S. Preventive Services Task Force. (2001). Screening for chlamydia: recommendations and rationale. *American Journal of Medicine* 20(35): 90–94.

7. U.S. Centers for Disease Control and Prevention. (2004). Sexually transmitted disease surveillance 2004. Retrieved January 7, 2006, from http://www.cdc.gov/std/stats/natoverview.htm.

8. Hatcher, R. A., et al. (2004). *Contraceptive Technology* (18th edition). New York: Ardent Media.

9. Harrell, W., Chesson, J., Blandford, J., Thomas, L., Gift, G., and Irwin, K. (2004). The estimated direct medical cost of sexually transmitted disease among youth, 2000. *Perspectives on Sexual and Reproductive Health* 36(1): 11–19.

10. United Nations. (2004). Report on the Global AIDS Epidemic. UNAIDS. Retrieved January 9, 2006, from http://www.unaids.org/bangkok2004/report.html.

11. U.S. Centers for Disease Control and Prevention. (2004). Trends in reportable sexually transmitted diseases in the United States. Retrieved January 4, 2006, from http://www.cdc.gov/stats/trends2004.htmref1.

12. Adderley-Kelly, B., and Stephens, E. (2005). Chlamydia—a major threat to adolescents and young adults. *Association of Black Nursing Faculty* May/June: 52–55.

13. U.S. Centers for Disease Control and Prevention. (2005). PID fact sheet. Retrieved January 7, 2006, from http://www.cdc.gov/std/PID/STDFact-PID.htm.

14. U.S. Centers for Disease Control and Prevention. (2005). Sexually transmitted disease surveillance 2004. Retrieved January 4, 2006, from http://www.cdc.gov/std/stats/womenandinf3.htm#figh.

15. U.S. Centers for Disease Control and Prevention. (1999). Adolescents and sexually transmitted diseases. *STD Surveillance 1999, Special Profiles*, 51–55.

16. Rein, D. B., Kassler, W. J., Irwin, K. L., and Rabiee, L. (2000). Direct medical cost of pelvic inflammatory disease and its sequelae: decreasing but still substantial. *Obstetrics and Gynecology* 95: 397–402.

17. Sutton, M. Y., Sternberg, M., Zaidi, A., St. Louis, M. E., and Markowitz, L. E. (2005). Trends in pelvic inflammatory disease hospital discharges and ambulatory visits, United States, 1985–2001. *Sexually Transmitted Diseases* 32(12): 778–784.

18. Bosch, F. X., Lorincz, A., Munoz, N., Meijer, C. J. L. M., and Shah, V. V. (2002). The causal relation between human papillomavirus and cervical cancer. *Journal of Clinical Pathology* 55(4): 244–264.

19. Moscicki, A. B. (2005). Impact of HPV infection in adolescent populations. *Journal of Adolescent Health* 37(6 suppl): S3–9.

20. Schiffman, M., and Castle, P. E. (2005). The promise of global cervical-cancer prevention. *New England Journal of Medicine* 353(20): 2101–2104.

21. Henry J. Kaiser Family Foundation. (June 2003). *Sexually Transmitted Diseases in America Fact Sheet.*

22. Corey, L., Wald, A., Patel, R., et al. (2004). Once-daily valacyclovir to reduce the risk of transmission of genital herpes. *New England Journal of Medicine* 350: 11–20.

23. U.S. Centers for Disease Control and Prevention. (2002). *Sexually Transmitted Disease Treatment Guidelines.* Retrieved January 6, 2006, from: http://www.cdc.govSTD/treatment/2-2002TG.htm#GenitalHerpes.

24. Holmes, K., Levine, R., and Weaver, M. (2004). Effectiveness of condoms in preventing sexually transmitted diseases. *Bulletin of the World Health Organization* 82(6): 454–461.

25. U.S. Centers for Disease Control and Prevention. (2005). Hepatitis B fact sheet. Retrieved January 6, 2006, from http://www.cdc.gov/ncidod/diseases/hepatitis/b/fact.htm.

26. U.S. Centers for Disease Control and Prevention. (2001). *National Hepatitis C Prevention Strategy.* Retrieved January 6, 2006, from http://www.cdc.gov/nicdod/diseases/hepatitis/c/plan/HCV_infection.htm.

27. U.S. Centers for Disease Control and Prevention. (2005). Hepatitis C fact sheet. Retrieved January 6, 2006, from http://www.cdc.gov/ncidod/diseases/hepatitis/c/fact.htm.

28. Schwebke, J. R. and Desmond, R. (2005). Risk factors for bacterial vaginosis in women at high risk for sexually transmitted diseases. *Sexually Transmitted Diseases* 32(11): 654–658.

29. Myer, L., Kuhn, L., Stein, Z. A., Wright, T. C., and Denny, L. (2005). Intravaginal practices, bacterial vaginosis, and women's susceptibility to HIV infection: epidemiological evidence and biological mechanisms. *Lancet Infectious Diseases* 5(12): 786–794.

30. Klebanoff, M. A., Schwebke, J. R., Zhang, J., et al. (2004). Vulvo-vaginal symptoms in women with bacterial vaginosis. *Obstetrics and Gynecology* 104: 267.

31. Zhang, J., Hatch, M. C., Zhang, D., et al. (2004). Frequency of douching and risk of bacterial vaginosis in African-American women. *Obstetrics and Gynecology* 104: 756–760.

32. U.S. Centers for Disease Control and Prevention. (2001). Fact sheet for public health personnel: male latex condoms. Retrieved January 9, 2006, from http://www.cdc.gov/hiv/pubs/facts/condoms.htm.

33. United Nations and World Health Organization. (2005). UNAIDS/WHO AIDS epidemic update. Retrieved January 4, 2006, from http://www.unaids.org/epi2005/index.html.

34. U.S. Centers for Disease Control and Prevention. (2005). HIV prevalence, unrecognized infection and HIV testing among men who have sex with men—five U.S. cities, June 2004–April 2005. *Morbidity and Mortality Weekly Report* 54(24): 597–601.

35. U.S. Centers for Disease Control and Prevention. (2004). *HIV/AIDS Surveillance Report #15.* Retrieved January 9, 2006, from http://www/cdc.gov/hiv/stats/hasrlink.htm.

36. U.S. Centers for Disease Control and Prevention. (2004). *HIV/AIDS Surveillance Report #16.* Retrieved January 9, 2006, from http://www/cdc.gov/hiv/stats/hasrlink.htm.

37. Anderson, R.N., and Smith, B.L. (2003). Deaths: leading causes for 2001. *National Vital Statistics Reports* 52(9): 32–33, 53–54. Retrieved January 10, 2006, from http://www.cdc.gov/nchs/data/nvsr/nvsr52/nvsr52_09.pdf.

38. The Global Business Coalition on HIV/AIDS. (December 2002). *Policy Update: Global Summary of the HIV/AIDS Epidemic.*

39. U.S. Centers for Disease Control and Prevention. (2005). *OraQuick Rapid HIV Test for Oral Fluid—Frequently Asked Questions.* Retrieved January 4, 2006, from http://www.cdc.gov/hiv/rapid_testing/oralfluidquandafin1_1.htm.

40. Bunders, M., Bekker, V., Scherpbier, H., et al. (2005). Haematological parameters of HIV-1 uninfected infants born to HIV-1-infected mothers. *Acta Paediatrica* 94(11): 1571–1577.

Chapter Eight

Menopause and Hormone Replacement Therapy

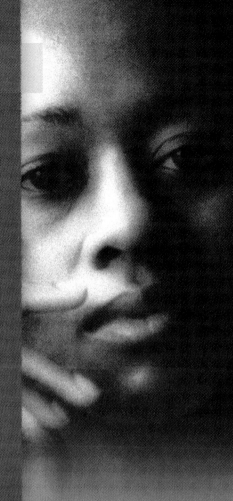

Chapter Objectives

On completion of this chapter, the student should be able to discuss:

1. The basic demographic aging trends in the United States.

2. The definition of menopause and the different stages that women go through before, during, and after menopause.

3. The ways in which cultural and societal attitudes about aging have influenced attitudes about menopause.

4. The positive effects that menopause can have in women's lives.

5. The basic biological sequence of events associated with menopause.

6. Health effects associated with menopause.

7. Hormone replacement therapy (HRT) as an option for menopause management.

8. Benefits of HRT for relieving symptoms associated with menopause.

9. Cardiovascular, osteoporotic, and neurological issues associated with HRT.

10. Other methods for managing menopause.

womenshealth.jbpub.com

Women's Health Online is a great source for supplementary women's health information for both students and instructors. Visit

http://womenshealth.jbpub.com

to find a variety of useful tools for learning, thinking, and teaching.

Introduction

Women today are living longer, and a growing proportion of the overall U.S. population consists of older adults. Nearly 13% of Americans are 65 or older; of those, more than half are women. By 2050, the U.S. Bureau of the Census estimates that nearly 21% of the population will be age 65 or older, with 55% of that group being female. This percentage represents a dramatic increase from 1900 (Figure 8.1). The most rapid population increase over the next decade will be among those age 85 and older. In 2000, this age group accounted for nearly 5 million people in the United States.[1]

Women, as they reach midlife, experience menopause. Consequently, as the aging trend continues, a higher proportion of women are experiencing or have experienced menopause. In 2000, an estimated 31.2 million American women were undergoing the transition into menopause.[2] The sheer size of this age group is profoundly influencing how society addresses a fundamental, natural facet of women's reproductive health. In particular, the once never discussed topic of menopause has gained recognition as a significant women's health issue. Menopause is now commonly recognized as a process that has a host of physical and emotional effects on women. This chapter provides an overview of both natural and surgically induced menopause, health effects of menopause, options for menopause management, and the controversy surrounding hormone replacement therapy.

Figure 8.1

Older population by age: 1900–2050.

Source: U.S. Bureau of the Census. Tables 42 and 45; Data for 1990 from 1990 Census of Population and Housing, Series CPH-L-74, Modified and Actual Age, Sex, Race, and Hispanic Origin Data. The 2000 data are from the 2000 Census. The figures for 2010 to 2050 are from NP-D1-A Census Projections issued January 13, 2000.

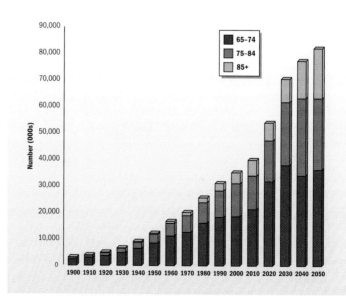

Perspectives on Menopause

Menopause has long been a source of confusion for women. The problems created by various myths and misinformation have been compounded, until recent years, by little coverage in lay or professional literature about this stage of life. Until relatively recently, menopause has been neglected as a research area. The paucity of research and interest in menopause cannot be blamed solely on historical neglect, however, because it is only since the turn of the century that the life expectancy of women has reached the point that took women into and beyond the age of menopause. Today most women will live a third or more of their lives postmenopausally.

In some non-Western cultures where women's status or role improves with age, aging and menopause are perceived as positive events. In the United States, women tend to be more concerned about aging. Menopause, also known as the "change of life," has traditionally been perceived as a difficult time for women during which they experience uncontrollable extreme moodiness, irritability, and depression. In the 1800s and early 1900s, popular stereotypes in the United States portrayed menopause as a major life tragedy that resulted in hypochondria, hysteria, and irritability. This view implied that solace to these conditions could be found only in a physician's office with pharmacological remedies or surgical intervention. In the 1940s and 1950s, "treatment" for menopause often focused on psychiatric conditions of depression and melancholy. The menopausal woman was portrayed as a burden to herself, to her family, and if she was married, to her suffering husband. In subsequent decades, menopause was examined as a "disease" entity because clinical concern focused on women reporting symptoms and seeking medical intervention.

Now menopause is being understood as a process of normal change. Open discussions about sexuality and life issues have fostered a foundation to continue delving into facets of menopause and aging without fear, embarrassment, or stigmatization. Many women, in contrast to the myths, either welcome or do not fear

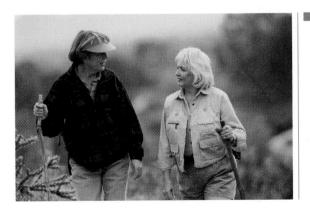

Women today are more open in their discussions about all aspects of their sexual well-being, including menopause.

menopause. The cessation of menses frees them from contraception concerns, in some cases leading to increased sexual satisfaction. Others appreciate the freedom from menstrual periods, which may have been inconvenient or uncomfortable. Social and cultural influences also have encouraged more positive attitudes toward menopause. Menopause may be a time of fewer obligations accompanied by increased opportunities in the workforce. This experience can be inviting and invigorating for women who are seeking added dimensions in their personal and professional lives. For some, this life stage is often more flexible in terms of leisure time and financial resources, increasing the opportunities for new forms of activity and self-expression. For others, it is merely the continuation of intense work, with many women taking on additional childcare responsibilities for grandchildren. In a study by the North American Menopause Society, more than half of postmenopausal women reported being happier and more fulfilled in their postmenopausal years as compared with earlier years.[3]

Economic and Global Dimensions

Attempts have been made to quantify the annual costs of menopause and its health repercussions. Findings suggest that total costs are approximately $2.2 billion, composed of the following elements:

- Urogenital tract health issues: $125 million
- Menopause and general physiological disturbances: $480 million
- Skeletal issues and osteoporosis: $540 million
- Cardiovascular and cerebral disease: $1.1 billion

These estimates are based on the combined indirect (e.g., disability, loss of productivity, and death) and direct costs (e.g., hospitalization, rehabilitation, and outpatient care) of menopause. In particular, the costs for elderly patients with urinary incontinence, mental disabilities, osteoporosis, and cardiovascular disease are all significant and lead to large socioeconomic challenges across the globe.

Until recently, a particularly strong economic factor associated with menopause was hormone replacement therapy (HRT). Over the 1998–2001 period, the HRT market grew from roughly $2.5 billion to $3.8 billion.[4] Of that amount,

- The United States accounted for $2.5 billion;
- Europe accounted for $900 million; and
- Latin America plus Canada accounted for approximately $300 million.

The vast majority of HRT is taken by women in more developed countries who have access to westernized pharmaceutical treatments. Women in less developed countries, especially those from very wealthy backgrounds, also had begun using HRT at growing rates. With the release of negative estrogen replacement therapy (ERT) and HRT study findings in 2002 and 2004, however, the use of these medications has declined sharply. Prevalence of HRT use varies significantly, however, even among more developed countries. For example, in 1999, 47% of eligible women took HRT in France, approximately 25% in the United States and Germany, 3% in Italy, and 2% in Japan.[4]

Menopause

Menopause refers to the cessation of regular menstrual periods. Also known as the climacterium or "change of life," it marks the end of menstruation and childbearing capability. Menopause can be considered to have four stages. **Premenopause** refers to the entirety of a woman's reproductive life—from first menstruation to menopause. This term is often mistakenly used interchangeably with **perimenopause**, the stage immediately prior to menopause, in which physical changes begin to accelerate and women are most likely to experience perceptible physical changes due to drops in hormone production. A woman is considered to be in menopause when she has gone through 12 months without menstruation. **Postmenopause** refers to life after the final menstrual period. In short, these stages describe the entirety of a woman's mature life in terms of her reproductive function. Although not a precise road map for menopause, they can provide important guideposts and markers for women as they age.

Most women enter and complete menopause between the ages of 45 and 55. Like the age of onset of a girl's first period, the age of onset of menopause varies widely. The average age of natural menopause—defined as one year without a menstrual period—is 51.[5] By age 58, 99% of women are postmenopausal.[6] The age at which a woman has her last period appears to be a result of many factors. Family history is one such factor. Increased body mass index and history of more than one pregnancy are linked to later menopause, whereas smoking and never being pregnant are related to earlier onset. Smokers generally experience menopause about two years earlier than nonsmoking women.

Natural Menopause

Natural menopause occurs when the ovaries begin to fail to respond to the luteinizing and follicle-stimulating hormones that are produced in the anterior pituitary, which is under the control of the hypothalamus. Although these hormones are still secreted into the bloodstream, the ovaries do not produce estrogen and progesterone in response. As a result, ovulation becomes somewhat erratic. The mechanisms underlying these changes are not well understood. Whatever the reasons, a woman beginning menopause will have more luteinizing and follicle-stimulating hormones present in the bloodstream and less estrogen and progesterone than she had during her regular cycling. For most women, menopause lasts from a few months to two or three years. Pregnancy remains a possibility because ovulation may occur in sporadic intervals during this time. Menopause is considered complete once monthly periods have ceased altogether for at least 12 months.

Generally in a woman's early to mid-forties—two to eight years before actual menopause—her menstrual cycle begins changing. The level of estrogen produced by the ovaries decreases, ovulation stops or becomes irregular, and the pattern of menstrual cycling changes. Although the pattern is not consistent for all women, initially the change may be characterized by heavier, more frequent periods, which later become less heavy and less frequent. Lack of ovulation may cause some light bleeding or spotting between periods.

I was well into my menopause before I realized what was happening. My symptoms were so minor and rather vague. I didn't understand all the hype about symptoms.

50-year-old woman

After menopause, women continue to produce estrogen, but far less is manufactured in the ovaries. Most postmenopausal estrogen is produced through a process in which the adrenal gland makes precursors of estrogen that are converted by stored fat to estrogen. Far less estrogen, however, is produced in this manner than was produced in the ovaries before menopause.

Surgically Induced Menopause

Hysterectomy performed in conjunction with the removal of both ovaries and the fallopian tubes, known as a **total hysterectomy** and **bilateral salpingo-oophorectomy,** has become increasingly common (Figure 8.2). When a woman's ovaries are surgically removed, a more abrupt and earlier menopause results. The pituitary gland continues to produce luteinizing and follicle-stimulating hormones, but the ovaries are not present to respond with ovulation. Estrogen and progesterone are no longer produced at the same level as prior to surgery because of the absence of the ovaries. Although hormones are still produced in the adrenal glands, the levels are considerably lower without the ovarian production. Studies have found that women who have had both ovaries removed before the onset of menopause experience more severe menopausal symptoms, and possibly an increased incidence of cardiovascular morbidity and mortality, than women who experience a natural menopause.[7–9]

Figure 8.2

Four types of hysterectomy.

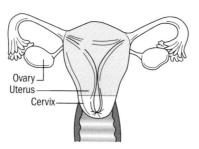

Partial hysterectomy: only the uterus is removed.

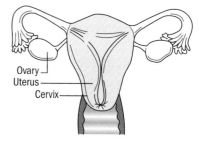

Total hysterectomy: both the uterus and cervix are removed.

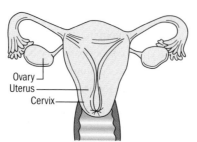

Total hysterectomy with bilateral salpingo-oophorectomy: both ovaries, the fallopian tubes, the uterus, and the cervix are removed.

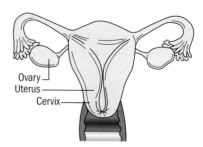

Radical hysterectomy: both ovaries, fallopian tubes, the uterus, the cervix, and the lymph nodes are removed.

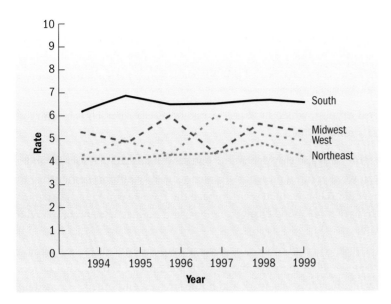

Figure 8.3

Hysterectomy rates, by geographic region: United States, 1994-1999.

Source: Keshavarz, H., Hillis, S., Kieke, B., and Marchbanks, P. (2002). Hysterectomy Surveillance—United States, 1994-1999. *Morbidity and Mortality Weekly Report* 51(SS05): 1-8.

Hysterectomy is the second most frequently performed surgical procedure, after cesarean section, in women of reproductive age in the United States. Approximately 600,000 hysterectomies are performed annually in the country, and approximately 20 million U.S. women have had a hysterectomy.[10] More than 25% of all women will have undergone a hysterectomy before they reach the age of 60.[11] This high prevalence has generated significant controversy regarding the risks and benefits of the procedure. The hysterectomy controversy is further fueled, as shown in Figure 8.3, by the national geographical variance that is present in the distribution of hysterectomy procedures.

Health Effects of Menopause

Hormonal changes during menopause often manifest themselves in both physical and emotional symptoms. Many women have only a few symptoms, while others experience everything from hot flashes to depression. A 2005 National Institute of Health State of the Science Conference on Management of Menopausal Symptoms revealed the latest scientific and clinical thinking regarding this stage of a woman's life.

Menopause-related symptoms vary greatly among women:[12]

- Roughly 85% of women have at least one or more symptoms. Of these women, about 10% will have symptoms severe enough to warrant a visit to their physician.

- At least 40% of women complain of hot flashes.

- As many as 29% of women experience some depression.

I was only 42 when I had my hysterectomy. Within two days, I discovered what "night sweats" were and I thought I would never survive the hot flashes. Thank goodness for hormone replacement therapy. As soon as I was put on estrogen, life became wonderful again. I am now 57, and every day I thank that little pill.

57-year-old woman

- As many as 45% of women experience some sleep disturbances, with more disturbances occurring in the later stages of menopause.

- Many women appear to suffer from some sexual dysfunction, although this seems to be correlated with hormonal variation experience throughout the stages of menopause.

- Vaginal dryness, which increases as menopause progresses, is a common complaint among women.

The symptoms also vary depending on the woman's cultural background. African American women often present with menopausal symptoms earlier than do white women, while Asian women seem to have the fewest symptoms. Hispanic women appear to have more mood changes, fatigue, and vaginal dryness compared to white women. [13]

As the researchers point out, however, it is often difficult for women to directly associate any or all of these symptoms with menopause. Often, other factors—such as family life, health issues, work and home stresses, and others—contribute to the process. Aging is certainly an important factor.

The most frequently reported physical symptom is the vascular response or instability known as **hot flashes** or hot flushes. Hot flashes are generally described as an uncomfortable sensation of internally generated heat beginning in the chest and moving to the neck and head or spreading throughout the body. Increased heart rate and finger temperature, shallow breathing, and sweating followed by chills are characteristic of hot flashes. Hot flashes may begin before a woman has stopped menstruating and may continue for several years after menopause. They are an early and acute symptom of estrogen deficiency.

Nearly 85% of menopausal women experience hot flashes.[14] Hot flashes often occur at night, resulting in sleep disruption, and therefore they are often credited with much of the insomnia associated with menopause. Sleep disturbances increase for many women in their forties and plateau during a woman's late fifties.[15] Many women find relief from hot flashes by changing their diets, reducing room temperatures, and wearing light-layered clothing; 25% of women experience enough discomfort to seek medical attention.[16]

Thinning of the vaginal lining, known as **vaginal atrophy,** is another physical symptom that occurs with some frequency following menopause. As estrogen levels decline, layers of the vaginal surface become drier and more sensitive. The vaginal wall becomes thinner, less elastic, and more vulnerable to infection. Some women experience pain or burning during intercourse, vaginal discharge, and more frequent vaginal infections. In addition, some may experience atrophy of the urinary tract. Diminished muscle tone may result in urinary incontinence. Some women also experience an increase in urinary tract infections. As many as one-third of women age 50 and older experience vaginal or urinary tract problems.[17] Physiological changes that affect the vaginal tract may affect a woman's sexual response as well. For example, lack of vaginal lubricant may affect sexual arousal. A change in hormone levels—specifically androgen production—may diminish libido.

Psychiatric syndromes have been linked to reproductive endocrine system changes at various stages of life, including postpartum psychosis and depression, premenstrual syndrome, post-hysterectomy depression, and menopausal psychiatric syndromes. Much of the current information on these conditions is based on myths, unwarranted assumptions, and conclusions derived from methodically flawed studies.[16] Perimenopausal changes in mental wellness and cognitive function are not well defined and remain an area of extensive research and debate. As with the physical symptoms associated with menopause, most women have few, if any, symptoms of psychological disturbances; most of the women who do experience these problems feel that these symptoms are manageable.[17]

Some women report irritability, mood swings, depression, and anxiety during menopause. These emotional changes may be due to the physical changes occurring in the body, but they also may be highly influenced by the normative traditional, cultural, and social expectations of a woman's worth expressed in relation to her reproductive capabilities. Significant psychosocial changes happen during the midlife transition, such as children leaving home, which eliminates some women's view of their primary role as mother and forces them to reevaluate their positions in life. For those who experience severe symptoms, medication or counseling may be indicated. Estrogen has been correlated with a positive effect on mood and overall sense of well-being, and is believed to be important for memory and mental functioning. As with all hormone-related issues, sensitivity and validation by a woman's physician is an important component of any treatment.

Other changes associated with menopause may include increased weight, breast changes, changes in hair growth, and changes in skin. Estrogen has a positive effect on collagen, so when estrogen levels decrease, a rapid loss of collagen occurs, causing the skin to become thinner and less elastic. The cycling levels of hormones also may cause a change in the prevalence or intensity of headaches. Women with a history of migraines during the menstrual period may find that their headaches worsen during perimenopause.

Long-Term Effects

Cardiovascular disease is the leading cause of mortality in women (see Chapter 10). Its incidence, which begins to rise in the perimenopausal years, continues to increase after menopause. Evidence shows that high levels of **HDL (high-density lipoprotein) cholesterol** and low levels of **LDL (low-density lipoprotein) cholesterol** are protective against the development of atherosclerosis. Research has also shown that the decrease in estrogen as a result of natural and surgical menopause is associated with changes in serum lipid profiles (blood cholesterol levels), such as a decline in HDL levels and an increase in LDL levels. These serum cholesterol changes may be factors in a woman's increased risk of developing postmenopausal cardiovascular disease.[18]

Another serious concern of many postmenopausal women is the development of **osteoporosis** or **osteopenia,** the loss of bone mass or bone density in which bones become brittle and more likely to fracture (see Chapter 11). The spine may

Figure 8.4

Prevalence of low femur bone density in U.S. women over 50, 1988–1994, by race.

Source: Centers for Disease Control and Prevention. (1996). *National Health and Nutrition Examination Survey III.*

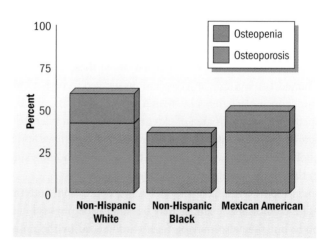

also lose flexibility and begin to curve. Osteoporosis is a major problem for many elderly women, and falls resulting from or leading to bone fractures constitute a leading health problem. Osteoporosis affects more than 30 million American women and causes approximately 300,000 hip fractures every year.[19] Estrogen deficiency is an important factor in bone loss, with approximately 20% of bone loss occurring within five to seven years of a woman reaching menopause.[18]

The prevalence of reduced bone density in older women varies by race and ethnicity (see Figure 8.4). Low bone density is most common among non-Hispanic white women (17% with osteoporosis and 42% with osteopenia), less common among Mexican American women (12% with osteoporosis and 37% with osteopenia), and least common in non-Hispanic black women (8% with osteoporosis and 28% with osteopenia).[20] Caucasian and Asian women have the highest incidence of low bone density, while women who smoke in all races have higher than average incidence and prevalence.

Estrogen loss that occurs with menopause may be a factor in the development of **Alzheimer's disease,** another disease associated with aging. Alzheimer's disease involves a slow, progressive loss of mental function caused by a neurodegenerative process in the brain (see Chapter 11). As the leading cause of lost independence and institutionalization, it is a major issue for older women for two reasons. First, women live longer than men and are therefore more likely to suffer from the disease. Second, Alzheimer's disease presents itself earlier in women than in men.

Menopause Management

Few topics in women's medicine today are as fraught with confusion and controversy as the question of appropriate treatment for menopausal symptoms and the prevention of long-term health problems associated with postmenopausal women.[21] Although it can be debated whether menopause is a medical condition or a "deficiency disease," the reality is that dozens of medications, herbal supplements, and other therapies are currently available for treating complaints associated with menopause. The widespread availability of these medications does not imply that all women should take them, however.

Hormone Replacement Therapy

Women naturally produce steroidal sex hormones including estrogens, progesterone, and androgens such as testosterone. During menopause, some may find that replacement of these hormones—particularly estrogen—can provide positive effects on their overall well-being. Beginning in the 1960s, physicians began prescribing hormone replacement therapy (HRT) with increased regularity for women affected by menopausal symptoms. Today, three types of HRT preparations are used:

- Estrogen alone (ERT)
- Estrogen and progesterone (often in the form of progestin, a synthetic form of progesterone)
- Estrogen, progesterone, and testosterone

"Estrogen" is often used as a general term, but it is actually a category of hormones. Of the many types of estrogen our bodies make, three are produced in major amounts: [22]

- *Estradiol* is the most potent form of estrogen, and the one produced in the largest amounts by a woman's ovaries before menopause. Estradiol levels fall after menopause. The brand-name drugs Estrace, Estraderm, Vivelle, and Climara all contain estradiol.
- *Estrone* is the predominant estrogen in a woman's body after menopause. When ovarian function declines, the fat cells in a woman's body take over the role of synthesizing estrone. Premarin and Ogen contain estrone (Premarin also contains other estrogens derived from the urine of pregnant horses).
- *Estriol* is known as the "weak" or "forgotten" estrogen. Produced in large amounts by the placenta during pregnancy, it is also converted in small amounts by the liver. Estriol is not commercially available in the United States, but must be compounded by a pharmacist.

Replacement hormones can be taken in a variety of different preparations, by various routes of administration, and in different dosages (see Table 8.1). There is no ideal regimen for every woman, so flexibility is the key to determining the correct dosage for each individual.

HRT can be given orally, vaginally, or transdermally (through skin patches). Oral preparations are prescribed most frequently.

Vaginal estrogen-containing creams can help women whose only symptom is vaginal dryness. Although estrogen does enter the bloodstream with such creams, the amount transferred is too small to provide all the benefits associated with estrogen, such as protection against osteoporosis.

I am so frustrated by the lack of definitive information about menopause and hormone replacement therapies. It's so confusing to wade between what seems to help and what could be potentially harmful down the road. How can it be that so little is known about such a basic and universal phenomenon?

45-year-old lawyer

Table 8.1

Types of HRT

Oral preparation
- Natural estrogen
- Synthetic
- Progestin
- Combination therapy
- Selective estrogen receptor modulators
- Natural dietary supplement

Vaginal cream

Vaginal ring

Transdermal patch

A vaginal ring is another form of estrogen and progestin delivery. A woman inserts this thin, transparent, flexible ring into the vagina. The vaginal ring was originally designed to provide contraception protection. The FDA approved Femring for treatment of menopause symptoms such as hot flashes and vaginal dryness. A single ring of this product provides continuous treatment of moderate or severe complaints associated with menopause for as long as three months.

A skin patch—that is, transdermal therapy—is another estrogen delivery mechanism. By feeding estrogen directly into the bloodstream via the skin, the liver is bypassed. This delivery method is a plus for some women whose livers respond to supplemental oral doses of estrogen by deactivating it with enzymes that also raise triglycerides, which contribute to heart disease. For women with low levels of HDL cholesterol, the "good" cholesterol, the oral pill form of estrogen is preferred because it increases HDL levels. Before deciding which form of estrogen therapy might better suit a particular woman, it is important to ascertain blood lipid levels.

A newer class of drugs called **selective estrogen receptor modulators (SERMs)** is also being investigated for its use in menopausal management. SERMs are called "designer estrogens" because they are designed to act like estrogen by providing the same beneficial effects, while eliminating this hormone's undesirable effects. (Benefits and side effects of estrogen are discussed later in this section.) Tamoxifen and raloxifene, for example, are both types of SERMs. Although it appears that tamoxifen protects against breast cancer and raloxifene protects against osteoporosis, both treatments are associated with a risk of blood clots similar to estrogen. Tamoxifen and raloxifene also can make hot flashes worse. Scientists are continuing to work on developing better SERMs for menopause management.

Known Positive Effects of HRT

ERT has been shown to provide relief from hot flashes, the most common and often earliest symptom of menopause. This type of therapy significantly improves symptoms related to urogenital changes such as atrophy, vaginal dryness, and infection, so it decreases the frequency of urinary tract infections and urinary stress incontinence in some women. Although many women initially begin ERT to relieve some of the more common complaints associated with menopause, some continue to use it after menopause ends in hopes of realizing long-term benefits. In addition to increasing bone density, ERT may protect women from bone loss and tooth loss that occur as a result of resorption of bone. Approximately 32% of U.S. women age 65 have no teeth.[23, 24] Another area of research for HRT is the association of estrogen with colon cancer: Several studies suggest that estrogen exerts a protective effect by either affecting the metabolism of bile acid or promoting tumor suppressor activity.[25] Age-related macular degeneration, the leading cause of legal blindness in the United States, also may be reduced by estrogen therapy.[26]

Decreased testosterone levels are believed to be responsible for the decreases in sex drive that many menopausal women experience. Adding testosterone supplements in pill or cream form may rejuvenate a woman's libido as well as her overall feelings of energy and well-being.

Known Negative Effects of HRT

Estrogen.   Estrogen use has been associated with endometrial cancer. Estrogen users who have an intact uterus have a two to eight times higher risk of developing this kind of cancer than women who are not using estrogen.[27] Researchers have found that the addition of a progestin to estrogen therapy can protect women against endometrial cancer by opposing the negative effects of estrogen—hence the terms "opposed estrogen" (estrogen given with progestin) and "unopposed estrogen" (estrogen given alone). Progestin appears to reduce uterine cancer risk by causing shedding of the estrogen-thickened endometrium, which lessens the chances of cancer development. When progestin is added to estrogen therapy, the treatment is considered to be "combined" and is often referred to as HRT or combined hormone therapy.[28] Many different types of estrogen and progestin exist, including both natural and synthetic versions. (See Table 8.2.)

Significant controversy has arisen regarding the association between estrogen therapy and breast cancer risk. Past analysis of numerous studies shows that short-term use of estrogen (five years or less) brings no increased risk, but there is a possible increased risk with long-term use of such therapy.[28] The Nurses' Health Study, an observational study,[29] showed no increased risk of breast cancer for past estrogen users, and the Iowa Women's Health Study showed no significant increase in former users or current users of estrogen therapy.[30] Recent results from the Women's Health Initiative (WHI) Estrogen-Alone Trial show no increased risk of breast cancer in postmenopausal women.[31]

Progestin.   Like estrogen, progestin has several side effects. Studies have suggested that this hormone diminishes estrogen's beneficial effects against heart disease, although debate continues over whether estrogen provides cardiovascular benefits (as discussed below).[2,32] Progestin also may increase the risk of breast cancer. Other possible side effects include menstrual-like bleeding, breast tenderness, mood swings, and bloating, similar to symptoms associated with premenstrual syndrome (PMS). The side effects of progestins vary according to the type and dosage used.

Estrogen/Progestin Combination.   Findings from the Breast Cancer Detection Demonstration Project (BCDDP), a nationwide breast cancer-screening program conducted by the National Cancer Institute, suggest that estrogen-progestin combination HRT may carry more risk for breast cancer than estrogen-only therapy. This increased risk was found mainly among current or recent users of HRT and dropped considerably over time. The same study also showed that the risk for developing breast cancer was only slightly increased for users of either type of HRT.[33]

Table 8.2 Different Brands of Estrogen and Progestins						
Estrogen oral preparation	Premarin	Cenestin	Estratab	Menest	Ortho-Est	Ogen	Estrace
Progestin oral preparation	Amen	Cycrin	Provera	Micronor	Nor-QD	Aygestin	Ovrette

Another concern regarding the use of HRT is the effect that the hormones may have on the usefulness of screening mammography. A recent study examined the effectiveness of screening mammograms in women with no history of confirmed or suspected breast cancer. HRT use was found to reduce the sensitivity of mammographic screening, which translates to approximately one missed case of breast cancer per 1,000 women taking HRT. The most likely explanation for this finding is the increased breast density among women using HRT and the difficulties in detecting lumps in higher-density breasts.[34]

Testosterone.   Testosterone replacement therapy remains controversial because it may bring on negative effects such as increased hair growth and heart disease. The FDA has not yet approved testosterone for menopause management.

Controversial Issues

The role of HRT in the prevention of heart disease and stroke remains unclear. To understand some of the complexities requires a basic understanding of clinical research studies, specifically observational and clinical trials (see Chapter 1). The research in this area continues to evolve, sometimes producing findings that appear conflicting or, at best, are not fully understood.

From the 1960s until 2000, HRT was believed to be an important medication in the fight against heart disease in menopausal women. Because animal and human observational studies showed that estrogen can slow the atherosclerotic process, physicians began prescribing ERT for their perimenopausal and postmenopausal patients. The original purpose of ERT was for the short-term treatment of perimenopausal symptoms, such as hot flashes and vaginal dryness. As more observational studies' findings were released, however, ERT became an important tool in the fight against heart disease. At the same time, studies showed that prescribing estrogen alone was not safe in women with a uterus—unopposed estrogen increases the risk of uterine cancer. Therefore, scientists concluded, a counteractive medication—a progestin—should be prescribed along with the ERT in women

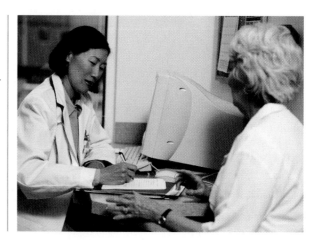

■ Replacement hormones can be taken in a variety of different preparations, by various routes of administration, and in different dosages. A woman should speak to her healthcare provider to determine what type of HRT will work for her.

with a uterus. In this way, the combination of estrogen and progestin (HRT) came into use.[35]

Scientists understood that while observational studies were important, they did not have the power of clinical trials in which the experimental medication was tested against a placebo (a pill that looks like the test medication, but that contains no medicine). The National Institutes of Health therefore began to fund clinical trials that examined the role of ERT and HRT as prevention against heart disease and stroke. Some of the first data released publicly came from ERT/HRT studies done in women who already had heart disease—the Estrogen Replacement and Atherosclerosis (ERA) Trial and the Heart and Estrogen Replacement Study (HERS). Both studies showed no significant difference in coronary heart disease risk reduction between users and nonusers. Furthermore, some women experienced an increase in coronary events in the first year of use and a modest decline thereafter. [36, 37]

During the 1990s, the first female director of the National Institutes of Health, Bernadine Healy, a cardiologist, initiated the Women's Health Initiative (WHI). The main purpose of this three-part study was to examine the role of ERT/HRT in several health areas in postmenopausal women: heart disease, stroke, dementia, breast and colon cancer, and osteoporosis. The study, which began in 1994, involved more than 67,000 postmenopausal women of all racial and ethnic groups across the United States. The ages of the participants ranged from those who had just entered the menopausal state to women who had been postmenopausal for more than 20 years. In 2002, the HRT portion of the study was stopped because of the apparent dangers of HRT use. The women taking HRT had higher rates of heart disease, strokes, blood clots, dementia, and breast cancer.[35] The ERT-alone portion of the study was stopped a year later with somewhat similar findings.

The release of these findings set off a storm of anxiety, distress, and action. The U.S. Food and Drug Administration officially declared that ERT/HRT was not to be used for cardiovascular disease (CVD) prevention and should be prescribed only for short periods in women suffering from perimenopausal symptoms. A number of other prestigious medical organizations agreed with the FDA's position. The press covered the findings with vigor. The end result was that the thousands of women who had been on ERT or HRT now had to make a decision about what to do. They were encouraged to discuss their next steps with their physicians. The only difficulty was that often the physicians were not entirely certain what to do. The observational studies had been so positive and now the clinical trials appeared so negative. Ultimately, a substantial number of women stopped taking ERT or HRT.

In 2003, a study was released comparing the findings from the observational studies and two of the clinical trials, HERS and WHI (Figure 8.5).[38] Clearly, there is both risk and benefit from taking HRT. Yet some scientists were not satisfied and so, early in 2006, some of the WHI investigators published a more in-depth examination of another long-term observational study, the Nurses' Health Study.[39] This latest analysis provided additional information regarding the WHI findings.

Figure 8.5

Observational versus clinical trial data on hormone replacement therapy's effect on risk for certain diseases.

Source: Grodstein, F., Clarkson, T. B., Manson, J. E. (2003). Understanding the divergent data on postmenopausal hormone therapy. *New England Journal of Medicine* 348: 645–650.

Disease	WHI	Amount of Risk HERS	Observational
Coronary heart disease	29% greater	No difference	49% less
Stroke	41% greater	20% greater	45% greater
Pulmonary embolism	113% greater	180% greater	110% greater
Breast cancer	26% greater	30% greater	115% greater
Colorectal cancer	37% less	N/A	54% less
Hip fracture	34% less	No difference	39% less

Basically, it appears that women who began taking ERT or HRT during the perimenopausal period—as many of the women in the earlier observational studies did—did not have as many negative effects from ERT/HRT as women who had been postmenopausal for five years or more when they started the therapy. The latest findings suggest that estrogen may have a positive effect when used continuously. In contrast, those women who had a break in estrogen exposure over time appear to be at increased risk for CVD. The reasons for this discrepancy are not entirely clear.

Another question also emerged: Might the study findings have differed if other forms of the medication had been used and/or administered? The medication given to the experimental group was the same as had been generally prescribed for the majority of women during the last several decades; however, it was administered in a manner that does not mimic the usual hormonal cycling. The same dosages of both estrogen and progesterone were taken every day throughout each month. In addition, it is not entirely clear what effect particular types of estrogen and progestin have on CVD as opposed to other formulas of those hormones.

This reexamination of the evidence has not changed the latest recommendations on ERT/HRT use. Further examination of current data and additional studies are required. All of these studies—both observational and clinical trials—have shed light on the importance of conducting studies, knowing how to interpret their results, and understanding what clinical applications should occur. This example also strongly underscores the importance of a woman's partnership with her physician. All women are not the same, and each should be treated as an individual. Each woman must understand her genetic history, her risk factors, and her lifestyle, and work with her physician to find the best healthy practices. Regarding ERT or HRT, women should consider several questions when deciding whether to take postmenopausal hormone therapy:

1. What are my risk factors for the particular diseases studied?

2. Am I more susceptible to the negative effects of ERT or HRT?

3. What type of ERT or HRT should I take?

4. In my case, do the benefits outweigh the risks?

Other Methods of Menopause Management

Good nutrition and regular exercise are important factors in maintaining well-being throughout premenopause and postmenopause. A diet rich in fruits, vegetables, and whole grains and low in saturated fat and cholesterol has been shown to be beneficial through most stages of life. Adequate calcium, vitamin D, and antioxidants such as vitamins E and C are also important for bone health and possibly prevention of CVD and cancer.

Exercise is critical in the menopausal years, a time when a woman is at increased risk for osteoporosis and osteoporosis-related fractures, heart disease, and chronic diseases such as diabetes. Weight-bearing exercise can increase bone density and improve balance and flexibility to decrease falls, thereby reducing fractures. Aerobic exercise can reduce a woman's risk for CVD by improving cardiac function, decreasing high body weight, and lowering LDL cholesterol levels. Regular exercise also may reduce the incidence and severity of hot flashes. Other symptoms associated with hormonal changes of menopause, such as insomnia, depression, other mood changes, weight gain, and headache, all may improve with exercise.[40]

Traditional herbal medicine has long offered a variety of treatments to address some of the symptoms of menopause. Few of these options have been sufficiently researched, but black cohosh (*Cimicifuga racemosa*) and vitex (*Vitex agnus-castus*), or chaste tree, have shown promise in relieving menopausal complaints; both of these supplements contain estrogen-like compounds. Further work is needed to determine how effective these herbal remedies are as actual substitutes for ERT. Dong quai (*Angelica sinensis*), an herb commonly used in traditional Chinese

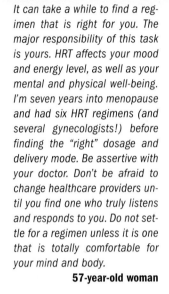

It can take a while to find a regimen that is right for you. The major responsibility of this task is yours. HRT affects your mood and energy level, as well as your mental and physical well-being. I'm seven years into menopause and had six HRT regimens (and several gynecologists!) before finding the "right" dosage and delivery mode. Be assertive with your doctor. Don't be afraid to change healthcare providers until you find one who truly listens and responds to you. Do not settle for a regimen unless it is one that is totally comfortable for your mind and body.

57-year-old woman

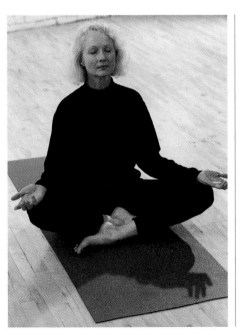

■ Symptoms associated with hormonal changes of menopause, such as hot flashes, may improve with regular exercise.

medicine, has been shown to relieve menopause symptoms in many women, but its mechanism of action is not clearly understood.[41]

North American Indians and eclectic physicians of the nineteenth century alike used black cohosh to treat gynecological problems. Today's herbalists and homeopaths suggest it as a hormone regulator and as a diuretic to relieve water retention. Studies carried out in Europe have verified black cohosh's effectiveness in reducing the secretion of luteinizing hormone, which has been implicated in causing hot flashes. Today in Germany, black cohosh is a main ingredient of three commercial drugs used for menopausal discomforts. A German governmental panel that studies and makes recommendations about medicinal herbs has found this herb to be a safe and reasonably effective treatment of nervous conditions associated with menopause. In 1986, however, the FDA found no pharmacologic evidence of therapeutic value in black cohosh and cautioned against its overuse.

Like black cohosh, vitex is lauded for its hormone-regulating action and often prescribed by herbalists to treat hot flashes, depression, and vaginal dryness associated with menopause. Vitex is believed to act on the hypothalamus and pituitary, regulating progesterone levels. In Europe, it has been used for about 40 years in a commercial alcohol-based tincture of the fruits known as Agnolyt.

Dong quai, long regarded as a blood-purifying tonic in traditional Chinese medicine, is one of the best-selling Chinese herbal products in North America. Western herbalists view it as having tonic and regulatory effects on the female reproductive system, and it is often used to treat menopausal symptoms. Scientific investigations have confirmed dong quai's pain-relieving, antispasmodic, and anti-inflammatory activity. It is generally believed to lower blood pressure and to soothe discomforts associated with menopause. Herbalists view dong quai as the "female ginseng," referring to its ability to revitalize and renourish the female body by correcting hormonal imbalances.[41] To date, the FDA has not issued any specific safety warnings about these supplements, nor has the agency overtly supported their use as safe and effective.

Informed Decision Making

Although it is commonly believed that health problems are inevitable as women age, many can actually be prevented or controlled. Clearly, it is best to have a full lifetime of healthy behaviors, but changing unhealthy behaviors, even in later years, can improve both the quality and the quantity of life. Health-promoting behaviors include cessation of cigarette smoking (it is best to never start), maintenance of good nutrition, loss of excess weight, and participation in regular physical exercise. For some women, menopause is a time of reflection and renewed determination to engage in healthier living. Protecting the body from heart disease and osteoporosis means not smoking, exercising throughout the life span, eating a healthy diet, and knowing one's body.

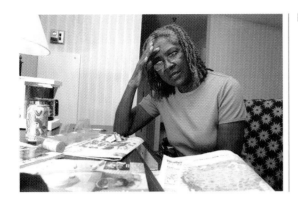

■ Rapidly changing information about the safety and effectiveness of HRT can be confusing for women deciding whether to use it to alleviate symptoms of menopause.

Many women remain uninformed about their health risks as they age and about options for decreasing these health risks. In a study looking at racial differences regarding menopause, 40% of African American women listed family members as their primary source of information about menopause, while one-third of white women cited television and magazines as their most common sources of information. Only 11% of African American women and 12% of white women listed health professionals as their primary source of information.[42] This study provides strong evidence that healthcare providers need to communicate better with their patients about menopause and provide helpful, practical, and informative advice to help women in their decision making regarding menopause.

The decision whether to take HRT is a personal one. No two women respond exactly the same way to the same therapy. Dosages, products, and regimens may require readjusting more than once to find an appropriate balance. Women with difficult menopause symptoms, those who have thin bones as measured by a bone density test, and those at high risk of heart disease are possible candidates for HRT. Women who have a history of liver disease, who are prone to blood clots, or who have had breast cancer are generally considered to be at too high a risk to begin HRT (Table 8.3).

I tried HRT but with all the contradictory news I decided that I preferred to not take "medicine" to get through a normal transition. Yes, I do have hot flashes, but they are manageable. It really is an individual decision.
61-year-old woman

Table 8.3	Conditions That May Preclude the Use of Hormone Replacement Therapy

Personal history of breast cancer

History of blood clots in legs, lungs, or eyes

Undiagnosed or abnormal vaginal bleeding

Preexisting cardiovascular conditions, such as blood clots, stroke, or uncontrolled hypertension

History of liver, gallbladder, or pancreatic disease; impaired liver function

Strategies for HRT Decision Making

The decision to use HRT is a personal and private one. Several factors should be carefully considered when making the decision:

1. Medical history
   - History of breast cancer
   - Blood clots in the legs, lungs, or eyes
   - Abnormal vaginal bleeding
   - Preexisting cardiovascular conditions, such as blood clots, stroke, or uncontrolled high blood pressure
   - Liver, gallbladder, or pancreatic disease
2. Menopausal symptoms and their severity
   - Hot flashes
   - Vaginal irritation and discomfort
   - Urinary tract problems
   - Emotional and mood changes
3. Review risks and benefits
4. Reevaluate decision periodically

Dr. Bobbie Gostout of the Gynecological Cancer Foundation notes that the unanswered questions about HRT are far more numerous than any answers we have to date:

> We don't know the effects of different doses or different medication schedules. We don't know the effects of the same estrogen with a different progestin or the same progestin with a different estrogen. It is not clear that the same risks pertain to estrogens and progesterones taken in the form of a skin patch instead of a pill. There may be cancer-causing or cancer-protective effects that only become evident years after these women stop taking hormone medication. These are among the many questions that must be answered by clinical trials.[43]

As with any form of medication, treatment, or procedure, the benefits must be carefully weighed and considered against the spectrum of associated risks before a decision is made (see Self-Assessment 8.1). In future years, it is hoped that women will have access to more information to help them better make these important health decisions.

Summary

Today menopause is no longer seen as the beginning of the end of life, but rather as the beginning of a second life, no longer confined or defined by procreative abilities. The phobia about aging and the myths and misconceptions

Profiles of Remarkable Women

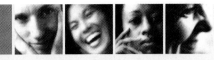

Gail Sheehy (1937–)

Gail Sheehy, the author of 15 books, has been tracking the stages of adult development for the last 20 years. A graduate of the University of Vermont, Sheehy received a fellowship to study under her mentor, Margaret Mead, at Columbia University in 1970. In 1974, she was awarded a grant from the Alicia Patterson Foundation to continue her studies in adult development. In 1976, Sheehy published the book *Passages,* which offered the perspective that adult life proceeds through predictable stages. *Passages* was eventually published in 28 languages and remained on the *New York Times* bestseller list for three years. A survey conducted by the Library of Congress placed it among the top 10 books that have most influenced people's lives.

Sheehy's next bestseller, *The Silent Passage: Menopause,* broke the silence around the previously taboo subject of menopause. Its author demystified issues surrounding menopause by presenting the facts, the myths, and the fears of women. *The Silent Passage* was revised, expanded, and released in paperback edition in 1993; this version remained on the best-seller list for 65 weeks. In July 1995, Sheehy published a newly revised paperback edition with a new introduction. The sequel to *Passages,* entitled *New Passages: Mapping Your Life Across Time,* discusses Sheehy's discovery of a shifting in all of the stages of adulthood. Through extensive research and surveys, Sheehy created a book that helps women to make sense of their lives by understanding other women's experiences.

Sheehy's other books have covered a wide range of topics based on portraits of people. For example, *Pathfinders* was created from a study of 60,000 American men and women; *Spirit of Survival,* a story of healing, is an account of a survivor of the Cambodian genocide. *Understanding Men's Passages: Discovering the New Map of Men's Lives* focuses on the fears and self-doubts of men over 40.

Sheehy has also published many magazine articles. She was one of the original contributors to *New York Magazine* and has revolutionized political writing through her role as contributing editor of *Vanity Fair.* Through her in-depth character portraits of national and world leaders, Sheehy has explored the psyches of Saddam Hussein, George Bush, Mikhail Gorbachev, Margaret Thatcher, Jesse Jackson, Gary Hart, Dan Quayle, Hillary Clinton, and Newt Gingrich.

In her newest book, *Sex and the Seasoned Woman: Pursing the Passionate Life,* Sheehy reports on Baby Boomer women, coverting topics such as sex, dating, divorce, remarriage, and living more passionately in the second half of life.

about the aging process need to be replaced with better knowledge and insight into the myriad opportunities that exist in the second half of a woman's life. Menopause is a time of change for many women. For some, it brings physical symptoms; for others, it inspires questions about changing roles. Menopause management—especially hormone replacement therapy—remains a controversial area that deserves ongoing research and requires individual choices by women and their physicians. For some women, this therapy is the ideal solution to their health issues associated with menopause. For other women, HRT may cause more health problems than it solves and leaves many women confused about their options. As a result, women must actively work with their physicians to understand the best course of action for themselves as it relates to menopause and their individual process of aging.

■■■■

Topics for Discussion

1. Why has medical research been slower to understand the physiological dimensions of menopause than those of other reproductive health matters?

2. What can be done to continue to change societal images of menopause, aging, and older women?

3. How can women understand menopause as a stage of life?

4. What can a woman do to maximize the effectiveness of her decision making about hormone replacement therapy?

5. What are some of the physical, emotional, and social dimensions of menopause?

■■■■

Web Sites

American College of Obstetricians and Gynecologists: http://www.acog.org

American Heart Association—Women and Cardiovascular Disease: http://www.goredforwomen.org

The Hormone Foundation: http://www.hormone.org

National Institute on Aging Information Center: http://www.nia.nih.gov

National Women's Health Information Center: http://www.womenshealth.gov

National Women's Health Resource Center: http://www.healthywomen.org

North American Menopause Society: http://www.menopause.org

Power Surge (an online community for menopausal women): http://www.power-surge.com

Society for Women's Health Research: http://www.womenshealthresearch.org

■■■■

References

1. U.S. Census Bureau. (2003). National Population Projections Summary File (NP-T3), Projections of the Total Resident Population by 5-Year Age Groups, and Sex with Special Age Categories: Middle Series, 1999 to 2100. Accessed online at http://www.census.gov/population/www/projections/natsum-T3.html.

2. Lobo, R. A. (1999). Menopause management for the millennium. *Medscape Women's Health. Clinical Management.* Vol. 1.

3. Utian, W. H., and Boggs, P. P. (1999). *The North American Menopause Society 1998 Menopause Survey. Part 1: Postmenopausal Women's Perceptions about Menopause and Midlife.* North American Menopause Society.

4. *The International Menopause Society Report on the 10th World Congress on the Menopause Climacteric.* (2002). 5: 219–228.

5. Hall, L. L. (1999). Taking charge of menopause. *FDA Consumer Magazine.* U.S. Food and Drug Administration.

6. Miller, A. M., Wilbur, J., and McDentt, J. (1997). Health promotion: the perimenopausal to mature years (45–64). In Allen, K. M., and Phillips, J. M. *Women's Health: Across the Lifespan.* Philadelphia: Lippincott-Raven.

7. Bachmann, G. A. (1999). Vasomotor flushes in postmenopausal women. *American Journal of Obstetrics and Gynecology* 180: 312–316.

8. Bush, T. (1990). The epidemiology of cardiovascular disease in postmenopausal women. *Annals of the New York Academy of Science* 592: 263–271.

9. Stampfer, M. J., Colditz, G. A., and Willett, W. C. (1990). Menopause and heart disease: a review. *Annals of New York Academy of Science* 392.

10. Keshavarz, M. D., Hillis, S. D., Kiekel, B. A., and Marchanks, P. A. (2002). *Hysterectomy Surveillance—United States, 1994–1999.* Division of Reproductive Health, National Center for Chronic Disease Prevention and Health Promotion, Epidemic Intelligence Service Program, Epidemiology Program Office.

11. Lepine, L. A., et al. (1997). Hysterectomy surveillance—United States, 1980–1993. *Morbidity and Mortality Weekly Report* 46(SS-4): 1–15.

12. Woods, N. F., and Mitchell, E. S. (2005). Symptoms during the menopause: prevalence, severity, trajectory, and significance in women's lives. *Journal of American Medicine* 118(12B): 14S–24S.

13. Ice, V. M. (2005). Strategies and issues for managing menopause-related symptoms in diverse populations: ethnic and racial diversity. *Journal of American Medicine* 118(12B): 142S–147S.

14. Oldenhare, A., Jaszmann, L. J. B., Haspels, A. A., et al. (1993). Impact of climacteric on well-being: a survey based on 5,213 women 39 to 60 years old. *American Journal of Obstetrics and Gynecology* 168: 772–780.

15. Owens, J. F., and Matthews, K. A. (1998). Sleep disturbance in healthy middle-aged women. *Maturitas* 30: 41–50.

16. Hammond, C. B. (1999). Confronting aging and disease: the role of HRT. *Medscape Women's Health.*

17. Samsoie, G. (1998). Urogenital aging: a hidden problem. *American Journal of Obstetrics and Gynecology* 178: S245–S249.

18. Stampfer, M. J., Colditz, G. A., Willett, W. C., et al. (1991). Postmenopausal estrogen therapy and cardiovascular disease: 10 year follow-up from the Nurses' Health Study. *New England Journal of Medicine* 325: 756.

19. National Osteoporosis Foundation (2006). *Fast Facts.* Washington, DC: National Osteoporosis Foundation. www.nof.org/osteoporosis/diseasefacts.htm.

20. Centers for Disease Control and Prevention. (1996). *National Health and Nutrition Examination Survey III.*

21. Office of Technology Assessment. (1992). The menopause, hormone therapy, and women's health—background paper. (S/N 052-003-01284-7). Washington, DC: U.S. Government Printing Office.

22. Women's Health Access. (2001). Estrogen and progesterone: the right regimen for you. *Women's Health America Fact Sheet.*

23. Jeffcoat, M. K., and Chestnut, C. H. (1993). Systemic osteoporosis and oral bone loss. *Journal of the American Dental Association* 124: 49–56.

24. Kribbs, P. J., Chestnut, C. H., Ottis, M., et al. (1990). Relationships between mandibular and skeletal bone in a population of normal women. *Journal of Prosthetic Dentistry* 63: 86–89.

25. Calle, E. E. (1997). Hormone replacement therapy and colorectal cancer: interpreting the evidence. *Cancer Causes Control* 8: 127–129.

26. Eye-Disease Case-Control Study Group. (1992). Risk factors for neovascular age-related macular degeneration. *Archives of Ophthalmology* 110: 1701–1708.

27. Collings, J. A., and Schlesselman, J. J. (1990). Hormone replacement therapy and endometrial cancer. In Lobo, R. A. (ed.) *Treatment of the Postmenopausal Women: Basic and Clinical Aspects,* 2nd ed. Philadelphia: Lippincott, Williams & Wilkins, 503–517.

28. Hulley, S., Grady D., Bush T., Furberg C., Herrington D., Riggs B., Vittinghoff E., et al. (1995). The use of estrogen and progestins and the risk of breast cancer in postmenopausal women. *New England Journal of Medicine* 332: 1589.

29. Colditz, G. A., Hankinson, S. E., Hunter, D. J., et al. (1995). The use of estrogen and progestins and the risk of breast cancer in postmenopausal women. *American Journal of Public Health* 85: 1128–1132.

30. Folsom, A. R., et al. (1995). Hormone replacement therapy and morbidity and mortality in a prospective study of postmenopausal women. *American Journal of Public Health* 85: 1128–1132.

31. Stefanick, M. L., Anderson, G. L., Margolis, K. L., Hendrix, S. L., Rodabough, R. J., Paskett, E. D., et al. (2006). Effects of conjugated equine estrogens on breast cancer and mammography screening in postmenopausal women with hysterectomy. *Journal of the American Medical Association* 295(14): 1647–1657.

32. Whitehead, M. I., Hillard, T. C., and Crook, D. (1990). The role and use of progestogens. *Obstetrics and Gynecology* 75(4 suppl): 695–765.

33. Schairer, C., et al. (2000). Menopausal estrogen and estrogen-progestin replacement therapy and breast cancer risk. *Journal of the American Medical Association* 283(4): 485–491.

34. Kavanagh, A. M., Mitchell, H., and Giles, G. G. (2000). Hormone replacement therapy and accuracy of mammographic screening. *Lancet* 355(9200): 270–274.

35. Writing Group for the Women's Health Initiative Randomized Controlled Trial. (2002). Risks and benefits of estrogen plus progestin in healthy postmenopausal women. *Journal of the American Medical Association* 288(3): 321–333.

36. Herrington, D., et al. (2000). Effects of estrogen replacement on the progression of coronary-artery atherosclerosis. *New England Journal of Medicine* 343(8): 522–529.

37. Hulley, S., et al. (1998). Randomized trial of estrogen plus progestin for secondary prevention of coronary heart disease in postmenopausal women. Heart and Estrogen/Progestin Replacement Study (HERS) Research Group. *Journal of the American Medical Association* 280: 605–613.

38. Grodstein, F., Clarkson, T. B., and Manson, J. E. (2003). Understanding the divergent data on postmenopausal hormone therapy. *New England Journal of Medicine* 348(7): 645–650.

39. Grodstein, F., Manson, J. E., and Stampfer, M. E. (2006). Hormone therapy and coronary heart disease: the role of time since menopause and age at hormone initiation. *Journal of Women's Health* 15(1): 35–44.

40. Burghardt, M. (1999). Exercise at menopause: a critical difference. *Medscape Women's Health* 4(1).

41. Hudson, T. (January–February 2000). Six paths to menopause wellness. *Herbs for Health Magazine* 6.

42. Grisso, J. A., et al. (1999). Racial differences in menopause information and the experience of hot flashes. *General Internal Medicine* 14: 98–103.

43. Gostout, B. (June 23, 2003). Women's hormones, women's cancers; gynecological cancer: what every women should know. *New York Times,* advertising supplement.

Chapter Nine

Nutrition, Exercise, and Weight Management

On completion of this chapter, the student should be able to discuss:

The importance of a healthful diet and an active lifestyle for disease prevention and health promotion.

The way in which nutrients fit into a balanced diet.

The building blocks of nutrition.

The concept of physical fitness and how it relates to health.

The physiological and psychological benefits of exercise.

The major components of physical fitness, total fitness, and their benefits.

Maximum and target-range heart rate.

Physical fitness concerns that are specific to women.

Myths and facts about exercise and fitness.

The ability of exercise to counter some of the natural conditions of the aging process.

Causes of athletic amenorrhea.

Reasons why women should maintain a healthy weight.

The cause of weight gain.

The effects of obesity and overweight on health.

Economic consequences of obesity and overweight.

Ways that women can achieve their weight-loss goals.

How body images of women have changed over time.

Sociocultural influences on body image.

Probable causes and health consequences of extreme underweight.

The effects of world hunger and malnutrition.

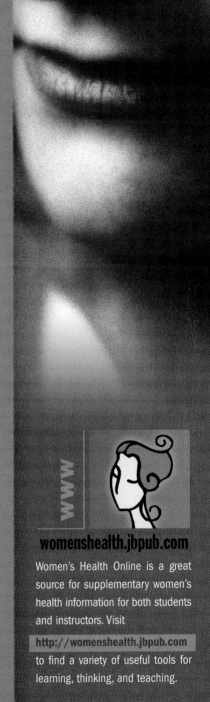

womenshealth.jbpub.com

Women's Health Online is a great source for supplementary women's health information for both students and instructors. Visit

http://womenshealth.jbpub.com

to find a variety of useful tools for learning, thinking, and teaching.

Introduction

A balanced diet and regular physical activity can help women to maintain or improve their health and weight. Despite scientific research documenting that healthful eating and regular exercise extend quantity and improve quality of life, many women continue to follow unhealthy eating patterns and lead sedentary lives. Together, these two behaviors are responsible for 400,000 deaths each year. These behaviors are the second leading preventable cause of death in the United States, just behind tobacco.[1]

Eating the proper foods in moderation and proportionality maximizes nutritional benefit. A well-balanced diet—one that is low in fat and high in fruits, vegetables, and fiber—can play a significant role in the prevention of cardiovascular disease, various cancers, diabetes, and other diet-related chronic conditions. Physical fitness greatly reduces the risk of developing heart disease, hypertension, colon cancer, and diabetes. Exercise promotes psychological well-being, controls body fat and fat distribution, and fosters healthy muscle, bones, and joints. Exercise also helps older adults maintain function and preserve independence. This chapter describes what is meant by healthful eating, how healthful eating and regular exercise are essential for weight control, how body image influences women and their eating (or dieting) and exercise decisions, and how women are especially vulnerable to an array of possible eating disorders and exercise abuse.

Nutrition and Healthful Eating

Nutrition is the science that explores the need for food and the role of food in nourishing the body and fostering good health. Nutritional needs change during different stages of a woman's life.

There are six groups of **nutrients,** which are categorized into three types:

- *Macronutrients,* which include carbohydrates, proteins, and fats, are needed in large amounts.
- *Micronutrients,* which include vitamins and minerals, are needed in smaller amounts.
- *Water,* a substance often overlooked as a nutrient, is indispensable for virtually every bodily function.

To achieve healthful eating, a woman should choose a diet that provides the right balance of carbohydrates, proteins, and fats; the necessary amounts of essential vitamins and minerals; and a constant supply of water.

Dietary Guidelines

The U.S. Department of Agriculture (USDA) has revised its dietary guidelines for Americans every five years since the guidelines' introduction in 1980. Based on current nutritional research, the 2005 guidelines identify unhealthy eating habits and a sedentary lifestyle as major causes of death and injury in the United States.

It's Your Health

Nutritional Jargon

Enriched: The replacement of nutrients in a product that may have been lost during processing; for example, bread may be enriched with iron, niacin, thiamin, and riboflavin.

Fortified: The addition of vitamins and minerals that were not originally present in a food product; for example, orange juice may be fortified with calcium.

Light or lite: A relatively meaningless descriptor that may refer to reduced calories, fat, or sodium, or even a "light" taste or fluffy texture.

Low-calorie: Term used for a food that has less than 40 calories per serving *and* less than 0.4 calorie per gram.

Low-fat: Term used for a food that has 3 grams or less of fat per serving.

Low-sodium: Term used for food that has 140 mg or less of sodium per serving.

Natural: A relatively meaningless descriptor that may refer to minimal processing or a product that is free of artificial ingredients. Many foods labeled as natural are highly processed, high in fat or sugar, or loaded with preservatives.

RDA: Recommended Dietary Allowance, the estimated amount of various nutrients needed each day to maintain good health. The guidelines were developed to address population-based dietary needs such as pregnant women; individual needs may vary owing to genetic, personal, and demographic factors.

Reduced-calorie: Term used for a food that has at least 25% fewer calories than regular preparations. The nutritional comparison must be displayed on the product label.

Sugarless and sugar-free: Another misleading descriptor because current FDA definition of "sugar" means sucrose but does not include other forms of sugar such as glucose, fructose, or sorbitol, which contain as many calories as sucrose.

It's Your Health

Dietary Guidelines for Americans

The USDA recommends the following for each of the six food groups as part of a healthy, 2,000-calorie per day diet:

Grains

Eat six ounces every day.

Make half of the grains you eat whole.

Vegetables

Vary the vegetables you eat.

Eat 2½ cups every day.

Vegetables to eat more of:

Dark green vegetables like spinach and broccoli.

Orange vegetables like carrots and sweet potatoes.

Dry beans and peas like kidney beans, pinto beans, and lentils.

Fruits

Eat a variety of fruit.

Eat 2 cups of fruit every day.

Try to consume whole fruits rather than fruit juices.

Dairy Products

Try to consume 3 cups of dairy products or other calcium-rich foods every day.

Try to consume low-fat dairy products when possible.

Consume fortified food or other sources of calcium if dairy products are unavailable or unpalatable.

Meat and Beans

Eat 5½ ounces of meat or beans every day.

Consume baked, broiled, or grilled meat products when possible.

Vary sources of protein, emphasizing fish, peas, beans, nuts, and seeds.

To promote health and prevent disease, the guidelines encourage Americans to participate in regular physical activity, to consume adequate nutrient requirements within a healthy caloric intake, to reach and maintain a healthy weight, and to adopt fats and sodium as a necessary but limited portion of their diets. The guidelines also highlight food choices that can help people meet their **Recommended Dietary Allowances.**[2] (See **It's Your Health:** Dietary Guidelines for Americans.)

Food Guide Pyramids

The 2005 dietary guidelines use a pyramid to symbolize the proportion of different foods that make up a healthy diet (see Figure 9.1). Unlike the 2000 USDA food guide pyramid, which featured different food groups as horizontal layers, the 2005 pyramid is divided into vertical slices. The 2005 pyramid replaces the traditional "four food groups" (breads and grains, fruits and vegetables, dairy products and meats) with six food groups: (1) grains; (2) vegetables; (3) fruits; (4) fats, sugars, and sodium; (5) meat and beans; and (6) dairy products. A figure climbing a flight of stairs along the side of the pyramid represents the importance that physical activity plays in a healthy lifestyle.[2] The different sizes of the food group "slices" in the pyramid represent the nutritional concept

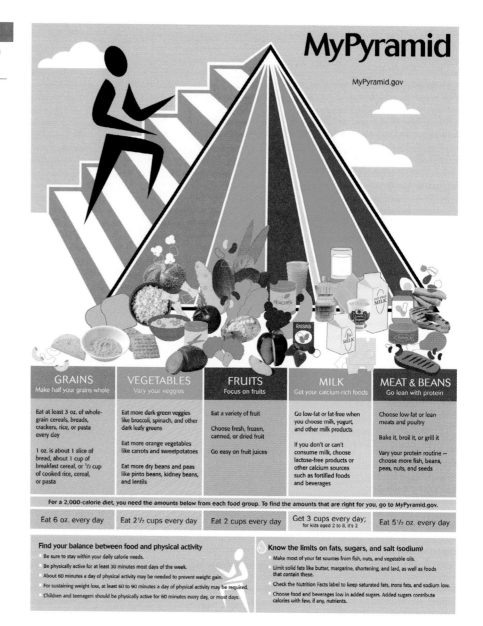

Figure 9.1

MyPyramid: The 2005 food guide pyramid.

of **proportionality**—eating different amounts from each of the food groups on a daily basis. Unfortunately, Americans "gobble huge amounts of added fats and sugars . . . and heaping plates of pasta and other refined grains [but] . . . are sorely lacking in the vegetables, fruits, low-fat milk products, and other nutritious foods in the middle of the pyramid.[2,3] More than 60% of young people eat too much fat and less than 20% eat the recommended five or more servings of fruits and vegetables each day. Poor eating habits are often established during childhood and carry into adulthood.[4] In fact, only 25% of U.S. adults eat the recommended five or more servings of fruit and vegetables each day.[5]

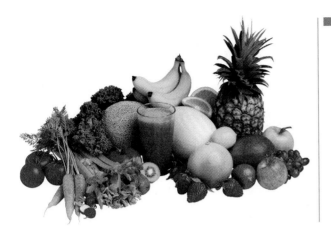

■ Fruits and vegetables contain numerous substances that could help prevent disease and promote good health.

Organizations have produced food guide pyramids that challenge or complement the USDA's food guide pyramid. In addition, pyramids have been developed for special populations, such as people older than 70 years of age and vegetarians. Culture-specific food pyramids have also been developed, including ones for Arabic, Chinese, Indian, Russian, and Mexican populations.

The Mediterranean food guide pyramid, based on the dietary traditions of Crete, much of the rest of Greece, and southern Italy has received much attention of late. Rates of chronic disease are among the lowest in the world and life expectancy is among the highest for these populations in this region. The food pyramid highlights the following characteristics of the Mediterranean diet:

- An abundance of food from plant sources, including fruits and vegetables, bread and grains, beans, nuts, and seeds
- Emphasis on fresh, locally grown foods
- Olive oil as the principal fat
- Moderate amounts of fish, poultry, cheese, and yogurt
- Moderate consumption of wine

Nutrition Facts Label

The Nutrition Facts label is designed to help people make healthful food choices and compare the nutritional quality of foods. The food label lists information on serving size, calories, nutrients, and vitamins and minerals, as well as other important facts relevant to a healthful diet (Figure 9.2). The Daily Value (%DV) section indicates how the nutrients in a serving of food contribute to satisfying one's total daily requirements for each nutrient. These values are based on recommendations for a 2,000-calorie diet. A woman under doctor's orders to eat a higher- or lower-calorie diet will need to recalculate these numbers to fit her own needs.[2]

Carbohydrates

Carbohydrates provide the basic fuel for the body and are available in two forms: simple carbohydrates (sugars) and complex carbohydrates (starches). Sugars provide

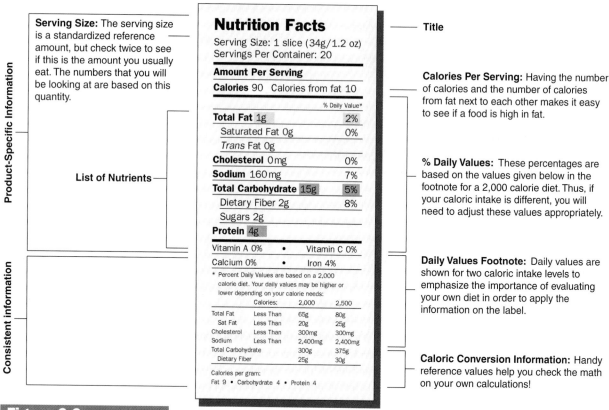

Product-Specific Information

Serving Size: The serving size is a standardized reference amount, but check twice to see if this is the amount you usually eat. The numbers that you will be looking at are based on this quantity.

List of Nutrients

Consistent information

Nutrition Facts

Serving Size: 1 slice (34g/1.2 oz)
Servings Per Container: 20

Amount Per Serving

Calories 90   Calories from fat 10

% Daily Value*

Total Fat 1g	2%
Saturated Fat 0g	0%
Trans Fat 0g	
Cholesterol 0mg	0%
Sodium 160mg	7%
Total Carbohydrate 15g	5%
Dietary Fiber 2g	8%
Sugars 2g	
Protein 4g	

Vitamin A 0%	•	Vitamin C 0%
Calcium 0%	•	Iron 4%

* Percent Daily Values are based on a 2,000 calorie diet. Your daily values may be higher or lower depending on your calorie needs:

	Calories:	2,000	2,500
Total Fat	Less Than	65g	80g
Sat Fat	Less Than	20g	25g
Cholesterol	Less Than	300mg	300mg
Sodium	Less Than	2,400mg	2,400mg
Total Carbohydrate		300g	375g
Dietary Fiber		25g	30g

Calories per gram:
Fat 9 • Carbohydrate 4 • Protein 4

Title

Calories Per Serving: Having the number of calories and the number of calories from fat next to each other makes it easy to see if a food is high in fat.

% Daily Values: These percentages are based on the values given below in the footnote for a 2,000 calorie diet. Thus, if your caloric intake is different, you will need to adjust these values appropriately.

Daily Values Footnote: Daily values are shown for two caloric intake levels to emphasize the importance of evaluating your own diet in order to apply the information on the label.

Caloric Conversion Information: Handy reference values help you check the math on your own calculations!

Figure 9.2

Example of the Nutrition Facts label.

little more than a quick spurt of energy, whereas starches are rich in vitamins, minerals, and other nutrients that provide more sustained fuel for the body. During digestion, all carbohydrates are broken down into sugar. The sugar enters the blood, increasing blood sugar levels. The body's normal response is to increase the production of insulin, which in turn uses the sugar for energy.

Simple Carbohydrates

Simple carbohydrates, or sugars, are consumed in four virtually identical forms: sucrose, glucose, fructose, and lactose. They are present in many foods, from fruit to milk to ice cream and ketchup. Processed foods are often much higher in sugar than their natural counterparts. A typical 12-ounce soft drink contains the equivalent of eight teaspoonfuls of sugar, and a typical chocolate bar contains about three teaspoonfuls of sugar per ounce. Foods high in sugar are often high in fat, and a high-fat diet is a major culprit in cardiovascular disease and obesity, as well as other chronic diseases. Sugar provides "empty calories"—that is, energy in the form of calories but with no other significant nutritional value. In addition, consumption of a sugared product, such as a soft drink, usually occurs in lieu of something else that may be nutritious, such as a glass of skim milk or water.

Foods high in sugar can have a particularly harmful effect on dental health, because sugar nourishes cavity-causing bacteria. The source of sugar can also affect the degree of damage it causes. Sugar in sticky foods, for example, clings to the teeth and encourages bacterial growth. Liberal use of sugar promotes the growth of plaque, the toxin-producing film that forms on teeth; plaque can lead to periodontal (gum) disease, the leading cause of tooth loss among American adults. Research has recently linked periodontal disease with an increased risk of heart disease.[6]

Complex Carbohydrates

Complex carbohydrates, or starches, are a good source of minerals, vitamins, and fiber. These substances are found in breads, cereals, legumes, rice, pastas, and "starchy" vegetables such as beans and potatoes. Digestion breaks down complex carbohydrates into simple sugars. Complex carbohydrates take longer to digest than simple carbohydrates and, therefore, are a good long-term source of energy. According to USDA dietary guidelines, complex carbohydrates should provide the major supply of calories in diets, approximately 55% to 60% of total calories consumed.

Fiber is not a single substance, but rather a group of widely different chemical substances with varied physical properties. It is derived from the parts of plants that cannot be digested by enzymes in the human digestive tract. Although not considered a nutrient because it cannot be digested, it is essential because it aids in digestion. Fiber was formerly called roughage or bulk, and was once thought of as a "filler food." It is found in foods composed of carbohydrates.

There are two kinds of fiber: soluble and insoluble. Both kinds benefit the body. Soluble fiber, once called crude fiber, absorbs water in the digestive tract and is easily fermented by bacteria in the large intestine. Oats, for example, are rich in soluble fiber, which helps lower blood cholesterol and manage blood sugar levels. In contrast, most insoluble fiber remains essentially unchanged during digestion. Wheat bran, whole-grain breads and cereals, broccoli, carrots, and pears are all rich in insoluble fiber, which tends to increase stool bulk. Studies now show an increased risk for heart disease when diets low in fiber are consumed.[7] Diets rich in dietary fiber also may help to prevent colon cancer, although data gathered on this point so far are inconclusive.

The recommended daily intake for total fiber for women 50 and younger is 25 grams; for women older than 50, it is 21 grams per day. A woman should increase dietary fiber by slowly adding fiber to her diet over time. When choosing sources of fiber, opt for less-processed food, such as an apple rather than applesauce. Eating the skin of fruits and vegetables also increases fiber consumption (see **It's Your Health**).

Glycemic Index

Recently, partly as a result of the newfound popularity of high-protein, low-carbohydrate diets, much attention has been given to the glycemic index of foods. The **glycemic index** is a measure of how fast glucose enters the bloodstream after a carbohydrate is eaten and thus how quickly the carbohydrate increases a person's blood sugar. In general, foods that are mostly simple sugars are highly processed, or contain refined sugars have a high glycemic index. This group includes refined breakfast cereals, white bread, white rice, white spaghetti, soft drinks, and sugar. Some complex carbohydrates, such as potatoes, behave just as simple carbohydrates

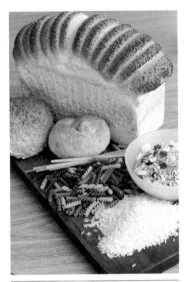

Complex carbohydrates are a good source of minerals, vitamins, and fiber.

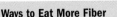

It's Your Health

Ways to Eat More Fiber

1. Eat whole fresh fruit instead of just drinking juice.

2. Eat the skins of fruits and vegetables, such as apples and potatoes.

3. Eat fruits with edible seeds, such as berries and kiwis.

4. Eat whole-grain foods.

5. Eat more of the stems when having broccoli or asparagus.

6. Peel citrus fruits and eat the sections with their membranes.

7. Eat more beans and peas.

do, elevating blood sugar to an excessive level. These complex carbohydrates have a high glycemic index, whereas complex carbohydrates that are high in fiber tend to have a lower glycemic index. Fiber aids in slowing digestion, so sugars tend to be absorbed into the bloodstream more slowly. Interestingly, ice cream has a fairly low glycemic index because the fat in ice cream tends to slow blood sugar absorption.

The rationale for avoiding high-glycemic-index foods relates to the resulting production of insulin. Avoiding high-glycemic-index foods and eating only low-glycemic-index foods may facilitate fat loss by reducing excess insulin. The weakness of this theory, however, is that obese and severely overweight individuals are already producing excess insulin; thus consuming a low-glycemic-index diet will not help them to achieve meaningful weight loss. And as nutrition expert Dr. Walter C. Willet notes, a food's glycemic index is only part of the larger picture. Many fruits, for example, have very high glycemic indexes but are high in desirable fiber and vitamins.[8]

Proteins

Protein provides the framework for muscles, bones, blood, hair, and fingernails. It is the main supply of amino acids—the building blocks that construct, repair, and maintain body tissues. The nine "essential" amino acids are the ones that the body cannot manufacture itself and must receive from dietary sources. Complete sources of protein contain all of the essential amino acids in their required amounts; incomplete sources of protein lack one or more of the essential amino acids. Complete proteins include meat, fish, poultry, and dairy products. Incomplete sources include beans, peas, peanuts, grains, and potatoes. Complementary proteins are protein sources that, when eaten together, supply the necessary amounts of all the essential amino acids. An example of complementary proteins is cooked dried beans eaten with rice. One difficulty for vegetarians or people eating a diet low in

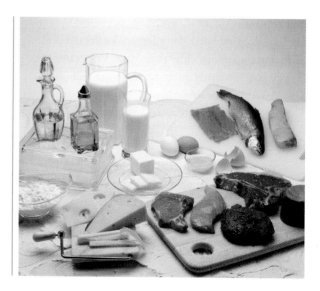

■ Complete proteins contain all the essential amino acids in their required amounts.

animal proteins is that the body cannot store amino acids. To benefit the body, a person must consume all the essential amino acids at the same meal. Interestingly, vegetarian foods that complement each other in essential amino acids also complement each other in taste. A peanut butter sandwich (containing wheat and peanuts), red (or black) beans and rice, or a bean burrito (beans wrapped in corn or wheat tortilla) are all complete sources of protein.

The National Academy of Science recommends that women consume 0.8 gram of protein per kilogram of body weight (0.36 gram per pound of body weight) on a daily basis.[9] Extra protein, like other excess calories, is stored as fat.

Many of the more recently publicized high-protein diets propose obtaining a significant percentage of daily calories from protein. A major problem with such diets is that their followers tend to consume proteins high in saturated fat, such as red meat and cheese, but eat fewer healthy carbohydrates such as fruit, vegetables, and fiber. Diets high in saturated fat increase a person's risk for heart disease and certain types of cancer. High-protein diets also may increase a woman's risk for osteoporosis. Excess dietary protein increases calcium loss in the urine.

Soy is a type of protein that is being studied to determine its health benefits. Soy-based foods may potentially lower cholesterol, ease hot flashes during menopause, prevent osteoporosis, and reduce the risk of breast and prostate cancer, all while helping a person lose weight. However, the evidence for these claims is still uncertain. While several studies have found that soy-based products can provide significant health benefits, others have found little to no difference between groups eating soy products and control groups. Soybeans contain products called phytoestrogens—plant products that act like estrogen in the human body. One phytoestrogen called isoflavone is present in particularly high levels in soybeans and soy products. Research still needs to be done on this topic, but some preliminary results have indicated that soy isoflavones may actually stimulate the production of breast cancer cells as well as lead to memory loss. However, soy-based products can still be a low-fat source of calcium, protein, and other nutrients. When consumed in moderation, soy-based products are probably not a major health risk.[8] The FDA has limited use of the soy-related health claim to foods containing intact soy protein—the claim does not extend to isolated substances from soy protein such as the isoflavones, so manufacturers of such products cannot include this claim on their food labels. Women are advised to use caution in consumption of soy isoflavones.

Fats

Fats perform many important bodily functions, such as storing energy, maintaining healthy hair and skin, carrying fat-soluble vitamins, supplying essential fatty acids, affecting levels of blood cholesterol, and creating a feeling of "fullness." Cholesterol is a type of fat produced by the liver. It is a vital constituent of cell membranes and nerve fibers and serves as a building block for estrogen, testosterone, vitamin D, and bile. Cholesterol is transported in the bloodstream in protein

■ Fats perform many bodily functions, such as storing energy, maintaining healthy hair and skin, carrying fat-soluble vitamins, and creating a feeling of "fullness."

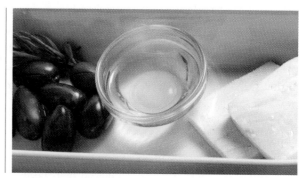

packages called lipoproteins, which are assembled in the intestinal tract and liver. **Low-density lipoproteins (LDLs)**—called the "bad" cholesterol—carry the cholesterol through the blood, dropping it off where it is needed for cell building and leaving any excess in arterial walls and other tissues. The excess accumulates in the arterial walls, causing blockage. **High-density lipoproteins (HDLs)**—known as the "good" cholesterol—pick up cholesterol deposits and bring them to the liver for reprocessing or excretion. Increased levels of LDLs are associated with an increased risk of heart disease, whereas increased levels of HDLs seem to have a protective effect against heart disease. The body normally produces all of the cholesterol that it needs, so dietary cholesterol (found in foods from animal sources such as eggs, meats, and dairy products) is actually unnecessary.

Fats are classified into three categories:

1. **Saturated fats** come primarily from animal sources such as meat, poultry, milk, cheese, and butter. Vegetable oils such as coconut, palm kernel, and palm oil also are saturated fats. From a chemical perspective, saturated fats are "saturated" with hydrogen atoms; each molecule holds as many as it can possibly carry. From a practical perspective, this means that saturated fats are generally solid at room temperature. They raise both LDL and HDL cholesterol, thereby increasing the risk of heart disease.

2. **Unsaturated fats** come from plants and include most vegetable oils. Carbon atoms in unsaturated fats have multiple bonds with each other. This prevents them from carrying the maximum number of hydrogen atoms they can carry (hence the name "unsaturated"). In turn, this configuration gives the molecules "kinks" that prevent unsaturated fat molecules from solidifying. They include two types:

   - **Monounsaturated fats,** such as those in olive, peanut, grapeseed, and canola oil
   - **Polyunsaturated fats,** such as those in safflower, sunflower, corn, and flaxseed oil

   Unsaturated fats lower LDL cholesterol and raise HDL cholesterol, which has a positive effect on overall blood cholesterol levels and can therefore lower the risk of heart disease.

3. Trans fats form when vegetable oils are processed into margarine or shortening. They are found in snack foods such as potato chips, commercial baked goods with "partially hydrogenated vegetable oil" or "vegetable shortening," many types of fast foods (french fries and onion rings), stick margarine, and some dairy products. Trans fats are solid or semi-solid at room temperature. These types of fats are worse for cholesterol levels than saturated fats because they not only raise LDL cholesterol, but also lower HDL cholesterol. A recent report on trans fats from the Institute of Medicine concluded that there is no safe level of trans fats in the diet. The FDA now requires that trans fats be listed on the Nutrition Facts food label used in the United States. The FDA estimates that the labeling requirement, which began in 2006, will prevent 600 to 1,200 coronary heart attacks and save 200 to 500 deaths per year by 2009.[10]

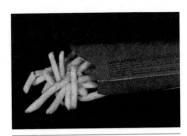

The fast-food industry is responding to consumer demand for more nutrition labeling about fats.

Lowering one's intake of saturated fat, trans fat, and dietary cholesterol has been identified as one of the major modifiable risk factors for coronary heart disease. Although it was once believed that dietary cholesterol alone was the culprit in heart disease, studies have since shown that lowering intake of dietary cholesterol has less effect on blood cholesterol levels than lowering intake of saturated fat.[11,12] In a study involving more than 80,000 female nurses, Harvard researchers found that increasing cholesterol intake by 200 mg for every 1,000 calories in the diet (about one egg per day) did not appreciably increase the risk for heart disease.[13]

It is recommended that 30% or less of daily calories come from fat, with 10% or less coming from saturated fat (Table 9.1). No daily limit has been set for trans fat (Table 9.2). Additionally, diets should contain less than 300 mg of cholesterol per day.[11] These guidelines, which parallel the dietary guidelines endorsed by the USDA and the U.S. Department of Health and Human Services, emphasize the importance to women of following careful eating patterns from early childhood to old age. Currently, few American women are meeting these standards. Self-Assessment 9.1 reviews the method for calculating daily fat intake.

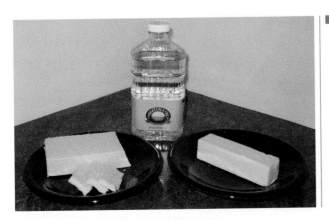

Fats are classified into three categories: saturated fats, which come primarily from animal sources; unsaturated fats, which come from plants; and trans fats, which form when vegetable oils are processed into margarine or shortening.

Table 9.1	Differences in Saturated Fat and Calorie Content of Commonly Consumed Foods

This table shows a few practical examples of the differences in the saturated fat content of different forms of commonly consumed foods. Comparisons are made between foods in the same food group (e.g., regular cheddar cheese and low-fat cheddar cheese), illustrating that lower saturated fat choices can be made within the same food group.

Food Category	Portion	Saturated Fat Content (grams)	Calories
Cheese			
▪ Regular cheddar cheese	1 oz	6.0	114
▪ Low-fat cheddar cheese	1 oz	1.2	49
Ground beef			
▪ Regular ground beef (25% fat)	3 oz (cooked)	6.1	236
▪ Extra lean ground beef (5% fat)	3 oz (cooked)	2.6	148
Milk			
▪ Whole milk (3.24%)	1 cup	4.6	146
▪ Low-fat (1%) milk	1 cup	1.5	102
Breads			
▪ Croissant (med)	1 medium	6.6	231
▪ Bagel, oat bran (4 inch)	1 medium	0.2	227
Frozen desserts			
▪ Regular ice cream	½ cup	4.9	145
▪ Frozen yogurt, low-fat	½ cup	2.0	110
Table spreads			
▪ Butter	1 tsp	2.4	34
▪ Soft margarine with zero trans fat	1 tsp	0.7	25
Chicken			
▪ Fried chicken (leg with skin)	3 oz (cooked)	3.3	212
▪ Roasted chicken (breast no skin)	3 oz (cooked)	0.9	140
Fish			
▪ Fried fish	3 oz	2.8	195
▪ Baked fish	3 oz	1.5	129

Source: U.S. Department of Agriculture. (2005). *Dietary Guidelines for Americans.*

Vitamins

Vitamins are organic substances that perform a variety of functions and are needed by the body in very small amounts. When a woman consumes a nutritious diet, she should have no need for vitamin supplements. Despite all the advertising claims, scientific evidence offers no indication that extra vitamins prolong life, enhance sexual pleasures, or enhance athletic performance. Although many people

Table 9.2 Trans Fatty Acid Content of Selected Foods

Food	Trans Fat as a Percentage of Total Fat
Bread, white	9.3%
Cake with chocolate frosting	18.3%
Cheesecake	12.0%
Cookies, chocolate chip	24.3%
Cookies, chocolate, cream filled	36.3%
Crackers, snack type	39.7%
Pastry, Danish	39.5%
French fries	23.9%
Granola bar	17.9%
Margarine, hard stick	29.4%
Shortening	22.2%
Popcorn, microwave	31.7%
Unprocessed vegetables, fruits, grains, nuts, vegetable oils, legumes, soy milk	0%

To find out whether a food contains trans fatty acids, look at the ingredient list. If the words "partially hydrogenated oils" are listed, it contains trans fats.

Source: U.S. Department of Agriculture, released on CD, 2001.

view vitamin supplements as a shortcut to good nutrition, vitamins cannot replace food or turn a junk-food meal into a healthy one. Vitamins are essential for life, promoting good vision, forming normal blood cells, creating strong bones and teeth, and ensuring proper functioning of the heart and nervous system. Although vitamins do not supply any energy, they do aid in the efficient conversion of foods into energy.

Scientific consensus is that 13 essential vitamins exist: A, C, D, E, K, and the eight vitamins of the B complex. Fat-soluble vitamins (A, D, E, and K) are stored in the liver for relatively long periods of time; water-soluble vitamins (B-complex

Self-Assessment 9.1

Calculating Daily Fat Limits

To determine the maximum number of daily grams of fat:

1. Calculate approximately how many calories are consumed on a daily basis: _____

2. Divide the answer above in (1) by 33: _____

Women who find that they are eating more grams of fat than the calculated number should work on achieving this desired amount. Women with an intake of greater than 30% of calories from fat are at greater risk for many chronic diseases as well as obesity.

vitamins and C) are stored for very short periods of time. Each vitamin carries out specific functions. The body generally cannot manufacture vitamins; instead, they must be derived from food sources. A particular disease usually results if a certain vitamin is lacking or is improperly used by the body. Table 9.3 summarizes facts known for each of the essential vitamins.

Folic Acid

Folate is a B vitamin found in foods such as chickpeas, spinach, strawberries, kidney beans, and citrus fruits and juices. Folic acid, a form of folate, is used to fortify grain-based foods, such as bread, flour, rice, pasta, and cereal. It is vital for cell growth and function and for the development of healthy neural tubes in fetuses. Neural tube defects, including spina bifida, are birth defects affecting the brain and spinal cord. Since fortification of cereal grains with folic acid began in the United States in 1998, the incidence of neural tube disorders has decreased by 20-30%. All women of childbearing age should include 400–600 micrograms (0.4–0.6 mg) of folic acid in their daily diet. A number of surveys have shown that as a group, women of childbearing age consume an average of 200 micrograms per day, only half of the recommended amount.[14] Folic acid also is important for maintaining levels of homocysteine, an amino acid found in the blood that builds and maintains tissues, but it can increase the risk of cardiovascular disease if it is consumed at excessive levels. Additionally, folic acid fortification is one of the few public health interventions besides immunization that actually saves money; one economic analysis concluded that folic acid fortification in the United States results in a cost savings of $88 million to $145 million annually and is associated with an overall economic benefit of $312 million to $425 million per year.[15]

Antioxidants and Phytochemicals

Antioxidants (substances such as vitamin E and vitamin C) and **phytochemicals** (substances such as carotenoids and flavonoids that appear to act as antioxidants) have been widely studied for their roles in disease prevention and health promotion. Evidence has shown that diets rich in fruits, vegetables, and grains—all of which are rich sources of antioxidants—are associated with a decreased risk of cardiovascular disease and cancer. Damage to cells from oxidation is associated with an increased risk of various diseases. Antioxidants are thought to block some of the oxygen-induced cell damage by stabilizing and neutralizing the effects of free radicals (toxic particles) in the body.

Some studies show that vitamin E protects against damage in the artery lining, thereby decreasing the risk of coronary artery disease. Many studies indicate that eating fruits and vegetables rich in vitamin C and beta-carotene (the carotenoid that is the precursor of vitamin A) is linked to a reduced risk of many cancers. Carotenoids and flavonoids, which are found in foods such as onions, broccoli, red wine, green tea, and black tea, appear to have a positive effect on heart disease; however, the association between phytochemicals and heart disease is still uncertain.

It is obvious that a healthy diet helps prevent disease. However, evidence for more specific claims, such as those that mention individual foods preventing specific

Table 9.3   Facts about Vitamins

Vitamin	Women's RDA*	Sources	What It Does
Vitamin A	700 μg	Liver, eggs, dairy products, carrots, bell peppers, green leafy vegetables, squash	Promotes good vision; helps form and maintain healthy skin and mucous membranes; helps fight infections
Vitamin B$_1$ (thiamin)	1.1 mg	Whole grains, dried beans, lean red meats, fish, sunflower seeds	Helps release energy from carbohydrates; necessary for healthy brain and nerve cells and for functioning of heart
Vitamin B$_2$ (riboflavin)	1.1 mg	Dairy products, liver, whole grains, spinach, broccoli	Aids in the release of energy from food; helps form antibodies and red blood cells
Vitamin B$_3$ (niacin)	14 mg	Nuts, dairy products, liver, enriched grains, poultry	Aids in the release of energy from food; involved in the synthesis of DNA; maintains normal function of skin, nerves, and digestive system
Vitamin B$_5$ (pantothenic acid)	5 mg	Whole grains, dried beans, eggs, nuts	Aids in the release of energy from food; essential for synthesis of numerous body materials
Vitamin B$_6$ (pyridoxine)	1.3 mg	Fortified breakfast cereals, meat, nuts, beans	Important in chemical reactions of proteins and amino acids; involved in normal functioning of brain and formation of red blood cells
Vitamin B$_{12}$ (cobalamin)	2.4 μg	Liver, beef, eggs, milk, shellfish	Necessary for development of red blood cells; maintains normal functioning of nervous system
Biotin	30 μg	Yeast, liver, eggs, milk	Important in the formation of fatty acids; helps metabolize amino acids and carbohydrates
Vitamin C[†] (ascorbic acid)	75 mg	Citrus fruits and juices, bell peppers, tomatoes, spinach, broccoli	Promotes healthy gums, capillaries, and teeth; aids iron absorption; maintains normal connective tissue; aids in healing wounds
Choline	425 mg[†]	Whole grains, egg yolks, legumes, liver, soybeans, green leafy vegetables	Manages cholesterol in body; important for brain function; involved in production of hormones; necessary for functioning of folic acid
Vitamin D (calciferol)	5 μg	Dairy products, mackerel, sardines, salmon and other cold-water fish	Promotes strong bones and teeth; necessary for absorption of calcium
Vitamin E (tocopherol)	15 mg	Nuts, vegetable oils, whole grains, margarine, dark green vegetables	Protects tissue against oxidation; important in formation of red blood cells; helps body use vitamin K
Folate (folic acid/folacin)	400 μg	Liver, fortified breakfast cereals, lentils, chickpeas, spinach, beans	Important in the synthesis of DNA; acts together with vitamin B$_{12}$ in the production of hemoglobin; vital to healthy fetal development
Vitamin K	90 μg	Leafy green vegetables, soybeans, broccoli, cauliflower	Aids in the clotting of blood

*Pregnant or breastfeeding women need additional levels of these vitamins.
†Smokers should consume an additional 35 mg daily of vitamin C.

Sources: Willet, W. C. (2002). *Eat, Drink and Be Healthy: The Harvard Medical School Guide to Healthy Eating.* New York: Simon and Schuster. Editors of the *University of California at Berkeley Wellness Letter.* (1995). *The New Wellness Encyclopedia.* Boston: Houghton Mifflin.

diseases, is uncertain at best. For now, experts recommend that people meet the RDAs by eating foods high in carotenoids, such as red, orange, and deep yellow fruits and vegetables (e.g., tomatoes, carrots, sweet potatoes) and dark green leafy vegetables (e.g., spinach, broccoli); foods high in vitamin E (e.g., vegetable oils, salad dressings, margarine, whole grains, peanut butter); and foods rich in vitamin C (e.g., citrus fruits, strawberries, broccoli). Eating a variety of fruits and vegetables promotes health by supplying the body not only with vitamins and fiber, but also with antioxidants that may reduce the risk of heart disease and some kinds of cancer.[8]

Minerals

Minerals are inorganic substances essential to bone formation (calcium), enzyme synthesis (iron), blood pressure maintenance (sodium), and normal functioning of

Table 9.4   Facts about Minerals

Mineral	Adult RDA*	Sources	What It Does
Calcium	1,000–2,500 mg*	Milk and milk products, sardines and salmon eaten with bones, dark green leafy vegetables, certain types of tofu and soy milk, fortified orange juice	Builds bones and teeth and maintains bone density and strength; helps prevent osteoporosis; plays a role in regulating heartbeat, blood clotting, muscle contraction, and nerve conduction; helps prevent hypertension
Chloride	700 mg	Table salt, fish, pickled and smoked foods	Maintains normal fluid shifts; balances pH of the blood; forms hydrochloric acid to aid digestion
Magnesium	310–320 mg*	Whole grains, raw leafy green vegetables, nuts (especially almonds and cashews), soybeans, tofu, hard water	Aids in bone growth; assists function of nerves and muscles, including regulation of normal heart rhythm; important in energy metabolism
Phosphorus	700 mg*	Meats, poultry, fish, egg yolks, dried peas and beans, milk and milk products, nuts; present in almost all foods	Aids bone growth and strengthening of teeth; important in energy metabolism
Potassium	4,700 mg†	Oranges and orange juice, melons, bananas, dried fruits, dried peas and beans, potatoes	Promotes regular heartbeat; active in muscle contraction; regulates transfer of nutrients to cells; controls water balance in body tissues and cells; contributes to regulation of blood pressure
Sodium	500 mg (estimated safe amount for dietary intake)	All from salt and foods containing salt	Helps regulate water balance in body; plays a role in maintaining blood pressure
Chromium	50–200 μg†	Meat, cheese, mushrooms, oysters, peanuts, brewer's yeast, potatoes	Important for glucose metabolism; may be a cofactor for insulin; regulates cholesterol production in liver; aids in digestion of protein

*These figures are not applicable to pregnant or breastfeeding women, who need additional vitamins.

†Although there is no RDA for these minerals, the Food and Nutrition Board recommends this value as an average healthy intake.

Sources: Willet, W. C. (2002). *Eat, Drink and Be Healthy: The Harvard Medical School Guide to Healthy Eating.* New York: Simon and Schuster. Editors of the *University of California at Berkeley Wellness Letter.* (1995). *The New Wellness Encyclopedia.* Boston: Houghton Mifflin Co.

the digestive process (potassium). Minerals make up the earth's surface. Carried into the soil, groundwater, and sea by erosion, they are taken up by plants and subsequently consumed by animals and humans. As components of the body, minerals are present in small amounts. Although more than 60 different minerals are found on earth, six of them (calcium, chloride, magnesium, phosphorus, potassium, and sodium) are generally designated as macrominerals, or major minerals. From a women's health perspective, calcium and iron are especially important.

Because of the complex interactions between minerals and the dangers of overdosing, self-administration of mineral supplements in doses greater than the RDAs should be avoided. Megadoses of certain minerals may do serious harm. The best way to ensure an adequate, but not excessive, supply of minerals is to eat a varied, balanced diet. Table 9.4 summarizes facts about each of the essential minerals.

Table 9.4   Facts about Minerals *(continued)*

Mineral	Adult RDA*	Sources	What It Does
Copper	900-10,000 $\mu g^\dagger$	Wheat, peanuts, shellfish (especially oysters), nuts, beef and pork liver, dried beans	Formation of red blood cells; cofactor in absorbing iron into blood cells; assists in production of several enzymes involved in respiration; interacts with zinc
Fluorine (Fluoride)	3.1 mg†	Fluoridated water, foods cooked with or grown in fluoridated water, fish, tea, gelatin	Contributes to solid bone and tooth formation; prevents dental cavities; may help prevent osteoporosis
Iodine	0.15 mg*	Primarily from iodized salt, but also seafood, seaweed food products, vegetables grown in iodine-rich areas, eggs, certain cheeses, whole milk	Necessary for normal function of the thyroid gland; essential for normal cell function; keeps skin, hair, and nails healthy; prevents goiter
Iron	18-45 mg*	Liver (especially pork liver), kidneys, red meats, egg yolks, peas, beans, nuts, dried fruits, green leafy vegetables, enriched grain products, blackstrap molasses	Essential to formation of hemoglobin, the oxygen-carrying factor in the blood; part of several enzymes and proteins in the blood
Manganese	320-350 mg†	Nuts, whole grains, vegetables, fruits, instant coffee, tea, cocoa powder, beets, egg yolks	Required for normal bone growth; helps maintain healthy skin; important for metabolism of glucose and fatty acids
Molybdenum	75-250 $\mu g^\dagger$	Peas, beans, cereal grains, organ meats, some dark green vegetables	Important for normal cell function
Selenium	50-55 μg	Fish, shellfish, red meat, egg yolks, chicken, legumes, whole grains	Protects cells against effects of free radicals that can damage cells; essential for normal functioning of the immune system and thyroid gland
Zinc	8-40 mg	Meat, liver, eggs, oysters, legumes, whole grain cereals, nuts	Essential for growth and skeletal development; important for immune system; assists in production of DNA and RNA

Calcium

As noted earlier, **calcium** is a mineral of special concern to women. Calcium is an integral component of bones and teeth, and consequently calcium deficiency is a major contributor to osteoporosis. When calcium levels in the blood fall too low, the body draws the mineral from the supply in the bones to meet its needs elsewhere. This process accelerates the gradual bone loss that occurs most dramatically in postmenopausal women. Calcium also plays a role in regulating heartbeat, blood clotting, muscle contraction, and nerve conduction. In addition, evidence suggests that this mineral helps prevent high blood pressure, is essential in the development of the fetus during pregnancy, and may play a role in preventing colon cancer.

The RDA's recommendation that women receive 1,000 mg of calcium per day is deceptive. Adolescents, young women (ages 11 to 24), and postmenopausal women are advised to consume 1,200 mg daily. However, many health experts believe that lower dosages may be adequate. Three to five cups of milk or servings of other calcium-rich foods such as collard greens, cheese, tofu, cornbread, or sardines can supply the 1,000 mg recommendation. (See **It's Your Health**.) Daily supplements can also be a viable calcium source.[8]

The 2005 food pyramid continues to emphasize dairy products as an important part of a healthy diet, and the first word that comes to many women's minds when

It's Your Health

Calcium Sources

Food	Amount	mg Calcium	Percent of RDA 1,000 mg/day	Percent of RDA 1,200 mg/day
Plain Yogurt	1 cup	415	41%	35%
Sardines with bones	3 oz	372	37%	31%
Skim milk	1 cup	302	30%	25%
Collard greens	1 cup	290	29%	24%
Swiss cheese	1 oz	262	26%	22%
Cheddar cheese	1 oz	213	21%	18%
Canned salmon, with bones	3 oz	167	17%	14%
Low-fat cottage cheese	1 cup	154	15%	12%
Blackstrap molasses	1 tbsp	137	14%	12%
Cooked broccoli	1 cup	136	14%	12%
Dried and cooked beans	1 cup	90	9%	7%
Orange	1 (medium)	54	5%	4%

thinking of calcium is "milk." Some nutrition experts, such as Walter C. Willett at the Harvard School of Public Health, believe that the U.S. dietary guidelines exaggerate the benefits and underestimate the dangers of a diet high in dairy foods. Dairy foods are an excellent source of calcium as well as protein, vitamin D, and other nutrients; however, they often contain large amounts of saturated fat and calories, and they are not an option for lactose-intolerant individuals. Women do not have to rely on dairy products for their calcium. A cup of collard greens, for example, has virtually the same amount of calcium as a cup of skim milk (see **It's Your Health**). In many Asian countries that have lower osteoporosis rates than the United States, dairy products are marginal to nonexistent in traditional diets.

People who cannot meet the daily calcium intake recommendations through consumption of calcium-rich foods may use calcium-fortified foods and calcium supplements. Women who are susceptible to kidney stones should avoid such supplements to prevent an increased risk of stone formation. Because large amounts of calcium may lead to constipation, kidney stones, and poor kidney function, as well as interfere with the absorption of other minerals, women should not consume calcium levels significantly beyond their RDA.

Iron

Iron is found in the human body primarily in **hemoglobin,** a key component of red blood cells and the oxygen-carrying protein that gives blood its red color. When hemoglobin is not produced, the body becomes fatigued and weak. Reduced levels of hemoglobin result in anemia, a serious risk for women whose diets are chronically deficient in iron. Symptoms of iron-deficiency anemia include headaches, fatigue, general weakness, and pallor. In severe cases, anemia can lead to an irregular or increased heart rate. Iron-deficiency anemia is relatively common in the United States today, with 12% of women age 12 to 49 experiencing some form of iron deficiency.[16] In addition to being found in hemoglobin, iron is stored in the liver, spleen, bone marrow, and other tissues.

Iron absorption is a complex process that varies with the types of foods consumed, the combination of foods, and the body's needs. Women can use several strategies to increase their dietary intake of iron. Eating lean red meats is an obvious strategy. Liver is one of the best sources of iron, but it should not be eaten more than once a week owing to its high cholesterol content. Chicken and fish typically contain one-third to one-half the iron of red meat. Vegetarian sources of iron include chickpeas, soybeans, kidney beans, and lentils. Choosing breads, cereals, and pasta labeled "enriched" or "fortified" and unrefined whole grains, such as whole-wheat bread, supplies a fair amount of iron. In addition, eating foods high in vitamin C helps facilitate the body's absorption of iron. For vegetarians, consuming vitamin C with meals is a must. Cooking in cast-iron cookware also helps to increase the iron content of foods. The more acidic the food (such as spaghetti sauce) and the longer it cooks, the higher the iron content. Other compounds, such as coffee, tea, and dietary fiber, block the body's ability to absorb iron.

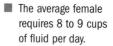

■ The average female requires 8 to 9 cups of fluid per day.

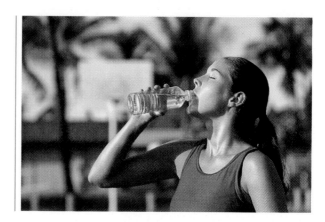

Water

The human body is approximately 50% to 70% water. Water is considered to be an essential nutrient because it is manufactured only in small amounts by the body and must be consumed in the form of liquids and solids to meet daily needs. Every system in the body depends on water to function. Water is responsible for regulating body temperature and chemical actions, disposing of waste, lubricating joints, cushioning the fetus during pregnancy, transporting nutrients, preventing bowel problems, and helping enzymes function properly.

The average female requires eight to nine cups of fluid per day; pregnant women have a slightly higher requirement due to the needs of the fetus. Some of this fluid comes from the food a woman eats; the rest must come from what she drinks. Drinking water by itself is one healthy option. Another is drinking skim milk or fruit juice, which can also supply the body with minerals, protein, and vitamins. Sweetened sodas and sports drinks are less healthy options because they are typically loaded with sugar and calories and provide no additional nutritonal benefit.

Water is so essential that the human body can survive only three days without it, even though the body can be denied food for a few weeks and still recover. As little as 2% to 5% loss of body weight from water loss results in symptoms of dehydration, including headache, fatigue, flushed skin, and excessive thirst. Greater need for fluids occurs during exercise and conditions of high temperature, high altitude, and low humidity, and when it is necessary to counter the effects of high intakes of caffeine and alcohol, which promote fluid loss. Many newer studies are examining the effects of water consumption on the risk of various conditions, including kidney stones, certain cancers, obesity, and oral health.

Exercise and Fitness

The United States has been a leader in understanding and promoting the benefits of physical activity. A national effort in the 1950s encouraged young Americans to join team sports so as to become physically active. The 1980s witnessed the emergence of a renewed national interest in physical fitness and exercise. During the 1990s, breakthrough findings reported the health benefits of moderate-intensity activities such as walking, gardening, and dancing. Despite these findings, physical inactivity remains a serious nationwide problem at the beginning of the twenty-first century. More than 60% of American adults do not get enough physical activity to provide health benefits. More than 25% of adults are not active at all. Men are more likely than women (21.3% to 16.9%) to engage in a high level of overall physical activity, but men and women are equally likely to engage in a medium-high level of overall physical activity (23%).[17] Physical activity decreases with age and is less common among those with lower incomes and less education.

Physical Fitness

"Physical fitness" means different things to different people. A dancer and a long-distance swimmer may both think of themselves as "fit" but they probably have different strengths, stretch different muscles, and have different workout goals. Fitness is also relative—a woman may be "more fit" this year than she was last year, and there is no clear endpoint at which fitness occurs. Fitness also can be defined as the ability to meet routine physical demands with a reserve to meet sudden challenges. The point is that if fitness is a goal, exercise is the means to get there. Fitness provides short-term and long-term benefits. Women who exercise just an hour per week or more are 33% less likely to die from cancer, 50% less likely to die from cardiovascular disease, and 66% less likely to die early than women who do not excercise.[18]

Benefits of Exercise

Regular exercise, whether recreational or work related, increases overall health and well-being. It offers many physical and psychological benefits that lead to greater quality and quantity of life (Table 9.5). Regular exercise reduces morbidity and mortality from heart disease, the leading cause of death in the United States. Physical activity not only improves overall cardiovascular status, but also affects other risk factors for heart disease. For example, regular physical activity lowers blood pressure, reduces body fat, builds lean body weight, improves blood cholesterol levels, and reduces stress. Colon cancer, type 2 diabetes, osteoporosis, and obesity are some of the other diseases in which the risk of developing the disease is lowered by exercise. This association also may be a consequence of exercise's ability to reduce the risk factors for various chronic diseases, such as high body fat and smoking behaviors.

Physical activity is extremely important for maintaining the health of muscles, bones, and joints; ensuring normal skeletal development; increasing bone mass and density; and slowing the rate of bone loss as women age—hence its role in reducing the risk of osteoporosis. Regular physical activity also improves balance and coordination, which reduce a woman's risk of fall-related fractures in later life.

The basic fact that exercise burns calories and increases lean body weight is important not only for the prevention of obesity (a major risk factor for many chronic diseases), but also for a woman's overall sense of well-being. Although

I really don't like to run so I have avoided exercise. I guess I believed that if it wasn't running, then it didn't count as exercise. A friend invited me biking a year ago and it sounded like fun. The next thing I knew I was seriously biking. Now I really look forward to my weekend trips. I'm planning a long trip for next summer. I learned that exercise does not have to be boring. I am doing this because it is fun. The exercise benefits are a great secondary gain.

22-year-old law student

Table 9.5	Benefits of Regular Physical Activity

- Reduces the risk of dying from coronary heart disease and of developing diabetes, high blood pressure, and colon cancer.
- Helps reduce blood pressure in people who already have high blood pressure.
- Helps maintain healthy bones, muscles, and joints.
- Helps control weight, build lean muscle, and reduce body fat.
- Helps control joint swelling and pain associated with arthritis.
- Reduces symptoms of anxiety and depression and fosters improvements in mood and feelings of well-being.
- May enhance the effect of estrogen replacement therapy in decreasing bone loss after menopause.
- Helps older adults to move about better without falling and risking fractures.

Source: U.S. Department of Health and Human Services. 2002. *Physical Activity Fundamental to Preventing Disease*. Atlanta, GA: Centers for Disease Control and Prevention, National Center for Chronic Disease Prevention and Health Promotion.

most individuals who exercise regularly report that they "feel better" when they exercise, until recently the scientific community has not been able to measure this phenomenon objectively. Many studies have confirmed the potential value of aerobic exercise, along with medication if necessary, as a complementary therapy for depression.[19,20] People who exercise regularly report feeling happier, feeling better about themselves, and in general experience a better quality of life than people who do not.[20] Regular exercise may also reduce the anxiety and depression that can appear during pregnancy.[21] Other studies have long suggested various psychological benefits from exercise, including decreased stress, increased sense of well-being, and improvements in cognitive function and mood.[22] Proper exercise during pregnancy also has many benefits, including improved psychological well-being, shorter labor, and speedier recovery after childbirth (see Chapter 6).

Components of Physical Fitness

Exercise physiologists usually define fitness in four major areas:

- Cardiovascular endurance
- Muscular strength
- Muscular endurance
- Flexibility

Modern lifestyles do not require much physical movement, and few American women are naturally fit as a result of day-to-day activities. Most women who wish to become fit in today's society will need to make a commitment of time and energy.

Cardiovascular endurance, the ability to carry on vigorous physical activity for an extended period of time, is the most vital element of fitness. It encompasses the

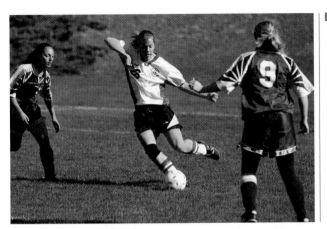

Organized sports are one form of exercise.

ability of the heart to pump blood efficiently through the body. The development of cardiovascular endurance enhances the ability of the heart, blood vessels, and blood to deliver oxygen to the body's cells and then remove waste products. Although muscles are able to draw on quick sources of energy for short-term exertion, when exercise lasts more than a minute or two, the muscles require oxygen from the blood. Such physical activity is called aerobic exercise. With repeated regular exercise, the heart becomes able to pump more blood and deliver more oxygen with greater efficiency. In addition, the muscles' capacity to use this oxygen improves. The coupled events are referred to as the "training effect." The heart rate, both at rest and exertion, decreases as a result of this regular exercise, and the heart acquires the ability to recover from the stress of exercise more quickly.

Muscular strength is the total force that muscle groups produce in one effort, such as a lift, jump, or heave. Working out with weights, either free weights or weight machines, is the best way to increase muscle strength. Strength gains come most quickly from heavy resistance and few repetitions.

Muscular endurance refers to the ability to perform repeated muscular contractions over a period of time without tiring. Although muscle endurance requires strength, it is not a single, all-out effort. The keys to increasing endurance are repetition, working at a moderate level, and building up to a specified goal. Sit-ups, push-ups, and pull-ups can be used to build endurance.

Flexibility refers to the ability of the joints to move through their full range of motion. It is best improved through static stretching exercises that apply steady pressure at the extreme range of motion without undue bouncing. Flexibility varies from person to person and from joint to joint. Women tend to be more flexible than men because of differences in their skeletons, muscle mass, and body composition. Good flexibility is thought to protect the muscles against pulls and tears because short, tight muscles may be more likely to be overstretched. Exercises intended to increase flexibility must be selected carefully, however, because some movements may actually cause injury to the lower back and knees. Some women find that stretching certain muscle groups helps relieve or prevent pain. Stretching

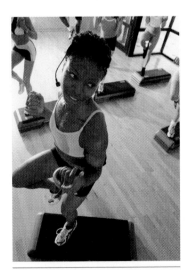

Strength training can help prevent or delay many of the declines associated with aging or inactivity.

hamstring and lower back muscles may alleviate lower back pain, and calf stretches may help prevent leg cramps.

Body composition, often considered a component of fitness, refers to the ratio of lean body weight (muscle and bone) to fat weight. It can be dramatically affected by exercise, which can help prevent and control obesity by reducing excess body weight through energy expenditure and increasing metabolic rate by changing the muscle-to-fat ratio. Calories are burned not only during the period of physical exercise, but also for several hours after the exercise ends (known as afterburn). The longer and more intense the exercise, the longer the **basal metabolic rate (BMR)** remains elevated. Regular exercise improves overall muscle tone, contributing to a less flabby appearance. Exercise can also improve balance, coordination (the ability to skillfully use different body parts and the senses together), and agility (the ability to coordinate multiple movements and to react quickly and safely).

Balance skills are frequently neglected and can be maintained only through regular use. Problems with balance are responsible for many falls and other accidents among the elderly. Exercise activities that can improve balance include dancing, tai chi, yoga, and skipping rope. Racket sports are particularly helpful in promoting coordination and agility.

Total Fitness

Activities to improve fitness are often referred to as conditioning programs or training regimens. A wide variety of fitness programs are possible, but they tend to fall into two categories: aerobic training and strength training. Aerobic training increases the body's ability to use oxygen and improves endurance. Strength training enhances the size and strength of particular muscles and body regions. The best fitness programs combine aerobic exercise with strength training. Both types of exercise provide unique benefits. Strength training builds muscle and bone, and aerobic exercise improves cardiovascular fitness. Together, aerobic and strength training provide better benefits than either form of exercise alone. Coupled with a healthy diet, the combination program also may be the most efficient way to lose weight. In addition to burning calories while working out, the resultant muscle mass from strength training boosts the basal metabolic rate further because muscle consumes more energy than does fat.

Warm-Up

A warm-up is essential before any aerobic or strength training session. Warming up prepares the body for exercise by gradually increasing the heart rate and blood flow, raising the temperature of the muscles, and improving muscle function. It may also decrease the chance of sports-related injury. Stretching is not a wise way to begin a workout, because stretching cold muscles increases the risk of injury. Sudden exercise without a gradual warm-up can lead to an abnormal heart rate and blood flow and changes in blood pressure, which can be dangerous, especially for older exercisers.

Activities such as jogging in place or stationary cycling are full body warm-ups that can be performed for 5 to 10 minutes to raise body temperature.

Strength Training

Strength training, like aerobic exercise, helps prevent or delay many of the declines associated with aging or inactivity. The "use it or lose it" adage applies with all muscle groups.

Strength training does not have to mean lifting massive weights to build bulging muscles. Instead, it often calls for working out against moderate resistance to tone muscles and build muscle endurance. Free weights, dumbbells, barbells, or weight machines can provide this resistance. Body weight can also be used as resistance, as in push-ups or pull-ups.

Strength training offers many benefits:

- Well-toned muscles help maintain good posture and may help prevent injuries.
- Muscle strength produces benefits in daily living, from lifting items to engaging in physical activity, by increasing stamina and self-confidence.
- Strength training increases bone density, thereby helping to delay or minimize osteoporosis and vulnerability to fractures.
- Injury prevention is another important benefit of strength training, especially for musculoskeletal injuries that are induced by exercise, such as runner's knee or shin splints. These injuries are due in part to muscle weakness and imbalances as well as joint instability. Such conditions are often corrected with strength training.
- Maintaining a strong back through strength training protects it from injury.

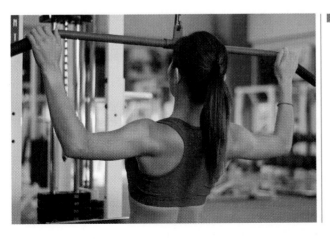

■ Maintaining a strong back through strength training protects it from injury.

Lower back pain often results from weakness of back and abdominal muscles, both of which help support the back.

- Strength training helps improve posture, a source of many back problems.

Women tend to have less muscle mass than men, especially in the upper body. This discrepancy has been attributed to hormonal differences, the fact that women are generally smaller than men, and the difference in men's and women's normal activities. Women who work out, however, gain strength at the same rate as men. Many women have avoided strength training out of fear of becoming "muscle bound." A moderate program will not create obvious muscle bulk in men or women but will result in a firmer, trimmer physique.

Aerobic Exercise

Aerobic exercise significantly raises the heart rate and provides different benefits than strength training. Aerobic exercise seems to lower body cholesterol levels and blood pressure more than strength training. It also improves cardiovascular fitness, the ability of the heart and lungs to supply the muscles with oxygen; strength training generally does not provide such a benefit. Examples of aerobic exercise include running, bicycling, and rollerblading.

Components of Exercise.   When exercising, there are three important variables to consider: intensity, duration, and frequency.

Exercise intensity is the work per unit of time. It can be monitored by measuring the target heart rate—the exercise heart rate needed to produce a training effect—for 20 to 30 minutes during each workout.

Exercise duration is the length of one exercise session. To benefit the heart, aerobic exercise must be intense enough to increase the heart rate and must continue for a minimum amount of time depending on the intensity of the workout: one hour for light-intensity activities, 30 to 60 minutes for moderate-intensity activities, and 30 minutes for high-intensity activities. See Table 9.6 for examples of exercises of different activity levels.

Exercise frequency measures the number of exercise sessions over the long term. Engaging in regular periods of exercise is essential for any exercise program. Exercising in three to five half-hour periods per week builds muscle and improves fitness faster and more safely than exercising for the same length of time in one long weekly workout.

The body responds best to a conditioning program that switches between light and heavy demands and that gives muscle groups time to recover after being worked. Alternating between "light" and "heavy" workouts or alternating between aerobic or strength-training sessions on a daily basis allows the body to repair itself between workouts, reducing the risks of injury, and makes individual sessions more relaxing.

Maximum and Target Range Heart Rates.   No aerobic exercise program will be beneficial unless it forces the heart to pump beyond its normal output. To determine this ideal pace, check whether the heart is beating within the target heart

Table 9.6 Examples of Light, Moderate, and Vigorous Activity

Light-Intensity Activities (require 60 minutes per session)

Walking slowly

Golfing using a powered cart

Swimming, slow treading

Gardening or pruning

Bicycling, very light effort

Dusting or vacuuming

Conditioning exercise, lightly stretching or warming up

Moderate-Intensity Activities (require 30 minutes per session)

Walking briskly

Golfing, pulling or carrying clubs

Swimming, recreational

Mowing lawn, power motor

Playing tennis, doubles

Bicycling 5 to 9 mph, level terrain, or with a few hills

Scrubbing floors or washing windows

Weight lifting, using Nautilus machines or free weights

High-Intensity Activities (require 20 to 30 minutes per session)

Racewalking, jogging, and running

Swimming laps

Mowing lawn, hand mower

Playing tennis, singles

Bicycling more than 10 mph or on steep uphill terrain

Moving or pushing furniture

Circuit training

Source: Physical Activity for Everyone: Measuring Physical Activity Intensity. Atlanta, GA: U.S. Department of Health and Human Services, Centers for Disease Control and Prevention. Retrieved December 20, 2005, from http://www.cdc.gov/nccdphp/dnpa/physical/measuring/examples.htm.

range—fast enough to ensure that the activity pushes the heart muscle to the point of improving fitness, but not so fast that it will become exhausted within too short a time or cause physical harm. (See Figure 9.3 to determine maximum and target heart rates.) Checking the pulse during or immediately after exercise is useful for determining if the exercise is at the appropriate intensity (see Self-Assessment 9.2). An exercise program that keeps the heart rate within the desirable range provides a training effect in as safe a manner as possible. If the heart does not reach the lower limit of the target heart range during an exercise activity, increase the intensity by exercising more vigorously. If the heart rate exceeds the upper limit of

Figure 9.3

Maximum and targeted heart rates.

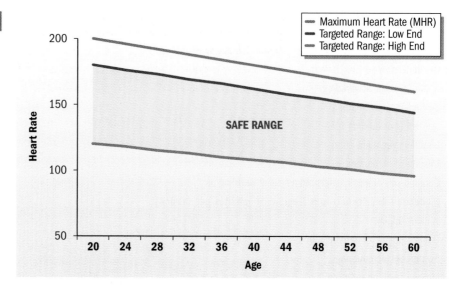

the target heart range, particularly in the early phases of an exercise program, reduce the intensity to stay within the range.

Many Options of Aerobic Exercise. Regular exercise is important. The form it takes is of secondary importance. Many women find that they are able to maintain their interest in exercise by changing their physical activity on a regular basis to avoid boredom. Seasonal variations and access to recreational facilities also influence exercise decision making. The following examples describe currently popular forms of aerobic exercise that are enjoyed by many women.

Moderate- to brisk-paced walking is an easy, safe, simple, and enjoyable way to stay healthy; walking for 30 to 45 minutes per day lowers the risk of heart disease, lowers blood pressure, helps control adult-onset diabetes, guards against osteoporosis, helps keep weight under control, and helps reduce stress. Most problems with walk-

Self-Assessment 9.2

How to Check Your Pulse

Each "pulse" you feel when you put your fingers on an artery represents the blood pushed by one pump of a person's heart. The easiest way to measure your pulse is to place your fingers on the carotid artery on your neck or the radial artery on your wrist.

1. To find the radial artery, place your first two or three fingers on the thumb side of your inner wrist. To find the carotid artery, place your fingers just below the edge of the jaw bone. Apply gentle pressure. Do not use your thumb.

2. Using a stopwatch or clock with a second hand, count the number of pulses in 30 seconds. Multiply by 2 to get the number of beats per minute.

Source: Limmer, D., O'Keefe, M. O., Dickinson, E. V., Grant, H., Murray, B., and Bergeron, J. D. (2004). *Emergency Care* (tenth edition). New York: Pearson Education.

ing can be avoided by simply wearing good walking shoes, warming up beforehand, practicing good walking technique, and working up slowly to the desired pace.

Jogging is aerobic exercise somewhere between a fast walk and a run. Technically it is defined as moving at a pace slower than a 9-minute mile. Jogging is the classic aerobic exercise because it strengthens the heart and lungs, boost stamina, and improves circulation.

Bicycling, whether on a stationary bike or outdoors, can be an excellent cardiovascular conditioner as well as an effective way to control weight. Stationary biking in aerobic settings, often referred to as "spinning," offers a variety of speed resistances to simulate biking a hilly course or race.

Stair climbing, either in buildings or on stair machines, offers the same fitness opportunity. A major advantage of stair climbing, particularly with the machines, is that it involves less impact on the joints and feet than many other forms of aerobic exercise. Step aerobics is another form of this exercise.

Swimming is an excellent way to strengthen and tone muscles as well as promote aerobic fitness. It does not, however, appear to be as effective an exercise modality for losing weight as other forms of exercise. A major benefit of swimming is that it places no excess stress on the joints, as do many other forms of aerobic exercise.

Aerobic dance is exercise combining music with kicking, stretching, bending, and jumping, to deliver the same benefits as running, cycling, or swimming. Aerobics can be especially good for cardiovascular fitness but presents risks to the joints and feet. Low-impact aerobics evolved in response to the many injuries incurred during traditional aerobic activities. This form of aerobics replaces jogging and jumping with steps that minimize the risk of injury or joint trauma. The third generation of aerobics, called "nonimpact aerobics," combines techniques of modern dance and martial arts with a focus on cardiovascular fitness.

In-line skating, also known as *rollerblading*, is a low-impact sport that improves cardiovascular development and lung capacity, as well as increases muscular strength and weight loss. Skating strengthens the muscles and connective tissues surrounding the ankles, knees, and hips, and it can burn nearly as many calories as running. In-line skating can be hazardous, however, if skaters neglect safety precautions such as wearing wrist guards and elbow pads, knee pads, and helmets.

Kickboxing is a sport that has recently evolved into a fitness activity for the general public. It combines martial arts and boxing skills with an aerobic workout to provide excellent benefits in strength, coordination, balance, speed, flexibility, and agility.

Cool-Down

A cool-down is as important as a warm-up. It is best to slow down from exercise gradually by exercising at a slow but steady rate for 5 to 10 minutes. This less intense activity helps to prevent muscle stiffness and potentially dangerous sudden drops in blood pressure that occur when vigorous activities stop abruptly. Stretching after exercise is essential to protect against injury.

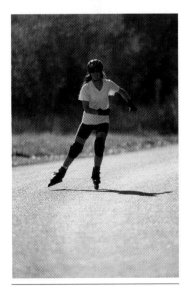

Aerobic exercise can take many forms. It is not limited to running or exercise classes.

Physical Fitness and Women

A variety of psychological, social, historical, and cultural factors all affect how women think about fitness and exercise. Historically, women were labeled "the weaker sex" and were not encouraged to become as fit as their male counterparts. Sociocultural prejudices have traditionally limited women's access to and full participation in sports. Self-esteem and self-confidence with physical activity are developmental tasks of childhood. Because young girls were traditionally not encouraged to excel or compete in the physical arena, they often lacked the self-esteem and confidence necessary to participate in sports as they grew older. It was not until 1978 that **Title IX** mandated that public schools provide equal funding for girls' sports. Even since its passage, opportunities, resources, and, perhaps most importantly, encouragement for physical fitness have not been equally distributed to children, regardless of gender. Groups like the Women's National Basketball Association and a new generation of popular women's sports stars are beginning to revise the societal rule that says only male athletes can be admired.

Traditionally, men have excelled in physical competition against women. In general, men are able to run longer and faster, jump higher and farther, lift more and longer, and so forth. The traditional assumption has been that men are inherently physically gifted whereas women are not. In recent years, however, women have become more competitive in all athletic arenas. Several questions naturally flow from these advances that seek to better define gender similarities and differences in sports and exercise. Nevertheless, resolving of these issues is difficult, because young girls and boys have not been raised with equivalent levels of emphasis, encouragement, and training in physical fitness.

Biologically, men and women are different. The influence of these differences on athletic performance is not yet well defined. No apparent differences exist between the muscles of men and women. Rather, the fact that men are stronger than women reflects the larger absolute quantity of their muscle mass. The individual muscle fibers do not appear to be different. From a strength perspective, women appear to be about half as strong as men in the upper body areas of the shoulders, arms, and backs and two-thirds as strong in the legs and lower body, primarily because men have larger muscle fiber areas and greater lean body weight (total weight minus body fat). Women's naturally higher percentage of body fat, essential for reproduction and general health, may have more of an effect on their physical performance than any other factor. Typically about 25% of a woman's body weight is fat, compared with 15% for men. Women's extra body fat may be a hindrance in sports such as running, but an advantage in sports such as swimming. In general, women also have a lower blood volume, about 5% less hemoglobin, smaller hearts, and less lung capacity than men.

In recent years, women's performances in endurance sports have dramatically improved. Women are increasingly being recognized as proficient athletes, whether in competition with each other or in mixed sports. The gender gap difference in

I always thought that exercise was for jocks. I have never felt comfortable in athletic clothes. I had been very self-conscious whenever I did anything physical. Then I started to read all this stuff about how important exercise was. I realized that it didn't matter what other people thought. At least I was going to take charge of myself. So I slowly ventured into public with my exercise program. In addition to all the benefits of exercise, an extra one happened—I am much more self-confident and I learned that I can really do what I need to do for me.

24-year-old student

such sports as biking is gradually shrinking. Female professional athletes may or may not reach the same levels of absolute performance as their male counterparts. In any case, it is important that women do not let prejudice or feelings or inferiority prevent them from reaching their own optimal fitness levels. Women's bodies respond to training as quickly as do men's. Reaching the level of fitness that best fits a person's individual preference and goals is the responsibility of an adult of either gender.

Exercise Myths and Facts

Fear and misinformation about fitness, workouts, or muscles cause many women to avoid exercise or to exercise inappropriately. Current medical knowledge shows that these fears are usually unfounded and that their resultant behaviors are often harmful.

Myth: Exercise increases the appetite.

Fact: Increased appetite is not necessarily a consequence of exercise. Some evidence suggests that exercise may even suppress the appetite for a short while. Those who do eat more when they exercise usually add fewer calories than they burn in their workouts. Exercise raises the basal metabolic rate, which remains elevated not only for the exercise period, but also for an extended time after the physical activity ends. Calories are thus consumed at a higher rate for an extended period of time.

Myth: Exercising special spots will reduce local fat.

Fact: There is no such thing as effective "spot reduction." Although gadgets and gimmicks such as weighted belts, body wraps, rubberized workout suits, and other specialized devices are widely advertised, none of them will fulfill the promise of delivering a "flat stomach" or "slender thighs" in return for just minutes of exercise a day (and, of course, a few dollars). Fat tissue cannot be converted into muscle. When a woman exercises, she uses energy produced by burning fat in all parts of the body—not just around the muscles that are doing the most work. Sit-ups will not take fat off the abdomen any faster than any other body area. Sit-ups can, however, strengthen the abdominal muscles, which may help hold the abdomen in more.

Myth: No pain, no gain.

Fact: Exercise does not have to hurt to provide benefits. During the initial phase or the beginning of an exercise program or when intensifying an exercise program, some muscle discomfort is probable. Once a regular routine has been established, however, there is no requirement to keep pushing beyond that level for benefit. It is best to avoid pain during and after exercise by intensifying workouts slowly and by beginning each session with a warm-up and ending it with a cool-down.

Myth: Lifting weights gives women a bulky masculine physique.

Fact: Because most women have relatively low levels of the hormone testosterone, it is difficult for them to build large muscles. Both men and women can build

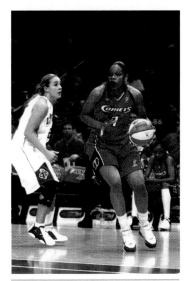

■ Women are increasingly being recognized as proficient athletes, whether in competition with one another or in mixed sports.

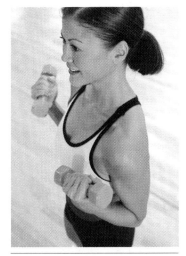

■ It is a myth that a woman will develop bulging muscles if she lifts weights.

firmer rather than bulkier muscles by lifting lighter weights more times rather than heavier weights fewer times.

Myth: The more sweat produced, the more fat lost.

Fact: Exercising in extreme heat or while wearing a plastic suit will, indeed, cause a person to sweat and lose weight. But sweat reflects the loss of water, not fat. Normal consumption of food and water will soon cause the weight to return. An individual who sweats too much during exercise without replenishing essential liquids runs the risk of developing heat exhaustion or dehydration. The amount of sweat produced is not a measure of energy expended. Sweating depends more on temperature, humidity, lack of conditioning, body weight, and individual variability.

Myth: Exercise is not good for trimming down because weight is gained in muscle.

Fact: Aerobic exercises, such as bicycling, jogging, and swimming, burn more fat than they add muscle. With exercises such as weight-lifting, muscle gain may indeed weigh more than burned-off fat. Usually, however, this tradeoff results in increased trimness because the added muscle is less dense and bulky than the lost fat. One added benefit is that the few extra pounds of muscle do not carry the health risks of excess fat. Another is that the body burns 15 to 20 times the calories to maintain a pound of muscle than it burns to maintain the same amount of fat.

Myth: Women cannot perform well athletically while menstruating.

Fact: Most women can perform physical activities consistently throughout their menstrual cycles. Researchers have found no significant differences in physical capabilities, such as oxygen intake, throughout the menstrual cycle. Evidence also shows that exercising during menstruation helps relieve pain and discomfort associated with the menstrual cycle.

Exercise and Aging

Exercise becomes more important with age. Many problems commonly associated with aging, such as increased body fat, decreased lean body weight (muscle mass), decreased muscle strength and flexibility, loss of bone mass, lower metabolism, and slower reaction times, are often signs of inactivity that can be minimized or even prevented by exercise. Reduced muscle strength is a major cause of physical disability in the elderly. Maintaining muscle strength and flexibility are critical components of maintaining the ability to walk and remain independent. For people 65 years and older, falls account for 80% of injuries requiring a hospital visit. When paired with calcium and vitamin D supplements, exercise can dramatically improve balance, coordination, and bone strength, greatly reducing the likelihood and severity of a fall.[23] In addition to improving physical fitness, exercise may aid in the prevention of osteoporosis (see Chapter 11). The combination of weight-lifting and aerobic exercise seems to be the best method for prevention of this chronic debilitating condition. Finally, exercise promotes a sense of well-being and reduces symptoms of depression, a common problem among aging women.

Exercise Abuse

The pressures to be svelte and physically attractive bombard women from many directions. Being healthy and fit are desirable and noble goals, but occasionally individuals become so zealous in the pursuit of fitness that injury results. Exercise abuse occurs when exercise or fitness becomes the "A number 1" priority, supplanting family, friends, work, and education in importance, or when athletic injuries are ignored. In an overuse syndrome, a body part or the entire body is exercised beyond its biological limit to the point of injury. Common overuse injuries affect the muscles, tendons, ligaments, joints, and skin. The most common causes of overuse injuries are excessive exercise, faulty technique, and poor equipment. "Going for the burn" is dangerous because the pain of overexertion is the body's message indicating that something is wrong; such a problem should be addressed, not ignored.

Some women may exercise so much that they stop menstruating. This condition, known as athletic amenorrhea, usually is the direct result of excessive exercise and an abnormally low ratio of body fat to body weight. The long-term consequences of prolonged athletic amenorrhea include the early onset of osteoporosis and its resultant risk for injury and debilitation. Athletic amenorrhea often affects adolescent female athletes who are involved in sports that emphasize slenderness, such as long-distance running, gymnastics, figure skating, and ballet.[24] The **female athlete triad** is the relationship between disordered eating, amenorrhea, and

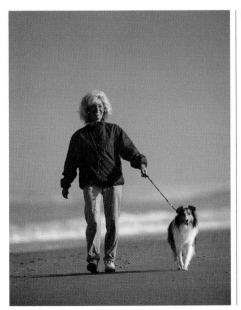

■ Exercise throughout the life span can help minimize or prevent many of the health problems associated with aging.

osteoporosis. This problem usually begins with disordered eating. The combination of poor nutrition and intense athletic training causes weight loss and a decrease in or shutdown of estrogen production. Consequently, amenorrhea occurs. The final condition in the triad, osteoporosis, may follow if estrogen levels remain low and the woman's diet continues to lack calcium and vitamin D. Although the triad can occur in any athlete, those at greatest risk are endurance athletes such as distance swimmers and runners, and athletes in appearance sports, such as gymnasts and figure skaters.

Anabolic steroid use is another form of exercise abuse. Anabolic steroids are synthetic derivatives of the male hormone testosterone. Although steroid use is particularly popular among teenage males, many women use these drugs as well. Men and women who take steroids in conjunction with heavy resistance training may increase their muscle and lean body mass, but may also experience severe physical and psychological side effects. The documented adverse physical effects of steroid use in women include enlargement of the clitoris, growth of facial hair, changes in or cessation of the menstrual cycle, deepened voice, and breast diminution. Other potential side effects include increased risk of heart disease and stroke, increased aggression, liver tumors and jaundice, aching joints, bad breath, and acne.

In adolescents, steroid use can halt growth prematurely. The AIDS epidemic has introduced another potential liability from steroid use: increased risk of human immunodeficiency virus (HIV) transmission from sharing needles. The psychological effects of long-term, high-dose anabolic steroid use may lead to a preoccupation (addiction) with drug use, difficulty stopping, drug cravings, and withdrawal symptoms when use of the drugs is stopped.[25] Hepatitis B and C, two diseases that can seriously damage the liver, are also easily spread by needle sharing. Clearly, anabolic steroids should be totally avoided.

Maintaining a Healthy Weight

To maintain a healthy weight, a woman should balance the number of calories she consumes as part of a healthy diet with the number of calories she burns through daily physical activities. Weight loss should occur at the level of no more than 0.5 to 1 pound per week. The USDA dietary guidelines no longer rely on the "desired weight tables" of the Metropolitan Life Insurance Company, which were originally developed in 1959. Adults are now advised to evaluate their weight-for-height ratio, or **body mass index (BMI).** (See **It's Your Health** and Self-Assessment 9.3.) Studies show that BMI is closely correlated with total body fat content for most people; however, a person who has a lot of muscle, a large body frame, and little fat may have a BMI above the healthy range but may still be considered healthy. Women who have a lot of fat and little muscle may have a BMI in the healthy range, but may not be at their most healthy weight. A BMI of between 25 and 29.9 is used to identify overweight and a BMI of 30 is used to identify obesity in adults.

It's Your Health

Evaluate Your Weight (Adults)

1. Weigh yourself and have your height measured. Find your BMI category in Self-Assessment 9.3. The higher your BMI category, the greater your risk for health problems.

2. Measure around your waist while standing, just above your hip bones. If it is greater than 35 inches for women or 40 inches for men, you probably have excess abdominal fat. This excess fat may place you at greater risk of health problems, even if your BMI is about right.

The higher your BMI and waist measurement, the more you are likely to benefit from weight loss.

Self-Assessment 9.3

Are You at a Healthy Weight?

Body Mass Index Table

BMI	Normal						Overweight					Obese										Extreme Obesity														
Height (inches)	19	20	21	22	23	24	25	26	27	28	29	30	31	32	33	34	35	36	37	38	39	40	41	42	43	44	45	46	47	48	49	50	51	52	53	54
	Body Weight (pounds)																																			
58	91	96	100	105	110	115	119	124	129	134	138	143	148	153	158	162	167	172	177	181	186	191	196	201	205	210	215	220	224	229	234	239	244	248	253	258
59	94	99	104	109	114	119	124	128	133	138	143	148	153	158	163	168	173	178	183	188	193	198	203	208	212	217	222	227	232	237	242	247	252	257	262	267
60	97	102	107	112	118	123	128	133	138	143	148	153	158	163	168	174	179	184	189	194	199	204	209	215	220	225	230	235	240	245	250	255	261	266	271	276
61	100	106	111	116	122	127	132	137	143	148	153	158	164	169	174	180	185	190	195	201	206	211	217	222	227	232	238	243	248	254	259	264	269	275	280	285
62	104	109	115	120	126	131	136	142	147	153	158	164	169	175	180	186	191	196	202	207	213	218	224	229	235	240	246	251	256	262	267	273	278	284	289	295
63	107	113	118	124	130	135	141	146	152	158	163	169	175	180	186	191	197	203	208	214	220	225	231	237	242	248	254	259	265	270	278	282	287	293	299	304
64	110	116	122	128	134	140	145	151	157	163	169	174	180	186	192	197	204	209	215	221	227	232	238	244	250	256	262	267	273	279	285	291	296	302	308	314
65	114	120	126	132	138	144	150	156	162	168	174	180	186	192	198	204	210	216	222	228	234	240	246	252	258	264	270	276	282	288	294	300	306	312	318	324
66	118	124	130	136	142	148	155	161	167	173	179	186	192	198	204	210	216	223	229	235	241	247	253	260	266	272	278	284	291	297	303	309	315	322	328	334
67	121	127	134	140	146	153	159	166	172	178	185	191	198	204	211	217	223	230	236	242	249	255	261	268	274	280	287	293	299	306	312	319	325	331	338	344
68	125	131	138	144	151	158	164	171	177	184	190	197	203	210	216	223	230	236	243	249	256	262	269	276	282	289	295	302	308	315	322	328	335	341	348	354
69	128	135	142	149	155	162	169	176	182	189	196	203	209	216	223	230	236	243	250	257	263	270	277	284	291	297	304	311	318	324	331	338	345	351	358	365
70	132	139	146	153	160	167	174	181	188	195	202	209	216	222	229	236	243	250	257	264	271	278	285	292	299	306	313	320	327	334	341	348	355	362	369	376
71	136	143	150	157	165	172	179	186	193	200	208	215	222	229	236	243	250	257	265	272	279	286	293	301	308	315	322	329	338	343	351	358	365	372	379	386
72	140	147	154	162	169	177	184	191	199	206	213	221	228	235	242	250	258	265	272	279	287	294	302	309	316	324	331	338	346	353	361	368	375	383	390	397
73	144	151	159	166	174	182	189	197	204	212	219	227	235	242	250	257	265	272	280	288	295	302	310	318	325	333	340	348	355	363	371	378	386	393	401	408
74	148	155	163	171	179	186	194	202	210	218	225	233	241	249	256	264	272	280	287	295	303	311	319	326	334	342	350	358	365	373	381	389	396	404	412	420
75	152	160	168	176	184	192	200	208	216	224	232	240	248	256	264	272	279	287	295	303	311	319	327	335	343	351	359	367	375	383	391	399	407	415	423	431
76	156	164	172	180	189	197	205	213	221	230	238	246	254	263	271	279	287	295	304	312	320	328	336	344	353	361	369	377	385	394	402	410	418	426	435	443

Source: Adapted from Clinical Guidelines on the Identification, Evaluation, and Treatment of Overweight and Obesity in Adults: The Evidence Report.

BMI measures weight in relation to height. The BMI ranges shown above are for adults. They are not exact ranges of healthy and unhealthy weights, but rather show that health risk increases at higher levels of overweight and obesity. Even within the healthy BMI range, weight gains can carry health risks for adults.

Directions: Find your weight on the bottom of the graph. Go straight up from that point until you come to the line that matches your height. Then look to find your weight group.

   Healthy Weight: BMI from 18.5 to 25.   **Overweight:** BMI from 25 to 30.   **Obese:** BMI 30 or higher.

Source: Adapted from Clinical Guidelines on the Identification, Evaluation, and Treatment of Overweight and Obesity in Adults: The Evidence Report. Available at http://www.nhlbisupport.com/bmi/bmicalc.htm.

Another way to define overweight is to measure the proportion of fat in the body, though it is a difficult measurement to perform accurately, even with professional training.

In addition to total weight, weight distribution is an important consideration. Women whose body-fat distribution favors the upper body ("apples") rather than the hips and thighs ("pears") are at higher risk of developing type 2 diabetes, coronary artery disease, hypertension, gallbladder disease, and polycystic ovarian syndrome.[26] Consequently, waist measurement has been used as a loose measure of one's chance of developing heart disease, cancer, or other chronic diseases. A waist larger than 35 inches for a woman and 50 inches for a man is considered to be a risk factor for the aforementioned diseases.

What Causes Weight Gain

For each individual, body weight is determined by a combination of genetic, metabolic, behavioral, environmental, cultural, and socioeconomic influences. Some people may have a genetic predisposition to gain weight or a genetic need to eat more than they need for energy. For the vast majority of individuals, however, overweight and obesity result from excess calorie consumption and/or inadequate physical activity. Simply put, when a woman takes in more calories than she burns, she will gain weight. Burning calories through physical activity helps to offset the amount of calories consumed and can help a person maintain or lose weight.

Recent studies have shown that environmental factors, such as portion size, price, and advertising, can influence the amount of food that an average person consumes. When moviegoers are given an extra-large tub of popcorn instead of a large tub, they will eat 40% to 50% more popcorn. Similarly, if high-fat food snack prices are increased and low-fat food snack prices are decreased in a vending machine, the purchase of low-fat food snacks increases. The U.S. food industry has used portion sizes and the concept of getting a better deal by purchasing larger quantities to increase its sales. As a consequence, serving sizes of many foods, such as fast-food burgers and fries, convenience-mart sodas, and muffins and bakery goods, have increased dramatically. Although it is ultimately the individual's responsibility to consume an appropriate amount of food without overindulging, society has made it difficult for people to understand portion size and portion control.[27] Table 9.7 provides examples of changes in portion size over the past 20 years.

Overweight and Obesity

Overweight is defined as a BMI of 25 to 29.9, with obesity beginning at a BMI of 30. **Obesity** is a medical term meaning the excessive storage of energy in the form of fat. Obesity is a complex, multifactorial chronic disease. Overweight and obesity are increasing in both genders and among all population groups. Today there are nearly twice as many overweight children and almost three times as many overweight adolescents as there were in 1980.[28] Overweight children and adolescents are more likely to become overweight or obese adults. Data collected from

Table 9.7 **Portion Distortion**

| Food Item | Size and Calories | | Ways to Burn the Extra Calories |
	20 Years Ago	Today	
Bagel	3-inch diameter/ 140 calories	6-inch diameter/ 350 calories	Rake leaves for 50 minutes to burn extra 210 calories
French fries	2.4 ounces/ 210 calories	6.9 ounces/ 610 calories	Walk 2 hours, 20 minutes to burn extra 400 calories
Soda	6.5 ounces/ 85 calories	20 ounces/ 250 calories	Garden for 35 minutes to burn extra 165 calories
Turkey sandwich	320 calories	820 calories	Bike for 1 hour, 25 minutes to burn extra 500 calories

Source: National Heart, Lung and Blood Institute. *Stay Young at Heart.* Retrieved January 2006 from http://hin.nhlbi.nih.gov/portion/index.htm.

1999 to 2002 reveal that 65.1% of U.S. adults are overweight or obese and 4.9% are extremely obese (see Figure 9.4). Approximately 16% of U.S. children are overweight and 31% are at risk of soon becoming overweight.[29] The prevalence of obesity is higher among African American women and Mexican American women than among women in any other ethnic group. This condition is also more common among people with low incomes and low education.[28]

It has been suggested that the major factor behind this increase in rates of obesity is the jump in average calorie intake between 1985 and 2000. In 2000, the average daily calorie consumption was roughly 300 calories more than the 1985 level. Of that 300-calorie increase,

- Grains (mainly refined grains) accounted for 46%;
- Added fats accounted for 24%;
- Added sugars accounted for 23%;

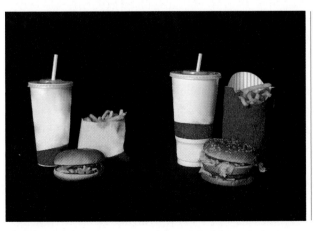

■ Food portions have become noticeably larger in the past 20 years, often providing enough food for at least 2 people.

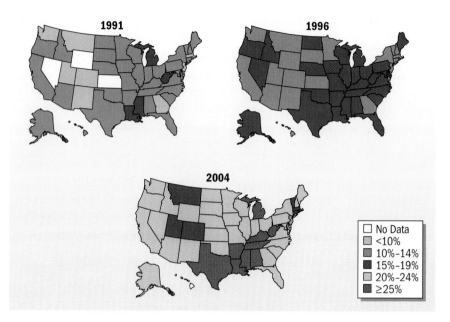

- Fruits and vegetables accounted for 8%; and

- Meat and dairy consumption declined by 1%.[3]

Being overweight or obese can lead to a wide range of health problems, including adult-onset diabetes, hypertension, coronary heart disease, certain cancers, gout, gallbladder disease, and certain arthritic conditions. Women suffer from additional obesity-related problems, including irregular menstrual cycles, amenorrhea, infertility, and polycystic ovarian syndrome. Studies show that the risk of death rises with increasing weight. Moderate weight excess (10 to 20 pounds for a person of average height), even for women who exercise, increases the risk of death, particularly among adults age 30 to 64 years. Obese women in general may be at a slightly higher risk of developing breast cancer, but researchers continue to investigate whether the effects of obesity on breast cancer depend on weight gained as an adult or as a child. The risk for endometrial cancer also goes up with increasing fat tissue. According to the American Cancer Society, being 30 pounds overweight can increase a woman's risk of endometrial cancer threefold and being 50 pounds overweight can increase her risk tenfold.[30] People who are obese also are subject to discrimination and social stigmatization, and consequently they may suffer from low self-esteem and depression.

It has been estimated that current obesity in the United States could account for 14% of all deaths from cancer in men and 20% of those in women.[31] Left unabated, overweight and obesity may soon cause as much preventable disease and death as cigarette smoking. The recognition of obesity as the second leading cause of preventable death in the United States was somewhat slow to develop. In the 1970s, controversy arose over the significance of obesity as an effect on general health. Not until 1985 at the NIH Consensus Development Conference was it acknowledged that obesity leads to increased morbidity and mortality.

The causes of obesity are complex, with the root causes lying in genetics, environment, economics, and culture. Although its development is complex, the benefits of treatment are certain. Obesity treatments often begin with weight loss, employing low-calorie diets in conjunction with physical activity, behavior therapy, and pharmacotherapy and weight-loss surgery for people who are severely obese (BMIs equal to or greater than 40). Recent developments in weight-loss medications are allowing the estimated 97 million adults in the United States who are obese to have a much better chance for decreased morbidity and mortality.

Economic Dimensions of Obesity and Overweight

The estimated annual cost of obesity and overweight in the United States is $117 billion.[32] This extremely high figure includes two types of costs: the direct medical costs to treat diseases associated with obesity such as diabetes, joint problems, and heart disease, and the indirect costs of morbidities associated with the condition.[33] These indirect costs are measured in terms of lost productivity, premature disability, and early death. Healthcare costs and the likelihood of complications from surgery for obese and overweight people are higher than those for people of normal weight. Additional costs may be felt at the individual or household level, when overweight or obese people need to purchase specially designed chairs and beds to support them, specialty clothes, and higher-than-average numbers of medications. Together these items can create a significant cost burden to families.

Americans spend billions of dollars every year addressing weight and weight concerns. In 2001, for example, they spent more than $12 billion per year at some 17,000 health clubs. In addition, close to $5 billion was spent on personal gym equipment, with treadmills being the biggest seller. More than $444 million worth of health- and diet-related books were sold in 2001 as well. Weight Watchers, along with Jenny Craig and LA Weight Loss Centers, tallied up more than $1 billion in annual business.[34]

How Women Can Lose Weight

To lose weight, it is necessary to burn more calories than are ingested. Fat contains nine calories per gram, whereas protein and carbohydrates have four calories per gram. The most important way that the body burns calories is through one's resting metabolism, or basal metabolic rate (BMR), the process that maintains body heat and controls automatic activities such as breathing and heartbeat. Nearly 75% of calorie use is devoted to these functions. When a woman attempts to lose weight by cutting calories, her body responds as it would to starvation, by burning fewer calories. Shifting from an intake of about 2,000 calories per day to a 1,200-calorie diet reduces resting metabolism by 5% to 10%, and a more stringent 800-calorie diet lowers it by 10% to 20%. Even after resuming a more normal calorie

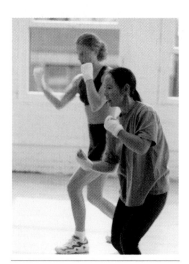

■ Regular exercise is an essential component of any weight-control program.

consumption, other changes keep the metabolic rate low. Much of the weight lost on a low-calorie diet can come from lost muscle tissue and lost water weight, and the muscles may shrink further as the woman stays at the lower weight because they do not have to work as hard to carry the body around. Less muscle tissue means a lower metabolic rate. The net effect is simple: The more weight that is lost through dieting, the more the metabolic rate will decline—and the greater the tendency to regain the weight that was lost. Although dieting still has a role in weight control, exercise provides some solution to the metabolic problem.

The key to successful weight loss is increasing the BMR by exercising, not by counting calories. Regular exercise is essential for any weight-control program. A vigorous 20- to 30-minute workout can easily burn 200 to 300 calories, and even brisk walking can have a significant impact. Equally important, exercise increases the metabolic rate by building muscle and by keeping muscle from shrinking as a result of weight loss. Because adding exercise to a diet program helps steady the metabolic rate, it makes it easier to keep the weight off.

Exercise alone does indeed burn up some calories, but the main advantage of exercise is that the metabolism remains higher for several hours afterward, so calories are burned at a higher rate, even during inactivity. Aerobic exercise burns calories faster than weight training, but weight training builds muscle, which is of critical importance in weight loss. A pound of muscle needs 30 to 50 calories per day just for maintenance, whereas fat needs only two maintenance calories per day. Substituting muscle for fat may therefore result in an increased daily caloric expenditure. Rather than simply promoting weight loss, exercise may actually affect the body in a more complex, integrated way, bringing appetite and energy expenditure into balance. In addition, exercise trims a physical profile even without weight loss. Muscle is denser than fat, so it is possible to appear thinner while the weight holds steady if a larger amount of fat is replaced with a smaller amount of muscle. Bathroom scales simply do not measure these changes. Regardless of its direct effects on weight and body fat, exercise serves to improve overall health by lowering blood pressure, improving cholesterol levels, strengthening the cardiovascular system, helping prevent type 2 diabetes, and reducing stress.

Keeping a food diary is helpful for some women because it enables them to better identify their eating and exercising patterns. Meals, snacks, and drinks should all be recorded in the diary. After a review of a few days of diary notes, a woman can objectively examine her own eating habits and set realistic goals that rely on a diet based on healthy foods. Progress can be monitored through the food diary and weekly (not daily) checks with the scale. Once the reasonable desired weight loss is achieved, the focus should be on maintenance, again through sensible eating and exercise.

Ways Not to Lose Weight

Women who need to lose weight for health reasons face the dilemma of how to do so. Popular media abound with conflicting guidance on weight-loss strategies for women.

It's Your Health

Helpful and Nonhelpful Weight-Loss Strategies for Women

Helpful

Allow occasional treats or servings of favorite foods.

Develop realistic goals that can be maintained.

Focus on long-term goals.

Stick with program even if there are lapses.

Plan meals and snacks to include more complex carbohydrates, more fruits and vegetables, and less fat.

Limit intake of fatty foods, oils, and dressings.

Avoid packaged snack foods.

Develop new interests that do not involve food.

Eat foods slowly.

Exercise regularly.

Join a support group or share the process with a friend.

Clean the pantry—give away foods that are not part of the new healthy eating plan.

Try a new low-fat recipe each week.

Eat small meals throughout the day to keep from getting too hungry.

Nonhelpful

Setting unrealistically high or short-term goals.

Choosing a program that makes eating unpleasant.

Any diet that promotes one particular food such as grapefruit or yogurt.

Unconventional theories to explain how food combinations add or decrease body weight.

Diets that omit any one food group.

Daily caloric intake less than 1,200 calories unless under medical supervision.

Any diet that promotes megadoses of vitamins to make up for nutritional deficits.

Fasting or starvation diets.

Any pill or potion that "melts fat."

Appetite-suppressant drugs.

Fiber supplements.

Giving up all sweets or breads.

Muscle stimulators.

Body wraps.

In any weight-loss effort, starvation or hunger is not the solution. Food substitution, in which a woman consumes twice as many calories from carbohydrates as she does from fat, is far better than food restriction. Foods such as pasta and whole-grain bread are nutritious, filling, and low in calories when they are not smothered in high fat products, such as butter, mayonnaise, and margarine. Alcohol should also be considered contraindicated in a weight-loss effort. Alcohol is a source of empty

I have tried every diet in the book. I have had times where I have eaten only grapefruit, only rice, or only salads. I have also tried all the gimmicks—pills, liquids, body wraps. You name it, I've tried it. But nothing has really worked. I quickly gain the weight back, sometimes more, within a short time after I lose it. I always swear I won't try another stupid method, but as soon as I read an ad or see a new product, I feel that I have to give it a try.

22-year-old woman

calories that contribute to weight gain without providing any nutritional benefit. Furthermore, alcohol affects the BMR because the body burns fat more slowly in the presence of alcohol; thus alcohol promotes the storage of body fat.

Dieting without exercise is the least effective way to lose weight. For 95% of dieters, lost pounds eventually return.[35] **Yo-yo dieting** is a term used to characterize the repeated, chronic pattern of dieting that describes most dieters' behavior. In addition to being frustrating, yo-yo dieting may be hazardous to health. Yo-yo dieting may be associated with a greater risk of coronary heart disease, although separating the direct physiological effects of the behavior and the resulting stress that comes with trying and failing to lose weight is difficult.[36] Yo-yo dieting may also weaken the immune system, making dieters more likely to become and stay sick.[37] It has been hypothesized that yo-yo dieters store more and more fat in the abdominal area with each failed diet, and, as noted earlier, abdominal fat has been shown to be more harmful to one's health than fat in other places.[27]

Diet supplements are another unhealthy way to lose weight. Weight-loss supplements often contain stimulants, which in high amounts may lead to an increased heart rate, heart attacks, nervousness, insomnia, headaches, seizures, or death. Many women have begun to use supplements such as Ephedra, which has recently been linked to adverse health outcomes and even possible mortality. Because the products are not subjected to the same testing standards as substances regulated by the FDA, supplements may have a higher rate of contamination or contraindications not stated on warning labels. Other weight-loss products, although not necessarily harmful, simply may be ineffective.

Other Weight-Loss Strategies

Many popular diets encourage different eating regimens to attain maximum weight loss. In the 1990s, diets typically focused on high-carbohydrate/very-low-fat daily regimens. And recently, the high-protein, high-fat, low-carbohydrate (Atkins) diet reemerged as a popular weight-loss strategy. Many people failed on these diets because they mistakenly believed that they could eat unlimited amounts of certain foods. In reality, excessive calories from most foods cause weight gain. Low-fat foods are often packed with sugar to make up for the loss of flavor when fat is removed. In contrast, several high-profile diets, including the Atkins diet and the Zone diet, identify high-protein/low-carbohydrate meals as being optimal. These diets have become financial empires unto themselves, with books, snacks, prepared meals, and energy drinks all being sold to the millions of people who are subscribing to them. A recent *Consumer Reports* analysis of clinical data found that people in Atkins and the Zone weight-loss programs were at least as likely as people in other top-rated weight-loss programs to lose weight in the short term but were more likely to drop out in less than a year. They were also more likely to eat too much saturated fat and not enough fruits and vegetables.[38]

For extremely overweight women, obesity drugs seemed to be the answer in the early to mid-1990s. In 1997, however, the most popular drug combination, fen/phen

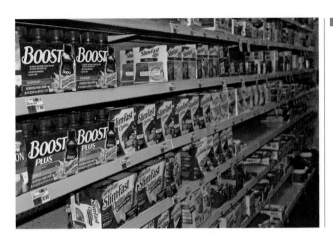

■ Weight-loss products should be used only when prescribed by a healthcare provider; in these selected patients, the products should be used in combination with lifestyle changes to increase the success of long-term weight loss.

(fenfluramine and phentermine), was linked to heart valve abnormalities and consequently taken off the market. Because fenfluramine was the culprit, doctors continued to prescribe phentermine either alone or combined with Prozac, an antidepressant that increases serotonin levels and is believed to decrease appetite. Other diet drugs, such as Xenical and Meridia, are more recent additions to the weight-loss market. Xenical (generic name orlistat) is a lipase inhibitor that works by reducing the amount of fat that the body absorbs. In one study, patients using orlistat with a mildly low-calorie diet lost significantly more weight than did patients who were treated with a placebo and ate the same diet. Weight-loss products should be used only when prescribed by a healthcare provider and should be used in combination with lifestyle changes to increase the success of long-term weight loss in selected patients.[39]

One increasingly popular option for severely overweight and obese people is weight-loss surgery. Gastrointestinal surgery for obesity, also called **bariatric surgery,** alters the digestive process. The operation promotes weight loss by closing off parts of the stomach to make it smaller. Operations that only reduce stomach size are known as "restrictive operations" because they restrict the amount of food the stomach can hold. Other operations, known as malabsorptive operations, combine stomach restriction with a partial bypass of the small intestine. These procedures create a direct connection from the stomach to the lower segment of the small intestine, literally bypassing portions of the digestive tract that absorb calories and nutrients. These operations often make eating and swallowing food extremely painful, literally making an ordeal out of every meal. All of these procedures are appropriate only for severely obese individuals who have not been able to control their weight with diet, exercise, and appropriate pharmaceutical interventions.

Body Image and Shape

Body image is a result of a complex interrelationship between self-perception, family attitudes toward bodies and food, social norms, and individual experiences. Standards for beauty and desirability are not absolute but vary over time and from

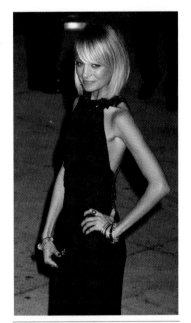

■ Women have been socialized to believe that an ultra-thin body shape is desirable.

culture to culture. The twentieth-century ideal promoted by Madison Avenue and Hollywood has ranged from images of emaciation to more recent images of perfectly toned women. In former times, big-bellied women were considered beautiful. In Greek and Roman representations of Aphrodite and Venus as well as in paintings by Titian, Rubens, and Rembrandt, "ideal" women often had ample thighs, hips, waists, and abdomens. The Venus de Milo, one of the most beautiful of the classical female torsos, is muscular and rounded. Contemporary society is weight conscious, fashion conscious, exercise conscious, diet conscious, and not very tolerant of perceived physical imperfection.

Women have been socialized to believe that their physical attractiveness determines their social value. The media have further distorted this message by use of airbrushing on images to produce flawless complexions, whitening and brightening of teeth and eyes, digital enhancement to increase breast size and decrease fat, and models and movie stars who are not representative of the average woman. A study examining physical measurements of Miss America contestants, models, and Playboy Playmates over the course of the twentieth century found that women in all three groups were likely to be underweight and were often thin enough to meet the World Health Organization's definition of anorexic. The weight and BMI of all three groups of women have also fallen even as the weight of the average American woman has increased over the past 50 years.[40] The gulf between what women see in the media and what they see in the mirror results in excessive dieting, eating disorders, a perceived need for plastic or cosmetic surgery, and feelings of self-loathing and inadequacy in many women, as seen in the following statistics:

- A 2003 poll by the Simmons Market Research Bureau found that 24% of the people who said they would try any diet to lose weight were obese women, while only 9% were obese men. Obese women were also much more likely than men to feel guilty about eating.[41]

- Females account for 90% of the estimated 8 million sufferers of eating disorders.[42]

- Nearly 12 million cosmetic surgical and nonsurgical procedures were performed in the United States in 2004, according to the American Society for Aesthetic Plastic Surgery (ASAPS). This represents an increase of 465% compared to the number of procedures performed in 1997. While the number of surgical procedures, such as liposuction, breast augmentation, and eyelid surgery, also grew, the biggest increase has been in procedures that do not require actual surgery, such as Botox injections and laser hair removals.[43]

Interestingly, this obsession was thought to be primarily an American phenomenon. In the early 1990s, it was noted that compared with women in other countries, girls and women in the United States dieted more and were less satisfied and more self-conscious about their bodies.[44] A 1997 international study of body image showed increased discontent with bodies, appearance, and weight by women across Western nations, suggesting a more global problem.[45] This phenomenon begins early, with inappropriate eating habits and high anxiety about being overweight prevalent among adolescent girls. In a large U.S. school-based study, one-third of adolescent girls believed they were overweight, and more than 60% of female adolescents were trying to lose weight.[46] Strategies used by high school girls to lose weight include starvation, fad diets, and purging methods, which can result in disordered eating behaviors. This finding is especially disturbing given the importance of high calcium intake for building healthy bones and developing critical bone mass, as well as the need for dietary fat to ensure healthy breast development in adolescents. Another concern is that a girl's preoccupation with body image and discontent with body shape during adolescence may persist for life.

Excessive dieting and bodily preoccupation among young women are believed to be causal factors in the millions of women who suffer from eating disorders. New research findings and growing numbers of activists are seeking to influence the women and girls who are alienated from their bodies and obsessed with dieting. Although the 1990s language of fat liberation has been replaced by the politically milder talk of "size discrimination" and "size acceptance," the goals remain the same: to empower women to accept themselves at their present sizes and to shatter the media image of the body ideal (Table 9.8).

Sociocultural Perspectives on Body Image

Women who grew up in largely African American communities often have a very different perspective on body ideals than women who grow up in white-dominated communities. Similarly, girls who grow up in families where their mothers had their own disordered eating habits or poor body images are more likely to internalize those signals and adopt similar attitudes. Religion also can influence a girl's or woman's concept of her body, either through doctrines of self-restraint, hard work, or negative viewpoints on sloth. Even when these attitudes are not specifically directed toward body size, these messages can translate into

I guess when I look in the mirror I see only the things that I feel are wrong. I wish I was thinner and taller, with a flatter stomach and a bigger chest. When I think about it, I realize that there are many things I actually like about myself but I can't seem to focus on them. When I look at other women, I notice their attributes. I wonder why I can't do that with myself.

25-year-old woman

Table 9.8	Comparison of the Average Woman with Unrealistic Models		
	Average Woman	**Barbie**	**Store Mannequin**
Height	5' 4"	6' 0"	6' 0"
Weight	145 lb	101 lb	Not available
Dress size	11–14	4	6
Bust	36–37"	39"	34"
Waist	29–31"	19"	23"
Hips	40–42"	33"	34"

Sources: *Health* magazine, September 1997; NEDIC, a Canadian eating disorders advocacy group; Anorexia Nervosa and Related Eating Disorders, Inc., 2003.

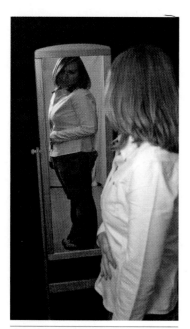

Women's perceptions about their bodies often are inaccurate.

feelings of blame for girls and women who struggle to control their weight. Finally, different communities have different food norms. For example, Southerners in the United States tend to eat more fried food and barbequed meat than their Northerner counterparts, and Asians tend to eat more rice than breads. These cultural norms can significantly influence weight management within these communities. A woman who wishes to change her eating habits may have to rebel against the traditions of her family or community.

Eating Disorders

When healthcare professionals speak of eating disorders, they generally mean **anorexia nervosa, bulimia nervosa,** or **binge eating disorder (BED).** Although eating disorders may seem to be modern afflictions, medical history indicates otherwise. A disease similar to anorexia was described as early as 1694, and the term "anorexia," meaning loss of appetite or desire, was first used in 1874.[47] Since that time, many other researchers have documented what is now referred to as anorexia nervosa. Bulimia, meaning "appetite like an ox," also has been described in historical writings. Ancient Egyptians believed that purging was a way to prevent disease, and women of the Middle Ages often purged for religious reasons.[48]

Today eating disorders are more prevalent among young, educated Western white and Hispanic females from middle to upper social classes than among females in other groups, with incidence rates peaking at age 18. Eating disorders can have roots in social, emotional, and even biological factors in women's lives; pressure to "fit in" with popular cliques or peers, a desire to avoid consumption as a way of dealing with strong emotions or maintaining control over one's life, and even feelings of euphoria that can occur when a person skips meals can all encourage a woman (or man) to adopt or conitnue an eating disorder. At the same time, these behaviors undermine one's health, self-esteem, and sense of competency. (For more on eating disorders, see Chapter 12.)

Global Perspectives on Hunger

Millions of people die each year from chronic hunger and malnutrition. **Hunger** is the painful or uneasy feeling caused by the continuous and involuntary lack of food. Chronic hunger results when a person's daily intake of calories is not enough for the individual to lead an active, healthy life. **Malnutrition** refers to an imbalance between the body's nutritional needs and the intake or digestion of nutrients. Malnutrition may result in disease or death and can be caused by an unbalanced diet, digestive problems, or absorption problems. Although most people think of malnutrition as **undernutrition,** this term also includes **overnutrition,** which results from overeating, insufficient exercise, and excessive intake of vitamins and minerals. Overnutrition can lead to overweight and obesity, epidemics that are growing around the world.

Hunger is everywhere. The World Hunger Organization notes that approximately 5 billion people live in the developing world. Economically, the constant securing of food consumes valuable time and energy of poor people, allowing less time for work and earning income. They estimate that 852 million people across the world are hungry. Today, across the world, 1.3 billion people live on less than $1 per day; 3 billion live on less than $2 per day; 1.3 billion have no access to clean water; 3 billion have no access to sanitation; and 2 billion have no access to electricity.[49]

In 2000, 33 million Americans—13 million children and 20 million adults—lived in families who suffered from hunger or lived on the edge of hunger. This population represents 10.5% of all U.S. households. Families who do not have access to nutritionally balanced and safe foods or who have limited access to nutritious and affordable food suffer from **food insecurity.** According to the U.S. Census Bureau, those at greatest risk of food insecurity live in households with the following characteristics:

- Headed by a single woman
- Hispanic or black
- Earning incomes below the poverty line[50]

Populations at risk of malnutrition include infants and children, women who are pregnant or breastfeeding, the elderly, vegetarians, fad dieters, alcoholics or substance abusers, and people with certain chronic diseases. Malnourishment magnifies the effects of every disease, causing malnourished children to be ill nearly 160 days each year, almost half of their daily lives. The most destructive form of malnutrition, which mainly affects infants and young children, is **protein-energy malnutrition (PEM).** Children have high energy and protein needs, and therefore they suffer most when protein is lacking in their diets. PEM affects more than one-fourth of the world's children. More than 70% of PEM-afflicted children live in Asia, 26% in Africa, and 4% in Latin America and the Caribbean.[51]

Other nutrients that are extremely important for health include the following:

- *Vitamin A.* Vitamin A deficiency (VAD) is the leading cause of preventable blindness, reduces the body's resistance to disease and infection, and can cause growth retardation in children. An estimated 250,000 to 500,000 children lose their sight every year due to VAD, and half of these children die within 12 months after becoming blind. This deficiency also poses a risk to pregnant women and their fetuses, causing night blindness, increased risk of maternal mortality, premature birth, low birthweight, and infection. Breastfeeding is the best way to protect babies from VAD, because breast milk is a natural source of vitamin A.

- *Iron.* Iron deficiency is the principal cause of anemia, which affects more than 30% of the world's population. Iron deficiency and anemia impose a heavy economic burden on society, because affected individuals are less able to work and be productive members of a community. In many developing countries, iron deficiency is aggravated by malaria and worm infections. Health consequences for pregnant women and their fetuses include premature birth, low birthweight, and increased risk of maternal death. Twenty percent of all maternal deaths have been attributed to anemia.

- *Iodine.* Iodine deficiency is primarily known for causing goiters (enlarged thyroid glands), a condition that can be dramatically disfiguring. Iodine deficiency disorders (IDD) threaten the mental health of children, representing the world's most prevalent cause of brain damage. Iodine deficiency during pregnancy may result in stillbirth, miscarriage, congenital abnormalities, and mental impairment in the baby. More than 13% (740 million) of the world's population is affected by this problem. Salt iodization has improved iodine status in numerous countries.[51]

■■■■

Informed Decision Making

Nutrition

Healthful eating is essential to health promotion and disease prevention. To develop sensible eating habits, women should eat balanced meals containing carbohydrates, fats, and proteins, as well as the essential vitamins and minerals. Understanding the nutrition facts label will help women choose foods based on their nutrient content. Women should also be aware of the dangers of nutrient deficiencies as well as nutritional excesses.

Maintaining a Personal Exercise Program

Women, like men, do not have difficulty starting exercise programs; unfortunately, like men, they have difficulty maintaining those regimens. The benefits of exercise are enormous—so enormous that public health experts believe that exercise should be not just a means to an end, such as "losing another five pounds," but a permanent part of a person's life. To stay fit, adults should participate in 30 minutes or more of moderate-intensity physical activity on most, if not all, days of the week (see Table 9.6). The form of exercise is not as important as the regularity with which it is undertaken. Exercise fads come and go, and it is possible to try them all. It is better to switch to a different form of exercise when one form becomes boring or dull than to give up exercising entirely.

A woman should select an exercise program that is right for her. Studies show that a lifestyle approach to exercise (incorporating walking, lifting, gardening, and other physical activities into one's daily routine) is equally as effective as a traditional structured exercise program for increasing the physical activity and cardio-respiratory fitness of a previously sedentary adult. Finding time is another important factor—when excuses dominate, it is time to reconsider the program or reprioritize commitments and obligations.

Common perceived barriers to exercise for women include lack of time to exercise, lack of encouragement from family and friends, not wanting to exercise alone, the desire to avoid exertion or soreness, and a fear of looking silly.[52] Staying committed to exercise can also be a challenge. About 50% of people who start structured exercise programs drop out in 6 to 12 months. However, there are habits that can make sticking with an exercise program easier:

- Keeping an exercise log
- Recording total calories burned in a workout, distance traveled, or improvements in performance
- Exercising with a friend or in a class
- Choosing activities that are personally enjoyable
- Switching to new programs or rotating between programs to maintain interest
- Giving oneself periodic rewards for continuing to exercise

Imagining exercise as a normal part of one's routine maintenance (like brushing one's teeth) can also help a woman stay on a program: A woman who misses an exercise session or who forgets to brush her teeth before going to bed one night should not give up on either activity, but should continue both habits the next day as if nothing unusual had happened.[52]

Body Image and Weight Management

A woman who decides to lose weight should begin by examining her diet and activity level to decide what changes would provide the most improvement. Before jumping into a weight-control program or joining a fitness center, however, it is important to "step back" and examine one's motives for losing weight. Some women want to lose weight to improve their health; some women want to lose weight to improve their physical appearance. Many women feel a combination of both desires. However, women who feel an especially powerful desire to lose weight may want to reflect on their own body image. Society places an enormous pressure on women to be thin and to conform to artificial body types that may be impossible to achieve. Developing a healthy body image, with the help of a medical professional if necessary, may benefit some women more than an Olympian-level fitness program.

Extra weight neither accumulates nor disappears overnight. Weight-loss programs that focus on slow-but-steady weight loss are healthier and more likely to keep weight off than programs that focus on dramatic short-term results. An average weekly loss of 1 pound is a realistic, safe goal for weight loss. Joining a group or making a serious arrangement for support with a friend can help sustain a long-term commitment.

A woman who adopts a healthy diet or starts an exercise program should not stop either activity once she reaches her initial weight-loss goal. A balanced diet and exercise continue to provide benefits only for as long as they are practiced. Reverting to unhealthy habits not only harms the body, but also is likely to result in the return of lost weight.

Profiles of Remarkable Women

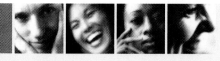

Shiriki K. Kumanyika, Ph.D., M.P.H. (1945–)

Shiriki K. Kumanyika, a native of Baltimore, Maryland, holds a B.A. from Syracuse University, an M.S. in social work from Columbia University, a Ph.D. in human nutrition from Cornell University, and a Master of Public Health (M.P.H.) from Johns Hopkins School of Public Health. Her background is interdisciplinary and involves the application of epidemiology and prevention approaches to address issues of nutrition, aging, prevention, minority health, and women's health. Kumanyika is professor of epidemiology and associate dean for Health Promotion and Disease Prevention at the University of Pennsylvania School of Medicine in Philadelphia. She is also a senior scholar in the Center for Clinical Epidemiology and Biostatistics and a senior fellow of the Institute on Aging and the Leonard Davis Institute for Health Economics. Prior to joining the University of Pennsylvania, Kumanyika was the Head of the Department of Human Nutrition and Dietetics at University of Illinois at Chicago.

Kumanyika has authored numerous research articles, focusing on the role of nutritional factors in the primary and secondary prevention of chronic diseases. Much of her work emphasizes the problems of obesity and sodium as they relate to health problems such as hypertension and diabetes, especially as found among African Americans. She has been a principal investigator or co-investigator on numerous randomized clinical trials of dietary behavior change for the improvement of cardiovascular risk factors.

Kumanyika has served on several national advisory committees, including the U.S. Dietary Guidelines Committees, the National Heart, Lung, and Blood Institute (NHLBI) Advisory Council, and the Women's Health Initiative advisory committees. She is a past Chair of the Food and Nutrition Section of the American Public Health Association and the Council on Epidemiology and Prevention of the American Heart Association, as well as a past member of the Board of Directors of the American Heart Association. She currently serves on the Institute of Medicine, Food and Nutrition Board and the Institute of Medicine Committee on Prevention of Obesity in Children. On an international level, she is a key member of the steering group of the International Obesity Task Force and has consulted with the World Health Organization on public health policy related to nutrition and obesity. Kumanyika is a member of the editorial board for *Ethnicity and Disease,* the journal of the International Society on Hypertension in Blacks, which addresses disease and health patterns among ethnic minority populations.

■ ■ ■ ■

Summary

The nutritional dimensions of women's health include a complex spectrum of topics. Dietary guidelines have been revised and will continue to change as scientists work to unlock the mysteries of diet and its relationship with health and illness.

American women spend most of their waking hours in sedentary activity. By incorporating regular exercise into their daily routine, women can improve their levels of fitness, improve their overall quality of life, and reduce their risk of chronic disease and premature death. These dramatic benefits to activity can also be pleasurable.

Profiles of Remarkable Women

Billie Jean King (1943–)

Billie Jean Moffit was born in Long Beach, California, and educated at Los Angeles State College (now California State College at Los Angeles). She started out playing softball, but knowing there was no significant future for women in the sport, she concentrated her efforts on tennis. In 1962, at the age of 18, King upset Margaret Smith Court, the world's leading women's tennis player, at Wimbledon. In 1967, after becoming the first woman player since 1939 to win the triple crown of singles, doubles, and mixed doubles in both the British and American championships, she was selected as "Outstanding Female Athlete of the World." By 1968, King had won three Wimbledon championships as well as the U.S. title and was the world's top-ranked women's amateur.

In 1972, King was named *Sports Illustrated*'s "Sportsperson of the Year," the first woman to win the award. In 1973, in front of a still-standing record crowd for the most people ever to attend a single tennis match, the 29-year-old King beat 55-year-old tennis professional Bobby Riggs in three straight sets. The "Battle of the Sexes" match was arranged after Riggs claimed that a woman player would never be able to beat a man. King continued winning competitions, and throughout her professional tennis career, she was ranked number one in the world five times and number one in the United States seven times. She holds 20 Wimbledon titles and was ranked in the top 10 in the world for 17 years.

King also became the first woman athlete to earn $100,000 in a single season. Even while displaying her outstanding athletic ability, she stayed committed to women's issues by speaking out and lobbying for women and their right to earn comparable money in tennis and other sports. She was founder and president of the Women's Tennis Association, a labor union for players; a founder of two leagues for professional women athletes, including the Women's Professional Softball League; and publisher, with her husband Larry King, of *WomenSport,* a magazine depicting women's progress as athletes. King established tennis camps, shops, and clinics across the country and created World Team Tennis, a league for professionals. As a coach for World Team Tennis, she became the first woman to coach male professional athletes. King has been inducted into the Women's Sports Foundation Hall of Fame and into the International Tennis Hall of Fame.

Topics for Discussion

1. How can an older sister best advise a younger sister about weight management? What are the important issues to be taken into consideration when talking to a girl about her weight?

2. What should a woman do if she has a friend whom she suspects to have an eating disorder but the friend denies it?

3. Women who are physically active are healthier and therefore at lower risk of chronic disease and early mortality than those who are inactive. Should they have to pay the same insurance rates as those women whose lifestyles place them at greater risk for illness?

4. Some believe that the physical fitness craze has been detrimental to the women's movement because it has added another layer of pressure to conform to an "ideal" body shape or size. Is that argument valid?

5. What can be done to improve women's attitudes toward exercise and physical fitness?

6. What are the biggest challenges to regular exercise and a healthy diet that you face? How are these challenges going to change over the next five years? How do they differ from the challenges your female friends have in these areas?

■■■■

Web Sites

American Council on Exercise: http://www.acefitness.org

American Dietetic Association: http://www.eatright.org

American Obesity Association: http://www.obesity.org

American Society of Bariatric Physicians: http://www.asbp.org

Center for Nutrition Policy & Promotion: http://www.usda.gov/cnpp

Dietary Guidelines: http://www.health.gov/dietaryguidelines

International Food Information Council Foundation: http://www.ific.org

National Eating Disorders: http://www.nationaleatingdisorders.org

National Institute Mental Health Center on Eating Disorders: http://www.nimh.nih.gov/publicat/eatingdisorders.cfm

Nutrition.gov: http://www.nutrition.gov

The President's Council on Physical Fitness and Sports: http://www.fitness.gov

U.S. Department of Agriculture: http://www.usda.gov

U.S. Food and Drug Administration: http://www.fda.gov

USDA: Center for Food Safety & Nutrition: http://www.cfsan.fda.gov

■■■■

References

1. Mokdad, A. H., Marks, J. S., Stroup, D. F., and Gerberding, J. (2004). Actual causes of death in the United States, 2000. *Journal of the American Medical Association* 291: 1238–1245.

2. U.S. Department of Health and Human Services and the U.S. Department of Agriculture. (2005). *A Healthier You—Dietary Guidelines for Americans*. Washington, DC: U.S. Government Printing Office.

3. Putnam, J., Allshouse, J., and Kantor, L. S. (2003). U.S. per capita food supply trends: more calories, refined carbohydrates, and fats. *FoodReview: Weighing in on Obesity* 25(3).

4. Lowry, R., Galuska, D. A., Fulton, J. E., Wechsler, H., and Kann, L. (2002). Weight management goals and practices among U.S. high school students: associations with physical activity, diet, and smoking. *Journal of Adolescent Health* 31(2): 133–144.

5. Centers for Disease Control and Prevention. (2003). Physical activity and good nutrition: essential elements to prevent chronic diseases and obesity. *At a Glance*.

6. Rufail, M. L., Schenkein, H. A., Barbour, S. E., Tew, J. G., and van Antwerpen, R. (2005). Altered lipoprotein subclass distribution and PAF-AH activity in subjects with generalized aggressive periodontitis. *Journal of Lipid Research* 46: 2752–2760.

7. James, S. L., Muir, J. G., Curtis, S. L., and Gibson, P. R. (2003). Dietary fibre: a roughage guide. *Internal Medicine Journal* 33(7): 291–296.

8. Willet, W. C. (2002). *Eat, Drink and Be Healthy: The Harvard Medical School Guide to Healthy Eating*. New York: Simon and Schuster.

9. Food and Nutrition Board, Institute of Medicine. (2002). *Dietary Reference Intakes for Energy, Carbohydrate, Fiber, Fat, Fatty Acids, Cholesterol, Protein, and Amino Acids (Macronutrients)*.

10. U.S. Department of Health and Human Services and the Food and Drug Administration. (July 9, 2003). FDA Backgrounder—FDA Acts to Provide Better Information to Consumers on Trans Fats. http://www.fda.gov/oc/initiatives/transfat/backgrounder.html.

11. Mensink, R. P., Zock, P. L., Kester, A. D., and Katan, M. B. (2003). Effects of dietary fatty acids and carbohydrates on the ratio of serum total to HDL cholesterol and on serum lipids and apolipoproteins: a meta-analysis of 60 controlled trials. *American Journal of Clinical Nutrition* 77(5): 1146–1155.

12. Caro, J., Huybrechts, K. F., Klittich, W. S., Jackson, J. D., and McGuire, A.; CORE Study Group. (2003). Allocating funds for cardiovascular disease prevention in light of the NCEP ATP III guidelines. *American Journal of Managed Care* 9(7): 477–489.

13. Hu, F. B., Stampfer, M. J., Rimm, E. B., Manson, J. E., Ascherio, A., Colditz, G. A., Rosner, B. A., Spiegelman, D., Speizer, F. E., Sacks, F. M., Hennekens, C. H., and Willett, W. C. (1999). A prospective study of egg consumption and risk of cardiovascular disease in men and women. *Journal of the American Medical Association* 281: 1387–1394.

14. Egen, V., and Hasford, J. (2003). Prevention of neural tube defects: effect of an intervention aimed at implementing the official recommendations. *Soz Praventivmed* 48(1): 24–32.

15. Grosse, S. D., Waitzman, N. J., Romano, P. S., and Mulinare, J. (2005). Reevaluating the benefits of folic acid fortification in the United States: economic analysis, regulation, and public health. *American Journal of Public Health* 95: 1917–1922

16. Iron deficiency—United States, 1999–2000. (2002). *Mortality and Morbidity Weekly Report* 51(40): 897–899.

17. Barnes, P. M., and Schoenborn, C. A. (2003). *Physical Activity Among Adults: United States, 2000. Advance Data from Vital and Health Statistics, no. 333.* Hyattsville, MD: National Center for Health Statistics.

18. Hu, F. B., Willet, W. C., Li, T., Stampfer, M. J., Colditz, G. A., and Manson, J. E. (2004). Adiposity as compared with physical activity in predicting mortality among women. *New England Journal of Medicine* 351(26): 2694–2703.

19. Moore, K. A., and Blumenthal, J. A. (1998). Exercise training as an alternative treatment for depression among older adults. *Alternative Therapies in Health and Medicine* 4: 48–56.

20. Elavsky, S., McAuley, E., Motl, R. W., Konopack, J. F., Marquez, D. X., Jerome, G. J., and Diener, E. (2005). Physical activity enhances long-term quality of life in older adults: efficacy, esteem, and affective influences. *Annals of Behavioral Medicine* 30(2): 138–145.

21. Da Costa, D., Rippen, N., Drista, M., and Ring, A. (2003). Self-reported leisure-time physical activity during pregnancy and relationship to psychological well-being. *Journal of Psychomatic Obstetrics and Gynecology* 24(2): 111–119.

22. U.S. Department of Health and Human Services. (1996). *Physical Activity and Health: A Report of the Surgeon General.* Atlanta, GA: Centers for Disease Control and Prevention, National Center for Chronic Disease Prevention and Health Promotion.

23. Kannus, P., Sievanen, H., Palvenen, M., Jarvinen, T. and Parkkari, J. (2005). Prevention of falls and injuries in elderly people. *Lancet* 366(9500): 1885–1893.

24. Warren, M. P., and Goodman, L. R. (2003). Exercise-induced endocrine pathologies. *Journal of Endocrinological Investigation* 26(9): 873–878.

25. Hall, R. C., Hall, R. C. W., and Chapman, M. J. (2005). Psychiatric complications of anabolic steroid use. *Psychosomatics* 46(4): 285–290.

26. Savard, M. and Svec, C. (2005). *The Body Shape Solution to Weight Loss and Wellness.* New York: Atria Publishers.

27. Goode, E. (July 22, 2003). The gorge-yourself environment. *The New York Times.*

28. U.S. Department of Health and Human Services. (2001). *The Surgeon General's Call to Action to Prevent and Decrease Overweight and Obesity.* Rockville, MD: U.S. Department of Health and Human Services, Public Health Service, Office of the Surgeon General.

29. Hedley, A. A., Ogden, C. L., Johnson, C. L., Carroll, M. D., Curtin, L. R., and Flegal, K. M. (2004). Prevalence of overweight and obesity among U.S. children, adolescents, and adults, 1999–2002. *Journal of the American Medical Association* 291: 2847–2850.

30. Calle, D., Rodriguez, C., Walker-Thurmond, K., and Thun, M. (April 23, 2003). Overweight, obesity, and mortality from cancer in a prospectively studied cohort of U.S. adults. *New England Journal of Medicine* 348: 1625–1638.

31. Calle, E., Rodriguez, C., Walker-Thurmond, K., and Thun, M. J. (2003). Overweight, obesity, and mortality from cancer in a prospectively studied cohort of U.S. adults. *New England Journal of Medicine* 348(17): 1625–1638.

32. U.S. Department of Health and Human Services, National Institutes of Health, National Institute of Diabetes and Digestive and Kidney Diseases. (January 31, 2006). Statistics Related to Overweight and Obesity. http://win.niddk.nih.gov/statistics/#econ.

33. Wolf, A. M., Manson, J. E., and Colditz, G. A., (2002). The economic impact of overweight, obesity, and weight loss. In Eckel R, ed. *Obesity: Mechanisms and Clinical Management.* New York: Lippincott, Williams and Wilkins.

34. Wapner, S. (March 4, 2003). Weight loss firms are fatter than ever. *CNBC News.*

35. Abdel-Hamid, T. K. (2003). Exercise and diet in obesity treatment: an integrative system dynamics perspective. *Medicine and Science in Sports and Exercise* 35(3): 400–413.

36. Ward, E. M. (1994). Researchers disagree on the dangers of yo-yo dieting. *Environmental Nutrition.* 17(6): 2.

37. Shade, E. D., Ulrich, C. M., Wener, M. H., Wood, B., Yasui, Y., Lacroix, K., Potter, J. D., and McTiernan, A. (2004). Frequent intentional weight loss is associated with lower natural killer cell cytotoxicity in postmenopausal women; possible long-term immune effects. *Journal of the American Dietetic Association* 104(6): 903–912.

38. Rating the diets from A to Z. (June 2005). *Consumer Reports* 70(6): 18–22.

39. Wyatt, H. R., and Hill, J. O. (2004). What role for weight-loss medication? Weighing the pros and cons for obese patients. *Postgraduate Medicine* 115(1): 38–42.

40. Byrd-Bredbenner, C., Murray, J., and Schlussel, Y. (2005). Temporal changes in anthropometric measurements of idealized females and young women in general. *Women and Health* 41(2): 13–20.

41. Yin, S. (2004). Size and gender. *American Demographics* 26(2): 14.

42. Rome, E. S. (2003). Eating disorders. *Obstetrics and Gynecology Clinics of North America* 30(2): 353–377, vii. Review.

43. American Society for Aesthetic Surgery National Survey (2004). http://www.surgery.org/press/proceduresfacts-asqf.php.

44. Rothblum, E. (1990). Women and weight: fad and fiction. *Journal of Psychology* 124: 5–24.

45. Garner, D. M. (January–February 1997). The 1997 body image survey results. *Psychology Today.* http://www.findarticles.com/p/articles/mi_m1175/is_nl_v30/ai_19013601.

46. Grunbaum, J., et al. (2002). Youth risk behavior surveillance—United States, 2001. *Morbidity and Mortality Weekly Report, Surveillance Summaries* 51(SS04): 1–64.

47. Hsu, L. K. G. (1990). *Eating Disorders.* New York: Guilford Press.

48. Crowther, J. H., Tennenbaum, D. L., Hobfoil, S. E., and Paris-Stephens, M. A. (1992). *The Etiology of Bulimia Nervosa.* Washington, DC: Hemisphere Publishers.

49. World Hunger Year Statistics. Retrieved January 2006 from http://www.worldhungeryear.org/info_center/just_facts.asp.

50. Food and Agriculture Organization of the United Nations. (2002). *The State of Food Insecurity in the World 2002.*

51. World Health Organization. (2003). *Nutrition.* Retrieved January 3, 2006, from http://www.who.int/nut/index.htm.

52. Harne, A. J., and Bixby, W. R. (2005). The benefits and barriers of strength training among college-age women. *Journal of Sport Behavior* 28(2): 151–166.

Chapter Ten

Understanding and Preventing Cardiovascular Disease and Cancer

Chapter Objectives

On completion of this chapter, the student should be able to discuss:

- The main components and functions of the circulatory system and blood.
- The processes leading to atherosclerosis and myocardial infarction.
- The conditions that contribute to congestive heart failure.
- Types of congenital heart disease and its associated prevalence and mortality rates.
- The cause and effects of rheumatic heart disease.
- The significance of angina pectoris.
- Conditions that lead to peripheral artery disease.
- The major causes of cerebrovascular accidents.
- The major modifiable risk factors for cardiovascular disease.
- Gender and race differences that determine risk for cardiovascular disease.
- The process of cancer development and metastasis.
- Cancer from an epidemiological perspective and racial, ethnic, and socioeconomic dimensions.
- Types of benign conditions of the breast, cervix, uterus, and ovaries.
- Risk factors, screening methods, and treatment modalities for breast, cervical, uterine, and ovarian cancer.
- The purpose of Pap smears and HPV tests and how they relate to benign cervical conditions as well as cervical cancer.
- Risk factors, screening methods, and treatment modalities for lung cancer, colorectal cancer, and skin cancer.
- Prevention of cardiovascular disease and cancer through lifestyle changes and health screening.

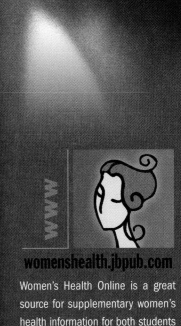

Introduction

Genetics and lifestyle are major contributors to chronic diseases. Genetics clearly plays a role in determining who is at highest risk for developing certain diseases and conditions. Lifestyle alone cannot totally counter a heavy genetic loading for certain conditions; among those who are genetically predisposed, however, changes in lifestyle may help make a difference. This chapter provides an overview of cardiovascular disease and cancer, which are the major killers of women today. Each disease is discussed in terms of epidemiological considerations, risk factors, screening, treatment, and personal decision making to reduce the risk of disease.

Cardiovascular Disease

Cardiovascular disease (CVD) comprises a group of diseases that includes two major categories: diseases of the heart and cerebrovascular disease (primarily stroke). Approximately 450,000 women die annually in the United States of CVD, equaling a rate of about one death per minute. Stroke accounts for approximately 22% of these deaths.[1] According to the Centers for Disease Control and Prevention (CDC)/National Center for Health Statistics (NCHS), if all major forms of CVD were eliminated, life expectancy would increase by almost seven years. More lives are claimed by CVD than by the next five leading causes of death combined. Cardiovascular deaths usually occur in later years when women are beset with a

Figure 10.1

Death rates for diseases of the heart for women, 45 and older.

Source: Centers for Disease Control and Prevention, National Centers for Disease Control. (2005). *Health United States.* Table 36.

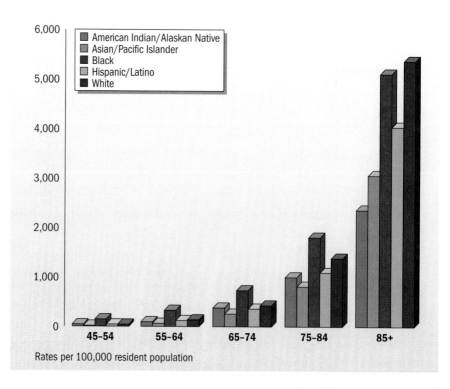

Rates per 100,000 resident population

variety of co-morbid conditions, such as high blood pressure, high blood cholesterol, osteoporosis, and diabetes. Figures 10.1 and 10.2 illustrate the rising death rates from CVD among women of different races as they age.

Cardiovascular disease is also among the leading causes of disability in women. Heart disease can be severely disabling, creating lifestyle limitations. Stroke can lead to paralysis, incontinence, language impairments, and loss of memory. Although it was once believed that heart conditions and stroke were an inevitable consequence of aging, it is now realized that these diseases are greatly influenced by negative lifestyle behaviors, such as cigarette smoking, poor nutrition, and lack of exercise.

Perspectives on Cardiovascular Disease

Epidemiology

Cardiovascular disease is the leading cause of death for women, regardless of racial or ethnic group. Of the various forms of CVD, coronary heart disease (CHD) is the leading cause of death, killing approximately 480,000 people in the United States annually, nearly equally divided between women and men. An estimated 250,000 of these deaths occur suddenly, within one hour of the onset of symptoms, many without warning. Stroke is the third leading cause of death (after heart disease and cancer), killing over 150,000 people annually. Sixty percent of stroke deaths occur in women.

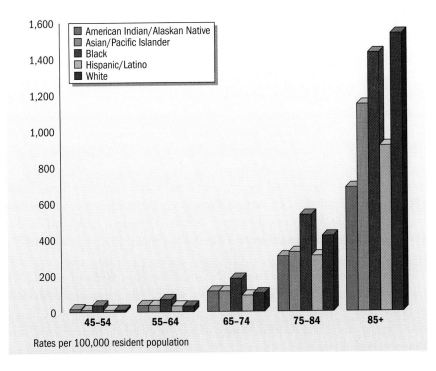

Rates per 100,000 resident population

Figure 10.2

Death rates for cerebrovascular diseases for women, 45 and older.

Source: Centers for Disease Control and Prevention, National Centers for Disease Control. (2005). *Health United States.* Table 37.

Although some cardiovascular diseases occur among children and adolescents, the majority are diseases of individuals who are middle-aged (50 years) and older. The incidence of CHD begins to rise for women between the ages of 55 and 60, about 10 years later than for men. The incidence of stroke begins to sharply rise in both women and men between the ages of 55 and 64.[1,2]

Economic Dimensions

Cardiovascular disease imposes a heavy burden on the medical care system in the United States, particularly on emergency medical departments and hospitals. Clinical care of CVD patients is costly and often prolonged. The estimated cost of cardiovascular disease and stroke in the United States in 2006 is $403.1 billion. This figure includes both direct and indirect costs.

- Direct costs: health expenditures including those for physicians and other professionals, hospital and nursing home services, medications, home health care, and other medical durables
- Indirect costs: lost productivity resulting from morbidity and mortality

An estimated $257.6 billion will be spent for the care of persons with cardiovascular diseases and stroke in 2006. The estimated indirect costs (those costs related to lost work days and lost future earnings) from these diseases include $35.6 billion for lost productivity due to morbidity and $109.9 billion for lost productivity due to mortality. Cardiovascular disease often affects individuals during their peak productive years at work, causing significant disruption to families who are dependent on the person's income.[1] The high rate of CVD also carries a burden for the countries that lose productive workers to disease. The emotional cost to women and their families and friends from such disease is incalculable.[3]

Global Dimensions

During the past century, CVD has been increasingly recognized as a leading cause of disability and death worldwide. With an ever-increasing life expectancy, countries that once were overwhelmed with infectious and communicable diseases, maternal and infant deaths, and malnutrition are now besieged with CVD. CVD is the leading cause of death among women worldwide.[4] The ability to acquire fast foods (which are often loaded with saturated fats and high in calories), the decrease in physical exercise, and the high rates of cigarette smoking have further contributed to the problem. Of particular concern is the increasing number of children in developing countries who engage in these dangerous health habits. The World Health Organization notes that obesity has tripled in China, Eastern Europe, and the Middle East.

The American Heart Association's *Statistical Fact Sheet for Populations* (2005) notes that death rates for CVD among women vary widely across the world: Russian Federation—53% of all female deaths are attributed to CVD; rural China—35%; Argentina—35%; United Kingdom—27%; United States—26%; and France—17%.[5]

Smoking among women has increased. Countries that have 20% to 30% of women smoking include Canada, the United States, Brazil, Colombia, the United Kingdom, Spain, many Eastern European countries, Greece, Turkey, and parts of India. In more developed countries, smoking rates are slowly declining as a result of widespread public health education. Nevertheless, they remain too high. The World Health Organization provides examples in smoking trends among women in three countries (see Table 10.1).[6]

Cultural attitudes affect lifestyle habits. In a number of developing countries, being overweight is seen as a sign of wealth and attractiveness. This attitude mirrors that held by many people in the United States in the nineteenth and twentieth centuries. Furthermore, women in many countries have moved from rural areas to urban areas—from physically active lifestyles such as farming to more sedentary work in offices and industry. Another concern is the "migration" effect that often occurs among women who migrate from developing to developed countries. As with migration from farm to city, women who migrate to more developed countries are exposed to different cultures and styles of living. Unhealthy foods may be convenient and present in greater quantities, while healthy foods and opportunities for physical activity may be more rare. These lifestyle changes put immigrant women at particularly high risk for obesity, high blood pressure, high blood cholesterol, and diabetes—all risk factors for CVD. Unfortunately, in many countries and for many women immigrants, disease prevention and health care remain fragmented.[7]

The Heart

Cardiovascular disease cannot be understood without an appreciation of the heart as a vital organ. Not only does the heart relentlessly pump blood throughout the body, but it has also served poets, writers, composers, lovers, and countless others as an object that has been assigned traits such as love, strength, courage, pain, warmth, fullness, and emptiness.

The heart is located in the chest behind the **sternum,** the breastbone. The **cardiovascular system** consists of the heart, arteries, veins, and capillaries (Figure 10.3). The heart has four major chambers: the **right atrium** and **right ventricle** and the **left atrium** and **left ventricle.** The right and left atria are the upper blood-receiving

Table 10.1	**Smoking Trends Among Women in Three Countries (%)**				
Country	**1960**	**1970**	**1980**	**1990**	**2000**
Japan	13	16	14	14	14
United Kingdom	42	44	37	29	26
United States	34	32	30	23	22

Source: Data from Mackey, J., Eriksen, M., Shafey, O. (2006). *The Tobacco Atlas*, 2nd edition. American Cancer Society.

Figure 10.3

Cardiovascular system.

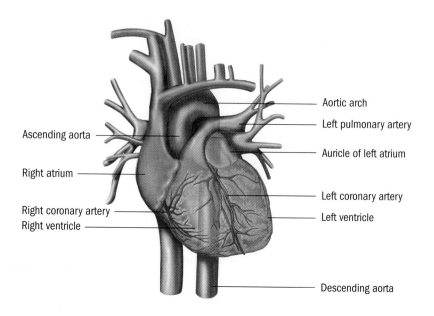

Aortic arch

Left pulmonary artery

Ascending aorta

Auricle of left atrium

Right atrium

Left coronary artery

Right coronary artery

Left ventricle

Right ventricle

Descending aorta

chambers, and the right and left ventricles are the lower blood-pumping chambers. The right atrium and ventricle and the left atrium and ventricle are each separated by a valve. The right atrium and ventricle are separated by the **tricuspid valve**; the left atrium and ventricle are separated by the **bicuspid** or **mitral valve.** Blood flows from the atrium through the valve to the ventricle below. A thick muscular wall known as the **septum** separates the right and left sides of the heart.

Oxygen-poor blood from throughout the body travels to the heart so that it can be pumped to the lungs for oxygenation. The oxygen-poor blood enters the right atrium of the heart from the **inferior** and **superior vena cava** (major veins). From the right atrium, blood flows through the tricuspid valve into the right ventricle, where it is pumped to the lungs via the **pulmonary arteries.** In the lungs, carbon dioxide and waste products are removed from the blood and exchanged for fresh oxygen. The newly oxygen-rich blood leaves the lungs via the **pulmonary veins** and flows into the left atrium. From the left atrium, it passes through the mitral valve into the left ventricle. The left ventricle contracts and forces the oxygen-rich blood through the **aortic valve** into the **aorta** (the main artery) and from there throughout the major arteries, flowing gradually into smaller and smaller arteries, **arterioles,** and finally **capillaries** throughout the body. The capillaries—microscopic vessels with thin walls—are the sites where the nutrients and oxygen in the blood are exchanged for waste and carbon dioxide at the cellular level. From the capillaries, the oxygen-poor but carbon dioxide–rich blood flows into the **venules** and veins as it makes its way back to the heart. The cycle then begins again.

For this system to function properly, the pump—the heart—must remain strong and forceful. It must contract forcefully and quickly when a woman runs a marathon, yet it must slow for rest during sleep. The heart is activated to perform its pumping function by electrical stimuli pulsed from specialized tissues called

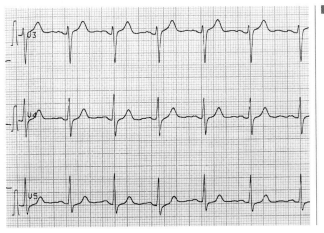

An electrocardiograph (ECG) can detect a normal heart rhythm or abnormalities such as a heart attack or a congenitally damaged tricuspid valve.

nodes buried in the cardiac muscle. This electrical stimulation can be detected by a special device known as an **electrocardiograph (ECG)**, sometimes known as an EKG. An ECG can detect a normal heart rhythm or abnormalities such as a heart attack or a congenitally damaged tricuspid valve.

Similar to the heart, the arteries have muscles and must expand and contract vigorously to meet the demands placed on the body, yet remain supple and open. Veins, although they must also remain supple and open, do not have muscles and must therefore rely on surrounding muscles to move the blood along through the venous system to its destination.

Blood is the vehicle for transporting the food and waste throughout the body. An average woman circulates about six quarts of blood per day. Blood consists of many critical components, which are all suspended in plasma. The primary components are as follows:

- The **red blood cells (erythrocytes)** carry oxygen and carbon dioxide. Hemoglobin is an important protein in the red blood cells that carries oxygen from the lungs throughout the body; it also gives blood its red color.

- The **white blood cells (leukocytes)** act as scavengers to rid the blood and body of bacteria and waste. Several types of white blood cells exist, each of which has its own role in fighting bacterial, viral, fungi, and parasitic infections.

- The **platelets (thrombocytes)** cause the blood to clot.

If the heart's electrical signal loses its regular pattern, the heart can begin to beat irregularly and less effectively, a condition called **arrhythmia.** Arrhythmias are very common and can occur in an otherwise healthy heart; in some cases, however, they may indicate a serious problem and can lead to heart disease. When the atria emit uncoordinated electrical signals, the condition is called **atrial fibrillation** (AF); when disordered electrical activity causes rapid, uncoordinated contractions of the ventricle, the condition is called **ventricular fibrillation** (VF). AF is not life-threatening in itself but can lead to other more serious conditions. For example, when the atrium doesn't pump blood evenly, some blood may remain in the atrium and form a clot. If this clot enters the bloodstream, it can travel to the brain and cause a stroke. In VF, little or no blood may be pumped from the heart, which can result in collapse and sudden death. Physicians can detect heart abnormalities and will first determine the origination of the arrhythmia and its severity before considering treatment.

Pathophysiology of the Heart

Cardiovascular disease encompasses both heart disease (coronary heart disease, congestive heart failure, rheumatic heart disease, angina pectoris, peripheral artery disease, hypertension) and cerebrovascular disease (stroke). Many of these diseases can be prevented or controlled with lifestyle modifications or medications (see "Risk Factors for Cardiovascular Disease").

Heart conditions, in general, can be diagnosed by a variety of tests. Which test is used often depends on a woman's risk factors, her history of heart problems, and her current symptoms. Types of tests include noninvasive tests such as electrocardiograms and magnetic resonance imaging (MRI), nuclear imaging tests that require a needle puncture, and possibly invasive imaging tests such as cardiac catheterization. (For more information on diagnostic tests, visit the Web sites listed at the end of this chapter.)

Treatment also varies greatly for each patient depending on the severity of the condition. This chapter describes the many medications, surgical interventions, and lifestyle changes that can be used to prevent and treat heart disease.

Coronary Heart Disease

Coronary heart disease (CHD) is a result of narrowed or clogged arteries. **Arteriosclerosis** is a generic term that describes any disease of the arteries that leads to thickening and hardening of the artery walls. **Atherosclerosis,** a form of arteriosclerosis, is the major culprit in CHD. It causes the heart vessels to become clogged, thereby impairing a woman's ability to function. This can happen in a variety of ways:

- The arteries can become clogged with waste, usually fat deposits (**plaques**). These waste deposits build up over years on the inner portion of the arteries, impeding the flow of blood.

- The arteries can become stiff with age or disease, rendering them less able to respond to the demands placed on them. If the blood flow is compromised, the area being fed by that particular artery or arteries does not receive proper nutrients and can become damaged or die.

Because the arteries surrounding the heart are so twisted and tortuous, they are particularly prone to developing atherosclerosis. When that occurs, a woman is at increased risk of suffering a **heart attack (myocardial infarction)**.

A heart attack, or death of a portion of the heart, occurs when one or more of the coronary arteries in the heart become damaged or clogged and, consequently, the arteries close off (Table 10.2). Such blockages can occur from a circulating blood clot called an **embolus.** As an embolus moves through the bloodstream, it can become lodged in an artery, blocking any further blood from getting through. The resulting blockage is called a **thrombus** (stationary blood clot). A clot can also form as a result of plaque (cholesterol) build-up within the arterial inner wall. Whatever the cause, blood cannot flow downstream from the blockage. As a result, the part of the body fed by the blocked artery does not receive blood carrying oxygen and nutrients and becomes severely impaired or dies. Blockages within different coronary arteries create different problems. For example, if the blockage occurs within the major artery feeding the left ventricle (the main pump of the heart), the entire ventricle can cease to pump. This stops blood flow to the rest of the body. If this situation is not reversed immediately, a woman can die or suffer irreversible brain damage within a matter of minutes from lack of oxygen to the brain. The heart also can become damaged from other diseases or conditions, such as rheumatic heart disease, or from injury, such as a heart attack, which can lead to congestive heart failure.

Atherosclerosis cannot be cured, but its progression can be slowed. Treatment often depends on which organs are involved. For heart conditions, cholesterol-lowering medications can be used to control high cholesterol levels and are a critical factor in treatment. **Balloon angioplasty** is a procedure used to open narrowed or blocked coronary arteries. A small, hollow tube called a catheter is inserted into an artery near the blockage, and then a balloon near the end of the catheter is inflated. This action helps to widen the vessel and allow blood to flow more freely. A wire mesh **stent** is usually placed at the site of the original narrowing to keep the artery open. In contrast, **coronary artery bypass surgery** (CABG) creates a "bypass" around the blocked part of the coronary artery to restore the blood supply to the heart muscle. When the brain is affected, antiplatelet medications, including aspirin, and anticoagulant medications, such as warfarin and heparin, may be

---

Table 10.2   Warning Signs of a Heart Attack

Uncomfortable pressure, fullness, squeezing, or pain in the center of the chest lasting two minutes or longer

Pain spreading to the shoulder, neck, or arm

Chest discomfort with lightheadedness, fainting, sweating, nausea, shortness of breath

Less Common Symptoms That May Present in Women

Atypical abdominal pain

Palpitations, cold sweat, paleness, dizziness

Unexplained fatigue

In the event of a heart attack, immediate action is required to prevent death or severe heart damage: Call 911 or the local emergency system and get medical help immediately.

used to prevent strokes. When atherosclerosis narrows arteries that supply the bowel, balloon angioplasty may be used or a bypass arterial graft may be performed.

Some of these treatments also may be useful in treating a patient after a heart attack. The ultimate goal of such treatment is to minimize damage by restoring blood flow to the heart muscle.

Research has shown that people with heart disease are more likely to suffer from depression than otherwise healthy people. Conversely, people with depression are at greater risk for developing heart disease. Furthermore, depression and low perceived social support after a heart attack are associated with higher morbidity and mortality. Data show that treating depression in recent heart attack patients does not reduce the risk of death or second heart attack; however, it may help the symptoms of depression and improve quality of life for the patients.[8]

Acute Coronary Syndrome

Acute coronary syndrome (ACS) is a term that is increasingly being used to describe individuals who present with specific cardiac symptoms: myocardial infarction (heart attack) or unstable angina (chest pain that is unexpected or unusual and may be more severe than usual). This important and relatively new diagnostic category seeks to identify individuals when they are moving toward a heart attack (unstable angina) or are in the early stages of a heart attack. The goal is to intervene before serious damage occurs.[9]

Congestive Heart Failure

Congestive heart failure (CHF) occurs when heart muscles are weak and flabby and cannot perform the pumping function with proper vigor. In such a case, the heart loses its ability to contract properly or sufficiently to meet the demands placed on it. Even if the arteries remain open, without a strong pumping action from the heart, the ability of the nutrient-rich and oxygen-rich blood to reach cells is hampered, and the cells may suffer damage or die. Additionally, the heart muscle itself depends on a rich blood supply from the coronary arteries, which must remain open and supple if the heart is to function with vigor. As a result, circulation suffers and fluids begin to accumulate in veins, causing breathing problems, kidney problems, and swelling in the extremities, particularly the legs. CHF may have many causes, but it is often a disease of older women who have suffered heart damage from high blood pressure, atherosclerosis, arteriosclerosis, or heart attack. In some cases, CHF occurs because of a congenital defect or damage to the heart from a bacterial disease, such as rheumatic heart disease.

In many cases, congestive heart failure can be prevented by controlling high blood pressure, treating underlying bacterial infections, and following lifestyle modifications that prevent other forms of CVD. Medication, salt reduction, and possibly surgery to alleviate blockages in coronary arteries may help to improve heart function once CHF has been diagnosed. CHF is the single most frequent cause of hospitalization for people age 65 and older, with women accounting for more than half of all cases.[1]

Congenital Heart Disease

Congenital heart disease is an abnormality of the heart that is present at birth. It can include one or more of the following:

- A hole in the septum
- Imperfectly formed blood vessels
- Valvular damage
- Left ventricular imperfections

Patent ductus arteriosus is a congenital condition in which the ductus arteriosus (passageway between the pulmonary artery and aorta) does not close. It is a common condition in premature babies. Another congenital heart disease, called **pulmonary stenosis,** occurs when the valve between the ventricle and the pulmonary artery is defective and does not open properly. Atrial or ventricular septal defects occur when an opening appears between the two upper or lower chambers of the heart. The majority of these imperfections can be corrected with surgery.

Nearly 40,000 babies are born each year with congenital heart defects; these defects claim the lives of approximately 4,300 young people per year. More than half of the deaths occur in infants less than one year old.[1] Mortality associated with congenital heart defects has been declining, however, due to advances in diagnosis and surgical treatments. From 1992 to 2002, for example, death rates declined 24%. Some 1 million American adults and children with congenital cardiovascular defects are alive today.[10]

Rheumatic Heart Disease

Rheumatic heart disease results from a bacterial infection (*Streptococcus*) that has been inadequately treated and causes damage to the heart valves. Rheumatic heart disease is a downward progression from an inadequately treated strep throat, which progresses to rheumatic fever and affects the entire body in an inflammatory process. The brain, heart, and joints can be adversely and permanently affected. In the heart, rheumatic heart disease can damage the valves by closing them off either completely or partially. This condition may require surgery and valve replacement. The best treatment is prevention—for example, treatment of the initial strep throat, which precludes further damage. Modern antibiotic therapy has sharply reduced mortality from rheumatic heart disease. In 1950, approximately 15,000 Americans died of this disease; in 2000, there were 3,582 deaths. Seventy percent of these deaths were in women.[1]

Angina Pectoris

Angina pectoris (or just *angina*) is chest pain resulting from an insufficient supply of blood, and thus oxygen, to the heart muscle. The symptoms can range in severity from a mild cramping ache to a crushing pain in the chest. The impairment of blood flow can result from atherosclerosis or a spasm of a normal artery. The estimated prevalence of angina is greater in women than in men, affecting more than 3 million women in the United States.[1] Angina is also a symptom of CVD and may be a predictor of future myocardial infarction. Depending on the cause of the impairment, the pain can be relieved by medication, often nitroglycerin, which is a strong vasodilator (opening the closed blood vessel).

Peripheral Artery Disease

Peripheral artery disease (PAD) is a disease of the extremities (hands, arms, but mainly legs and feet) in which the blood supply is diminished and sufficient oxygen and nutrients do not reach these areas properly. Because waste is not removed from these areas sufficiently, a woman can experience symptoms that range from cramping and numbness to gangrene (tissue death), which may require amputation of the extremity. The cause of PAD is related to atherosclerosis and arteriosclerosis and is particularly associated with diabetes, smoking, and hypertension. Of all the known risk factors, smoking is the most strongly related to PAD. Treatment options include lifestyle modifications, such as smoking cessation, anticoagulant or antiplatelet medications, angioplasty, or bypass surgery.

Metabolic Syndrome

Metabolic syndrome is the name for a group of diseases that can occur together and create a greater risk for CVD. The National Heart, Lung, and Blood Institute and the American Heart Association note that the presence of three or more of the following diseases predisposes a woman to an increased risk for metabolic syndrome:

- Elevated waist circumference—high levels of fat around the abdomen equal to or greater than 35 inches (88 centimeters) or an "apple" appearance
- High blood lipid levels—especially high triglycerides, equal to or greater than 150 mg/dL (milligrams per deciliter)
- Low HDL ("good") cholesterol—less than 50 mg/dL in women
- High blood pressure—equal to or greater than 130/85 mm Hg (millimeters of mercury)
- Elevated fasting blood glucose (sugar)—equal to or greater than 100 mg/dL

The principal factors contributing to metabolic syndrome appear to be central obesity and insulin resistance—factors that are increasingly common among women. Both organizations recommend weight loss and control, healthy eating, and increased physical activity as ways to prevent metabolic syndrome.[11]

Cerebrovascular Disease (Stroke)

Cerebrovascular accident, commonly called **stroke,** is a condition in which blood vessels leading to and within the brain become damaged. The process of blood flow blockage that occurs in the coronary vessels of the heart is similar to that which occurs in the brain. The other major process involved in stroke is vessel rupture, often resulting from atherosclerotic vessels. When the blood vessel either is blocked or bursts, part of the brain cannot get blood and therefore oxygen, which it needs to survive. The most common type of stroke, **ischemic stroke,** is caused by blockage; the clot in such cases is called a cerebral thrombus or cerebral **embolism. Hemorrhagic strokes** are caused by ruptured blood vessels.

An **aneurysm** is one type of weakened blood vessel that can cause a stroke. It entails a ballooning of a weakened region of a blood vessel resulting from several factors including a congenital defect, chronic high blood pressure, or an injury to the brain. If left untreated, the aneurysm will continue to weaken until it ruptures and bleeds in the brain (Figure 10.4).

Warning signs (Table 10.3) may precede a stroke in the form of a **transient ischemic attack (TIA).** In a TIA, the artery may close momentarily in a spasm, and the woman may have a brief memory lapse or garbled speech. Such an event often occurs very quickly, and the woman may have little memory of it.

To diagnose a stroke, a variety of tests are used to examine the brain and outline the injured brain area:

- Imaging tests, such as a CT (computed tomography) or CAT (computerized axial tomography) scan, produce a picture of the brain similar to X rays.
- Electrical tests, such as an EEG (electroencephalogram) or an evoked response test, record the electrical impulses of the brain.
- Blood flow tests, such as B-mode imaging, Doppler testing, duplex scanning, and angiography (arteriography or arteriogram), show any problem that may cause changes in blood flow to the brain.

Surgery, drugs, acute hospital care, and rehabilitation are all accepted stroke therapies. Treatment of an ischemic stroke focuses on removing the obstruction and restoring blood flow. The most promising medication for ischemic stroke is the clot-busting drug tissue plasminogen activator (tPA). For maximum benefit, tPA therapy must be started within three hours of the onset of stroke symptoms. Generally, only 3% to 5% of people who suffer a stroke reach the hospital in time to be considered for this treatment. Although tPA carries a risk of bleeding in the brain, its benefits generally outweigh the risks when an experienced doctor uses it properly. A five-year study by the National Institute of Neurological Disorders and Stroke (NINDS) found that stroke patients who received tPA within three hours of the start of stroke symptoms were at least 30% more likely to recover with little or no disability after three months.[12]

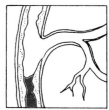

Thrombus

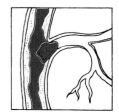

Embolism

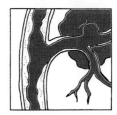

Aneurysm (ruptured)

Figure 10.4

Types of cerebrovascular accidents.

Table 10.3	**Warning Signs of a Stroke**

Temporary weakness or numbness of the face, arm, or leg, especially on one side of the body

Temporary confusion, loss of speech, trouble speaking, or trouble understanding speech

Temporary loss of vision or dimness in one or both eyes

Unexplained dizziness, unsteadiness, or loss of balance or coordination

In the event of a stroke, immediate attention is required: Call 911 or the local emergency system and get medical help immediately.

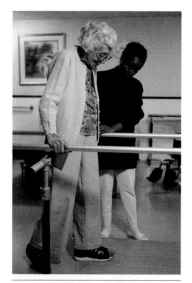

■ Recovery from a stroke can be very difficult.

Doctors sometimes use balloon angioplasty and the implantable steel screens called stents to remedy fatty build-up clogging a vessel. When the carotid artery (a neck artery) is partially blocked by a fatty build-up, surgery might be performed to remove the plaque—a technique called carotid endarterectomy. Antiplatelet agents, such as aspirin, and anticoagulants, such as warfarin, interfere with the blood's ability to clot and can play an important role in preventing ischemic stroke.

To treat a hemorrhagic stroke, an obstruction needs to be introduced to prevent rupture and bleeding of the affected blood vessel. Surgical treatment is often recommended to either place a metal clip at the base of the aneurysm or to remove the abnormal vessels. Endovascular procedures are less invasive and involve the introduction of a catheter through a major artery in the leg or arm; the catheter is then guided to the aneurysm, where it deposits a mechanical agent, such as a coil, to prevent rupture.

After a stroke, rehabilitation is often necessary to help survivors relearn skills that are lost when part of the brain is damaged and learn new ways of performing tasks to compensate for any disabilities. Therapy begins in the acute-care hospital after the patient's medical condition has been stabilized, often within 24 to 48 hours after the stroke. Post-stroke rehabilitation requires the services of physicians; rehabilitation nurses; physical, occupational, recreational, speech-language, and vocational therapists; and mental health professionals.

The types and degrees of disability that follow a stroke depend on which area of the brain is damaged. Generally, stroke can cause five types of disabilities:

- Paralysis is one of the most common disabilities resulting from stroke. It usually appears on the side of the body opposite the side of the brain damaged by stroke, and may affect the face, an arm, a leg, or the entire side of the body.

- Stroke patients may lose the ability to feel touch, pain, temperature, or position. Some experience pain, numbness, or odd sensations of tingling or prickling in paralyzed or weakened limbs. The loss of urinary continence and/or bowel control is fairly common immediately after a stroke and often results from a combination of sensory and motor deficits. Permanent incontinence after a stroke, however, is uncommon.

- At least one-fourth of all stroke survivors experience language impairments, involving the ability to speak, write, and understand spoken and written language. Interestingly, sex-related differences have been noted depending on which portion of the brain is affected. Functional MRI scans have shown that males predominantly rely on areas of the left hemisphere of the brain, whereas females activate both the left and right regions for certain aspects of language. A stroke that occurs in the left hemisphere can therefore have disastrous results for men in terms of speech, whereas women can use the other, unaffected side to regain speech. This knowledge helps to explain why women seem to be more resilient to the effects of such injury and are more likely than males to recover language ability after suffering a left-hemisphere stroke.[13]

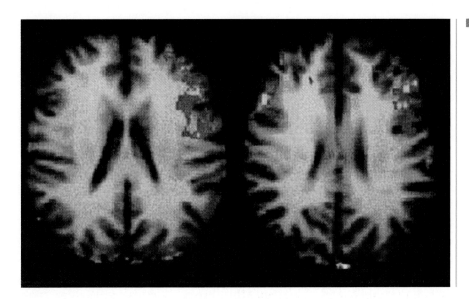

Functional MRI scans show that male subjects predominantly rely on areas of the left hemisphere of the brain, while females activate both the left and right regions for certain aspects of language. (Image courtesy of Dr. Sally Shaywitz.)

- Stroke can damage parts of the brain that are responsible for memory, learning, and awareness. Stroke survivors may have dramatically shortened attention spans or may lose their ability to make plans, comprehend meaning, learn new tasks, or engage in other complex mental activities.

- Survivors of stroke often feel fear, anxiety, frustration, anger, sadness, and a sense of grief for their physical and mental losses. The physical effects of brain damage are responsible for some of these emotional disturbances and personality changes. Clinical depression appears to be the emotional disorder most commonly experienced by stroke survivors.

Whatever the cause of the stroke, the damage to the artery prevents oxygen and nutrients from reaching a particular area of the brain, and as a result that portion dies. Depending on where the stroke occurs in the brain, speech, memory, thought, and movement can be affected or lost. Stroke is the leading cause of serious, long-term disability in the United States. The length of time it takes a person to recover depends on the severity of the stroke:[1]

- 50% to 70% of survivors regain their functional independence.

- 15% to 30% are permanently disabled.

- 20% require institutional care within three months after onset.

Although a stroke can happen at any time to anyone, it is generally a condition that occurs in older individuals. The incidence of a stroke doubles each decade for people older than 55. Of those women with an initial stroke, 25% die within a year. Those who suffer a stroke at age 65 or older have an even greater chance of dying. Among women younger than 65, 53% of those who have a stroke will die within eight years.[1]

Risk Factors for Cardiovascular Disease

Cardiovascular diseases result from a complex interaction of genetics, lifestyle, and environmental factors that lead to different pathological conditions of the cardiovascular system. The major risk factors (those that make a significant contribution to the development of a disease) for CHD that can be modified or controlled include cigarette smoking, high blood pressure, high blood cholesterol, diabetes, obesity, and sedentary lifestyle (see Self-Assessment 10.1). The major risk factors for stroke that can be modified or controlled are high blood pressure, cigarette smoking, and diabetes. Risk factors that cannot be changed or controlled include increasing age, family history of CVD, and being African American. Although these factors can contribute to a person's risk of disease, they are not perfect predictors of disease. A woman with normal cholesterol levels, for example, may have heart disease. Conversely, a woman with high cholesterol may

Self-Assessment 10.1

Personal Risk Factors for Cardiovascular Disease

Age
A woman's risk of cardiovascular disease increases as she gets older, most noticeably after menopause.

Genetics
A family history of cardiovascular disease increases a woman's risk.

Race
Until age 75, African American women are twice as likely to die of cardiovascular disease as white women; after age 75, white women are more likely to die of cardiovascular disease.

Obesity
Being 20% over recommended body weight is a risk factor for cardiovascular disease.

Smoking
For women, smoking is the most significant risk factor for cardiovascular disease.

Hypertension
Elevated blood pressure is a risk factor for cardiovascular disease. A woman's blood pressure is likely to rise after menopause.

Elevated cholesterol
Elevated cholesterol is a major risk factor for cardiovascular disease.

Sedentary lifestyle
Failure to achieve adequate levels of physical activity predisposes an individual to cardiovascular disease.

Diabetes
Diabetes is more prevalent in women and is a major risk factor for cardiovascular disease.

Menopause (natural or surgical)
A woman's risk of heart disease rises as she approaches menopause (loss of estrogen) and continues to rise thereafter.

Having one or more of these risk factors increases the risk of developing heart disease. The more risk factors a woman has, the greater her risk.

not have heart disease even though she does have one of the factors that put her at risk.

Cigarette Smoking

As discussed in detail in Chapter 13, cigarette smoking is the greatest preventable cause of death in the United States. Not only does it increase the risk of several kinds of cancers, but it also sharply increases the risk of heart attack (especially sudden death from heart attack), stroke, and PAD. While smoking rates have declined sharply since the 1960s, too many women still smoke. The estimate is at least 18.5%. Furthermore, smoking is highest among women with little education and lowest among women with a bachelor's degree or higher.[14]

Certain components in cigarette smoke act as **vasoconstrictors,** meaning they close down the blood vessels. One such compound is carbon monoxide, a gas in tobacco smoke that reduces the amount of oxygen that red blood cells can carry. This poor oxygen-carrying ability decreases the amount of oxygen available to the heart, brain, muscles, and every organ in the body. Nicotine is another vasoconstrictor. By narrowing the blood vessels, it increases the likelihood of a blood clot forming. Over time in a chronic smoker, vasoconstriction contributes to the increased fragility and brittleness of arteries, which in turn contributes to atherosclerosis.

The good news is that when a woman stops smoking, her risk for heart disease begins to decline within months. According to the World Health Organization, one year after quitting, the risk of coronary heart disease decreases by 50%; within 15 years, the relative risk of an ex-smoker dying from CHD approaches that of a lifetime nonsmoker.[6]

Secondhand smoke, also known as **environmental tobacco smoke (ETS),** comes from nearby tobacco products that are burning. The toxins contained in secondhand smoke include more than 60 cancer-causing agents, nicotine, and carbon monoxide.[15, 16] Secondhand smoke is associated with a number of potentially lethal conditions: lung cancer, sinus cancer, lung conditions (such as asthma, or impaired lung function, especially in young children), and heart disease, low birthweight in babies (especially when mothers smoke during pregnancy), and others. Repeated exposure to secondhand smoke almost doubles the risk of heart disease.[17]

Hypertension

Blood pressure is the pressure exerted against the walls of the arteries when the heart pumps, specifically when the left ventricle contracts. This pressure is crucial in maintaining equilibrium throughout the vascular system as different forces affect this system. For example, when an athlete runs a race, the heart must pump faster and harder to meet the demands of the cells for oxygen. As part of this process, the arteries must constrict to keep the pressure constant to accomplish the task of running.

Blood pressure is measured with a **sphygmomanometer.** This cuff device is connected to a hose, which is in turn connected to a measuring device. The cuff is

I know that I shouldn't smoke cigarettes, but what the heck, it's cool and I look more sophisticated. I know that I can quit any time I want to. Besides, a few years of smoking won't hurt.
15-year-old student

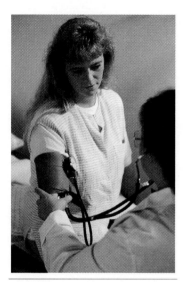

■ All women should know their personal risk for hypertension and regularly monitor their blood pressure.

wrapped around the woman's upper arm (or in rare instances the leg) and inflated, thereby constricting the underlying artery and stopping the blood flow and with it the sound of the heartbeat. Gradually the pressure in the cuff is released, and the blood begins to flow back through the artery and the sound of the heartbeat returns. The first sound heard as the blood begins to flow back into the artery is called the **systolic,** and the last sound heard before it disappears again is called the **diastolic.** The measurement is shown as millimeters of mercury (mm Hg) and is expressed as a fraction, such as 115/75 mm Hg, or 115 mm Hg systolic and 75 mm Hg diastolic. The first number, which expresses the systolic pressure, represents the amount of force the blood exerts against the wall of the artery when the heart contracts. The second number, which expresses the diastolic pressure, represents the amount of pressure the blood exerts against the wall of the artery when the heart rests between beats.

Hypertension, also known as high blood pressure, is a blood pressure that remains elevated above what is considered a safe level. Hypertension is not the same as excessive stress or tension, as some individuals mistakenly imagine. Although numbers such as 120/80 mm Hg have been noted over the years as "normal" blood pressure, there is no true normal number because blood pressure varies throughout the day and during different activities. A young woman may have a blood pressure of 90/70 mm Hg during a visit to the doctor, whereas an older woman may have a blood pressure of 138/80 mm Hg during her doctor's visit. Both may be deemed appropriate. The numbers used by the National Heart, Lung, and Blood Institute's National High Blood Pressure Education Program and by the American Heart Association to indicate high blood pressure are 140 mm Hg systolic and 90 mm Hg diastolic. Although blood pressure can reach heights such as 140/90 mm Hg or greater in a healthy adult during exercise, these levels return to a lower level after exercise. Continuing levels of blood pressure at 140/90 mm Hg or higher, however, are considered high blood pressure and, as such, increase an individual's risk for heart disease and stroke (see Table 10.4). One out of every three adults in the United States has high blood pressure.[1]

Table 10.4	Classification of Blood Pressure for Adults	
BP Classification	**Systolic Blood Pressure (mm Hg)**	**Diastolic Blood Pressure (mm Hg)**
Normal	Less than 120	And less than 80
Prehypertension	120–139	Or 80–89
Stage 1 hypertension	140–159	Or 90–99
Stage 2 hypertension	Equal to or greater than 160	Or equal to or greater than 100

Source: U.S. Department of Health and Human Services, National Institutes of Health, National High Blood Pressure Education Program. (2003). *The Seventh Report of the Joint National Committee on Prevention, Detection, Evaluation, and Treatment of High Blood Pressure.*

Over time, high blood pressure exerts a damaging effect on small arteries, known as arterioles. Arterioles become thicker and less elastic, resulting in arteriosclerosis. This condition, coupled with the effects from atherosclerosis, creates an explosive situation. When faced with the demands of heavy exertion (such as running or shoveling snow), arterioles, particularly in the brain, heart, or kidneys, can close off, rupture, or leak, causing a stroke, heart attack, or renal accident (in kidneys). About half of the people who have a first heart attack and two-thirds of people who have a first stroke have blood pressures higher than 160/95 mm Hg.[1]

The highest rates of high blood pressure occur among African American and Hispanic women; those who are older, overweight, or obese; and those who are poor or near poor.[1] The risk of high blood pressure increases with age. More than half of women older than age 55 have elevated or high blood pressure. With the rise in blood pressure comes a higher risk of heart disease and death. According to the American Heart Association, the estimated death rate associated with high blood pressure was 14.5 per 100,000 for white women and 40.8 per 100,000 among black women.[1]

Women who are obese tend to have higher levels of blood pressure than do women who are more slender. In many cases, high blood pressure can be brought under control by diet, weight control, and weight maintenance. In some women, especially African American women, salt sensitivity appears to be important in the development and control of high blood pressure. To counter this problem, women may have to limit the intake of salt in their diet. When necessary, medication can be used to lower elevated blood pressure. A woman with high blood pressure should be under the supervision of a healthcare provider. Blood pressure should be checked periodically, especially as a woman ages.

High Blood Cholesterol

Cholesterol is a fatty substance found in all cells that is essential for the manufacture and maintenance of cells, sex hormones, and nerves throughout the body. In most individuals, the body manufactures an appropriate amount of cholesterol to serve its needs. In some individuals, however, blood cholesterol levels may be excessively high, due to obesity, poor diet, or genetic abnormalities. High blood levels of cholesterol (greater than 240 mg/dL) are associated with an increased risk of mortality and morbidity from CHD.

When an excessive amount of cholesterol is present, the body can become overwhelmed, and the unused cholesterol is deposited on the inner walls of the arteries. Over time (usually decades), these deposits gradually accumulate, slowly narrowing the artery (Figure 10.5). The inner walls become clogged and brittle, and pieces of the artery tear, leaving jagged edges. These jagged edges stick up and catch material that flows by in the bloodstream, thereby adding more waste deposits to the wall. The artery is gradually closed off either by a fatty plaque or by a transient embolus, which may become lodged in the narrowed artery. Another type of smaller plaque, called an unstable plaque, also may cause blood to clot. If the plaque bursts within the artery wall, its contents are released into the bloodstream and can trigger

Figure 10.5

Narrowing arteries.

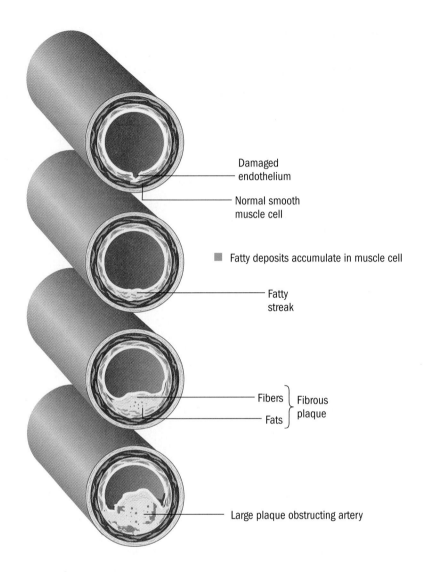

Damaged endothelium

Normal smooth muscle cell

■ Fatty deposits accumulate in muscle cell

Fatty streak

Fibers ⎫
        ⎬ Fibrous plaque
Fats ⎭

Large plaque obstructing artery

a blockage. In any case, the blood does not reach a part of the body, and that part will die unless the artery is once again opened. If this blockage happens in a coronary artery, a heart attack occurs.

Cholesterol is made in the liver and small intestine and is transported throughout the body in a **lipoprotein.** Lipoproteins consist of fats and protein bound together in a chemical structure that enables them to be transported in the blood. They are made up of the following key elements: low-density lipoproteins (LDL), high-density lipoproteins (HDL), very-low-density lipoproteins (VLDL), and triglycerides. Everyone has each of these substances in varying amounts in each lipoprotein molecule.

- LDL cholesterol is often referred to as "bad" cholesterol because of its affinity for sticking to the wall of the artery and lodging there.

- HDL cholesterol is often referred to as "good" cholesterol because it functions somewhat like a trash collector, taking the LDL cholesterol out of the body.

- **VLDL** is associated with the transport of fats known as triglycerides.
- **Triglycerides** are a form of fat that comes from food and is also made in the body. High triglycerides are often a sign of high total cholesterol.

When speaking of cholesterol levels in the blood, healthcare professionals generally refer either to the total blood cholesterol level, or to the LDL cholesterol and HDL cholesterol levels. Cholesterol levels are measured from a small amount of blood (about one teaspoonful) drawn from a vein. To obtain a total blood cholesterol measurement, the person does not have to fast for 12 hours before the drawing. If the physician wishes to obtain an accurate measurement of the LDL cholesterol and the HDL cholesterol, however, the person must fast for 12 hours before the sample is drawn. The measurement is shown in milligrams per deciliter (mg/dL). As with blood pressure measurements, there is no one "normal" level for blood cholesterol. Table 10.5 summarizes the cholesterol-related recommendations from the National Heart, Lung, and Blood Institute's National Cholesterol Education Program.

Table 10.5 **What Do Cholesterol Numbers Mean?**

Level	Category
Total Cholesterol	
Less than 200 mg/dL	Desirable
200–239 mg/dL	Borderline high
240 mg/dL or greater	High
LDL Cholesterol	
Less than 100 mg/dL	Optimal
100–129 mg/dL	Near optimal/above optimal
130–159 mg/dL	Borderline high
160–189 mg/dL	High
190 mg/dL or greater	Very high
HDL Cholesterol	
Less than 40 mg/dL	Major risk factor
40–59 mg/dL	Borderline
60 mg/dL or greater	Protective factor
Triglyceride	
Less than 150 mg/dL	Desirable
150–199 mg/dL	Borderline high
200 mg/dL or greater	High

*Cholesterol levels are measured in milligrams (mg) of cholesterol per deciliter (dL) of blood.

Source: National Heart, Lung, and Blood Institute, National Cholesterol Education Program. (2001). *High Blood Cholesterol: What You Need to Know.* NIH Publication No. 01-3290.

A low level of HDL has been found to be a predictor of mortality from CHD in both young and older women, and is a stronger predictor in women than in men.[1] Women, particularly those who are fit and slender and who have not experienced menopause, tend to have slightly elevated HDL cholesterol levels compared with men or with postmenopausal women. Elevated HDL cholesterol levels are shown to be protective against heart disease. Indeed, after menopause, a woman's hormone levels begin to drop and so do her HDL cholesterol levels—sometimes by as much as 10% to 20%. During this time, a woman's risk for heart disease continues to rise.[18] Research has shown that elevated triglyceride levels sharply increase a person's risk of dying from a heart attack, even if a person's blood cholesterol is normal.[19]

As discussed in Chapter 9, cholesterol levels can usually be controlled by diet. A diet low in cholesterol and saturated fat is crucial in maintaining a low overall total cholesterol level. Saturated fats eaten in food actually have a greater effect on blood cholesterol than cholesterol eaten in food. Eating saturated fats increases the total blood cholesterol, particularly the LDL cholesterol—the "bad" cholesterol. This does not mean that a woman should not limit the amount of cholesterol she consumes; rather, she should be careful to limit both the dietary cholesterol and the dietary saturated fat she eats. A diet that is low in cholesterol and saturated fat should not limit essential nutrients.

Despite cholesterol being a strong predictor of potential heart attack or stroke, almost half of people who have heart attacks have normal levels of cholesterol. Studies have shown that levels of **C-reactive protein** (CRP), a protein found in the blood when inflammation is present, may actually be a stronger predictor of potential cardiovascular disease than cholesterol levels. CRP levels can be measured by a simple blood test.[20] In January 2003, the American Heart Association and the Centers for Disease Control and Prevention issued guidelines for the use of such testing; the guidelines recommend that CRP screening should be reserved for people with moderate cardiovascular risk and that it should not replace assessment for major risk factors. If CRP levels are high, treatment that is used to lower cholesterol—such as exercise, aspirin, and **statins**—can also be used to lower CRP. Although CRP can be useful as a predictor, high levels of this protein can indicate a number of other acute and chronic conditions, including arthritis, tuberculosis, cancer, pneumonia, or the common cold. Positive CRP also can occur during the last half of pregnancy or with the use of oral contraceptives. More research is needed to determine whether reducing CRP actually reduces heart attacks.

Another substance found in the blood is **homocysteine,** an essential amino acid. Increased levels have been shown to harm the arterial lining and increase the risk for heart disease. Folic acid and vitamins B_6 and B_{12} can lower homocysteine levels. Whether such efforts reduce the rates of heart disease is not yet clear. Until the studies are more clear, women at high risk for heart disease should make certain that their diet is rich in folic acid and vitamins B_6 and B_{12} (fruits and green leafy vegetables).[21]

Lp(a), a lipoprotein, is one variation of LDL cholesterol. To date, it is not clear how Lp(a) contributes to heart disease but it is known to be a strong risk factor. No effective treatment for high Lp(a) levels is presently available.[22]

Diabetes

Diabetes is a disorder of the pancreas in which naturally occurring insulin (a hormone that is used to convert sugar, starches, and other types of food into energy—mainly glucose) is not properly manufactured or used. The most common form of diabetes is diabetes mellitus, or type 2 diabetes. In women with diabetes mellitus, these sources of energy cannot be moved from blood into the cells. This creates many serious problems and can lead to life-threatening situations. Nearly 9% of women have diabetes, although some are not aware of their disease. The risk of heart disease for women with diabetes has risen more than 23% in the past 30 years. When diabetes interacts with other CVD risk factors, the threat of CVD rises again. Women who develop diabetes during pregnancy (gestational diabetes) also are at much higher risk of having the disease.[23]

The prevalence of diabetes is two to four times greater in black, Hispanic, American Indian, and Asian American women.[24] The reasons for this greater prevalence are not entirely clear, although higher rates of overweight and obesity certainly contribute to the risk. Scientists are exploring whether certain genes might predispose certain groups to diabetes. The critical issue for anyone with diabetes is to keep the disease under control with proper nutrition, exercise, and medication as needed.

Overweight and Obesity

Overweight and obesity are two major risk factors for a number of diseases, especially heart disease. Overweight is defined as having a body mass index (BMI) of 25 or greater; obesity is having a BMI of 30 or greater, or being more than 20% over desirable body weight. More than 61% of U.S. women are considered overweight and 32% are obese. The highest rates of both are in African American and Hispanic women.[25] This condition is considered a major factor in the development of CHD. It is also associated with high blood pressure, high blood cholesterol, and diabetes, all of which are major risk factors for CHD. Obesity is correlated with other risk factors for CHD, such as sedentary lifestyle and poor nutrition. Eating an excess of saturated fat and cholesterol leads to clogged arteries, which place a strain on the heart, compromise the efficiency of the pump, and can lead to heart attacks.

Evidence suggests that how fat is distributed on a woman's body may prove to be an indicator for heart disease. Truncal distribution of fat (stomach and upper body) as opposed to hip and thigh fat distribution appears to place a woman at greater risk for heart disease. This distribution has been referred to as "apple" (truncal obesity) versus "pear" (hip and thigh) fat distribution. More information on obesity can be found in Chapter 9.

Sedentary Lifestyle

Sedentary lifestyle is another important modifiable risk factor for cardiovascular disease. Sedentary lifestyle simply means that a woman is not getting enough regular aerobic exercise—any movement that raises the heart rate significantly for an extended period of time. More than 30% of women do not participate in the recommended amount of leisure-time activity. For all races, women are less physically active than men on average. Aerobic exercise is a critical factor in keeping

I am overweight and know that I need to lose weight, but how can I afford all those expensive weight-loss foods in the supermarket? My kids need the fat in their diet, and I can't afford to buy and fix two separate meals.

35-year-old mother

the heart and other muscles strong and in good working condition. Regular exercise also aids in controlling weight, helping to raise HDL cholesterol levels, and both controlling and reducing the risk of developing diabetes. The Nurses' Health Study, a large ongoing study observing female nurses, showed similar protective effects against coronary heart disease for brisk walking and vigorous exercise.[26] See Chapter 9 for more information.

Other Factors Affecting CVD Risk

Menopause.   After menopause (the cessation of menses), the risk for heart disease and stroke increases significantly for women. Coronary heart disease rates in women after menopause are two to three times higher than those in women of the same age who have not yet reached menopause. One reason appears to be related to the loss of natural estrogen. Scientists believe that during and after menopause, women experience a decrease in HDL cholesterol and an increase in LDL cholesterol and triglycerides. Increased plaque is noted in the arteries, and heart attacks and strokes begin to occur. Research also has shown that the decrease in estrogen as a result of natural and surgical menopause is associated with these changes in serum lipid profiles (blood cholesterol levels).[27]

Estrogen loss during menopause and the use of hormone replacement therapy (HRT) are issues that have inspired tremendous debate in the last several years. Observational studies in both animals and humans, carried out largely in the 1970s and 1980s, showed that HRT could be beneficial in slowing the onset of heart disease. More recent clinical trials, carried out in the 1990s and early 2000s, however, showed that HRT was neutral in effect or even dangerous. Recent examination of some of those clinical trials has shown where some of the differences in findings may lie. Women who started HRT after they had been menopausal for a number of years and those with established heart disease had a greater number of heart disease events and death on a particular regimen of HRT. Women who started HRT during or immediately after cessation of menstrual periods generally did not show an increased risk. (See Chapter 8 for more information.)

Oral Contraceptives.   The high doses of estrogen and progestin in early oral contraceptives were associated with an increase in risk for CVD; however, newer oral contraceptives containing lower doses of hormones have reduced the risk of cardiovascular events associated with earlier high-dose formulations. Using oral contraceptives may somewhat increase one's risk of heart attack, but this higher risk is largely limited to older women who smoke or have high blood pressure. Combining birth control pill use with other risk factors for heart disease—particularly smoking, hypertension, and long-term or uncontrolled diabetes—raises the risk of myocardial infarction substantially. Recent studies have suggested no increased risk of myocardial infarction among users of newer oral contraceptives without any other risk factors.

Oral contraceptive users without other risk factors do have an increased risk of stroke. Those who smoke, have a history of hypertension, or are older than age 35 have an even greater risk.

Pill users also may have an increase in blood pressure, although women who are nonsmokers and take low-dose oral contraceptives have the lowest risk of an increase in blood pressure. Older women and obese women have the highest risk of increased blood pressure from oral contraceptives.

Concerns also have been raised regarding thromboembolism, also known as deep-vein thrombosis (VTE), with oral contraceptive use. The estimated risk of VTE is low with all modern low-dose oral contraceptives.[28]

Several studies have found that oral contraceptive users with a history of migraine are two to four times more likely to have an ischemic stroke than women with a history of migraine who do not use this form of birth control. Studies suggest the risk is greater among women who have severe migraine headaches with "aura"—focal neurologic symptoms such as blurred vision, temporary loss of vision, seeing flashing lights or zigzag lines, or trouble speaking or moving. Experts now recommend that a woman who has migraine headaches with focal neurologic symptoms should not start combined oral contraceptives and a woman age 35 or older should choose another method if possible if she has migraine headaches even without focal neurologic symptoms. Mild or severe headaches that are not migrainous do not rule out use of birth control pills.[29]

Because the risk of cardiovascular disease increases in oral contraceptive users with other risk factors, women should have a complete medical checkup before choosing oral contraceptives as their method of birth control.

Alcohol and Illicit Drugs.   Research has shown that consuming modest levels of wine or other alcohol has a beneficial effect on CVD risk—namely, a daily intake of no more than one drink per day can reduce the risk of coronary heart disease in women. Research is being conducted to find out whether these benefits are due to an increased intake of antioxidants, which can be found in red wine; the increase in HDL cholesterol that alcohol produces; or the prevention of platelets sticking together due to certain substances in alcoholic beverages. There is, however, an increase in risk of stroke and other causes of morbidity and mortality with moderate to heavy consumption of alcohol.[30] Therefore, nondrinkers should not take this as a recommendation to begin drinking, and those who are drinking more than the recommended amount should cut back. One "drink" equals

- 1 to $1/2$ fluid once (fl oz) of 80–100 proof alcohol *or*
- 4 fl oz wine *or*
- 12 fl oz beer.

Illicit drugs, such as cocaine, LSD (acid), and heroin, may cause short-term cardiovascular effects as well as long-term cardiovascular complications. Cocaine and LSD both increase heart rate and blood pressure while constricting the blood vessels. Cocaine can lead to medical complications such as ventricular fibrillation (disturbances in heart rhythm) and heart attacks. Cocaine-related deaths are often a result of cardiac arrest.[31] Heroin slows down cardiac function during use. Its long-term effects include scarring and collapsing of the veins and bacterial infections of

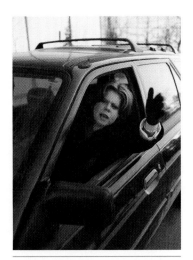

■ Continuous stress is associated with cardiovascular disease.

the blood vessels and heart valves, often leading to death. These drugs also are associated with many other short- and long-term negative effects. See Chapter 13 for more details.

Stress.   Stress is a normal part of everyday life and, in fact, is essential to proper functioning of the body. External stimulation can push a person to action—to study for a test, or to sprint the final lap in a race. A kiss from a loved one can also create stress, but most would not want to do without it. Distress can have negative side effects. The extent to which these negative side effects influence a person's sense of self and well-being differs greatly. A number of studies have associated heart disease with job stress, defined as low job control and high job demands. Researchers are also investigating the link between anger in stressful conditions and increased risk of premature cardiovascular disease. Whether women manifest stress differently from men requires additional study. What does seem clear is that women are affected by negative stress, which can make them more susceptible to heart disease.

Compounding Risk Factors

Cardiovascular risk factors play a crucial role in the development of CVD. The existence of multiple risk factors has a cumulative effect. For example, consumption of a diet high in cholesterol and saturated fats leads to high blood cholesterol and deposition of fatty plaques in the arteries. That same diet, which is often also high in calories, leads to overweight and obesity, which strain the heart and arteries and contribute to high blood pressure and diabetes. These factors place additional strain on arteries already carrying increasing amounts of plaques. The addition of cigarette smoking compounds the problem, making the arteries fragile and more constrictive. Arteries become clogged with waste, and the supreme pump—the heart—becomes sluggish and weak. In short, the combination of these risk factors produces a scenario for disaster: heart attack, stroke, CHF, and peripheral vascular disease.

Such disaster events are not always fatal. If a woman survives the heart attack or stroke, she may be severely limited by a damaged heart or the effects of the stroke, such as impaired vision, memory, speech, or movement. Thus, even though she may be alive, the quality of her life and that of her family may be seriously diminished. Although no one can predict what will happen, this scenario can usually be prevented or controlled by establishing and maintaining good health habits early in life.

Sex/Gender Differences in Cardiovascular Disease

Cardiovascular disease, especially heart attack, has rarely been thought of as a woman's disease by women, their families, and some healthcare professionals. Part of the reason may be the fact that women present with signs and symptoms of the diseases about 10 to 15 years later than men do. Indeed, between the ages of 25 and 34, CVD is twice as prevalent in men as in women. By ages 45–54, however, the two sexes are equal in their CVD prevalence. After that, women take over as leaders in CVD prevalence.[1] These differences in prevalence may in part stem from estrogen loss in women as they age. Estrogen has been shown to have a positive effect on the cardiovascular system. As women approach menopause, their rates of CVD begin to climb. Overall, more women than men die of CVD: In 2002, for example, 456,064 women died from CVD, while 403,455 men died from this cause. In addition, while heart disease is the leading cause for both women (356,024 deaths) and men (340,933 deaths), stroke is the third leading cause of death for women (100,050 deaths) but the fourth leading cause for men (62,622 deaths).[32]

The signs and symptoms of an acute myocardial infarction (heart attack) in women may differ from those observed in men. Both men and women may experience the following symptoms:

- Pain or discomfort in the chest region, *and/or*
- Pain or discomfort in the upper torso (body), which includes both front and back as well as arms and stomach, *and/or*
- Shortness of breath, *and/or*
- Cold sweat, nausea, and dizziness.

Women often experience angina pectoris (chest pain or discomfort) as the first symptom of heart attack, whereas crushing chest pain is more frequently the initial symptom in men. In fact, some women may not even be aware that they are experiencing a heart attack. The fact that women's symptoms may differ from the "usual" heart attack symptoms presents a challenge to healthcare providers. They may not suspect a heart attack but rather address the "stomach" or "gas" as a gastrointestinal problem, when a heart attack may actually be occurring. Further complicating the issue is that women may have a "silent" heart attack in which there are no signs or symptoms. Approximately 38% of women—compared to 25% of men—will die in the year following a heart attack. Within the period of six years post heart attack, roughly 46% of women will develop heart failure, a debilitating disease that severely compromises quality of life.[33]

Women are 55% less likely to participate in rehabilitation following heart attack than men are, and the older the woman is, the less likely she is to participate.[34] Furthermore, 11% of women who have a heart attack may go on to have a stroke.

The reason for these sex-related differences is not entirely clear. Certainly women tend to have more chronic conditions and be older than men when they have their first obvious evidence of disease. With the heightened research focus on sex/gender differences in health, clearer information is emerging. However, a great deal more research is required before we will fully appreciate these differences and healthcare providers can understand how to appropriately diagnose and treat CVD in women.

Racial Differences in Cardiovascular Disease

The adjusted death rates for CVD vary significantly among the five major U.S. ethnic groups: American Indian/Alaskan Native: 123 per 100,000; Asian/Pacific Islander: 108 per 100,000; black: 263 per 100,000; white: 192 per 100,000; and Hispanic: 150 per 100,000. While the rates for CVD are highest among black

I started having chest pains, but I thought they were just due to stress. I didn't want to make a big deal of it. My doctor didn't suspect anything either—I guess I look pretty healthy. But when they did the tests, they found that I had had a "silent heart attack." I wish I had paid closer attention to the pain, and I wish that my doctor had been more sensitive about the possibility of my having a heart attack.

60-year-old woman

women, white and Hispanic women also have high rates. The adjusted death rates for stroke also vary: American Indian/Alaskan Native: 38 per 100,000; Asian/Pacific Islander: 45 per 100,000; black: 71 per 100,000; white: 53 per 100,000; and Hispanic: 38 per 100,000. (These data are shown graphically in Figures 10.1 and 10.2.) Thus, the highest death rates for both CVD and stroke are found among black women, while the lowest death rates for CVD occur among Asian/Pacific Islander women. American Indian/Alaskan Native and Hispanic women have the lowest death rates from stroke.

The reasons for these disparities are not fully understood. Examination of CVD risk factors shows that black women have the highest rates of high blood pressure, obesity, and diabetes. These risk factors are also interrelated for obesity (in itself an important risk factor for CVD), which also leads to high blood pressure and diabetes—other important risk factors for CVD.[35]

High blood pressure (defined as blood pressure greater than 140/90 mm Hg) is a particular problem for black women. Higher rates of related problems exist among blacks with elevated blood pressure compared with whites: 1.5 times greater risk of heart disease death, 4.2 times greater risk of end-stage renal disease, 1.3 times greater risk of nonfatal stroke, and 1.8 times greater risk of fatal stroke. The death rate from high blood pressure in black women was 40% compared with 14% for white women. In an obese woman of any race who is taking oral contraceptives, the risks of high blood pressure rise markedly.

Overweight and obesity begin early. Among pre-schoolers, 13% of Mexican American children, 8.8% of black children, and 8.6% of white children are overweight. By adolescence, 22.5% of Mexican American children are overweight, as well as 21% of black children and 13.7% of white children. Rates of overweight and obesity are rising as more people do less physical activity.[36]

Diabetes rates are rising along with the obesity and high blood pressure rates. From 1994 to 2002, the prevalence of diabetes among adults in the United States rose 54%. One of the greatest increases was observed among Native Americans/Alaskan Natives.[37] The 2003 death rates from diabetes were 47 per 100,000 for

▪ African American women bear a disproportionate burden of stroke disability and death.

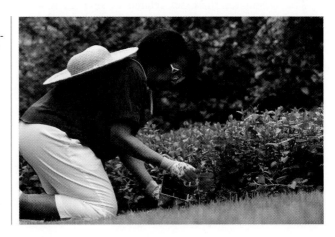

black women and 20 per 100,000 for white women. The risk of CVD among diabetic women is double that among nondiabetic women.

The presence of two or more CVD risk factors compounds this risk. For example, women who are obese and smoke lose about seven years of life expectancy compared with non-obese nonsmokers.[38] Black and American Indian/Alaskan Native women had the highest rates of multiple risk factors for CVD.

Other, less obvious factors play a role in the development of CVD in women. When examining women of comparable socioeconomic status, one study showed that black and Mexican American women still have higher rates of risk factors for CVD.[39] Yet another study showed that at younger ages, women of lower socioeconomic status had higher rates of CVD. By 60 years of age, however, those differences had disappeared.[40] Other factors that have not been fully studied but that appear to have an important impact are culture and neighborhood environments. The force of a community or culture can have an important effect on how a woman sees herself—fat, thin, just right—what she eats, and how she maintains her health.[40, 41]

Cancer

Cancer is a disease characterized by uncontrolled cellular growth and reproduction. It is not a new disease. The term **carcinoma,** meaning a cancerous growth, was coined by Hippocrates in the fourth century B.C. There are more than 100 different diseases categorized as "cancer." Table 10.6 provides a summary of the major

Table 10.6 Types of Cancer

Main Groups of Cancer

Carcinoma: the most common of all tumors—accounting for approximately 90% of all cancers; affects cells that cover the body, line the organs, and form glands.

- Adenocarcinoma—cancer that originates in an organ or gland.
- Squamous cell carcinoma—cancer that originates in the skin.

Sarcoma: rare type of cancer that originates in the connective tissue, such as muscle and bone.

Leukemia: cancer that originates within the blood and blood-producing organs.

Lymphoma: cancer that originates from lymph tissue, which is part of the body's immune system.

Other Types of Cancer

Hepatoma: a cancer that originates from liver cells.

Melanoma: a cancer that originates within the melanocytes (skin cells that produce the pigment melanin).

Neuroblastoma: a cancer that originates from cells in the nervous system.

types of cancer. Many distinctions may be made between these types of cancer, although they all follow similar basic processes.

A **tumor,** also referred to as a neoplasm or "new growth," is any abnormal growth of cells. Some tumors are solid, whereas others known as cysts consist of a thin-walled sac filled with fluid. A **benign tumor** is one that remains localized and confined in its original growth site; that is, it does not invade the surrounding tissue or spread to distant body sites. Examples of benign tumors include skin warts or cysts. Because benign tumors are confined and localized, they often are left alone, drained, or surgically removed. Usually benign tumors are not life threatening unless they are located in a surgically inaccessible location.

In contrast to benign tumors, **malignant tumors,** also called malignant neoplasms, are capable of spreading to other tissues and organs and invading adjacent tissue, the definition of a cancerous growth. The process of cancer cell invasion and spreading is known as **metastasis.** Cancer cells circulate through the blood or lymphatic system and can invade healthy cells in other parts of the body. These circulating cells often become trapped in the first network of capillaries that they encounter, which are usually the lungs. Blood leaving every organ other than the intestines travels to the lungs to get oxygenated, so the lungs are the most common site for metastasis. Blood leaving the intestines goes to the liver, the second most common site of metastasis. Some cancer cells have an affinity for other receptors and, therefore, may metastasize to certain types of tissues. Once metastasis has occurred, localized surgical treatment is usually impossible.

Two kinds of **carcinogens** (cancer-causing substances) appear to lead to cancer: carcinogens that damage genes that control cell reproduction and migration and carcinogens that enhance the growth of tumor cells. **Carcinogenesis** is promoted by a range of agents, including chemical substances, viral or bacterial carcinogens, physical agents, and natural substances in the blood. Smoking is one of the major causes of carcinogenesis. Smoking cigarettes is associated with increased risk for cancers of the lung, mouth, nasal cavities, pharynx, larynx, esophagus, stomach, pancreas, liver, cervix, kidney, and bladder. The frequency of smoking, tar content, and duration of the habit all play important roles in the initiation and promotion of cancer-cell growth.

Factors in the diet also affect the development of cancer. What a woman consumes as part of her diet is just as important as what she avoids. Saturated fat; nonnutrient food additives such as salt, nitrates and nitrites; and alcohol all have been associated with increased risk of cancer. In contrast, vegetables and fruits containing phytochemicals (see Chapter 9) may act as protective factors against cancer.

Radiation, occupational carcinogens such as asbestos, and even certain drugs or medications can cause cancer. Viral carcinogens also have been recognized as contributors to cancer. For example, the human papillomavirus (HPV) and hepatitis B virus are responsible for a majority of cancers in the anal-genital region and the liver, respectively. Scientific evidence suggests that approximately one-third of the 556,500 cancer deaths expected to occur in 2005 will be related to nutrition, physical inactivity, obesity, and other lifestyle factors and could be prevented.[40]

Perspectives on Cancer

Epidemiological Overview

Cancer is the second leading cause of death for women in the United States, with an estimated 273,560 women dying from this disease in 2006.[42a] When examined by racial and ethnic group, cancer is the second leading cause of death for black, white, and Hispanic women; for American Indian/Alaskan Native and Asian women, however, it is the leading cause.[42b] According to the CDC/NCHS, if all forms of cancer were eliminated, life expectancy would increase by three years. Although anyone can develop cancer, most cases affect adults beginning in middle age. More than 75% of cancers are diagnosed in people age 55 and older.[43]

Although lung cancer is the leading cause of cancer deaths in women, breast cancer has the highest prevalence among new cancer cases among women in the United States (Figure 10.6). Breast cancer is estimated to have caused more than 40,000 deaths among women in 2005. The vast majority of new cases and deaths are in women aged 40 and older. The rates for new cases of breast cancer in women have remained fairly constant at about 0.4% per year since 1987. Death rates, however, appear to be declining since 1990 at about 2% per year, with the greatest decline among women younger than 50 years of age. White and black women have higher rates of new cases and deaths than all other racial and ethnic groups.[44]

Cancer of the lung is the second most commonly diagnosed cancer among both men and women. Although fewer new cases of lung cancer are diagnosed each year

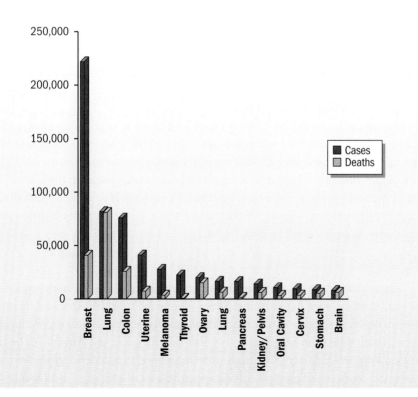

Figure 10.6

Estimated cancer cases and deaths in women, 2005.

Source: *Surveillance Epidemiology and End Results 2006*, National Cancer Institute, U.S. National Institutes of Health.

in women than are cases of breast cancer, annual lung cancer deaths surpass breast cancer deaths in women. The mortality rates are steadily increasing for women even as they decrease for men. Decreasing lung cancer incidence and mortality rates most likely result from decreased smoking patterns over the past 30 years; women lag behind men in terms of smoking cessation trends, however. Although the death rate from lung cancer has increased for women, so has the one-year survival rate for both men and women, largely due to improvements in surgical techniques. In 1973, only 32% of people diagnosed with lung cancer survived one year. By 2000, 49% of people met this survival benchmark. The five-year survival rate for lung cancer is low (15%), and early detection of this disease is difficult because symptoms often do not appear until it has reached advanced stages.[45]

Colorectal cancer is the third leading cancer diagnosed in women, although the number of cases declined sharply in the 1990s. Nevertheless, an estimated 56,290 deaths from colorectal cancer in women occurred in 2005. The death rate also has declined over the past 20 years. When diagnosed at an early stage, the death rates from this type of cancer are low. The five-year survival rates are as high as 90% if diagnosed at a localized stage and as low as 9% if diagnosed at a distant stage.[46]

Endometrial cancer is the fourth most common cancer in women. Cases of endometrial cancer for 2005 were expected to total over 40,100 in the United States, with 7,800 deaths. Death rates are twice as high in African American women as in white women. Ovarian cancer causes more deaths than any other cancer affecting the female reproductive system. While there are fewer cases of ovarian cancer, more than twice as many deaths are attributable to this cause than to endometrial cancer. If diagnosed and treated early, there is a 95% survival rate. Only 19% of cases are diagnosed at an early stage, however. Approximately 10,370 cases of cervical cancer were expected to be diagnosed in 2005, despite the fact that cervical cancer is nearly 100% preventable. The significant decline in the death rate from cervical cancer over the past 40 years is largely attributed to widespread cervical cancer screening programs using the Papanicolaou (Pap) test.[43]

Skin cancer is one of the 10 most common cancers in women. Approximately 1 million cases of basal cell and squamous cell carcinomas were expected to be diagnosed in 2005, along with 26,000 cases of melanoma in women. Since 1974, the rate of skin cancer has been increasing about 6% per year; however, the rate of increase has recently slowed to a little less than 3% per year. If detected at a localized stage, the five-year survival rate for skin cancer is 98%. Some 7,800 deaths in women from skin cancer occurred in 2005.[43]

Racial/Ethnic and Socioeconomic Dimensions

The morbidity and mortality of cancer and chronic diseases are not evenly distributed across women in the United States. The extent to which African American women experience higher cancer mortality than white women is striking. Although overall death rates from cancer have dropped for both white and African American women since 1973, African American women continue to experience greater overall cancer incidence rates, breast cancer death rates, colorectal and lung cancer incidence rates, and colorectal cancer death rates compared with women of any other racial and ethnic group. Although white women have higher rates of breast cancer, African American women have the highest mortality rate from breast cancer.[44] These racial differences in breast cancer mortality rates may be due to a combination of factors, including the lower likelihood of African American women with breast cancer being diagnosed in the early disease stages and a lower survival rate in women whose disease has advanced.

Although incidence and mortality rates for cervical cancer have declined markedly during the last several decades, the numbers still remain too high. African American women have the highest mortality rates from cervical cancer, while Hispanic women have the highest incidence rates. The racial disparity is even more pronounced in the incidence and mortality rates among older (age 65-plus) women of color as compared to older white women.[47]

Because cancer risk is strongly associated with lifestyle and behavior, differences in ethnic and cultural groups—such as dietary patterns, alcohol and tobacco use, and sexual and reproductive behaviors—can provide clues to factors involved in development of the disease. Cultural values and belief systems can also affect attitudes about seeking medical care or following screening guidelines. Screening programs are particularly important for early detection of cancer. Socioeconomic factors, such as lack of health insurance, transportation, or child care, can impede women's access to care and lead to late diagnosis and poor survival. Lack of participation in and reduced access to screening have been hypothesized as possible contributors to the disproportionate cancer burden in minority women. For example, mammography use has been found to be higher among nonminority women with a higher income and more education. To be effective, screening programs must be culturally sensitive and readily available. Language barriers, lack of health insurance, lack of availability and access to health care, and mistrust of the medical profession all have been identified as significant barriers to effective prevention programs in minority populations.

Economic Dimensions

The National Institutes of Health (NIH) estimated overall costs for cancer in 2004 at $189 billion, with $60.9 billion for direct medical costs and over $120 billion in lost productivity.[48] There is also a great economic burden placed on the individual cancer patient and family in terms of time, reduced employment opportunities, and payments for cancer treatments not covered by insurance. The emotional costs to the patients and their friends and families are incalculable.

Global Perspective

Cancer knows no boundaries. Women across the world are affected, but better prevention, early detection, and improved treatment have helped many nations lower cancer incidence and mortality rates. Yet, in many developing countries, cancer rates continue to rise, especially in those where Western lifestyles—cigarette smoking, high-fat diets, and less physical activity—have been adopted. Eastern Europe has some of the highest rates of cancer worldwide. Among women, Northern America has the highest cancer incidence rates, while Northern Europe has the highest cancer mortality rates. The highest rates for lung cancer are among Northern American women, followed by Northern European and Chinese women. Breast cancer incidence is highest in North America and Western Europe, with the lowest rates being found in Africa and China. Breast cancer mortality rates are highest in Western and Northern Europe. The highest incidence and mortality rates for cervical cancer are among East African women, and the lowest among Western Asian women.[49]

Breast Conditions

More than half of all women who menstruate regularly go through the frightening experience of finding a lump in a breast. In more than 90% of these cases, the lump is benign and needs no treatment. Being able to understand the issues and concerns about breast conditions is an important dimension of women's health.

Benign Breast Diseases

Most breast lumps are not cancer. **Fibrocystic breast disease,** also called **cystic mastitis,** is the most common breast disorder and the most frequent cause of a breast lump in women younger than age 25. This disease is most prevalent in women between the ages of 30 and 50. Typical symptoms of this condition include lumpy, tender breasts, particularly during the week before menses. Fibrocystic changes also may cause pain and swelling. Several modalities have been used to treat fibrocystic breast disease, including hormonal therapy and vitamin E, but none has emerged as the definitive treatment. Restricting dietary fat and eliminating caffeine intake can decrease symptoms. Although fibrocystic breast changes are not a medical problem, affected women may find it more difficult to detect lumps during breast self-exams. Only a small subgroup of women with fibrocystic breast disease is at increased risk for breast cancer. These women have an atypical cell condition known as **hyperplasia,** which can be diagnosed by a breast **biopsy,** a procedure in which a small sample of breast tissue is removed and examined under a microscope.

Another nonmalignant form of breast tumor is **fibroadenoma,** which is common in women in their twenties and thirties. This type of tumor produces a firm, movable, nontender lump. Fibroadenomas are usually removed both to confirm the

■ Breast cancer survivors and advocates have raised awareness and billions of dollars for research.

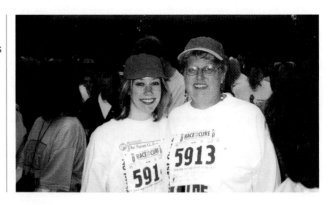

diagnosis and to prevent further damage to breast tissue from continued localized tumor growth.

Breast Cancer

Breast cancer is a frightening condition for women. Before 1974, when U.S. First Lady Betty Ford underwent a mastectomy, breast cancer was not considered to be a public news item. Since then, news reports about breast cancer victims and breast cancer research have become more common. Women, however, still feel that information can be frightening, conflicting, and sometimes misleading. An understanding of breast cancer is important for all women, because this disease is one of the most treatable cancers if it is detected early.

The classification system for breast cancer consists of five levels:

- In situ stage breast cancer can be diagnosed by mammogram, but the tumors are usually too small to be felt. The five-year survival rate for in situ tumors is nearly 100%.
- Stage I breast cancer remains localized to the breast, generally is smaller than 2 cm in size, and has not spread to the lymph nodes.
- Stage II breast cancer tumors generally are larger—2 to 5 cm in size—and have not spread to the lymph nodes. Stage II tumors also may be smaller than 2 to 5 cm but have spread to nearby lymph nodes.
- Stage III tumors are growths that are larger than 5 cm in size or that have grown into the chest wall, skin, or distant lymph nodes.
- Stage IV tumors are classified as growths that have spread to other parts of the body.

Five-year breast cancer survival rates decline with increasing size and invasiveness of the tumor.

Risk Factors

Several major risk factors have been identified for breast cancer. The greatest risk factor is simply being a woman, and the second most important risk factor is age. Most breast cancer cases occur in women older than 50 years of age.[42]

Family history also plays a role in breast cancer risk. Women with mothers or sisters who had breast cancer are at greater risk themselves. Approximately 10% of all cases are hereditary. Most of these hereditary cases result from mutations in two breast cancer genes, BRCA1 and BRCA2. These genes are protective against breast cancer, but an inherited mutated gene can make a woman more susceptible to breast cancer and increase her risk of developing ovarian cancer. Mutated BRCA1 and BRCA2 account for approximately 5% to 10% of all cases of breast cancer. Eighty-five percent of women with BRCA1 or BRCA2 mutations will develop cancer by the age of 70.[50] Mutations of the p53 tumor suppressor gene also can increase a woman's risk of developing breast and other cancers.

Women with a family history of breast cancer may choose to have their DNA analyzed (through a blood sample) to look for mutations. If the test is positive, some women may choose tamoxifen (hormone therapy used as treatment for breast cancer) as a preventive measure or a prophylactic mastectomy and removal of the ovaries. Recent findings suggest that prophylactic removal of the breasts in carriers of these mutated genes decreases the risk of breast cancer considerably. Raloxifene, a hormone therapy typically used for osteoporosis treatment, has been shown to have breast cancer risk reduction properties similar to those associated with tamoxifen. Some women may choose these measures after having breast cancer in one breast, being that they are at increased risk of developing a new cancer in the other breast.

Women who never had children or women who delayed having their first child until after the age of 30 are also at increased risk of developing breast cancer. In addition, early menarche (before 12) and late menopause (after 55) are associated with increased risk for this disease. Because long-term exposure to estrogen is believed to contribute to one's risk of developing breast cancer, many studies have looked at the long-term effects of oral contraceptive use and HRT. A number of studies have shown some effect of oral contraceptives on the risk for breast cancer, while others have shown little risk. An international study of more than 100,000 women found that while there was a slight increase in risk, after 10 years of being off oral contraceptives, the risk of breast cancer was reduced. Newer low-dose contraceptives are now on the market and are generally considered even less risky for healthy young women. Any woman considering taking oral contraceptives should be advised carefully. A woman with risk factors for heart disease—smoking, high blood pressure, or family history of thromboembolism (tendency to develop blood clots)—should be advised not to take the medication.[51,52]

Other factors associated with an elevated risk of breast cancer include consumption of a high-fat diet, alcohol consumption, environmental factors, and obesity. Scientists have yet to reach a consensus on whether these factors are significant risk factors.

Screening and Diagnosis

Many of the identified risk factors for breast cancer cannot be modified by lifestyle behaviors. Early detection of breast cancer, however, can be lifesaving. Indeed, the prognosis for breast cancer strongly depends on the stage at which it is detected (Table 10.7). There are three basic methods for early detection of breast cancer, all of which are important prevention behaviors for women to reduce their risk of breast cancer:

- **Breast self-examination** (BSE) consists of the systematic palpation of the breast tissue of each breast while lying on one's back. The most common sign of breast cancer is a new lump or mass in the breast, although other signs, such as swelling of the breast, skin dimpling, or nipple changes, may be present as well. The American Cancer Society recommends that women over the age of 20 years examine their breasts monthly after menses and at the same time each month. For women who have reached menopause, regular BSE should be done on a scheduled monthly basis. In addition to examining for

Table 10.7 Breast Cancer Survival Rates

Stage*	Tumor Size	Five-Year Survival Rates
I	Less than 2 cm or about 1 inch—no metastasis	98%
IIA IIB	2–5 cm with no or lymph node involvement in the same side of the breast—no metastasis	81–92%
IIIA IIIB	More than 5 cm with lymph node involvement on same side of breast—no metastasis	54–67%
IV	Not applicable because of metastasis	20%

*The stages are expressed in Roman numerals: I = 1, II = 2, III = 3, and IV = 4.
Source: The 2002 American Joint Committee on Cancer TNM System. Revised 9/2/2005.
http://www.cancer.org.

lumps, women should check for breast discharge. Figure 10.7 provides detailed guidance on the BSE procedure.

- Clinical breast examinations (CBE) are conducted by a woman's healthcare provider and should be performed every three years for women age 20–39 and every year for women age 40 and older. The exam consists of observing the breasts for signs such as dimpling, feeling the breast and underarm for abnormal areas or swollen lymph nodes, and squeezing the nipples to check for discharge.

- **Mammography,** a low-dose radiograph of the breast tissue, can detect smaller breast lesions that cannot be felt through BSE or CBE. This technology has the potential to detect breast cancer at its earliest stages of development. Mammography involves compressing the breast between two flat disks. Two radiographs are taken of each breast, and one is taken from above the breast. Although mammograms can detect some breast cancers before they can be felt, other tumors may be felt through BSE or CBE that could not be detected by a mammogram. For this reason, it is extremely important to perform regular BSEs and have regular CBEs. The use of mammography is recommended by several major medical and health organizations as part of an early detection program for breast cancer, in conjunction with regular physical examinations. The National Cancer Institute and the American Cancer Society recommend screening mammograms for women age 40 years and older every one to two years. Women with a family history of breast cancer should discuss when to begin mammograms with their healthcare provider.

Although a breast tumor may be suspected with an examination or mammography, the ultimate diagnosis is made by biopsy. The biopsy removes a sample of tissue, which is then examined for abnormal cell growth.

Treatment and Reconstruction

Surgery is the primary treatment for breast cancer, although it may be combined with radiation therapy or hormone therapy. Breast cancer surgery may be performed immediately following a positive biopsy, thereby avoiding the need for a second

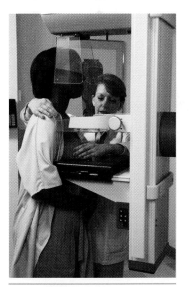

Mammography is the best screening method currently available for detecting nonpalpable tumors in the breast.

Breast Self-Examination

Breast self-examination should be done once a month so you become familiar with the usual appearance and feel of your breasts. Familiarity makes it easier to notice any changes in the breast from month to month. Early discovery of a change from what is "normal" is the main idea behind BSE. The outlook is much better if you detect cancer in an early stage.

If you menstruate, the best time to do BSE is 2 or 3 days after your period ends, when your breasts are least likely to be tender or swollen. If you no longer menstruate, pick a day such as the first day of the month, to remind yourself it is time to do BSE.

Here is one way to do BSE:

1. Stand before a mirror. Inspect both breasts for anything unusual, such as any discharge from the nipples or puckering, dimpling, or scaling of the skin.

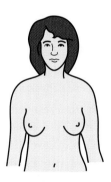

The next two steps are designed to emphasize any change in the shape or contour of your breasts. As you do them, you should be able to feel your chest muscles tighten.

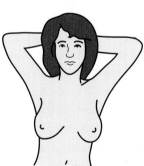

2. Watching closely in the mirror, clasp your hands behind your head and press your hands forward.

3. Next, press your hands firmly on your hips and bow slightly toward your mirror as you pull your shoulders and elbows forward.

Some women do the next part of the exam in the shower because fingers glide over soapy skin, making it easy to concentrate on the texture underneath.

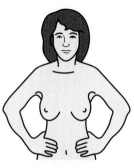

4. Raise your left arm. Use three or four fingers of your right hand to explore your left breast firmly, carefully, and thoroughly. Beginning at the outer edge, press the flat part of your fingers in small circles, moving the circles slowly around the breast. Gradually work toward the nipple. Be sure to cover the entire breast. Pay special attention to the area between the breast and the underarm, including the underarm itself. Feel for any unusual lump or mass under the skin.

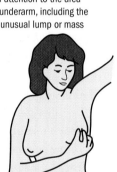

5. Gently squeeze the nipple and look for discharge. (If you have any discharge during the month–whether or not it is during BSE–see your doctor.) Repeat steps 4 and 5 on your right breast.

6. Steps 4 and 5 should be repeated lying down. Lie flat on your back with your left arm over your head and a pillow or folded towel under your left shoulder. This position flattens the breast and makes it easier to examine. Use the same circular motion described earlier. Repeat the exam on your right breast.

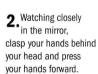

Figure 10.7

Breast self-exam.

round of anesthesia and procedure. Most women, however, prefer a two-step procedure in which the biopsy and the necessary surgery are separate events. The two-step process enables the woman to review her options better and make her decision carefully.

A number of different types of breast removal surgical procedures are used to treat breast cancer.

- A **lumpectomy** is often used for early-stage localized tumors when it is possible to remove only the tumor and some surrounding tissue. A separate incision may be made to remove the axillary lymph nodes (lymph nodes in the armpit area). In women with early cancer, a lumpectomy with subsequent radiation therapy has become the primary alternative to modified radical mastectomy. Lumpectomies are usually limited to those breast tumors that are well defined and less than one to two inches in total diameter.

- A **partial** or **segmental mastectomy** involves the removal of some breast tissue and some of the lymph nodes.

- A **simple mastectomy** involves the complete removal of the breast but not the lymph nodes under the arm or the chest wall muscles.

- A **radical mastectomy** is the removal of the entire affected breast, the underlying chest muscles, and the lymph nodes under the arm. Although once a very common surgery, this procedure is used less often today because of the disfigurement and the side effects it causes.

- A **modified radical mastectomy** has become the standard surgical procedure for most breast cancers that require removal of the entire breast. It involves removing the breast, some of the lymph nodes, and the lining over the chest muscles. This procedure has survival rates comparable to those with the radical mastectomy, but it is more conducive to breast reconstruction and results in greater mobility and reduced swelling.

Adjuvant therapies—treatments that enhance surgical effectiveness—include **chemotherapy,** hormone therapy, and **radiation therapy.** Chemotherapy and hormone therapy may be used in the treatment of localized tumors, as well as for the control of metastatic conditions. Hormone therapy is used to block the effects of estrogen, which promotes the growth of some breast cancers. Tamoxifen is the most commonly used antiestrogen drug. It is also being studied as a chemopreventive agent to reduce the risk of breast cancer in high-risk women. Although studies from the Breast Cancer Prevention Trial have shown that tamoxifen is beneficial in reducing breast cancer incidence among high-risk women, serious side effects have been reported in some users, including endometrial cancer and blood clots in the lungs. Raloxifene's ability to block the effect of estrogen on breast tissue has been shown to reduce a woman's risk of breast cancer.

After mastectomy, a woman faces the decision of whether to undergo breast reconstruction. Reconstruction of breast tissue may be an important part of breast cancer recovery for some women. The degree of difficulty associated with reconstruction varies with the extent of surgery.

In addition, emotional support and social support are important components of recovery. Local support groups may provide valuable information and assistance with physical and psychological breast cancer recovery issues.

Gynecological Conditions

The term "gynecological conditions" refers to any disease process in a woman's upper or lower reproductive tract. This section provides an overview of the major gynecological conditions of the cervix, uterus, and ovaries. Malignant and non-malignant conditions are discussed in terms of their risk factors, screening, and treatment.

Benign Cervical Changes

Polyps are small benign growths that develop in the endocervical canal, often after the onset of menstruation. Polyps usually produce mild symptoms such as abnormal vaginal bleeding or discharge. Although they are rarely cancerous, the growths should still be examined. Treatment of a cervical polyp consists of removing the polyp and examining the tissue to rule out malignancy.

Cervical dysplasia, which involves abnormal changes in the cells of the cervix, also is a benign condition. It is considered precancerous, however, because severe untreated **dysplasia** can result in invasive cervical cancer. Low-grade or mild dysplasia usually occurs in women from the ages of 25 to 35 years and usually can be detected with a Pap smear. High-grade or moderate to severe dysplasia refers to the presence of a large number of precancerous cells covering the surface of the cervix. Also referred to as **carcinoma in situ,** severe dysplasia is more likely to become cancerous but can be successfully cured if detected and treated rapidly. Treatment varies depending on the severity of the dysplasia.

Cervical Cancer*

Cervical cancer is a type of uterine cancer affecting the lower part of the uterus, which is referred to as the cervical canal. Most cancers of the cervix originate on the cells lining the surface of the cervix. Cervical cancer is classified into five stages, 0 through IV:

- In its localized first stage or stage 0, cervical cancer involves only the outer layer of skin.
- Stage I cancer has spread throughout the cervix.
- Stage II cancer has spread beyond the uterus but not to the pelvic wall.
- Stage III cancer has spread to the pelvic wall and the vagina, and may affect the kidney.

*AUTHOR'S NOTE. The cervix is technically part of the uterus, but because the characteristics and risk factors for uterine and cervical cancer are distinctive, they are discussed separately.

- Stage IV cancer affects the regional nodes and has spread past the pelvic wall. It also may be found on the bladder or rectum.

As with other forms of cancer, survival rates decline as the condition becomes more invasive.

Risk Factors.   Cervical cancer is primarily caused by persistent infection with certain high-risk strains of the human papillomavirus (HPV). These high-risk types of HPV that are associated with cervical cancer are not the same types that produce genital warts, however. HPV infection is a sexually transmitted disease that most sexually active women contract during their twenties. In fact, nearly 80% of women will have HPV at some point in their lives. Most women who become infected with HPV will clear the virus on their own, through their body's natural immune response. A few women will not clear the virus, however, and instead develop a long-term persistent infection. These women are at higher risk for developing cervical cancer. Factors that may contribute to whether a woman develops a long-term persistent infection with high-risk HPV include smoking and infection with other sexually transmitted diseases. Women with weakened immune systems, such as those with HIV infection or those taking immunosuppressant drugs, and daughters of women who took diethylstilbestrol,* are also at risk. Women aged 30 and older can now be tested for HPV when they get their Pap smear.

Invasive cervical cancer rarely occurs in women who have regular gynecological examinations. When it does, however, symptoms may include bleeding between menstrual periods, spotting after intercourse, and increased vaginal discharge. By the time symptoms of cervical cancer appear, a tumor is usually quite large and may have already invaded nearby tissue.

Screening and Diagnosis.   Cervical cancer is preventable through regular screening; it is one of the few cancers with a truly effective screening modality. The **Pap smear,** also referred to as a Pap test, provides a method of screening for the cellular changes before cancer develops and to detect cancer at its earliest stages. The Pap test has played a significant role in reducing cervical cancer rates and deaths in the United States. This screening test is usually performed during a routine gynecological examination (see Chapter 7). A sample of cells is obtained from the cervix and then sent to a laboratory for microscopic analysis. A Pap smear can be done in one of two ways: the collected cells can be smeared on a slide or they can be put in a liquid solution.

A newer screening method, the HPV test, looks for the DNA of cancer-causing types of HPV. The HPV test was first approved in the United States by the FDA for follow-up evaluation in women whose Pap results are uncertain—typically referred to as ASC-US (atypical squamous cells of undetermined significance). More

*Diethylstilbestrol (DES) was prescribed from 1938 to 1971 to prevent miscarriages or premature deliveries in pregnant women. In 1971, the FDA advised physicians to stop prescribing DES because it was linked to a rare vaginal cancer.

recently, it has been approved for cervical cancer screening in women age 30 and older. The HPV test can be done at the same time as the Pap test using a similar method of collecting cervical cells. Once collected, the cell sample is sent to the laboratory for analysis and detection. Studies show that when used in conjunction with the Pap test, the HPV test's ability to identify a woman needing early intervention to stop the disease is nearly 100%.

The American College of Obstetricians and Gynecologists and the American Cancer Society have released new guidelines for cervical cancer screening.[53,54] Both guidelines recommend that women begin cervical cancer screening within three years of becoming sexually active or at age 21, whichever comes first. Women should be screened every year with a conventional Pap test and every two years with a liquid-based Pap test until age 30. Women age 30 and older can have a Pap test with an HPV test; if both are normal, she can safely wait to have a repeat test in three years. Having a positive HPV test does not mean that a woman will get cervical cancer; it just means that she should be followed more closely by her healthcare provider. If a Pap smear is abnormal, regardless of the results of the HPV test, the clinician will want to perform a colposcopy and possibly a biopsy to view the cervical cells more closely. If Pap test results are inconclusive (also referred to as ASC-US), the HPV test can help the clinician clarify a woman's risk of cervical cancer. A negative HPV test means a woman is not at risk of developing cervical cancer in the next few years. Even when results are negative, all women should still continue to visit their healthcare provider for an annual exam.

In addition, the HPV vaccine will likely protect future generations against ever acquiring certain types of the cancer-causing virus. Since only some HPV types are covered by the vaccine, cervical cancer will remain important for all women.

Treatment.   Treatment following an abnormal Pap smear depends on the results of the cervical biopsy. Inflammation of the cervix, known as **cervicitis,** may be associated with a vaginal infection or discharge that requires only local treatment with specific vaginal creams or suppositories. Treatment for dysplasia depends on its severity and usually consists of cryosurgery, cone biopsy, or laser cone biopsy.

Cryosurgery is a procedure that destroys tissue by a freezing process. It is most often used to treat mild or moderate dysplasia. As a procedure, cryosurgery has the advantage of producing little or no discomfort. It also presents few risks for complications, such as bleeding, further infection, or infertility from scarring. A watery vaginal discharge is common for about two weeks after cryosurgery. It is generally recommended that women avoid intercourse, douching, or tampons during this recovery time.

A cone biopsy (or **conization**) is considered to be both a diagnostic and a therapeutic procedure because it provides tissue for an accurate diagnosis while removing the abnormal tissue. Cone biopsy procedures are less common today than they were a few years ago because of the widespread use of **colposcopy.** Colposcopy is performed in the physician's office using a colposcope, a special microscope that permits close examination of the cervix and vagina as well as biopsy.

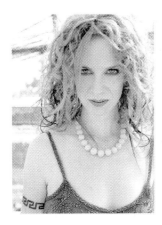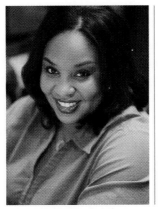

Cervical cancer survivors Christine Baze (*left*) and Tamika Felder (*right*) have created nonprofit organizations to educate women about HPV and cervical cancer. They spread the message that through screening with Pap tests and HPV tests, as well as immunizing with the new HPV vaccine, no woman should suffer or die from cervical cancer. Christine shares her message through her music via The Yellow Umbrella Tour (www.popsmear.org), while Tamika Felder conducts educational "House Parties" on HPV and cervical cancer (www.tamikaandfriends.org).

Treatment of cervical cancer depends on the tumor's stage when diagnosed. Carcinoma-in-situ may be treated with cone biopsy in a woman who wishes to have more children. Surgery to remove abnormal tissue in or near the cervix will remove the tumor but leave the uterus and the ovaries intact. Definitive treatment of carcinoma-in-situ, however, may require a hysterectomy, surgical removal of the uterus, to ensure complete removal of the cancerous cells. Lymph nodes, as well as the fallopian tubes and ovaries, may also need to be removed. Depending on the stage of the cancer, radiation therapy or chemotherapy may be used as adjuvant therapy. Even after hysterectomy, a small percentage of women experience a recurrence of cancer in the vagina, so lifelong gynecological follow-up is important.

Benign Uterine Conditions

Fibroids are benign tumors composed of muscular and fibrous tissue in the uterus (see Figure 10.8). They often begin developing in women between the ages of 25 and 35. Fibroids are the primary cause of an abnormally enlarged uterus and one of the most common reasons for hysterectomy. Although single fibroid tumors occur, multiple tumors are more common. Symptoms depend on the size and location of the tumors and may include the following:

- Irregular vaginal bleeding
- Vaginal discharge
- Pain in the lower back
- Pain during sexual intercourse
- Frequent urination

Fibroids may increase in size under the influence of estrogen produced during pregnancy, from oral contraceptives, or from HRT. They often shrink and disappear with menopause. These tumors are usually detected during routine pelvic examinations because they create an enlarged and irregular uterus.

Hormone-based treatments are useful for temporarily reducing the size of the fibroid and relieving symptoms. A gonadotropin-releasing hormone (GnRH)

Figure 10.8

Uterine fibroids. Uterine fibroids are classified according to their location within the uterus. They may develop in the outer portion of the uterus, within the uterine wall, or under the lining of the uterine cavity; some fibroids grow on a stalk inside or outside of the uterus.

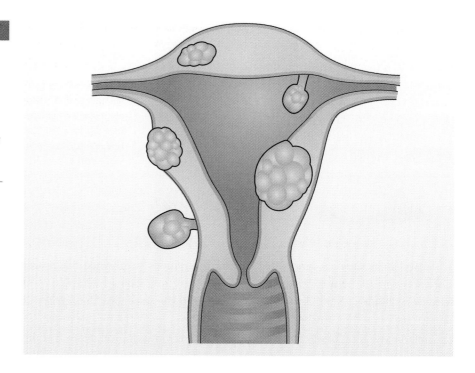

agonist may be used to block the production of hormones, particularly estrogen, by the ovary. The most commonly used GnRH agonist in the United States is Lupron, which is given by an injection either once a month or every three months. Fibroids usually regrow, however, once treatment stops.

Surgery may be indicated for fibroids if they cause severe pain or bleeding. Surgery involves removing either the fibroid alone (**myomectomy**) or the entire uterus (hysterectomy). A hysteroscopic resection may be used for certain types of fibroids; in this procedure, a fiber-optic scope is inserted through the vagina while a dilation and curettage is used to remove the fibroid. Uterine artery embolization is a newer procedure in which small particles of plastic or gelatin sponge are injected through a catheter that is placed in the uterine artery. The particles block the blood supply to the fibroid, resulting in the death of the fibroid tissue. The fibroid shrinks and symptoms are usually relieved without the need for surgery.

Endometriosis is another benign condition of the uterus. In this condition, tissue that looks and acts like endometrial tissue begins to grow outside the uterine lining. When it grows directly into the muscle wall of the uterus (**myometrium**), the condition is termed **adenomyosis**. This progressive condition is most common in women age 30 to 40 years. Because endometrial tissue responds to hormonal influences during the menstrual cycle, women who have this disorder often feel pain just before or during menstruation. Endometriosis also may cause abdominal upset during menstruation and abnormal vaginal bleeding. Many women, however, have advanced lesions without any symptoms. About 16% of cases of infertility are caused by endometriosis.[56]

Treatment of endometriosis involves hormones to prevent ovulation. When hormonal drugs fail to relieve symptoms of pain or when the endometriosis has progressed to the point of forming large cysts, surgery may be indicated. Through operative **laparoscopy,** deposits of endometriosis as well as more extensive disease involving cysts and adhesions can be removed using either electrocautery (burning of tissue) or a laser. The most radical surgery as well as a more definitive cure for endometriosis involves a complete hysterectomy. If diseased tissue remains after surgery, the pain of endometriosis may continue to affect a woman.

Endometrial hyperplasia is an increase in the number of normal cells lining the uterus. Although the condition is not cancer, it may develop into cancer in some women if left untreated. Hyperplasia is caused by a constant production of estrogen and a lack of progesterone, which results in an abnormal thickening of the endometrium. Its most common symptoms are heavy menstrual periods and bleeding between periods. Treatment depends on the extent of the condition (mild, moderate, or severe) and on the age of the woman. Young women are usually treated with progesterone, and the endometrial tissue is checked often. Hyperplasia in women near or after menopause may be treated with hormones if the condition is not severe. Hysterectomy is the usual treatment for severe cases.

Malignant Uterine Tumors

Uterine cancer typically begins in the tissue lining of the uterus, the **endometrium.** Endometrial cancer is most common in women between the ages of 45 and 74. With the decline in the use of estrogens and changes in the composition of replacement hormones used in postmenopausal women, the incidence of endometrial cancer has declined.

Carcinoma-in-situ is found only on the surface layer of the endometrium. As the cancer progresses to stage I, it spreads to the muscle wall of the uterus. Stage II cancer spreads to the cervix and, possibly, regional glands (tissue supporting the cervix). By stage III, cancer has spread to the vagina, pelvic lymph nodes, and other membranes or organs in the pelvic cavity. The final stage of cancer involves the bladder, rectum, and possibly the abdominal lymph nodes.[57]

Risk Factors.   Endometrial cancer accounts for most uterine cancers. The greatest risk factor for endometrial cancer is being older than 50 years of age. Risk factors of uterine cancer in general are believed to involve excess stimulation of endometrial cell proliferation by estrogen in the absence of progesterone. Obesity is believed to increase endometrial cancer risk, perhaps owing to estrogen production in fat cells. Other risk factors that may be a result of high levels of estrogen in the body include high blood pressure, diabetes, early menarche (before age 12), and late menopause (after age 55). Failure to ovulate and a history of infertility also increase risk and may be associated with an estrogen imbalance. Other risk factors include postmenopausal long-term, high-dose estrogen replacement therapy.

In addition to hormonal risk factors, cigarette smoking has been linked to an increased risk for endometrial cancer. Family history of endometrial cancer and personal history of breast, ovarian, or colon cancer increase a woman's risk as well. Finally, risk is increased for women using tamoxifen treatment for breast cancer. Further research is needed to ascertain the mechanisms and roles of all these risk factors for endometrial cancer.

Screening and Diagnosis.   Because endometrial cancer affects the inside of the uterus, the tumor initially cannot be seen or felt during a pelvic examination. Unfortunately, a pelvic exam and Pap smear are only partially effective in the diagnosis of endometrial cancer and the disease is not usually detected until symptoms become manifest. The most common symptom of endometrial cancer after menopause is vaginal bleeding. Other symptoms may include pain in the pelvic area, difficult or painful urination, pain during intercourse, and change in bowel patterns.

The American Cancer Society recommends that women at increased risk for endometrial cancer (i.e., those with a history of infertility or obesity) have an endometrial biopsy at menopause. Women on unopposed estrogen replacement therapy should have such biopsies repeated on a regular basis. A **transvaginal ultrasound** also has proven useful as a screening tool for endometrial cancer.

Diagnosis of endometrial cancer is by biopsy, ultrasound, dilation and curettage (D&C), or **hysteroscopy**. These procedures permit the evaluation of the tissue and cells lining the uterine cavity.

Treatment.   Treatment of endometrial cancer depends on a number of factors, including the stage of the disease. Because uterine cancer may spread rapidly, treatment of early-stage disease involves removal of the uterus as well as the fallopian tubes and ovaries. A combination of surgery and radiotherapy is effective in the treatment of localized disease. Regional spread of the cancer outside of the uterus is treatable by radiation. Advanced, metastatic endometrial cancer is generally treated by the administration of progesterone, which results in prolonged survival but not cure. Treatment for later-stage disease includes removal of not only the uterus, fallopian tubes, and ovaries, but also the cervix, part of the vagina, and lymph nodes.

Benign Ovarian Growths

Cysts are fluid-filled growths that are extremely common. Ovarian cysts are usually benign and rarely cause discomfort or pain. If symptoms do occur, they often include pain or pressure in the pelvic cavity, irregular periods, and pain during intercourse.

A number of different types of cysts exist, which are differentiated by the tissue that makes up the cyst. The most common type results from the follicle that surrounds a mature egg. If the follicle does not rupture to release the egg during ovulation, it becomes a cyst. Many of these cysts go away without treatment within a few months. Other types of cysts include the following:

- Hemorrhagic cysts formed by blood
- Epithelial cysts formed by epithelial cells from the ovary
- Dermoid cysts formed from skin precursor cells

Epithelial cysts and dermoid cysts must be removed surgically to avoid continued growth. Birth control pills are often used as a form of treatment for women who have recurrent cysts.

Polycystic ovarian syndrome, a condition that affects women of reproductive age, causes the formation of numerous cysts in the ovaries. The disorder results from increased levels of hormones, including estrogen and testosterone. Women with polycystic ovarian syndrome are often obese (an effect of excess estrogen) and have excess body or facial hair (an effect of testosterone).

Ovarian Cancer

Ovarian cancer, the fourth most common cancer in women, causes more deaths than any other cancer of the female reproductive system. This cancer usually affects women around the time of menopause or later (ages 50 to 70). Stage I ovarian cancer is limited to the ovaries. Spreading to areas elsewhere in the pelvis is representative of stage II cancer. Stage III cancer spreads to the lymph nodes or other areas inside the abdominal cavity. Once the cancer has spread to distant sites, stage IV has been reached.

Risk Factors. Most cases of ovarian cancer cannot be explained by any currently known risk factors. The risk of ovarian cancer does appear to be related to reproductive history, indicating the importance of hormonal factors. Women who have not borne children have about a twofold increased risk of developing ovarian cancer, but the risk decreases to below average in women who have experienced several pregnancies. Early menstruation (before age 12), late menopause (after age 55), and pregnancy after age 30 also appear to increase risk, due to the body's longer exposure to estrogen. Oral contraceptives, which—like pregnancy—prevent ovulation, also appear to decrease the risk of ovarian cancer.[58] Conversely, a history of previous cancer, particularly of the breast, increases a woman's risk. Another possible risk factor is long-term use of the fertility drug clomiphene citrate, especially if used without success in achieving pregnancy.[59]

Screening and Diagnosis. Ovarian cancer, often called the "silent cancer," usually remains asymptomatic until it is relatively advanced. It is not detected by Pap smears. Early detection is best accomplished through regular pelvic examinations, transvaginal ultrasound, and a laboratory test for an ovarian tumor marker in the blood, called CA-125. Elevated levels of CA-125 are associated with ovarian cancer, but also may indicate other conditions.

Early symptoms of ovarian cancer may include pelvic pressure, abdominal swelling, gas pains, indigestion, and vague abdominal discomfort. Rarely, however, are any of these symptoms attributed to ovarian cancer because they are all symptoms of other common benign conditions. Diagnosis of ovarian cancer is confirmed through ultrasound or biopsy.

Treatment. Definitive treatment for ovarian cancer consists of surgery, radiation, and chemotherapy. Surgical treatment involves removal of the uterus, fallopian tubes, and ovaries. If a woman desires to have children and has a slow-growing

My mom died of lung cancer at the age of 50. She never smoked a day in her life. But my dad smoked, my uncle who lived with us smoked, all her friends smoked, and many of her co-workers smoked in her office before her workplace became smoke free. It makes me so angry when I see people smoking. Don't they realize that they're not just killing themselves but they're also killing their family and friends?

32-year-old woman

tumor, her doctor may remove only the affected ovary. Chemotherapy and radiation therapies are used after surgery to kill remaining cancer cells and improve survival.

Other Cancers of Special Concern to Women

Women are susceptible to cancer anywhere in their bodies. Lung cancer, colorectal cancer, and skin cancer, however, all deserve special consideration in terms of women's health issues. Each of these cancers is discussed next in terms of its risk factors, screening guidelines, and treatment.

Lung Cancer

Since 1987, more women have died each year from lung cancer than from breast cancer, and lung cancer remains the leading cause of cancer deaths among women. This disease is deadly, with overall five-year survival rates of only 15% for patients at all stages of diagnosis. If detected in early states, the survival rate is 49%; however, only 15% of lung cancers are detected at this early stage.[45]

Most cases of lung cancer start in the lining of the bronchi, but the disease can originate anywhere. Lung cancer is believed to develop over many years, and it often spreads before it can be detected radiographically. Causes of lung cancer vary, but most cases share a common factor—a persistent exposure to lung irritants, particularly those that are inhaled such as cigarette smoke.

Risk Factors.   Although exposure to radon, asbestos, radioactive materials, and some industrial compounds has been associated with lung cancer, cigarette smoking is clearly the most significant risk factor for lung cancer. This risk factor has been estimated to be responsible for more than 80% of lung cancer cases and almost 90% of lung cancer deaths. A diagnosis of cancer usually reflects the cumulative effect of many years of smoking. Lung cancer mortality rates are about 22 times higher for current male smokers and 12 times higher for current female smokers compared with lifelong nonsmokers.

Secondhand smoke is also a risk factor. A nonsmoker married to a smoker has a 30% greater risk of developing lung cancer than the spouse of a nonsmoker. Each year, approximately 3,000 nonsmoking adults die of lung cancer as a result of breathing secondhand smoke. A family history of lung cancer may increase a person's risk, although this increase may be associated with exposure to secondhand tobacco smoke from smoking family members as opposed to being a hereditary factor.

Another major risk factor is exposure to asbestos. It increases a person's risk of developing lung cancer sevenfold. Asbestos workers who smoke have a 50–90 times greater risk than people in general.

Diagnosis.   Early detection of lung cancer is difficult because symptoms do not appear until the disease has reached an advanced stage. A persistent cough may then present as a predominant symptom. Along with cough, common symptoms of lung cancer include weight loss, bloody **sputum,** recurring bronchitis or pneumonia, and chest pain. There are no specific screening techniques or guidelines for the early detection of lung cancer. Newer tests, such as low-dose helical CT scans and molecular markers in sputum, have the potential to detect early lung cancer. A person with symptoms may have a chest radiograph, sputum tests, and fiberoptic examination of the bronchial passages for a more definitive diagnosis.

Treatment.   Because most lung cancers are not diagnosed until they are in advanced stages, treatment options are usually limited. Treatment typically includes surgical removal of the affected regions, followed by radiation and chemotherapy. A **lobectomy** removes a lobe of the lung; a **pneumonectomy** removes an entire lung; and a **segmentectomy** removes a section of a lobe of a lung.

Colorectal Cancer

Colorectal cancer is the third most common cancer in men and women. This type of disease develops in a gradual, progressive manner and may present anywhere in the colon and rectal areas. Cancer affecting different areas of this anatomical region often presents with different symptoms. More than 95% of colorectal cancers develop in the glandular cells that line the inside of the colon and the rectum (**adenocarcinoma**).[46] Carcinoma-in-situ, or stage 0 cancer, is found in the lining of the colon or rectum. Stage I cancer spreads to other layers of the lining, whereas stage II disease spreads to nearby tissue. Lymph node involvement indicates stage III cancer, and spreading to the parts of the body indicates stage IV cancer. Colon cancer is about twice as common as rectal cancer.

Risk Factors.   Increasing age is the primary risk factor for colorectal cancer. Ninety percent of people with colorectal cancer are older than 50 years of age. The risk of developing colon and rectal cancers is about twice as high for individuals with an immediate family member who has had colorectal cancer or certain conditions such as **familial adenomatous polyposis (FAP).** FAP is characterized by the presence of hundreds of polyps in the colon and rectum (see Figure 10.9). Likewise, a history of inflammatory bowel disease is associated with a high risk of developing colon cancer. An individual who has developed a polyp or carcinoma in the past is also at increased risk of developing a second carcinoma.

Dietary factors are thought to be an important determinant of colon and rectal cancer risk. An increased incidence of these cancers appears to be associated with diets that are high in fat and low in fiber or other components of fruits and vegetables. In particular, the most definitive dietary risk for colorectal cancer is a high-fat diet.

Recent studies have suggested that estrogen replacement therapy and nonsteroidal anti-inflammatory drugs such as aspirin may reduce colorectal risk.

Screening and Diagnosis.   In its early stages, colorectal cancer usually causes no symptoms. Warning signs for advanced colorectal cancer include rectal bleeding, blood in the stool, a change in bowel habits, and cramping in the lower abdomen.

Similar to other forms of cancer, early detection of colorectal cancer greatly improves the likelihood of complete recovery. Approaches to the detection of colorectal

Colon polyps. An individual who has a history of polyps in the colon is at increased risk of developing colorectal cancer.

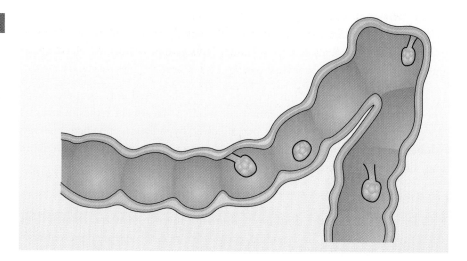

cancer include **digital rectal examination, sigmoidoscopy, fecal occult blood testing,** and **colonoscopy.** In contrast to breast cancer and cervical cancer studies, there are fewer and more limited studies demonstrating the efficacy of these measures in terms of reducing mortality, although studies do support the efficacy of screening in terms of earlier cancer detection.

Each of these tests for colorectal cancer screening has inherent advantages and disadvantages:

- Digital rectal examination is a simple part of a routine physical examination; however, it is relatively insensitive as a screening test because very few colorectal lesions develop within the range of the examining finger.

- Sigmoidoscopy entails examination of the rectum and lower part of the colon with a thin, lighted tube. Although more tumors can be detected with this procedure, a significant disadvantage is discomfort for the patient.

- Screening for tumors by fecal occult blood testing has the potential advantage over the other two methods to detect a tumor in any part of the colon. This type of test employs a simple procedure of smearing a small sample of stool on a slide containing a chemical that changes color in the presence of hemoglobin. Developing tumors cause minor bleeding, which results in the presence of occult blood (small amounts of blood in the stool). Unfortunately, the testing process is plagued by a significant number of false-positive and false-negative findings.

- Colonoscopies are often used when a sigmoidoscopy detects a polyp or abnormality, or the person is at high risk for colorectal cancer. While sigmoidoscopies screen only the rectum and lower portion of the colon, a colonoscopy examines the entire colon. If an abnormality is detected, the physician can use the colonoscope to remove all or part of the polyp or inflamed tissue by passing tiny instruments through the scope. Medicines, lasers, and heat probes also can be passed through the scope to stop any bleeding.

I am a 65-year-old woman who for years was terrified of getting a colorectal screening. I went for mammograms, monitored my blood pressure and cholesterol, and exercised regularly. But the thought of a colorectal exam seemed so uncomfortable and painful. When my daughter showed me the statistics, I realized that I needed to take care of myself. Now, both my husband and I have gone for screening and it's so good to know we're healthy.

65-year-old grandmother of two

Despite the limitations of each of these methods, screening for colorectal cancer is important for early detection. The American Cancer Society recommends that all individuals age 50 and older have yearly fecal occult blood tests, sigmoidoscopy every three to five years, and a colonoscopy every 10 years. Screening should begin earlier if there is a strong family or personal history of polyps, colorectal cancer, or chronic inflammatory bowel disease.

Treatment.   Surgical removal of the colorectal tumor is the primary treatment modality. Segmental resection or partial colostomy involves removing the tumor and healthy tissue surrounding it. If a large amount of tissue is removed and the healthy tissue cannot be repaired, the procedure is called a colostomy. Surgery is sometimes combined with radiation and chemotherapy. When detected at an early localized stage, the five-year survival rate is 96%; after regional spread, this rate drops to 55%; and with distant metastases, the rate is 5%.

Skin Cancer

Cancer of the skin—the most common of all cancers—can be classified as either nonmelanomas or melanomas. The nonmelanoma skin cancers are the most common skin cancers and include two types:

- **Basal cell carcinomas.** Approximately 75% of all skin cancers are basal cell carcinomas, with more than 1 million cases occurring annually. Basal cell carcinomas usually develop in areas exposed to the sun, such as the head and neck. The growth rarely spreads, but, if left untreated, it can invade other tissues. Many people with basal cell carcinomas will have recurring growths in the same or other places on their body.

- **Squamous cell carcinomas.** Squamous cell carcinomas also appear on areas of the body commonly exposed to sun. These growths are more likely to spread and invade other tissues than the basal cell carcinomas, although very few affect other areas of the body if treated promptly.

Melanoma is a cancer arising from pigment-producing cells in the skin, called **melanocytes.** Although not nearly as common as basal and squamous cell carcinomas, it is a much more serious condition. Melanoma often appears as brown or black growths on the legs of fair-skinned women, although the growths can form on people with darker skin. This form of skin cancer is curable in its early stages, but if left untreated, it will metastasize to other areas of the body.

Risk Factors.   The major risk factor for melanoma is ultraviolet radiation from sunlight. The rates of melanoma are 20 times higher in whites than in African Americans.[43, 60] It is believed that the greater pigmentation of dark skin affords more protection against radiation. The presence of moles is also an indicator of increased risk of melanoma. Although they are benign, certain types of moles, such as **dysplastic nevi**, can increase a person's risk. Dysplastic nevi is the term for irregular moles (*nevi* is the medical term for multiple moles), and this condition often runs in families. Moles are considered irregular when they

■ The American Cancer Society emphasizes four warnings of melanoma: Asymmetry; Border irregularities; Color irregularities; and Diameter.

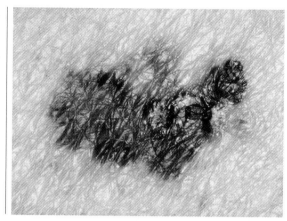

have an uneven border or color. A family history of melanoma is another important risk factor; individuals with a first-degree relative who has had melanoma are eight times more likely to develop melanoma themselves.

Similar to melanomas, nonmelanoma skin cancers are caused by solar ultraviolet radiation. Fair skin and male gender also increase the risk of nonmelanoma skin conditions. All forms of sun tanning and sun exposure are potentially hazardous to the skin. In fact, the American Cancer Society considers the sun to be the greatest single cause of cancer in the United States. Basal cell carcinoma and squamous cell carcinoma are associated with frequent exposure to the sun over many years. In contrast, melanoma has been associated with a single, blistering sunburn early in life. Occupational exposure to coal tar, pitch, creosote, arsenic compounds, or radium is also a risk factor.

Preventive measures for skin cancer include limiting or avoiding sun exposure during midday hours (10 A.M. to 4 P.M.), using sun lotion with a sun protective factor (SPF) of 15 or greater, and avoiding tanning beds and sun lamps. According to the American Cancer Society, if everyone used sun protection, 1 million cases of skin cancer could be prevented each year.

Screening and Diagnosis. Early detection of all skin cancers is critical and is essential to the outcome of melanoma. Recognition of changes in skin growths or the appearance of new growths is the best way to find early skin cancer.

Screening is best accomplished by skin examination. Basal cell carcinomas often appear as flat, scaly red areas or small, raised, translucent areas. Squamous cell carcinomas are growing lumps or flat, reddish patches. Melanomas may develop within a mole or as a new mole-like growth. They are characterized by increasing size and changes in color. The American Cancer Society emphasizes four warnings of melanoma (the ABCD system):

- Asymmetry—the shape of one half of a lesion or mole is different from the other.

- Border irregularities—the edge may be uneven, ragged, or blotched.

I had so many sunburns as a child. My mom has had basal cells removed from her face and my grandfather had melanoma, so I know I'm at high risk for skin cancer. I get checked regularly by a dermatologist, but so far, the moles that she has removed from my back have been normal. I finally understand how important it is to protect myself from the sun.

30-year-old fair-skinned woman

- Color irregularities—different colors may be present in the mole or lesion.
- Diameter—the mole or lesion is usually greater than 6 mm (about 1/4 inch) in diameter.

If a skin growth looks suspicious, diagnosis will be performed through a skin biopsy (sample of the growth). A woman should check her own body on a monthly basis for new skin growths or changes. A cancer check by a dermatologist is recommended every three years for women age 20 to 40 years, and every year for those older than age 40.

Treatment.   There are five primary treatment modalities for nonmelanoma skin cancer. Surgery is used in 90% of the cases.[60] Radiation therapy, electrodesiccation, cryosurgery, and laser therapy are also employed for early forms of nonmelanoma skin cancer. Treatment for melanoma usually consists of surgical removal of the mole or lesion and possibly regional lymph nodes. Advanced cases of disease are treated with chemotherapy, radiation therapy, or immunotherapy. Survival rates are high for localized lesions, but metastatic disease is not responsive to therapy. Because melanomas are able to metastasize quickly, early detection is the major determinant of survival.

Informed Decision Making

There are several things that a woman can do to try to reduce her risk of CVD and cancer. The first step is to develop a plan of action. The second step is to implement preventive measures. The old adage, "An ounce of prevention is worth a pound of cure," is still correct. It is much smarter to do everything you can to reduce your risk of suffering a life-threatening or disabling heart attack at 55 by never smoking, eating a prudent diet, and exercising—all behaviors that should begin in childhood. Although it's better to begin these behaviors earlier in life rather than later, it is never too late to change your ways.

Prevention Through Lifestyle

Lifestyle is a critical part of maintaining a woman's health and preventing disease. Such efforts also help to minimize problems when a woman is affected by a disease. Prevention and health enhancement include quitting smoking (or never starting), limiting alcohol intake, avoiding illegal and dangerous substances, practicing safe sex, being physically active, using sunblock while in the sun, maintaining an appropriate weight, and eating a proper diet. Enjoying life and maintaining a positive mental outlook are other important factors. These activities should be put in place as children and maintained throughout life. Another important part of maintaining health and preventing disease is for each woman to work in partnership with her physician or other healthcare provider. This is a partnership for health.

It's Your Health

Quitting Tobacco

The positive effects of quitting begin very soon after you stop using tobacco and continue long after you've quit.

Short-Term Benefits

- Your blood pressure, pulse, and body temperature, which were abnormally elevated by nicotine, return to normal. Persons taking blood pressure medication should continue doing so until told otherwise by their physician.

- Your body starts to heal itself. Carbon monoxide and oxygen levels in your blood return to normal.

- Your chance of having a heart attack goes down.

- Nerve endings start to regrow. Your ability to taste and smell improves.

- Your breathing passages (bronchial tubes) relax, lung capacity goes up, and your breathing becomes easier.

- Your circulation improves.

- Your lungs become stronger, making it easier to walk.

- In your lungs, the cilia (hairlike structures on the lining) begin to regrow, increasing the ability of your lungs to handle mucus, to clean themselves, and to reduce infection.

- Coughing, sinus congestion, fatigue, and shortness of breath decrease. Your overall energy level increases.

Long-Term Benefits

- As a former smoker, your chance of dying from lung cancer is less than it would be if you continued to smoke. Your chance of getting cancer of the throat, bladder, kidney, or pancreas also decreases.

Source: National Cancer Institute, U.S. National Institutes of Health. Available at (http://www.cancer.gov/cancertopics/ factsheet/Tobacco/quitting-benefits).

I had a lump in my breast, and it had been there for some time. It didn't hurt. I guess that I was hoping it was nothing and would go away. I waited too long. This has been a rough year, but I am trying to tell other women not to make the same mistake. If you feel a lump, regardless of the size, have it checked right away.

42-year-old woman

Prevention Through Health Screening

Cardiovascular disease prevention involves getting screened and knowing the numbers. A woman should know her family history of heart disease and stroke. When she visits the doctor, she should discuss her smoking, alcohol, and dietary status. Her blood pressure, blood cholesterol and triglycerides, and fasting blood glucose should be measured. In addition, her waist circumference should be measured to assure that she is not developing excess fat around her waist.[61]

It has been estimated that breast cancer death rates could be reduced by 19% to 30% if guidelines for regular breast cancer screening were followed.[62] Mammography is the best way to detect breast cancer in its earliest, most treatable stage—an average of 1.7 years before a woman can feel the lump. Clinical breast exams and monthly breast self-exams are recommended for women younger than age 40 and should supplement mammograms for women older than age 40. Any breast lumps; skin changes, such as flaking or crusting, or weeping eruptions around the nipple; discharge from the nipple; or dimpling or retraction of the skin should be evaluated by a physician.

Pap smears and HPV testing are screening methods that can greatly reduce invasive cervical cancer morbidity and mortality rates. Because cervical cancer is a slow-growing disease, screening programs started at age 21 dramatically decrease the risk of developing advanced disease. In fact, when cervical cancer is detected at its earliest stage, the five-year survival rate is more than 90%. Pelvic exams are also essential for women to detect any abnormal changes of the reproductive system.

Self-examination of one's skin enables a woman to detect early forms of skin cancer. Women should become familiar with their bodies to be able to recognize any of the warning signs of cancer.

Table 10.8 summarizes the current cancer screening recommendations.

Summary

Cardiovascular disease and cancer together represent the greatest risks to women's health. The underpinnings of disease causality and progression have been shown to be a complex interrelationship between an individual's family history, environment, lifestyle, and co-morbid conditions. Though family history is not the only risk factor, it has been shown that women with genetic predispositions to cardiovascular disease and certain types of cancers are at increased risk for developing disease. Recognizing that these diseases affect women of all ages should be an incentive for women to begin making lifestyle changes in diet, physical activity, tobacco use, and health screening as early as possible.

Adopting healthy lifestyle choices can have a dramatically positive effect in minimizing a woman's risk. Women must challenge themselves to become familiar with

Table 10.8	Screening Tests

Most Americans Do Not Know When or How Often To Get Cancer Screening Tests.

- While most Americans know that mammograms, pap smears, and colonoscopies are screening exams for cancer, the majority of Americans do not know the appropriate age at which initiation of these tests is recommended, according to the latest brief from the Health Information National Trends Survey (HINTS).

- A recent analysis of HINTS 2005 data found that 57% of American women are unaware that they should receive mammograms to screen for breast cancer beginning at age 40. The survey also revealed more positive results: Three-quarters of women reported that their health care providers had recommended mammograms, and 74% reported having received a mammogram within the recommended timeframe.

- A larger majority of women are unaware that they did not need a Pap test every year to screen for cervical cancer; current general guidelines advise women to get Pap tests at least once every three years. A large proportion of women—87% of those who had ever received a Pap test—said they did so as part of an annual exam. Another finding was that 61% of women surveyed had never heard of human papillomavirus (HPV), which causes most cases of cervical cancer.

- While there are several tests available to screen for colorectal cancer, including fecal occult blood tests (FOBT), sigmoidoscopy, and colonoscopy, 40% of HINTS respondents could not name one when asked. However, 54% did know that screening for colorectal cancer is recommended for men and women age 50 or older, according to general recommendations. Knowledge of different screening options is important; research shows that being offered a choice may improve the chance that people get screened and that they continue to get screened as recommended.

- Knowledge of screening recommendations varied by race and ethnicity. When asked when screening for colorectal cancer is recommended, 79% of Hispanic respondents did not know the recommended age, compared to 75% of African Americans, 70% of American Indians/Alaskan Natives, and 38 percent of whites. Similar levels of misinformation were reported among women of all ethnicities who were asked when it is recommended that they should begin to receive mammograms, with only 32% of all women responding that mammograms should begin at age 40. The U.S. Preventive Services Task Force recommends screening mammography, with or without a clinical breast exam, every one to two years for women age 40 and older.

Source: Adapted from the National Cancer Institute, U.S. National Institutes of Health. Available at (http://www.cancer.gov/newscenter/pressreleases/HINTS).

the risk factors for cardiovascular disease and cancer, and their changing risk status as they age. Women should be vigilant about following prevention recommendations and screening guidelines for disease. By working cooperatively with healthcare providers, women can diminish their risk of developing disease, and most effectively deal with treatment should the need arise. Knowledge, personal preventive measures, and lifestyle modifications are the best ways for a woman to reduce her chances of morbidity and mortality associated with these diseases.

Profiles of Remarkable Women

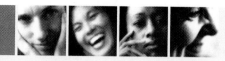

Elizabeth Barrett-Connor, M.D. (1935–)

Dr. Elizabeth Barrett-Connor is a world-renowned epidemiologist who has greatly increased the knowledge base regarding cardiovascular disease, diabetes, cancer, and osteoporosis, and the relationships of these diseases to lifestyle and behavior. Among her many accomplishments, she is widely recognized for conducting the Rancho Bernardo study, a long-term observational study of a group of largely middle-class women and their lifestyles and behaviors. This study has provided substantial knowledge about women as they age, particularly in the area of menopause.

Barrett-Connor attended Mount Holyoke College, and then received her medical degree from Cornell University Medical College. After completing her internship and residency at the University of Texas, Southwestern Medical School, and University of Miami School of Medicine, she completed post-doctoral studies in Clinical Medicine of the Tropics at the London School of Hygiene and Tropical Medicine. She then received a certificate in Advanced Epidemiology from the University of Minnesota and a Certificate in Genetics from John Hopkins University.

In 1970, Barrett-Connor became an Assistant Professor of Community Medicine at the University of California, San Diego. In 1974, she was appointed Chief of the Division of Epidemiology. Barrett-Connor moved on to become Professor of Family and Preventive Medicine, then was appointed Chair of the Department of Family and Preventive Medicine in 1982. She has been honored numerous times and has been the recipient of grants from various organizations for her research in areas ranging from heart disease to diabetes to aging. Barrett-Connor is a member of numerous professional societies, a reviewer of 14 journals, and has been on the editorial boards of more than 10 journals.

Long an advocate for studies that bring exacting science to women's health issues, Barrett-Connor is noted for her work in chronic diseases that are common in older women. Her studies and her advocacy have advanced women's health knowledge substantially. For example, her studies on the role of hormone replacement therapy in the possible prevention of heart disease are internationally recognized. Barrett-Connor entered medicine at a time when few women had followed this path. She persevered and became a leader in the field. Over the years, Barrett-Connor has established herself as a role model through her leadership in medicine and her dedication to mentoring other women physicians and healthcare professionals.

■ ■ ■ ■

Topics for Discussion

1. What factors can influence younger women to adopt healthier lifestyles and engage in preventive behaviors so as to reduce their risks of cardiovascular disease and cancer?

2. What actions can women take to increase their general awareness of cardiovascular problems?

3. Dramatic differences are apparent in the racial distribution of cancers and chronic diseases. What are some possible reasons for this variation, and how can society and researchers address the problem?

4. Prolonged involuntary smoking is one risk factor for lung cancer. How can the situation be handled when someone is being exposed to passive smoke?

5. How can academic institutions take a more active role in disease prevention for young women?

Profiles of Remarkable Women

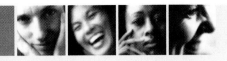

Nanette K. Wenger, M.D. (1930–)

Dr. Nanette Wenger is a Professor of Medicine (Cardiology) at Emory University School of Medicine. She received her B.A. from Hunter College and her M.D. from Harvard University School of Medicine. Wenger interned and became a resident at Mt. Sinai Hospital, before moving on to Emory University in Atlanta, Georgia. At Mt. Sinai, she was the only woman cardiology fellow in the internal medicine training program. At Emory University School of Medicine, she moved from Senior Resident in Medicine, to Fellow in Cardiology, to Instructor and Associate in Medicine, to current Professor of Medicine (Cardiology). She is now also the Director of Cardiac Clinics, Chief of Cardiology, and Director of the Ambulatory Electrocardiography Laboratory at Grady Memorial Hospital in Atlanta, and a consultant at the Emory Heart Center.

Wenger has been honored and recognized numerous times, including being the recipient of the Atlanta Woman of the Year in Medicine award, the American College of Sports Medicine 1994 citation, the Best Doctor in America award for 1994–1998, and the Physician of the Year award from the American Heart Association in 1998. She has also been cited in *Time* magazine's "Women of the Year" issue for her accomplishments in cardiac rehabilitation and international medical teaching.

Wenger has been appointed as a member and chair on numerous boards and committees. At present, some of her appointments include member of the review board for the National Heart, Lung, and Blood Institute's Cardiovascular Health Study, a member of the Expert Advisory Panel in Cardiovascular Disease for the World Health Organization, Editor-in-Chief of the *American Journal of Geriatric Cardiology,* and consultant, editor, or reviewer for numerous journals.

Much of Wenger's work has highlighted gender and age differences in clinical outcomes. She has been involved in cardiac rehabilitation and education of heart disease in women for many years.

Web Sites

American Cancer Society: http://www.cancer.org

American Heart Association: http://www.heart.org

CDC: Cancer Prevention and Control: http://www.cdc.gov/cancer/index.htm

The Gilda Radner Familial Ovarian Cancer Registry:
  http://www.ovariancancer.com

Gynecological Cancer Foundation: http://www.wcn.org/gcf

LungCancer.org: http://www.lungcancer.org

Lung Cancer Online: http://www.lungcanceronline.org

National Alliance of Breast Cancer Organizations: http://www.nabco.org

National Cancer Institute: http://www.cancer.gov

National Cervical Cancer Coalition: http://www.nccc-online.org

National Heart, Lung, and Blood Institute: http://www.nhlbi.nih.gov

National Ovarian Cancer Coalition: http://www.ovarian.org

The Skin Cancer Foundation: http://www.skincancer.org

Profiles of Remarkable Women

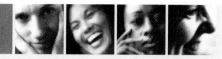

Mary-Claire King (1946–)

Mary-Claire King is an American Cancer Society Professor in the Departments of Medicine and Genetics at the University of Washington in Seattle. She did her undergraduate work at Carlton College in Minnesota and received her Ph.D. in Genetics from the University of California, Berkeley. She also took post-doctoral courses at the University of California, San Francisco.

King has received many honors, including election to the American Epidemiological Society, fellow in the American Association for the Advancement of Science, and election to the American Academy of Arts and Sciences. She has participated in numerous public advisory committees, including the Breast Cancer Program Review Group with the National Cancer Institute, the Board of Scientific Consultants at Memorial Sloan Kettering Cancer Center, the National Institutes of Health Office of Women's Health Scientific Advisory Committee, and the United Nations War Crimes Tribunal. King has been politically active since the Vietnam War, working with Ralph Nader's consumer-interest group, and consulting on a project to reunite kidnapped children from the Argentinean civil war with their grandparents.

King was the first person to suggest the idea that familial breast cancer could be traced to a particular gene. In 1990, she proved the existence of the gene for hereditary breast cancer, now known as BRCA1. She later found that the same gene could stop and in some cases reverse breast and ovarian cancers. King is also working on genetic research focused on AIDS and inherited deafness.

The Susan Komen Breast Cancer Foundation: http://www.komen.org

Women's Cancer Network: http://www.wcn.org

Y-Me National Breast Cancer Organization: http://www.y-me.org

■■■■

References

1. American Heart Association. (2006). *Heart Disease and Stroke Statistics—2006 Update.* Dallas, TX: American Heart Association. www.americanheart.org.

2. National Center for Health Statistics. (2005). *Health United States,* Tables 36–37. Hyattsville, MD: National Center for Health Statistics.

3. Psychological Factors and Cardiovascular Diseases. (2005). *Annual Review of Public Health* 25: 469–500.

4. World Heart Federation Fact Sheet. (2002). http://www.worldheart.org.

5. American Heart Association. (2002). Death rates for total cardiovascular disease, coronary heart disease, stroke, and total death in selected countries, 2002. *Heart and Stroke Statistical Update.* Dallas, TX: American Heart Association.

6. World Health Organization. (2005). Female smoking. *Smoking Trends: 1960–2000.* Geneva, Switzerland: World Health Organization. http://www.who.int/en/.

7. American Heart Association. (2005). Biostatistical update. *International Cardiovascular Disease Statistics.* Dallas, TX: American Heart Association.

8. Writing Committee for the ENRICHD Investigators. (2003). Effects of treating depression and low perceived social support on clinical events after myocardial infarction: the Enhanced Recovery in Coronary Heart Disease Patients (ENRICHD) Randomized Trial. *Journal of the American Medical Association* 289: 3106–3116.

9. Diop, D., and Aghababian, R. V. (2001). Definition, classification, and pathophysiology of acute coronary ischemic syndromes. *Emergency Medicine Clinics of North America,* 19(2): 259–267.

10. American Heart Association. (2006). *Congenital Cardiovascular Defects: Statistics.* Dallas, TX: American Heart Association.

11. American Heart Association. (2006). *Metabolic Syndrome.* Dallas, TX: American Heart Association.

12. National Institute for Neurological Disorders and Stroke. Review of the t-PA Review Committee. (August 24, 2004). http://www.ninds.nih.gov/funding/review_committees/t-pa_review_committee/t-pa_committee_report.pdf.

13. Shaywitz, B.A., et al. (1995). Sex differences in the functional organization of the brain for language. *Nature* 373: 607–609.

14. National Center for Health Statistics. (2005). *Health United States, 2005,* Table 64. Hyattsville, MD: National Center for Health Statistics.

15. U.S. Department of Health and Human Services. (2005). *Report on Carcinogens* (eleventh edition). Research Triangle Park, NC: U.S. Department of Health and Human Services, Public Health Service, National Toxicology Program. http://ntp.niehs.nih.gov/ntp/roc/toc11.html.

16. National Cancer Institute. (2004). *Cancer Progress Report 2003.* Public Health Service. National Institutes of Health, U.S. Department of Health and Human Services. http://progressreport.cancer.gov/.

17. U.S. Environmental Protection Agency. (1992). *Respiratory Health Effects of Passive Smoking* (also known as *Exposure to Second Hand Smoke or Environmental Tobacco Smoke—ETS*). Washington, DC: U.S. Environmental Protection Agency. http://cfpub2.epa.gov/ncea/cfm/recordisplay.cfm?deid=2835.

18. LaRosa, J.C. (1997). Triglycerides and coronary risk in women and the elderly. *Archives of Internal Medicine* 157: 961–968.

19. Austin, M.A., et al. (2000). Cardiovascular disease mortality in familial forms of hypertriglyceridemia: a 20-year prospective study. *Circulation* 101: 2777.

20. Ridker, P.M., et al. (2002). Comparison of C-reactive protein and low density lipoprotein cholesterol levels in the prediction of first cardiovascular events. *New England Journal of Medicine* 347(20): 1557–1565.

21. American Heart Association. (2005). *Homocysteine, Folic Acid, and Cardiovascular Disease.* Dallas, TX: American Heart Association.

22. American Heart Association. (2005). *Cholesterol.* Dallas, TX: American Heart Association.

23. Ohio State University Medical Center. (2006). http://medicalcenter.osu.edu/patientcare/healthinformation/diseasesandconditions/diabetes/statistics/.

24. American Diabetes Association. (2006). *All about Diabetes.* Alexandria, VA: American Diabetes Association.

25. National Center for Health Statistics. (2005). *Health United States, 2005,* Table 73. Hyattsville, MD: National Center for Health Statistics.

26. Hu, F., et al. (2000). Physical activity and risk of stroke in women. *Journal of the American Medical Association* 283: 2961–2967.

27. Stampfer, M.J., and Colditz, G. A. (1991). Estrogen replacement therapy and coronary heart disease: a quantitative assessment of the epidemiologic evidence. *Preventive Medicine* 20: 47–63.

28. Population Information Program, Center for Communication Programs. (2000). Oral Contraceptives. *Population Reports*, vol. XXVIII, no. 1, series A, no. 9.

29. Becker, W.J. (1999). Use of oral contraceptives in patients with migraine. *Neurology* 53(suppl 1): 519–525.

30. Gorelick, P.B., et al. (1999). Prevention of a first stroke: a review of guidelines and a multidisciplinary consensus statement from the National Stroke Association. *Journal of the National Medical Association* 281: 1112–1120.

31. American Heart Association. (2005). *Cocaine, Marijuana, and Other Drugs.* Dallas, TX: American Heart Association.

32. National Center for Health Statistics. (2005). *Health United States, 2005,* Table 31. Hyattsville, MD: National Center for Health Statistics.

33. National Heart, Lung, and Blood Institute. (2005). *The Healthy Heart Handbook for Women.* Bethesda, MD: National Institutes of Health. http://www.nhlbi.nih.gov/health/public/heart/other/hhw/hdbk_wmn.pdf.

34. Witt, B.I., et al. (2004). Cardiac rehabilitation after myocardial infarction in the community. *Journal of the American College of Cardiology* 44(5): 988–996.

35. Centers for Disease Control and Prevention. (2001). Major cardiovascular disease (CVD) during 1997–1999 and major CVD hospital discharge rates in 1997 among women with diabetes—United States. *Morbidity and Mortality Weekly Report.* 50(MM43): 948. http://www.cdc.gov/mmwr/.

36. Peeters, A., et al. (2003). Obesity in adulthood and its consequences for life expectancy: a life-table analysis. *Annals of Internal Medicine* 138(1): 24–32.

37. Centers for Disease Control and Prevention. (2005). Racial/ethnic and socioeconomic disparities in multiple risk factors for heart disease and stroke—United States, 2003. *Morbidity and Mortality Weekly Report*, 54(5).

38. Winkelby, M.A., et al. (1998). Ethnic and socioeconomic differences in cardiovascular disease risk factors: findings for women from the third National

Health and Nutrition Examination Survey, 1988–1994. *Journal of the American Medical Association* 280(4): 356–362.

39. Lee, J.R., Paultre, F., and Mosca, L. (2005). The association between educational level and risk of cardiovascular disease fatality among women with cardiovascular disease. *Women's Health Issues* 15(2): 80–88.

40. Finkelstein, E.S., et al. (2004). Racial/ethnic disparities in coronary heart disease risk factors among WISEWOMAN enrollees. *Journal of Women's Health* 13(5): 503–518.

41. Sharma, S.M., et al. (2004). Racial, ethnic and socioeconomic disparities in the clustering of cardiovascular disease risk factors. *Ethnicity and Disease* 14(1): 43–48.

42A. Jemal, A., et al. (2006). *Cancer statistics, 2006. CA: A Cancer Journal for Clinicians* 56: 106–130.

42B. Jemal, A., et al. (2006). *Cancer statistics, 2005. CA: A Cancer Journal for Clinicians* 55: 10–30.

43. American Cancer Society. (2005). *Cancer Facts & Figures, 2005.* Atlanta, GA: American Cancer Society.

44. American Cancer Society. (2005). *Breast Cancer Facts & Figures, 2005–2006.* Atlanta, GA: American Cancer Society.

45. Centers for Disease Control and Prevention. (2002). *Lung Cancer Statistics, 2002.* Atlanta, GA: Centers for Disease Control and Prevention. http://www.cdc.gov/lungcancer/statistics/index.htm.

46. American Cancer Society. (2005). *Colorectal Cancer Facts & Figures, Special Edition 2005.* Atlanta GA: American Cancer Society. http://www.cancer.org/downloads/STT/CAFF2005CR4PWSecured.pdf.

47. American Cancer Society. (2005). *What Are the Key Statistics about Cervical Cancer?* Atlanta, GA: American Cancer Society. http://www.cancer.org/docroot/CRI/content/CRI_2_4_1X_What_are_the_key_statistics_for_cervical_cancer-8.asp?sitearea=.

48. American Cancer Society. (2005). *Preventing and Controlling Cancer: The Nation's Second Leading Cause of Death, 2005.* Atlanta, GA: American Cancer Society. http://www.cdc.gov/nccdphp/publications/aag/pdf/aag_dcpc2005.pdf.

49. Parkin, D.M., et al. (2006). Global cancer statistics, 2002. *CA A Cancer Journal for Clinicians* 55: 74–108. http://caonline.amcancersoc.org/cgi/content/full/55/2/74.

50. Petrucelli, N., et al. (2005). BRCA1 and BRCA2 hereditary breast/ovarian cancer. *GeneReviews.* http://www.ncbi.nlm.nih.gov/books/bv.fcgi?rid=gene.chapter.brca1.

51. Speroff, L. (1999). Modern low-dose contraceptives are very safe. *Journal of Clinical Endocrinology and Metabolism* 84(6): 1823–1825.

52. Marchbanks, P., et al. (2002). Oral contraceptives and the risk of breast cancer. *New England Journal of Medicine* 346(26): 2025–2032.

53. American College of Obstetricians and Gynecologists. (2003). Cervical cytology screening. *Obstetrics and Gynecology* 102: 417–427.

54. Saslow, D., et al. (2002). American Cancer Society guidelines for the early detection of cervical neoplasia and cancer. *CA A Cancer Journal for Clinicians* 52: 342–362.

55. National Institute of Allergy and Infectious Diseases. (2005). Pelvic Inflammatory Disease. http://www.niaid.nih.gov/factsheets/stdpid.htm.

56. Centers for Disease Control and Prevention, American Society for Reproductive Medicine, Resolve. (1998). *1996 Assisted Reproductive Technology Success Rates: National Summary and Fertility Clinic Reports.*

57. American Cancer Society. (2005). *Endometrial (Uterine) Cancer.* Atlanta, GA: American Cancer Society. http://documents.cancer.org/140.00/140.00.pdf.

58. American Cancer Society. (2005). *Ovarian Cancer.* Atlanta, GA: American Cancer Society. http://documents.cancer.org/114.00/114.00.pdf.

59. Carson, S.A., and Casson, P.R. (1999). *The American Society for Reproductive Medicine Complete Guide to Fertility.* Chicago, IL: Contemporary Books.

60. Ries, L.A.G., et al. (2002). *SEER Cancer Statistics Review, 1975–2002.* Bethesda, MD: National Cancer Insitute. http://seer.cancer.gov/csr/1975_2002.

61. Pearson, T., et al. (2002). American Heart Association guidelines for the primary prevention of cardiovascular disease and stroke. *Circulation* 106: 388–391.

62. Blackman, D.K., et al. (1999). Trends in self-reported use of mammograms (1989–1997) and Papanicolou tests (1991–1997); behavioral risk factor surveillance system. *Morbidity and Mortality Weekly Report* 48(SS-6).

Chapter Eleven

Other Chronic Diseases and Conditions

On completion of this chapter, the student should be able to discuss:

- Prevalence and incidence of various chronic diseases and their effects on women.

- Differences between racial and ethnic groups in the incidence rates of chronic diseases.

- The individual and societal costs of various chronic diseases.

- Risk factors, screening tests, and preventive and treatment measures for osteoporosis.

- The process of bone resorption, bone formation, and osteoporosis development.

- The two major forms of arthritis that disproportionately afflict women.

- Risk factors and symptoms of arthritis and methods for pain management.

- The differences between the two major types of diabetes.

- The special risks that pregnancy presents to the diabetic mother.

- Diabetes management and responding in emergency situations.

- Autoimmune diseases that most commonly affect women.

- Types of lupus and the clinical manifestations of the disease.

- The basics of Hashimoto's disease and Graves' disease.

- The development of Alzheimer's disease and the resulting symptoms.

- Methods for diagnosing Alzheimer's disease and ways to treat symptoms of the disease.

- Ways that a woman can recognize symptoms of a disease so as to seek treatment and prevent future disease-related complications.

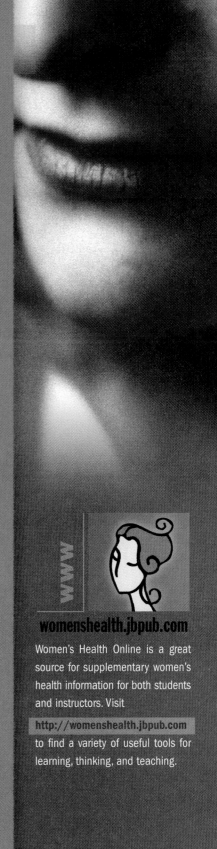

WWW

womenshealth.jbpub.com

Women's Health Online is a great source for supplementary women's health information for both students and instructors. Visit

http://womenshealth.jbpub.com

to find a variety of useful tools for learning, thinking, and teaching.

Introduction

Chronic diseases are diseases or conditions that persist or progress over a long time. Chronic diseases develop slowly. Chronic illnesses are prolonged, do not resolve spontaneously, and are rarely cured completely. Many of these diseases manifest themselves in young women, creating health issues that these individuals must learn to live with for the rest of their lives. Living with a chronic disease can become an encompassing process, especially when the disease causes frequent illness and necessitates many visits to physicians. Some women begin to consider the management of their illness to be a full-time job. Others try to live as they did before diagnosis, not wanting their condition to become central to their lives. Women's responses to chronic disease are as individual as the women themselves. In all cases, however, active support networks via family, friends, healthcare providers, disease support groups, or therapy can help ease the burden of disease management. Support can help the woman cope with the physical and emotional ramifications of having a chronic disease.

Lifestyle factors greatly influence some chronic diseases. Chronic diseases of lifestyle share similar risk factors as a result of exposure, over many decades, to unhealthy diets, smoking, lack of exercise, and possibly stress. These lifestyle risk factors contribute to high blood pressure, high cholesterol levels, diabetes, and obesity, which in turn lead to conditions such as stroke, heart attack, tobacco- and nutrition-induced cancer, chronic bronchitis, and emphysema, culminating in high mortality and morbidity rates.

Internationally, these diseases are also called "noncommunicable diseases" or "degenerative diseases." According to a recent World Health Organization (WHO) report, chronic diseases are by far the leading cause of death in the world and their impact is steadily growing. The WHO report projects that approximately 17 million people die prematurely each year as a result of the global epidemic of chronic disease.[1]

This chapter provides a brief review of osteoporosis, arthritis, diabetes mellitus, certain autoimmune diseases, and Alzheimer's disease—chronic diseases that have dramatic effects on the health of women in the world today. Other chronic diseases, such as herpes, cardiovascular disease, and cancer, are reviewed in other chapters.

Dimensions of Chronic Diseases

Epidemiological Overview

Understanding, preventing, and managing chronic conditions are important steps for maintaining satisfactory health. The prevalence of chronic conditions is difficult to ascertain because of differences and inconsistencies in diagnostic criteria and the lack of national reporting systems. Many chronic diseases affect women more often than they do men.

- Of the 10 million Americans estimated to have osteoporosis, 8 million are women and 2 million are men.[2]

- Osteoarthritis and rheumatoid arthritis, two of the most common health problems in the United States, are far more prevalent in women than in men.

- Diabetes affects nearly 8.9% of all American women. Two to five percent of women are affected by gestational diabetes during pregnancy, putting both the women and their babies at risk.[3]

- About 75% of autoimmune diseases occur in women and most often present during women's childbearing years. Table 11.1 shows the disproportionate female-to-male ratios in autoimmune diseases. Reproductive hormones are thought to play a role in their development, because some autoimmune illnesses present more frequently after menopause, others suddenly and dramatically improve during pregnancy, with flare-ups occurring after delivery, while still others get worse during pregnancy.[4]

- There is some evidence that women may be at greater risk for developing Alzheimer's disease (AD). The fact that women live longer than men puts women at higher risk for AD. More evidence is showing that genes are likely to play a role in determining who develops AD. Even when they are not affected by the disease itself, women are affected by AD when they are the primary care providers for their parents, spouses, and other family members.

Table 11.1	Female–Male Ratios in Autoimmune Diseases
Hashimoto's Disease/hypothyroiditis	10:1
System lupus erythematosus	9:1
Sjögren's syndrome	9:1
Antiphospholipid syndrome—secondary	9:1
Primary biliary cirrhosis	9:1
Autoimmune hepatitis	8:1
Grave's disease/hyperthyroiditis	7:1
Scleroderma	3:1
Rheumatoid arthritis	2.5:1
Antiphospholipid syndrome—primary	2:1
Autoimmune thrombocytopenic purpura	2:1
Multiple sclerosis	2:1
Myasthenia gravis	2:1

Source: American Autoimmune Related Diseases Association (http://www.aarda.org). Autoimmune Disease in Women—The Facts. Retrieved February 1, 2006, from http://www.aarda.org/women.html. Reprinted with permission.

Racial/Ethnic and Socioeconomic Dimensions

Racial differences in chronic disease statistics are inconsistent. White and Asian American women have osteoporosis more often than African American women do, owing to African Americans' higher bone mineral density. As they age, however, African American women's risk of osteoporosis changes to resemble that of white women, and their risk for hip fracture doubles approximately every seven years. African American women are more likely than white women to die following a hip fracture. Although it is not clear why this discrepancy exists, studies show that a woman's age, her health status, and the time frame in which she receives medical attention for the fracture are important predictors for a positive outcome following a hip fracture. Women who are older, have preexisting medical conditions, and have a delay in surgery for a fracture are much more likely to die. Asian American women are at high risk for osteoporosis, possibly as a consequence of their low calcium intake. Perhaps this is due to general lactose intolerance, which affects approximately 90% of Asian Americans.[5] Although they have lower hip fracture rates than white women, Asian American women have rates of vertebral fractures that are as high as those for white women. In recent decades, a significant increase in hip fracture incidence has been noted in the Far East.

Racial differences are also evident with arthritis. U.S. survey data indicate that while blacks have a prevalence of arthritis similar to that of whites, blacks have a higher proportion of activity limitations attributable to arthritis and thus a higher prevalence of arthritis-attributable activity limitations (10.1% versus 7.9%). Overall, blacks with doctor-diagnosed arthritis have a higher prevalence of severe pain attributable to arthritis, compared with whites (34.0% versus 22.6%).[6]

Diabetes is another chronic disease that is more prevalent among non-white populations. As seen in Figure 11.1, American Indians and Alaska Natives have the highest prevalence rates of diabetes in the United States, followed by Hispanics and non-Hispanic blacks.[7]

Figure 11.1

Age-adjusted total prevalence of diabetes in people aged 20 years or older, by race/ethnicity—United States, 2002.

Data from 1999–2001 National Health Interview Survey and 1999–2000 National Health and Nutrition Examination Survey estimates projected to year 2002. 2002 outpatient database of the Indian Health Services.

Source: Centers for Disease Control and Prevention. (2005). National Diabetes Fact Sheet. Retrieved February 2, 2006, from http://www.cdc.gov/diabetes/pubs/estimates.htm#prev4.

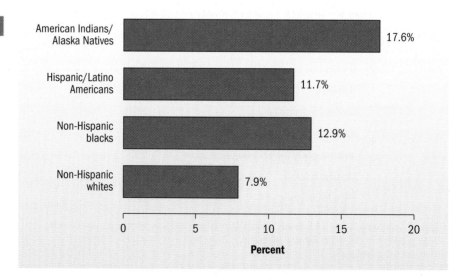

Economic Dimensions

Chronic diseases have a dramatic impact on both the national economy and individual lives. According to the CDC, more than 90 million Americans live with chronic diseases, and chronic diseases account for 70% of all deaths in the United States. Overall, the medical care costs for chronic diseases account for more than 75% of America's $1.4 trillion in medical care costs. Chronic diseases decrease life expectancy and account for one-third of the years of potential life lost before age 65.[8]

Costs associated with specific chronic diseases are also staggering. Diabetes costs an estimated $132 billion per year. Arthritis costs are more than $22 billion, and $300 billion is spent on cardiovascular disease.[8] National direct and indirect annual costs of caring for individuals with Alzheimer's disease are at least $100 billion.[9]

Clearly, the magnitude of these diseases' impact on the health system is huge. Individuals with chronic diseases sometimes struggle with paying for appropriate care, often having to turn to public insurance programs such as Medicaid or Medicare for coverage. Keeping a full-time job may become increasingly difficult for those with a chronic disease, so the option of employer-sponsored health insurance may be lost for them. Others experience costs in their personal relationships as the strain of dealing with chronic disease often negatively affects marriages or other interpersonal relationships.

Women are also disproportionately affected by caregiving associated with chronic disease. Whether they or someone in their family is suffering, women carry the majority of the burden of care and support for patients.

Osteoporosis

Osteoporosis is an age-related, debilitating disorder characterized by a general decrease in bone mass and structural deterioration of bone tissue. Bone is living, growing tissue that changes throughout life. **Bone remodeling** is the process that removes older bone (resorption) and replaces it with new bone (formation) so as to maintain a healthy skeleton. Until a woman's mid-twenties, new bone forms faster than resorption occurs until peak bone mass is reached. After age 30, bone resorption begins to exceed bone formation. The first few years after menopause are the most significant for bone loss. As bone is lost, the skeletal structure weakens, leading to an increased risk of fracture. Osteoporosis develops when bone resorption occurs too quickly or bone replacement occurs too slowly (Figure 11.2).

Osteoporosis is a major cause of bone fractures in postmenopausal women and a leading cause of frailty. It affects approximately 8 million women, with millions more at increased risk of developing osteoporosis due to low bone mass. This translates to one in two women older than age 50 having an osteoporosis-related fracture in her lifetime. Osteoporosis is responsible for more than 1.5 million fractures per year, including 300,000 hip fractures, 700,000 vertebral fractures, 250,000 wrist fractures, and more than 300,000 fractures at other sites.[2]

Hip fractures are especially serious. Women have two to three times as many hip fractures as men, and white, post-menopausal women have a one in seven chance

Figure 11.2

Left to right, healthy bone versus osteoporotic bone.

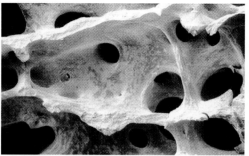
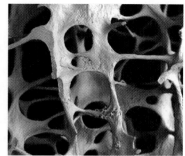

of hip fracture during their lifetime. The rate of hip fracture increases at age 50, doubling every five to six years. Nearly one-half of all women who reach age 90 have suffered a hip fracture.[10] Hip fractures present long-term problems when they occur. Only 25% of hip fracture patients will make a full recovery; 40% will require nursing home care; 50% will need a cane or walker; and 24% of those over age 50 will die within 12 months.[10]

Osteoporosis is often classified into three categories: primary, secondary, and fractures. Primary osteoporosis, the most common form of osteoporosis, is diagnosed when other disorders known to cause osteoporosis are not present. Primary osteoporosis is also classified according to the age group of the patient:

- Juvenile osteoporosis affects prepubescent boys and girls.
- Idiopathic osteoporosis describes the condition in young adults when the cause is not related to another disease.
- Postmenopausal osteoporosis occurs in women within 15 to 20 years after menopause.

Postmenopausal osteoporosis, the most common form of primary osteoporosis, is characterized by low bone mass. Factors contributing to low bone mass are outlined in Table 11.2. The use of alcohol and caffeine-containing beverages is inconsistently associated with decreased bone mass. Late menarche, early menopause, and low endogenous estrogen levels are also associated with low bone density.[11]

Secondary osteoporosis is diagnosed when the condition is related to another illness or to the use of medications or drugs. A variety of factors contribute to secondary osteoporosis, including congenital conditions, diet, drugs, endocrine disorders, and other systemic disorders.

Diet or nutritional disorders contributing to secondary osteoporosis include vitamin C deficiency, calcium or vitamin D deficiency, high-protein diet, high phosphate intake, and iron overload.

Risk Factors

Smoking is especially detrimental to bone health. Smoking is known to cause early menopause and to cause faster deterioration of the bones. The effects of smoking on bone health have been difficult to analyze in more detail due to possible confounding factors, such as lifestyle differences between smokers and nonsmokers. Smokers are often thinner, have higher alcohol intake, are more likely

Table 11.2   Risk Factors for Osteoporosis

Risk Factors That Are Not Modifiable

- Being female
- Increased age/postmenopausal
- Small frame and thin-boned
- White or Asian race
- Family history of osteoporosis or fractures

Risk Factors That Are Modifiable

- Diet low in calcium and vitamin D
- Sedentary lifestyle
- Cigarette smoking
- Estrogen deficiency
- Low weight and body mass index
- Certain medications, such as glucocorticoids, some anticonvulsants, and thyroid hormones
- Abnormal absence of menstrual periods (amenorrhea)
- Anorexia nervosa or bulimia

Having one or more of these risk factors increases the risk of developing osteoporosis. The more risk factors a woman has, the greater her risk.

to lead sedentary lifestyles, and tend to have earlier menopause than nonsmokers do—all of which are risk factors for poor bone health.

Some medications may also cause bone loss. For example, long-term use of glucocorticoids (medicines prescribed for a wide range of diseases including arthritis, asthma, Crohn's disease, and lupus) can lead to a loss of bone density and fractures. Antiseizure drugs, gonadotropin-releasing hormone (GnRH) analogs, excessive use of aluminum-containing antacids, certain cancer treatments, and excessive thyroid hormone also may cause bone loss. This possibility of bone loss is not a reason for women to stop taking these medications, however. Women using these medications should discuss their options for osteoporosis prevention with their healthcare providers.

Certain medical conditions may lead to bone loss, including diseases of the thyroid gland such as hyperthyroidism and hypothyroidism. Amenorrhea (lack of menstrual periods) or diseases that lead to amenorrhea, such as anorexia nervosa, cause estrogen deficiencies, which in turn lead to accelerated bone loss (Table 11.2).

Signs and Symptoms

Osteoporosis is often called a "silent disease" because neither pain nor specific symptoms are associated with this condition. Three times as many women have osteoporosis than report having the condition.[12] Some women notice a loss of height as the vertebrae weaken, collapse, and consequently fracture. When the bones in the spine fracture, a woman loses a small amount of height. The spine also begins to curve as multiple fractures occur.

My mother just found out that she has osteoporosis. I have watched my grandmother shrink with it. The doctor says that my mother can do some things to prevent further bone loss. The message for me is to prevent it from happening. I am now much more interested in diet and exercise.

26-year-old woman

Screening and Diagnosis

The diagnosis of osteoporosis is often made when a patient is treated for a fractured bone that is the result of minimal trauma. To test for osteoporosis, a bone mass measurement (also referred to as a bone mineral density test) must be taken. Methods for measuring bone mineral density are painless, noninvasive, and safe. Traditional tests measure bone density in the areas most susceptible to fractures due to osteoporosis: the spine, the hip, and the wrist. Newer machines measure density in the finger, the kneecap, the shinbone, and the heel (Table 11.3).

Women who should be tested include the following groups:

- All postmenopausal women younger than age 65 who have one or more additional risk factors for osteoporosis besides menopause.
- All women age 65 and older.
- Postmenopausal women with fractures.
- Women who are considering therapy for osteoporosis or who want to monitor the effectiveness of certain osteoporosis treatments.

Prevention and Treatment

In the absence of a cure for osteoporosis, prevention is the best strategy currently available to women. Lifestyle and personal behaviors are the key osteoporosis prevention strategies. A woman should not start smoking and she should quit if she already smokes. While data on alcohol and caffeine consumption and osteoporosis risk are inconclusive, common sense dictates that moderate consumption levels are healthier than excessive levels.

An inadequate supply of calcium over a woman's lifetime is a major risk factor for developing osteoporosis. Calcium plays an important role in achieving peak bone mass, maintaining bone mass prior to menopause, and preventing bone loss in the

Table 11.3 Bone Mineral Density Tests

- DXA (dual energy X-ray absorptiometry) measures the spine, hip, or total body.
- pDXA (peripheral dual energy X-ray absorptiometry) measures the wrist, heel, or finger.
- SXA (single energy X-ray absorptiometry) measures the wrist or heel.
- QUS (quantitative ultrasound) uses sound waves to measure density at the heel, shin bone, and kneecap.
- QCT (quantitative computed tomography) is most commonly used to measure the spine, but can be used at other sites.
- pQCT (peripheral quantitative computed tomography) measures the wrist.
- RA (radiographic absorptiometry) uses an X-ray of the hand and a small metal wedge to calculate bone density.
- DPA (dual photon absorptiometry) measures the spine, hip, or total body (used infrequently).
- SPA (single photon absorptiometry) measures the wrist (used infrequently).

Source: National Osteoporosis Foundation. (2006). Retrieved January 28, 2006, from http://www.nof.org/osteoporosis/bonemass.htm.

postmenopausal years. Vitamin D is necessary for intestinal absorption of calcium. Studies show that supplemental calcium and vitamin D reduce the risk of fracture of the spine, hip, and other sites. Dietary calcium is preferable; however, supplements should be used if a woman cannot meet a daily intake of 1,000–1,200 milligrams per day (see Chapter 9). The typical diet of American women contains less than 600 milligrams of calcium per day. Vitamin D is synthesized in the skin through exposure to sunlight and also can be provided through diet via vitamin D–fortified milk, cereal, egg yolks, saltwater fish, and liver. Those people who cannot obtain enough vitamin D naturally should include 200–600 IU (International Units) in their diets per day.

Participating in weight-bearing and muscle-strengthening exercises on a regular basis is important for both osteoporosis prevention and overall health. These exercises improve agility, strength, and balance, thus reducing a woman's risk of

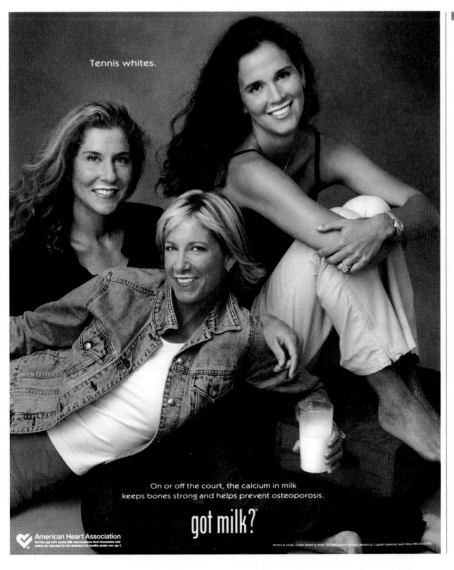

Calcium and vitamin D, both found in fortified milk, are essential for achieving peak bone mass, maintaining bone mass, and preventing bone loss.

falls and thereby decreasing her risk of fractures. Weight-bearing exercises (types of exercise in which bones and muscles work against gravity) include walking, hiking, jogging, stair-climbing, dancing, and tennis. Muscle-strengthening exercise, such as weight lifting, is useful for improving muscle mass and bone strength.

Bone loss accelerates after menopause, and long-term estrogen replacement therapy is reported to be effective in preventing osteoporosis and fractures in women by reducing bone resorption and slowing postmenopausal bone loss.[13]

The treatment of osteoporosis involves management of osteoporosis-associated fractures, universal prevention measures, and medical treatment of the underlying disease. The currently approved medications include alendronate (Fosamax), risedronate (Actonel), and raloxifene (Evista) for prevention and treatment of osteoporosis; teriparatide (Forteo) and nasal calcitonin spray (Miacalcin) for treatment only; and estrogens or combinations of hormones (hormone replacement therapy [HRT]) for prevention only. Current osteoporosis recommendations indicate that all persons who have had osteoporotic vertebral or hip fractures and those with a bone mineral density diagnostic of osteoporosis should receive treatment. In those with a bone mineral density above the osteoporosis range, treatment may be indicated depending on the number and severity of other risk factors.[14]

In addition to prevention of osteoporosis, prevention of fall-related fractures is a special concern for those with osteoporosis. Many factors can cause falls, including impaired vision or balance, certain chronic diseases, and certain medications. A woman should be aware of any of these factors that may potentially affect her balance or gait, and should discuss these changes with her healthcare provider. Additionally, environmental factors can lead to falls; however, some of these factors can be easily prevented as shown in Table 11.4.

Table 11.4   Tips for Fall Prevention

Outdoors
- Use a cane or walker for added stability.
- Wear rubber-soled shoes for traction.
- Walk on grass when sidewalks are slippery.
- In winter, carry salt to sprinkle on slippery sidewalks.

Indoors
- Keep rooms free of clutter, especially on the floors.
- Be careful on highly polished floors that become slick and dangerous when wet.
- Avoid walking in socks, stockings, or slippers without rubber soles.
- Be sure carpets and area rugs have skid-proof backing or are tacked to the floor.
- Keep stairwells well lit.
- Attach handrails on both sides of all stairwells.
- Install grab bars on bathroom walls near tub, shower, and toilet.
- Use a rubber bath mat in shower or tub.
- Keep a flashlight with fresh batteries beside the bed.

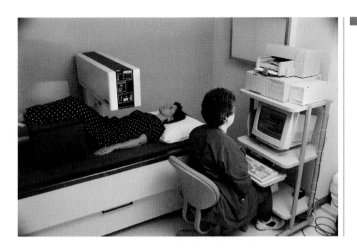

Bone mineral density tests are painless, noninvasive, and safe. Bone density may be measured in the spine, hip, wrist, finger, kneecap, shin bone, or heel, depending on the machine.

Arthritis

Arthritis, defined as any inflammation of the joints, encompasses more than 100 diseases and conditions that affect joints, the surrounding tissues, and other connective tissues. The most common forms of arthritis are osteoarthritis, rheumatoid arthritis, and gout. Regardless of the form of arthritis, similar processes occur as the disease develops. Scientists do not yet fully understand the causes of arthritis. All joints are encased in a capsule that contains lubricating fluid; if swelling and inflammation occur within the joint capsule, stiffness, rigidity, and pain during movement may result. Eventually a scar between the bones may develop, resulting in joint deformity. Recurrent joint pain in women is usually caused by arthritis.

Arthritis and other rheumatic conditions (conditions affecting the joints and muscles) are among the most common chronic conditions and the leading causes of disability in the United States. Arthritis affects an estimated 43 million Americans—nearly one out of every six people.[6] The prevalence of arthritis is higher among women than among men. As the number of older Americans grows, so will the prevalence of arthritis, due to the high frequency of the disease among older adults. Although aging is a risk factor, nearly three of every five people with arthritis are younger than 65 years of age. Arthritis significantly affects quality of life, limiting the ability of more than 7 million people in the United States to participate in their usual daily activities. By 2030, an estimated 64.9 million Americans 18 and older will have doctor-diagnosed arthritis.[15]

Osteoarthritis

Osteoarthritis, also called degenerative joint disease, is a common chronic health problem, affecting more than 21 million people. A milder form of arthritis than rheumatoid arthritis, it is seen in all age groups but is most common among older adults. After age 50, osteoarthritis is more common in women than in men.[16]

In osteoarthritis, the surface layer of cartilage erodes, causing bones under the cartilage to rub together. This friction results in joint pain, swelling, and loss of

I am twenty-three, and I have arthritis. Sometimes I am frightened that I will end up with gnarled hands like my grandmother. I am hopeful that new treatments will prevent my disease progression.

23-year-old student

movement of the joints. This disease most often affects the hips, knees, hands, neck, and lower back, but it may affect other joints as well. Joint stiffness and pain occur at the end of the day with osteoarthritis, and other body parts are usually not affected. Hip and knee osteoarthritis are the leading causes of arthritis disability and the primary reasons for joint replacement surgery.

Rheumatoid Arthritis

Rheumatoid arthritis is a chronic inflammatory disease with increasing prevalence among older adults. It currently affects more than 2.1 million people in the United States.[17]

With this disease, inflammation occurs in the joint lining but may extend to other tissues and cause bone and cartilage erosion, joint deformities, movement problems, and activity limitations. Connective tissue and blood vessels also may be affected by inflammation; if inflammation affects other organs, such as the lung and the heart, a person may be at increased risk of mortality from respiratory and infectious diseases. Rheumatoid arthritis generally occurs in a symmetrical pattern, meaning that it will involve both the left and right hands, not just one of them. The disease varies significantly between individuals: some people have flare-ups followed by periods of remission, whereas others have severe disease that is continuously active.

Rheumatoid arthritis is an autoimmune disease, meaning that the person's immune system attacks the body's own cells. In this condition, the cells inside the joint capsule are attacked, causing inflammation and affecting the cells of the synovial (thin membrane inside the joint capsule). The abnormal synovial cells eventually invade and destroy cartilage and bone within the joint (Figure 11.3), which can lead to severe disability.

Gout

Gout is a painful and potentially disabling form of arthritis that was first described in the days of Hippocrates. Treatments are now available to control most cases of gout, but diagnosing gout can be difficult and treatment plans often must be

Figure 11.3

Left to right, healthy joint, joint affected by osteoarthritis, and joint affected by rheumatoid arthritis.

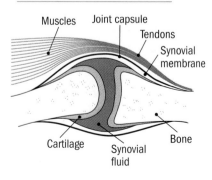
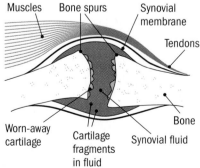
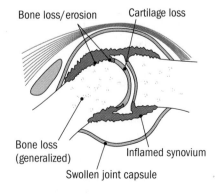

individualized. Gout is caused by an excess of uric acid in the body. This excess can result from an increase in the production of uric acid in the body or the inability of the kidneys to adequately clear uric acid. It has been suggested that consumption of certain foods (such as shellfish) and an excess of alcoholic beverages may increase uric acid levels and precipitate gout attacks, but studies are not conclusive on these associations. Some medications, such as hydrochlorothiazide (a fluid pill) and some transplant drugs (cyclosporine and tacrolimus), can also increase uric acid levels. With time, elevated levels of uric acid in the blood may be deposited around joints, especially in the feet and toes. Eventually, the uric acid may form needle-like crystals in joints, leading to acute painful gout attacks. Uric acid may also collect under the skin, where it is known as tophi, or in the urinary tract as kidney stones.

In the United States, gout afflicts an estimated 21 million people.[18] While gout and its complications occur more commonly in men, the disease also presents in women after menopause and in people with kidney disease. Gout is strongly associated with obesity, hypertension, hyperlipidemia, and diabetes. Some families have a genetic predisposition to gout. African Americans and people with poor kidney function are more likely to have gout attacks.

Diagnosis of gout can be tricky because several other kinds of arthritis can mimic a gout attack. Given that its treatment is specific to gout, proper diagnosis is essential. The definitive diagnosis of gout is dependent on finding uric acid crystals in the joint fluid during an acute attack. However, uric acid levels in the blood alone are often misleading and may be transiently normal or even low. Additionally, uric acid levels are often elevated in individuals without gout.

Treatments for gout are limited. Since the 1800s, colchicine has been a standard treatment for acute gout. While colchicine is very effective, its side effects may include nausea, vomiting, diarrhea, and other adverse events. Because of the unpleasant side effects of colchicines, nonsteroidal anti-inflammatory drugs (NSAIDs) have become the treatment of choice for most acute attacks of gout. Indomethacin is the NSAID most commonly prescribed for gout. NSAIDs may also have significant toxicity, but if used over a short term, are generally well tolerated. However, some people are unable to take NSAIDs because of other medical factors such as ulcer disease, poor kidney function, or use of blood thinners. Elderly patients often cannot tolerate NSAIDs because of their multiple side effects. High doses of aspirin and aspirin-containing products should be avoided during acute attacks, but low-dose aspirin can be continued. Corticosteroid-type medications are also used to treat gout attacks and can be given as pills or by injection. Decisions about which treatment is appropriate must be tailored to the individual and depend on his or her kidney function and other medical factors. With correct treatment, gout should be well controlled in almost all cases.

Risk Factors

Arthritis is the leading chronic condition among women and a major cause of activity limitation.[21] Two to three times more women than men are affected by rheumatoid arthritis.[22] Risk of arthritis also increases with age, with nearly half of the elderly population being affected by some form of arthritis. Some people are genetically predisposed to arthritis, placing them at higher risk for developing the disease. Other risk factors associated with arthritis are modifiable, although altering these factors does not necessarily decrease a person's risk. This is because the mechanism through which these factors increase the risk of developing arthritis is not clearly understood. Obesity is one such factor. In 1971, obese people were approximately 20% more likely to develop arthritis than those who were not overweight. In 2002, that number jumped to 60%. These findings suggest that obesity has contributed to more cases of arthritis in recent years than in previous decades.[21] Joint injuries from sports, infectious diseases such as **Lyme disease,** and certain occupations that require repetitive joint use and knee bending are other factors that increase a person's risk of arthritis.

Because women are more likely than men to have rheumatoid arthritis, researchers have been studying the role of hormones in the development of the disease. The investigations conducted to date have produced contradictory results.

Certain factors have been shown to be associated with a greater risk of arthritis. According to the CDC, some of these risk factors are modifiable, while others are not. These risk factors are summarized in Table 11.5.

Arthritis is not uniformly distributed across the United States. The reasons for the inequitable distribution are unclear but are the subject of ongoing research. As seen in Figure 11.4, arthritis cases are the highest in the middle eastern states and less prevalent in most other states.

Table 11.5   Risk Factors for Arthritis

Risk Factors That Are Not Modifiable

› Age: The risk of developing most types of arthritis increases with age.

› Gender: Most types of arthritis are more common in women, who account for 60% of all cases. Gout is more common in men.

› Genetic: Genes have been identified that are associated with a higher risk of certain types of arthritis, such as rheumatoid arthritis (RA) and systemic lupus erythematous (SLE).

Risk Factors That Are Modifiable

› Overweight and Obesity: Excess weight can contribute to both the onset and the progression of knee osteoarthritis.

› Joint Injuries: Damage to a joint can contribute to the development of osteoarthritis of that joint.

› Infection: Many microbial agents can infect joints and potentially cause the development of various forms of arthritis.

› Occupation: Certain occupations involving repetitive knee bending are associated with osteoathritis of the knee.

Source: Centers for Disease Control and Prevention. (2005). Retrieved January 26, 2006, from http://www.cdc.gov/arthritis/arthritis/risk_factors.htm.

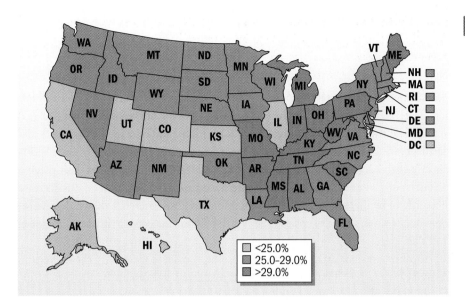

Figure 11.4

Percentage of adults with arthritis,* 2003.

Source: Centers for Disease Control and Prevention. (2005). *At a Glance— Targeting Arthritis: Reducing Disability for 43 Million Americans.* Atlanta, GA.

*People 18 or older with self-reported doctor-diagnosed arthritis.

Legend:
- <25.0%
- 25.0–29.0%
- >29.0%

Symptoms

Arthritis has many consequences, including physical and psychological symptoms as well as effects on one's social well-being. Osteoarthritis evolves slowly. Early in the disease, joints may ache after physical work or exercise. Small bony knobs may appear on the joints of the fingers, causing the fingers to become enlarged, gnarled, achy, stiff, and numb. Osteoarthritis in the knees or hips may make it difficult for a person to walk or bend.

Rheumatoid arthritis is regarded as the most painful and the most disabling form of arthritis in women. Symptoms, such as pain, stiffness, and swelling of multiple joints, may improve or worsen with or without treatment. As a result of these symptoms, people with arthritis typically lead inactive lives, placing them at greater risk for other diseases, including heart disease, hypertension, diabetes, colon cancer, obesity, depression, and anxiety.

Diagnosis

No single test can diagnose arthritis. Instead, a medical and family history and a physical exam to check the joints, reflexes, and muscle strength are the first steps in diagnosis. Radiographs may be used to determine the amount of damage done to a joint by showing cartilage loss, bone damage, and bone spurs. In the early stages of arthritis, before damage is evident, radiographs are not useful; however, they are helpful for monitoring the progression of the disease. Blood tests to determine the cause of the symptoms, a test for rheumatoid factor (an antibody present in most rheumatoid arthritis patients), and a joint aspiration (drawing fluid from the joint for examination) are other methods that may be used for diagnosing arthritis.

Prevention and Treatment

Maintaining an appropriate weight is an important preventive measure. Losing weight through healthful eating and regular exercise also can help reduce the effects of osteoarthritis. To avoid injuries during any type of physical activity, certain precautions should be taken. Women should participate in warm-ups, strengthening exercises, and cool-downs when performing any type of exercise or sports-related activities. Other methods for preventing joint injury and damage to ligaments and cartilage, which in turn can prevent osteoarthritis, include avoiding contact sports and repetitive joint motion; wearing braces, pads, and proper shoes; and playing certain sports or exercising on appropriate surfaces. Exercise in general can decrease impairment by increasing muscle and joint function. Research has shown that weakness in a woman's quadriceps muscle is a risk factor for osteoarthritis of the knee, and that exercise can significantly benefit knee osteoarthritis pathology.[23]

Another cause of arthritis is Lyme disease, a disease caused by the bacterium *Borrelia burgdorferi*. These bacteria are transmitted to humans by the bite of infected deer ticks and cause 24,000 infections in the United States each year.[24] After several months of being infected, more than half of people who are not treated with antibiotics experience recurrent attacks of painful and swollen joints. About 10% to 20% of these people develop chronic arthritis.[25] Strategies to prevent Lyme disease include using insect repellants, wearing long-sleeved shirts and pants when walking in wooded areas, and checking one's body for ticks immediately upon return.

In 1998, the U.S. Food and Drug Administration (FDA) approved a new Lyme disease vaccine, under the brand name of LYMErix, for Americans aged 15 to 70 years. However, in 2002, the manufacturer of LYMErix announced that it would no longer make the vaccine available commercially. Concerns had been raised that the vaccine was actually causing some of the arthritis symptoms that it had been designed to prevent, although the manufacturer reported that the vaccine was safe and it was being withdrawn due to low demand.

The goals of treating arthritis are to decrease pain, improve joint care by slowing down or stopping joint damage, and improve a person's sense of well-being and ability to function. Exercise is one of the best treatments for arthritis. Such physical activity maintains healthy and strong muscles, preserves joint mobility, and maintains flexibility. It is important to exercise when pain is least severe and to recognize when rest is necessary. Resting the body helps to reduce active joint inflammation and pain and to prevent pain from over-exercising. Canes, splints, or braces may be used to temporarily take pressure off joints or to provide extra support. Controlling body weight through a healthful diet is also an important way to reduce stress on weight-bearing joints and limit further injury.

Many people with osteoarthritis or rheumatoid arthritis use medications to reduce pain and inflammation, as well as prevent joint damage:

- NSAIDs, either in prescription or over-the-counter form, are used to reduce pain, swelling, and inflammation.

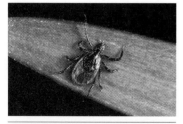

■ Infected deer ticks can transmit bacteria by biting humans, causing Lyme disease, which has many possible adverse outcomes, including arthritis.

- Topical pain-relieving creams, rubs, and sprays, such as those containing capsaicin, are applied directly to the skin to relieve pain.

- Corticosteroids (anti-inflammatory hormones) may be used for short-term pain relief, stiffness, and swelling and to reduce the risk of joint swelling.

- Hyaluronic acid, a new medication for joint injection, is useful for relieving pain associated with osteoarthritis of the knee.

- For rheumatoid arthritis, disease-modifying anti-rheumatic drugs (DMARDs) may produce significant improvement. DMARDs are used to alter the course of rheumatoid arthritis and to prevent joint and cartilage destruction. Serious side effects can occur, however, so the medications are not appropriate for everyone.

- Biologic response modifiers (BRMs) inhibit proteins called cytokines that contribute to inflammation and joint damage in rheumatoid arthritis. BRMs must be injected under the skin or given as an infusion into a vein.

- Immunosuppressants appear to be very effective in restraining the active immune system, the key to the disease process. These medications can cause side effects, however, and their effectiveness appears to diminish over time.

Another option for treatment is surgery. Surgery may be performed to resurface and reposition bones, replace joints, remove loose pieces of bone or cartilage, reconstruct tendons, or remove inflamed synovial tissue. Some people may find alternative treatments helpful, such as acupuncture, nutritional supplements, relaxation techniques, and biofeedback. Although most of these approaches are not harmful, studies have not been conducted to prove that they offer a definite benefit.

Diabetes Mellitus

Diabetes mellitus is a disease characterized by abnormal glucose production or metabolism. A person with diabetes has either a deficiency of insulin (the hormone produced by the pancreas and needed to convert glucose to energy) or a decreased ability to use insulin. As a result, glucose builds up in the bloodstream and, without treatment, will damage organs and contribute to heart disease. There are two major types of diabetes: **insulin-dependent diabetes mellitus (IDDM)** and **non-insulin-dependent diabetes mellitus (NIDDM).** IDDM is also called type 1 diabetes or juvenile diabetes because it often appears in childhood or adolescence. This type of diabetes is considered an autoimmune disease because the immune system attacks the insulin-producing beta cells in the pancreas and destroys them. Thus, the pancreas produces little or no insulin. NIDDM, also referred to as type 2 diabetes or adult-onset diabetes, is the most common type of diabetes. About 90% to 95% of people with diabetes have NIDDM. In cases of NIDDM, the pancreas usually produces insulin but the insulin is not used effectively.

Most people with type 1 diabetes develop the disease early in life, while type 2 diabetes generally occurs later in life; however, the rise in childhood obesity is leading

Dramatic new evidence signals the unfolding of a diabetes epidemic in the United States. With obesity on the rise, we can expect the sharp increase in diabetes rates to continue. Unless these dangerous trends are halted, the impact on our nation's health and medical care costs will be overwhelming.

Jeffrey P. Koplan, M.D., M.P.H.
Director, Centers for Disease
Control and Prevention,
1998–2002

to a dramatic surge in the incidence of type 2 diabetes among children and adolescents.

Diabetes affects 18.2 million people in the United States, or about 6.3% of the population, and is the fifth leading cause of death in the country.[7, 26] According to the CDC's most recent analysis of the effects of diabetes on women:[26]

- Of the approximately 18 million people with diabetes in the United States, about half (9 million) are women.

- Minority racial and ethnic groups are the hardest hit by type 2 diabetes; the prevalence is at least two to four times higher among black, Hispanic, American Indian, and Asian/Pacific Islander women than among white women.

- The risk of diabetic ketoacidosis (DKA), often called diabetic coma, is 50% higher among women than men.

- Heart disease is the leading cause of diabetes-related deaths. Adults with diabetes have heart disease rates and risk for stroke rates about two to four times higher than adults without diabetes.

Gestational diabetes is a form of diabetes that develops in 2% to 5% of all pregnant women, but usually disappears when the pregnancy is over. Women who have had gestational diabetes are at increased risk of developing type 2 diabetes later in life. Approximately 40% of women with gestational diabetes who are obese before pregnancy develop type 2 diabetes within four years.[26]

Risk Factors

Several risk factors for diabetes have been identified, including having a first-degree relative (mother, father, or sibling) with diabetes, being overweight, and having hypertension or abnormal high-density lipoprotein (HDL) or triglyceride levels. Certain racial and ethnic groups are at increased risk for type 2 diabetes, including African Americans, Hispanics, and American Indians/Alaska Natives. American Indians have the highest rate of diabetes in the United States—for example, 14.9% of American Indians and Alaska Natives aged 20 years and older and receiving care from the Indian Health Services have diabetes.[7] **It's Your Heath** provides a checklist of factors to ascertain personal risk of diabetes.

Symptoms and Complications

Symptoms of type 1 diabetes (IDDM) usually develop over a short period of time. They may include increased thirst and urination, constant hunger, weight loss, blurred vision, and extreme tiredness. If not treated with insulin, a person can lapse into a coma and eventually die. Symptoms of type 2 diabetes (NIDDM) develop gradually. Although they are not as noticeable as symptoms of type 1 disease, type 2 symptoms are similar and include frequent urination, unusual thirst, weight loss, blurred vision, feelings of fatigue or illness, frequent infections, and slow healing of sores.

It's Your Health

Am I at Risk for Diabetes?

- I am 45 or older.
- I am overweight.
- I have a parent, brother, or sister with diabetes.
- My family background is Alaska Native, American Indian, African American, Hispanic/Latino American, Asian American, or Pacific Islander.
- I have had gestational diabetes, or I gave birth to at least one baby weighing more than 9 pounds.
- My blood pressure is 140/90 mm Hg or higher, or I have been told that I have high blood pressure.
- My cholesterol levels are not normal. My HDL cholesterol ("good" cholesterol) is below 35 mg/dL or my triglyceride level is above 250 mg/dL.
- I am fairly inactive. I exercise fewer than three times per week.
- I have polycystic ovary syndrome (PCOS) (women only).
- On previous testing, I had impaired glucose tolerance (IGT) or impaired fasting glucose (IFG).
- I have other clinical conditions associated with insulin resistance (acanthosis nigricans).
- I have a history of cardiovascular disease.

The more items you checked, the higher your risk.

Anyone 45 years old or older should consider getting tested for diabetes. If you are 45 or older and overweight, getting tested is strongly recommended. If you are younger than 45, are overweight, and have one or more of the risk factors above, you should consider testing. Ask your doctor for a fasting blood glucose test or an oral glucose tolerance test. Your doctor will tell you if you have normal blood glucose, pre-diabetes, or diabetes.

Source: NIH, NDIC. (2006). Am I at Risk for Getting Diabetes? Available at http://diabetes.niddk.nih.gov/dm/pubs/riskfortype2/.

The most alarming part of diabetes is the severity of the complications associated with the disease (Table 11.6). Diabetes is the leading cause of new cases of blindness in adults 20 to 74 years of age. Each year, an estimated 12,000 to 24,000 people become blind because of diabetic eye disease. Early detection and treatment can prevent 90% of these cases of blindness.[26] Diabetes is also the leading cause of end-stage renal disease (ESRD) or kidney failure, accounting for about 44% of new cases.[26] At least half of the new cases of diabetes-related kidney failure could be prevented each year.

Because unregulated diabetes causes thickening of blood, circulation issues are common. As a result, many people have trouble with wound healing, especially in their extremities. About 60% to 70% of people with diabetes suffer mild to severe forms of damage to their nervous system, including impaired sensation or pain in the feet. If severe, the nerve damage can lead to lower-limb amputation. More than 60% of nontraumatic lower-limb amputations occur among people with diabetes.[26]

Table 11.6	Complications of Diabetes

- Heart disease, including peripheral vascular disease, coronary heart disease, and cardiac failure
- Stroke
- High blood pressure
- Retinopathy (broken blood vessels in retina)/blindness
- End-stage renal disease (kidney failure)
- Damage of the nervous system
- Lower-extremity amputations
- Periodontal disease
- Congenital malformations/spontaneous abortions
- Neonatal mortality
- Macrosomia (large-birthweight babies)
- Diabetic ketoacidosis (coma)
- Susceptibility to infections and illness, such as pneumonia

Amputations are also caused by infection related to nonhealing diabetic foot ulcers. New treatments for nonhealing diabetic foot ulcers include genetically engineered replacement dermis, growth hormone products, and better wound management programs.

Adults with diabetes are two to four times as likely to develop heart disease or stroke as those without diabetes. In fact, heart disease is the leading cause of diabetes-related deaths. Women with poorly controlled diabetes also are at risk of diabetic ketoacidosis. The association of diabetes and mental function has also been studied. Diabetes is known to affect brain function, cognitive decline, dementia, depression, and stroke. These complications frequently occur together, leading to poor quality of life with considerable social and economic implications. While the results of different studies may be contradictory, the overall conclusion is that diabetes, often associated with high blood pressure, contributes to cognitive decline in elderly diabetics as well as to increased frequency and severity of cerebral vascular events.[27, 28]

Pregnancy presents special risks to diabetic women. The likelihood of a good pregnancy outcome is enhanced if the mother's diabetes is well controlled before she becomes pregnant and throughout the pregnancy. The risk of serious congenital malformations and macrosomia (large birthweight) in babies born to mothers with diabetes is greater than in the general population. Due to the increased incidence of babies with large birthweights, women with diabetes are three to four times more likely to have a cesarean delivery than are women without diabetes. In addition, 3% to 5% of pregnancies among women with diabetes result in death of the newborn, compared with 1.5% for women who do not have diabetes.[26]

Diagnosis

The routine test for diagnosing diabetes is a fasting plasma glucose test. A doctor may choose to perform an oral glucose tolerance test, which involves a fasting blood sample followed by numerous blood samples after glucose syrup is ingested. The "gold standard" for diagnosing diabetes is an elevated blood sugar level after an overnight fast (not eating anything after midnight). A value above 126 mg/dL on at least two occasions typically means a person has diabetes. People without diabetes have fasting sugar levels that generally run between 70 and 110 mg/dL. A fasting glucose level of 100 to 125 mg/dL indicates a form of pre-diabetes called impaired fasting glucose (IFG), meaning that the person is more likely to develop type 2 diabetes but does not have it yet.[29]

Prevention and Treatment

Type 1 diabetes is managed through a strict regimen of multiple daily insulin injections, a carefully calculated diet, planned physical activity, and home blood glucose testing several times a day. Treatment of type 2 diabetes is also based on diet control, exercise, and blood glucose testing, and for some people may entail oral medications or insulin. Daily management is important to control blood sugar levels from going too high or too low. **Hypoglycemia** (low blood sugar levels) can cause a person to become nervous, shaky, and confused and can result in the person passing out. Consumption of food or drink with sugar in it can counteract low blood sugar. If levels rise too high, as in **hyperglycemia,** a person may become very ill. Early signs of hyperglycemia include high blood sugar, high levels of sugar in the urine, frequent urination, and increased thirst. Hyperglycemia should be treated as an emergency situation and emergency services (such as 911) should be called immediately.

I was diagnosed with diabetes at the age of five. I still remember being in the hospital and how scared I was. My father died young from diabetes complications. I am determined to learn as much as I can to take care of myself.

32-year-old woman

Autoimmune Diseases

Autoimmune diseases, in which the immune system attacks normal components of the body, are more common among women than among men. More than 80 serious, chronic illnesses are collectively referred to as autoimmune diseases, and these diseases involve the nervous, gastrointestinal, and endocrine systems, as well as skin and other connective tissue, eyes, blood, and blood vessels. Approximately 75% of autoimmune diseases occur in women, most frequently first manifesting during the childbearing years.[30] Such diseases include multiple sclerosis, type 1 diabetes, scleroderma, rheumatoid arthritis, thyroid disorders, Sjögren's syndrome, and systemic lupus erythematosus (SLE). Rheumatoid arthritis, diabetes, SLE, and thyroid disease are the most common autoimmune diseases. As a whole, autoimmune diseases represent the fourth largest cause of disability among women in the United States.[30]

Lupus

Lupus is a complex chronic inflammatory disorder in which the immune system forms antibodies that target healthy tissues and organs. It can be a mild, moderate, or severe disease. Although lupus may affect men and women of any age, it is primarily a disease of young women of childbearing age. This condition affects women 10 to 15 times more often than it does men, and it affects African American women two to three times more often than it does white women.[31]

Lupus presents in three forms. Discoid lupus, also known as cutaneous lupus, only affects the skin and causes a rash that usually appears on the face and upper body. Only about 10% of people with discoid lupus will progress to the systemic form of lupus, which can involve any organ or system of the body. Systemic lupus erythematosus (SLE) is the most common and more severe form of the disease; it is characterized by unpredictable periods of disease activity and periods of symptom-free remission. SLE can affect many parts of the body, including joints, skin, kidneys, lungs, heart, blood vessels, nervous system, blood, and brain. Drug-induced lupus is a reaction to some prescription medicines. The symptoms of this type of lupus are similar to SLE, but do not affect the kidneys or central nervous system. Drug-induced lupus usually disappears when the medication is discontinued.[32]

Risk Factors

The cause of lupus is unknown, although it is hypothesized that genetic, hormonal, and environmental factors play a role. Lupus is known to occur within families, although no specific gene for it has been found. Environmental factors, including infections, exposure to sunlight, stress, and certain medications, play a role in triggering flare-ups of the disease. Because the cause of lupus is unknown, it has been difficult to determine its risk factors.

Symptoms

The two most common symptoms of lupus are painful, swollen joints and a skin rash. Lupus has been called "The Great Imitator" due to its array of varied symptoms that often mimic other, less serious illnesses. Symptoms can range from mild to life-threatening. Lupus is characterized by periods of remission where no symptoms are present. Although lupus can affect any part of the body, most people experience symptoms in only a few organs. The many symptoms of lupus and their presentation in percentages of cases are summarized in Table 11.7. Because lupus can affect any organ system, symptoms can vary significantly from patient to patient.

The etiology of lupus remains a mystery and is the subject of considerable speculation and research. Cigarette smoking is one of many environmental exposures, including infectious agents, silica exposure, and hormonal and dietary factors, such as vitamin D, hypothesized to be linked to the development of SLE.[33, 34]

Table 11.7 Lupus Symptoms

Symptom	Percentage of Cases
Achy joints (arthralgia)	95%
Frequent fevers of more than 100°F	90%
Arthritis (swollen joints)	90%
Prolonged or extreme fatigue	81%
Skin rashes	74%
Anemia	71%
Kidney involvement	50%
Pain in the chest on deep breathing (pleurisy)	45%
Butterfly-shaped rash across the cheek and nose	42%
Sun or light sensitivity (photosensitivity)	30%
Hair loss	27%
Abnormal blood clotting problems	20%
Raynaud's phenomenon (fingers turning white and/or blue in the cold)	17%
Seizures	15%
Mouth or nose ulcers	12%

Source: Courtesy of Robert G. Lahita, MD, PhD from the LFA brochure, "What Is Lupus?" Reprinted with permission from the Lupus Foundation of America, Inc. All rights reserved.

Diagnosis

The clinical diagnosis of systemic lupus involves taking note of symptoms of lupus, such as skin rash, joint pain, chest pain, seizures, and photosensitivity, and reviewing a person's history of medications. A complete blood count and urinalysis may provide evidence of the involvement of the kidneys and blood vessels.

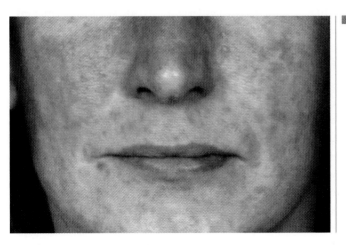

A rash is a common symptom of lupus.

The antinuclear antibody test (ANA) may be used to rule out a diagnosis of lupus. It is positive in virtually all people with lupus and is the best diagnostic tool for lupus available. ANA is not a definitive test, however, because a positive ANA result can be found in people with certain other illnesses and conditions, people using certain medications, or even people in the general population without any illnesses.

Treatment and Prevention

Lupus is characterized by periods of symptoms called "flare-ups." The symptoms are unpredictable and inconsistent when they present.

To reduce flare-ups, women with lupus can take certain preventive measures. People who are photosensitive should avoid sun exposure and regularly use sunscreen to prevent rashes. Exercise is important to prevent muscle weakness and fatigue, while stress reduction can be achieved through support groups and counseling. Treatment usually involves nonsteroidal anti-inflammatory drugs (NSAIDs) to ease muscle and joint pain. Corticosteroids are used on a short-term basis to treat skin rashes. Some people find antimalarial agents, such as Plaquenil or Aralen, helpful for skin and joint symptoms, as well as oral ulcers. Immunosuppressant drugs and steroids work by suppressing inflammation in more severe cases of lupus. These agents are used in serious cases of lupus, when major organs are losing their ability to function. Immunosuppressant drugs suppress the immune system to limit the damage to the organ. Examples are azathioprine (Imuran) and cyclophosphamide (Cytoxan). Serious side effects may occur with their use, including nausea, vomiting, hair loss, bladder problems, decreased fertility, and increased risk of cancer and infection.

Thyroid Disease

The thyroid is a small gland, shaped like a butterfly, located in the middle of the lower neck. Its primary function is to control the body's metabolism—the rate at which cells perform duties essential to living. To control body metabolism, the thyroid produces two hormones, T_4 and T_3, that regulate cell energy.

A properly functioning thyroid will maintain the right amount of hormones needed to keep the body's metabolism functioning at a steady state. The quantity of thyroid hormones in the bloodstream is monitored and controlled by the pituitary gland, which is located in the center of the skull below the brain. When the pituitary gland senses either a lack of thyroid hormones or a high level of thyroid hormones, it will adjust its own thyroid-stimulating hormone (TSH) and send messages to the thyroid to regulate hormone production.

Thyroiditis is an inflammation of the thyroid gland (Figure 11.5). When the thyroid produces too much hormone, the body uses energy faster than it should; this condition is called hyperthyroidism. When the thyroid doesn't produce enough hormone, the body uses energy slower than it should; this condition is called hypothyroidism. The American Association of Clinical Endocrinologists estimates

Figure 11.5

Thyroiditis.

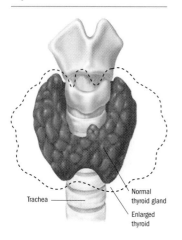

Trachea — Normal thyroid gland
Enlarged thyroid

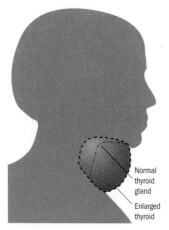

Normal thyroid gland
Enlarged thyroid

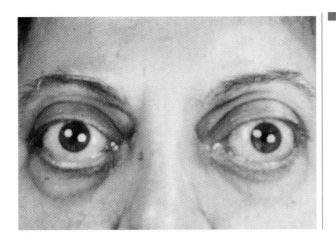

■ There are many symptoms of Graves' disease, including increased appetite, weight loss, nervousness, insomnia, and bulging appearance of the eyes.

that more than 27 million Americans have overactive or underactive thyroid glands, but more than half are undiagnosed.[35]

Hypothyroidism, which results from an underactive thyroid, is most commonly known as Hashimoto's disease or Hashimoto's thyroiditis. It is estimated that 8 million Americans are affected by this condition.[36] Hypothyroidism is most often seen in middle-aged women. It is caused by a reaction of the immune system against the thyroid gland. Disease onset is slow, and many people are asymptomatic or remain undiagnosed because their symptoms are often confused with aging processes. The symptoms of Hashimoto's disease are outlined in Table 11.8. Chronic thyroiditis is most common in women and individuals with a family history of thyroid disease. It is estimated to affect between 0.1% and 5% of all adults in Western countries.[37]

Hyperthyroidism results when an overactive thyroid creates increased body metabolism—sometimes by as much as 60% to 100%.[38] Hyperthyroidism is 8 to 10 times more common in women than in men.[39] Graves' disease causes up to 80% of hyperthyroid cases in the United States. About 5% of patients with Graves' disease also have some involvement with their eyes, in which the eyes may become inflamed and appear enlarged.

Risk Factors

Both Hashimoto's disease and Graves' disease are inherited conditions. Risk factors include being a woman over 20 years old, although the disorder may occur at any age and may affect men. Risk factors for thyroid disorders include factors that do not seem to be a direct cause of the disease, but seem to be associated with it in some way. Having a risk factor for thyroid disorders makes the chances of developing a condition higher but does not inevitably lead to a thyroid disorder. Also, the absence of any risk factors or the existence of a protective factor does not necessarily guarantee that a person will not develop a thyroid disorder.

Risk factors for thyroid conditions include the following:

- Family history of thyroid disease
- Previous thyroid concerns, nodules, enlargement, or goiter
- Previous transient thyroid condition during a pregnancy

Symptoms

Clinical manifestations of both Hashimoto's disease and Graves' disease are summarized in Table 11.8. However, many people have no symptoms, and symptoms rarely occur all at once.

Screening and Diagnosis

Thyroid disease can be difficult to diagnose because its symptoms are easily confused with other conditions. A comprehensive history and physical examination are integral to a diagnosis of thyroiditis. Such an examination would include weight

Table 11.8   Symptoms of Hypothyroidism and Hyperthyroidism

Hypothyroidism	Hyperthyroidism
Many people may have no symptoms.	
· Feeling tired and listless	· Weight loss
· Fatigue	· Heat tolerance
· Difficulty concentrating	· Shakes and tremors of hands
· Sensitivity to cold	· Feeling nervous and irritable
· Dry skin	· Increased energy expenditure
· Dry, coarse hair and hair loss	· Diarrhea
· Constipation	· Sweating more than normal
· Heavy and irregular menses	· Fingernails growing faster
· Slow-growing and brittle fingernails	· Muscle weakness, especially thighs and upper arms
· Feeling of fullness in throat	· Faster heart rate, sometimes irregular rhythms and an erratic pulse
· Hoarse voice	
· Slow heart rate	· Diarrhea
· Leg cramps	· Vision problems, eye irritation
· Difficulty swallowing	· For women, lighter periods, as well as difficulties in becoming pregnant or in carrying the child to term
· Sore muscles	
· Depression	· For men, loss of interest in sex, erectile dysfunction
· For men, loss of interest in sex, erectile dysfunction	· Sleep disturbances
· Weight gain due to fluid retention, but usually no more than 3–4 pounds	· Eyes that appear larger than normal
· Goiter	

and blood pressure, pulse rate and cardiac rhythm, thyroid palpation and auscultation (to determine thyroid size, nodularity, and vascularity), neuromuscular examination, eye examination (to detect evidence of exophthalmos or ophthalmopathy), dermatologic examination, cardiovascular examination, and lymphatic examination (nodes and spleen).[40]

Laboratory testing is also important. The thyroid-stimulating hormone (TSH) test is generally used as a screening test because it can often identify thyroid disorders before the onset of symptoms. Blood tests measuring levels of thyroxine (T_4) are also used to confirm the presence of thyroid disease.

Thyroid nuclear medicine tests are sometimes included in a comprehensive diagnosis. There are two types of thyroid nuclear medicine tests. A thyroid scan produces a picture of the gland to help evaluate any lumps or inflammation or to investigate the cause of an overactive thyroid. A radioactive iodine uptake test is performed to determine whether the thyroid is functioning normally and to determine why thyroid hormone levels may be elevated. For both types of tests, a small amount of a radioactive substance, known as radionuclide, is either injected into a vein or given as a pill. A thyroid scan is usually ordered when a physical examination or laboratory finding suggests that the thyroid is enlarged. If laboratory tests show an overactive thyroid, a radioactive iodine uptake test may be ordered at the same time. The latter test measures the amount of radioactivity in the thyroid after the patient ingests a small dose of radioactive iodine. The thyroid gland absorbs iodine and uses it to make hormones. Therefore, the amount of radioactive iodine detected in the thyroid gland corresponds to the amount of hormone produced by the thyroid.

When thyroid disease is caught early, treatment can control the disorder even before symptoms become evident.

Treatment

Treatment for Hashimoto's disease is based on determining the correct amount of thyroid hormone (thyroxine) needed to stimulate the thyroid gland. Gradually increasing doses of thyroxine are given until a person's blood levels become normal. Annual check-ups are necessary to confirm that the prescribed dose is still appropriate. During pregnancy, doses of thyroxine usually increase; as a person ages, doses usually decrease. Overtreatment of hypothyroidism with thyroid hormone can result in bone loss. Graves' disease is treated with antithyroid drugs to prevent the thyroid gland from manufacturing thyroid hormone.

Alzheimer's Disease

Alzheimer's disease is an irreversible, progressive brain disorder that evolves gradually and results in memory loss, behavior and personality changes, and a decline in cognitive abilities. It is one of a group of disorders that cause **dementia** (cognitive decline). The changes result from the death of brain cells and the breakdown of the connections between them. The progression of Alzheimer's disease and the resulting cognitive decline vary from person to person. On average, people with this disease live years after first experiencing symptoms, but the duration varies from 3 to 20 years.[41] Alzheimer's disease is the most common cause of dementia among people age 65 and older, with approximately 4 million people currently suffering from it. As the population ages, its incidence will undoubtedly increase.[42] The risk of developing Alzheimer's disease increases with age, although the disease and symptoms of dementia are not a part of normal aging.

The main characteristics of the brain in a person with Alzheimer's disease include amyloid plaques and neurofibrillary tangles. Plaques are dense deposits of protein and cellular material that form outside and around the brain's neurons. Researchers are not certain whether the plaques cause the disease or are simply a by-product of the disease process. Tangles are insoluble twisted fibers that build up inside neurons. A form of a protein called tau is the main component of the tangles. In healthy neurons, tau proteins help stabilize a cell's structure. In brains affected by Alzheimer's disease, the tau protein is chemically altered and cannot hold the structure together. The resulting collapse is responsible for malfunctions in communication.

Risk Factors

It is not fully understood what causes Alzheimer's disease, but it is clear that its onset can be triggered by a number of factors that interact differently in people. Researchers believe that age, genetic background, and possibly lifestyle all are contributing factors. Some studies have implicated female gender, severe or repeated head injuries, lower education levels, and environmental agents as risk factors; however, more studies are needed to determine the exact relationship among these risk factors and the development of Alzheimer's.

Familial Alzheimer's disease (FAD) follows a pattern of inheritance. It often has an early onset, meaning that it occurs most often in people younger than 65. FAD often progresses faster than the more common form of Alzheimer's disease, which typically occurs in people age 65 and older. As many as 50% of FAD cases are caused by defects in three genes located on three different chromosomes.

■ Alzheimer's disease is a devastating disease that results in memory loss, behavior and personality changes, and a decline in cognitive abilities.

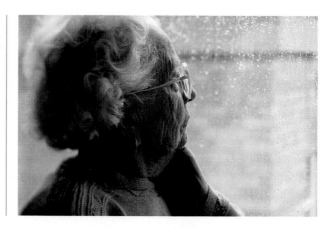

Even if only one of these mutations is inherited from a parent, a person will inevitably develop a form of early-onset Alzheimer's. Genetics play a role in late-onset disease as well; however, a person can inherit the gene associated with late-onset Alzheimer's and not get the disease. Similarly, people with late-onset Alzheimer's may not have any genetic factor.

The risk of developing Alzheimer's increases with age. One out of every 10 persons 65 years and older is a victim of Alzheimer's disease, although early-onset victims may be in their forties and fifties. Approximately 20% of Americans between the ages of 75 and 84, and almost half of those 85 years and older, suffer from Alzheimer's disease.[43]

Symptoms

In people with Alzheimer's disease, three key processes in the brain are disrupted—nerve cell communication, metabolism, and repair. This disruption ultimately causes many nerve cells to stop functioning, lose connections with other nerve cells, and die. The disease advances by stages, from early, mild forgetfulness to severe loss of mental function (i.e., dementia). As noted earlier, symptoms usually first appear after age 65.

The disease first destroys neurons in parts of the brain that control memory; as a result, a person's ability to do easy and familiar tasks begins to decline. People in the initial stages of disease often think less clearly and forget the names of familiar people and common objects. Later in the disease, they may forget how to do simple tasks, such as brushing their teeth. The cerebral cortex, particularly the area responsible for language and reasoning, is affected next, disrupting a person's language skills and ability to make judgments. Personality changes also may occur. Emotional outbursts and disturbing behavior, such as wandering and agitation, become more frequent as the disease runs its course. Eventually, many other areas of the brain are involved. All of these brain regions atrophy, and the person becomes bedridden, incontinent, totally helpless, unresponsive to the outside world, and susceptible to a variety of illnesses and infections. People with Alzheimer's disease often die from pneumonia.

Diagnosis

At this time, there is no definitive diagnosis for Alzheimer's disease. The only way to conclusively diagnose it is through autopsy, by examining the characteristic plaques and tangles in the brain.

Currently, several tools are used to diagnose possible Alzheimer's disease in a person who is having difficulties with memory or other mental functions. A health-care provider will examine a person's history, do a complete physical exam, run various laboratory tests and brain scans, and perform a series of tests that measure memory, language skills, and other abilities related to brain functioning. Using these special tests, clinicians can now diagnose Alzheimer's with up to 90% accuracy.[44] It is important to rule out other illnesses or medications that can cause dementia; severe depression in the elderly is often accompanied by memory loss and therefore is often confused with Alzheimer's. Depression and Alzheimer's disease do coexist in many patients.

Researchers are currently studying various brain imaging techniques in an effort to improve their diagnostic ability in detecting biological changes or signs of dysfunction in the brain. The earlier an accurate diagnosis of disease can be made, the better the chance of managing symptoms and helping patients and their families plan for future care while the patient is still able to take part in the decision-making process.

Treatment and Research

There is no cure for Alzheimer's disease, but the FDA has approved several medications for its treatment. These drugs may temporarily delay memory decline for some individuals, but none of the currently approved drugs stop the underlying degeneration of brain cells. Research is producing new insights into many Alzheimer's concerns. Studies are showing how drug and nondrug approaches to treatment can improve daily functioning and maximize quality of life. While medications cannot stop the deterioration associated with Alzheimer's disease, sometimes they can slow the progression of symptoms. A number of drugs are prescribed for specific manifestations of Alzheimer's such as aggressive behavior and agitation, depression, and insomnia. While drug therapy is important and beneficial, especially in early stages of the disease, the management of Alzheimer's has evolved to include nonpharmacological therapies as integral aspects of care. These therapies include the management of problematic behaviors, home or "environmental" modifications, and the use of appropriate communication techniques. Support and education for caregivers and family members are also crucial to the best care of people with Alzheimer's.

The care of a person who has Alzheimer's disease is challenging on many fronts. More than 70% of people with Alzheimer's live at home, where family and friends provide their care.[41] Care can be emotionally devastating, physically demanding, and a financial burden. Caregivers are subject to high levels of chronic stress, and caregiver burnout is a major factor in the inability to continue caring for a person with Alzheimer's at home.

Physical activity, good nutrition, and social interaction are important for keeping Alzheimer's patients as functional as possible. Maintaining a calm, safe, structured environment also helps patients feel better and remain independent longer. Drugs can help soothe agitation, anxiety, depression, and sleeplessness, and may help boost participation in daily activities. Newer medications can also improve or preserve thinking skills, at least temporarily.

Genetic research is an important area of Alzheimer's disease study. Scientists have found genetic links to the two forms of Alzheimer's disease. Early-onset Alzheimer's is a very rare form of the disease that can occur in people between the ages of 30 and 60. In the 1980s, researchers found that mutations (or changes) in certain genes on

My grandfather has Alzheimer's disease. My mother tries to take care of him but it is very difficult. Sometimes my sisters and I feel angry that she does not have time for us even when we understand that he needs her attention.

20-year-old woman

three chromosomes cause early-onset disease. A person has a 50% chance of developing early-onset disease if one parent has any of these genetic mutations.

Late-onset Alzheimer's disease, the more common form, develops after age 65. In 1992, researchers found that certain forms of the apolipoprotein E (APOE) gene can influence this Alzheimer's disease risk. Scientists are now intensively searching for other genes that may be linked to Alzheimer's. Discovering these genes is essential for understanding the disease's etiology and identifying targets for new drug development and other prevention or treatment strategies.

In 2003, a major expansion of Alzheimer's genetics research efforts began. The Alzheimer's Disease Genetics Study is collecting genetic material and cell lines from individuals in families with more than two living siblings who have late-onset Alzheimer's disease. This program will allow geneticists to speed up the discovery of additional risk factor genes.[45]

Informed Decision Making

In some cases, lifestyle changes can be the first step toward chronic disease prevention. A healthy diet, regular exercise, and avoidance of harmful substances are standard methods for health promotion. Other important approaches toward disease prevention include being knowledgeable about chronic diseases and their symptoms and visiting one's healthcare provider regularly. A woman who knows her body can recognize changes or problems readily and prevent or slow progression of disease before symptoms begin or complications arise.

For osteoporosis prevention purposes, a woman usually only needs to have a bone mineral density test two or three times during her lifetime. If her bone density is decreasing, preventive measures such as medication may be an appropriate option.

A significant aspect of arthritis treatment involves learning ways to ease pain and perform daily activities. A diagnosis of arthritis should encourage women to become more active in their own health care and learn better ways to manage their diseases.

Some diseases can cause significant damage if left undiagnosed and therefore untreated. Uncontrolled diabetes, for example, can lead to serious illness and possibly death. With appropriate treatment, however, women with diabetes can live complete and satisfying lives.

A disease such as Alzheimer's presents different issues. Early diagnosis appears to have little effect on treatment or management of the disease. It does, however, afford both the patient and family members time to arrange for who will make future healthcare, financial, long-term care, and any other decisions necessary for the patient. Many issues need to be considered with Alzheimer's disease because as the disease progresses, a person will no longer be able to make rational decisions or care for himself or herself. A woman who is considering becoming a caregiver for a person with this disease needs to understand the time and commitment involved before making such a decision. Early diagnosis assists people in this preparation.

Today, the Internet is playing an important role for patients and their families in dealing with the issues that arise from managing a chronic disease. It provides individuals with access to large networks of patients who may share their condition or situation. Sharing tales of common experiences is often very comforting, as is having a large, informal network for information dissemination. In addition, the Internet has provided a massive educational venue for chronic disease, acting as a resource on disease symptoms, diagnostic options, treatments, and support tools. Of course, there are some risks to information received on the Internet, including inappropriate claims for supposed "miracle cures" for certain disorders. As with all other topics, women should make every effort to go to trusted sources to get information about chronic diseases. (See the Web sites listed at the end of this chapter.)

■ ■ ■ ■

Summary

Knowledge, personal preventive practices, and lifestyle modifications are the best measures by which a woman can reduce her chances of developing certain chronic conditions and be proactive in seeking early diagnosis, treatment, and care. In the cases of chronic disease that are genetically triggered, women can better understand their risks by learning about their family history. Health screenings can alert a woman to an increased risk of disease, allowing her to make decisions on lifestyle changes and treatment options. Although prevention is the first step, chronic diseases can affect a woman who has followed a healthy lifestyle and has adhered to screening guidelines for various conditions. The next step is understanding how to control or treat a condition, through both lifestyle modifications and treatment options.

■ ■ ■ ■

Topics for Discussion

1. What type of ethical issues may arise with testing for genetic predisposition to various chronic diseases?
2. How can lifestyle changes affect chronic disease management?
3. How can chronic disease affect a woman's day-to-day life?
4. What differences exist between chronic diseases that occur early in life versus those that manifest later in life?
5. In what ways does early diagnosis help a woman and her family to cope with her disease?

Profiles of Remarkable Women

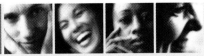

Mary Tyler Moore (1936–)

Mary Tyler Moore began her career as a dancer and actress in TV commercials. After a series of unsuccessful TV series and specials, she landed a role on *The Dick Van Dyke Show* in the early 1960s. From that point, Moore's career took off. *The Mary Tyler Moore Show* ran from 1970 to 1977 and was followed by *Mary* (1978), *The Mary Tyler Moore Hour* (1979), and *Mary* (1985-1986). Moore won five Emmy awards for her roles on *The Dick Van Dyke Show* and *The Mary Tyler Moore Show*. Her career has continued with roles in movies and on Broadway.

Moore has overcome many obstacles in her personal life. Her son committed suicide at the age of 24; soon thereafter, she divorced her husband. She later checked herself into the Betty Ford Clinic with alcohol abuse problems.

Since early adulthood, Moore has also had diabetes. Over the course of her disease, she has experienced several flare-ups of diabetic retinopathy that have been kept under control with laser surgery. As the International Chairwoman of the Juvenile Diabetes Foundation (JDF), Moore has advocated for diabetes education, awareness, and increased funding for diabetes research. She has been featured in a series of public service announcements for the JDF. In June 1999, Moore led 100 child delegates in the first Juvenile Diabetes Foundation Children's Congress before the Senate Committee on Appropriations, Subcommittee in Labor, Health and Human Services, and Education. She and the children, as well as other advocates, called on lawmakers to increase funding for diabetes research to help speed up the discovery of a cure. Moore has continued to lead the Children's Congress to Capitol Hill every other year, making the event one of the largest media and grassroots efforts held in support of finding a cure for juvenile diabetes, raising national awareness, and representing personal advocacy. Moore continues her fight against the disease that affects her life and the lives of the more than 16 million people with diabetes.

Web Sites

Alzheimer's Association: http://www.alz.org

Alzheimer's Disease Education and Referral Center (ADEAR): http://www.alzheimers.org

American Diabetes Association: http://www.diabetes.org

Arthritis Foundation: http://www.arthritis.org

Lupus Foundation of America: http://www.lupus.org

National Institute of Arthritis and Musculo-skeletal and Skin Diseases: http://www.niams.nih.gov

National Institute of Diabetes & Digestive & Kidney Diseases: http://www.niddk.nih.gov

National Institutes of Health, Osteoporosis and Related Bone Diseases National Resource Center: http://www.niams.nih.gov/bone

National Multiple Sclerosis Society: http://www.nmss.org

National Osteoporosis Foundation: http://www.nof.org

■■■■

References

1. World Health Organization. (2005). *Preventing Chronic Diseases: A Vital Investment.* Department of Chronic Diseases and Health Promotion. WHO Library ISBN 92 4 156300 1. Geneva, Switzerland: WHO Press.

2. National Osteoporosis Foundation. (2006). Osteoporosis Fast Facts. Retrieved January 26, 2006, from http://www.nof.org/osteoporosis/diseasefacts.htm.

3. U.S. Food and Drug Administration. (2002). Diabetes Facts. Retrieved January 26, 2006, from http://www.fda.gov/womens/taketimetocare/diabetes/fswomen.html.

4. National Institutes of Health. (2005). Progress in Autoimmune Disease Research: Report to Congress. Retrieved January 26, 2006, from http://www.niaid.nih.gov/dait/pdf/ADCC_Final.pdf.

5. National Institutes of Health. (2005). Osteoporosis and Asian American Women Fact Sheet. NIH Osteoporosis and Related Bone Diseases National Resource Center. Retrieved January 26, 2006, from http://www.osteo.org/newfile.asp?doc=r601i&doctitle=Osteoporosis+and+Asian+American+Women&doctype=HTML+Fact+Sheet.

6. Centers for Disease Control and Prevention. (2005). Racial/ethnic differences in the prevalence and impact of doctor-diagnosed arthritis—United States, 2002. *Morbidity and Mortality Weekly Report* 54(05): 119–123.

7. Centers for Disease Control and Prevention. (2005). National Diabetes Fact Sheet. National Center for Chronic Disease Prevention and Health. Retrieved January 26, 2006, from http://www.cdc.gov/diabetes/pubs/estimates.htm#prev4.

8. Centers for Disease Control and Prevention. (2005). Chronic Disease Overview. Retrieved January 26, 2006, from http://www.cdc.gov/nccdphp/overview.htm.

9. Alzheimer's Association. (2006). Statistics about Alzheimer's Disease. Retrieved January 26, 2006, from http://www.alz.org/AboutAD/statistics.asp.

10. American Academy of Orthpaedic Surgeons. (2001). Falls and Hip Fractures. Retrieved January 28, 2006, from http://orthoinfo.aaos.org/fact/thr_report.cfm?Thread_ID=77&topcategory=Hip.

11. National Institutes of Health. (2000). Osteoporosis Prevention, Diagnosis, and Therapy. Consensus Development Conference Statement. March 27–29, 2000. Retrieved January 28, 2006, from http://consensus.nih.gov/2000/2000Osteoporosis111html.htm.

12. U.S. Department of Health and Human Services. (2004). *A Report of the Surgeon General: Bone Health and Osteoporosis.* Washington, DC: U.S. Government Printing Office.

13. Delaney, M. F. (2006). Strategies for the prevention and treatment of osteoporosis during early menopause. *American Journal of Obstetrics and Gynecology* 194(2 suppl): S12–S23.

14. Cosman, F. (2005). The prevention and treatment of osteoporosis: a review. *Medscape General Medicine* 7(2):73.

15. Centers for Disease Control and Prevention. (2005). Arthritis Related Statistics. Retrieved January 29, 2006, from http://www.cdc.gov/arthritis/data_statistics/arthritis_related_statistics.htm#1.

16. Arthritis Foundation. (2005). Osteoarthritis Fact Sheet. Retrieved January 29, 2006, from http://www.arthritis.org/conditions/fact_sheets/OA_Fact_Sheet.asp.

17. Arthritis Foundation. (2005). Newly Diagnosed Fact Sheet. Retrieved January 29, 2006, from http://www.arthritis.org/conditions/diseasecenter/ra/ra_newly_diagnosed.asp.

18. Arthritis Foundation. (2005). Gout Fact Sheet. Retrieved January 29, 2006, from http://www.arthritis.org/AFStore/StartRead.asp?idProduct=3323.

19. American College of Rheumatology. (2003). Exercise and Arthritis. Retrieved January 29, 2006, from http://www.rheumatology.org/public/factsheets/exercise.asp.

20. Harrison, M. J. (2003). Young women with chronic disease: a female perspective on the impact and management of rheumatoid arthritis. *Arthritis and Rheumatology* 49(6): 846–852.

21. Leveille, S. G., Wee, C. C., and Iezzoni, L. I. (2005). Trends in obesity and arthritis among baby boomers and their predecessors, 1971–2002. *American Journal of Public Health* 95(9): 1607–1613.

22. Messier, S. P., Loeser, R. F., Miller, G. D., et al. (2004). Exercise and dietary weight loss in overweight and obese older adults with knee osteoarthritis: the Arthritis, Diet, and Activity Promotion Trial. *Arthritis and Rheumatology* 50(5): 1501–1510.

23. Miyaguchi, M., Kobayashi, A., Kadoya, Y., Ohashi, H., Yamano, Y., and Takaoka, K. (2003). Biochemical change in joint fluid after isometric quadriceps exercise for patients with osteoarthritis of the knee. *Osteoarthritis and Cartilage* 11: 252–259.

24. Centers for Disease Control and Prevention. (2004). Lyme disease—United States, 2001–2002. *Morbidity and Mortality Weekly Report* 53(05): 365–369.

25. National Institutes of Health. (2005). *Lyme Disease: The Facts, the Challenge.* National Institute of Allergies and Infectious Diseases and National Institute of Arthritis and Musculoskeletal and Skin Diseases. NIH Publication #05-7045.

26. U.S. Food and Drug Administration. (2002). Diabetes Facts: Women and Diabetes. Retrieved February 1, 2006, from http://www.fda.gov/womens/taketimetocare/diabetes/fswomen.html.

27. Bauduceau, B., Bourdel-Marchasson, I., Brocker, P., and Taillia, H. (2005). The brain of the elderly diabetic patient. *Diabetes Metabolism* 2: 92–97.

28. Kumari, M., and Marmot, M. (2005). Diabetes and cognitive function in a middle-aged cohort: findings from the Whitehall II study. *Neurology* 65(10): 1597–1603.

29. National Institutes of Health. (2005). Diagnosis of Diabetes. National Diabetes Information Clearing House. Retrieved February 1, 2006, from http://diabetes.niddk.nih.gov/dm/pubs/diagnosis/.

30. American Autoimmune Related Diseases Association. Autoimmune Disease in Women—the Facts. Retrieved February 1, 2006, from http://www.aarda.org/women.html.

31. Lupus Foundation of America. (2001). Lupus Fact Sheet. Retrieved February 2, 2006, from http://www.lupus.org/education/factsheet.html#4.

32. U.S. Department of Health and Human Services. (2003). Lupus Fact Sheet. Retrieved February 2, 2006, from http://www.4woman.gov/faq/lupus.htm.

33. Kamen, D. L., Cooper, G. S., Bouali, H., Shaftman, S. R., Hollis, B. W. and Gilkeson, G. S. (2006). Vitamin D deficiency in systemic lupus erythematosus. *Autoimmune Review* 5(2): 114–117.

34. Costenbader, K. H., and Karlson, E. W. (2005). Cigarette smoking and systemic lupus erythematosus: a smoking gun? *Autoimmunity* 38(7): 541–547.

35. American Association of Clinical Endocrinologists. (2006). Thyroid Awareness Month—March 2006. Retrieved February 3, 2006, from http://www.aace.com/public/awareness/tam/2006/.

36. Thyroid Foundation of America. (2004). Thyroid Disorders and Treatments. Retrieved February 2, 2006, from http://www.tsh.org/disorders/index.html.

37. National Institutes of Health and the National Library of Medicine. (2004). Chronic Thyroiditis (Hashimoto's Disease). Retrieved February 2, 2006, from http://www.nlm.nih.gov/medlineplus/ency/article/000371.htm.

38. MayoClinic.Com. (2005). Hyperthyroidism. Retrieved February 2, 2006, from http://www.mayoclinic.com/health/hyperthyroidism/DS00344.

39. Thyroid Foundation of America. (2004). Racing the Engine—Hyperthyroidism. Retrieved February 2, 2006, from http://www.tsh.org/disorders/hyperthyroidism/hyperthyroidism.html.

40. AACE Thyroid Task Force. (2002). American Association of Clinical Endocrinologists medical guidelines for clinical practice for the evaluation and treatment of hyperthyroidism and hypothyroidism. *Endocrinology Practice* 6: 457–469.

41. Alzheimer's Association. (2005). Fact Sheet—Alzheimer's Disease. Retrieved February 3, 2006, from http://www.alz.org/Resources/FactSheets/FSADFacts.pdf.

42. Answers 4 Families. (2004). Alzheimer's Disease and Other Dementias: Satatistics on Alzheimer's Disease (AD). Retrieved February 3, 2006, from http://nncf.unl.edu/alz/info/alz.stats.html.

43. American Health Assistance Foundation. (2005). Alzheimer's Disease: Risk Factors. Retrieved February 3, 2006, from http://www.ahaf.org/alzdis/about/adrisk.htm.

44. Alzheimer's Disease Education and Referral Center (2005). Alzheimer's Disease—Diagnosis. Retrieved February 3, 2006, from http://www.alzheimers.org/diagnosis.htm.

45. Alzheimer's Disease Education and Referral Center. (2005). Can Alzheimer's Disease Be Prevented? Retrieved February 3, 2006, from http://www.alzheimers.org/pubs/PreventingAD/Learning.htm.

Chapter Twelve

Mental Health

Chapter Objectives

On completion of this chapter, the student should be able to discuss:

The gender differences and patterns of mental disorders.

The economic, legal, and political dimensions of mental health.

Types of mental disorders, their symptoms, and treatment.

Risk factors for suicide among adults, adolescents, and children.

The factors that contribute to a woman's overall mental health.

Strategies for coping with life's daily stresses and improving mental health in general.

Factors to consider before seeking treatment for a mental disorder.

Different methods of treating mental disorders, including pharmaceutical treatments and counseling.

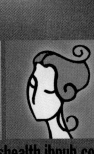

womenshealth.jbpub.com

Women's Health Online is a great source for supplementary women's health information for both students and instructors. Visit

http://womenshealth.jbpub.com
to find a variety of useful tools for learning, thinking, and teaching.

Introduction

Mental health problems cause a significant amount of morbidity and disability. The World Health Organization identifies both the "undefined" and "hidden" burden of mental problems. The *undefined burden* of mental problems refers to the economic and social burden for families, communities, and countries. Although obviously substantial, this burden has not been efficiently measured because of a lack of quantitative data and difficulties in measuring and evaluating its impact. The *hidden burden* refers to the stigma and violations of human rights and freedoms associated with mental problems. Like the undefined burden, the hidden burden is difficult to quantify. Mental health disorders cause significant—and often under-reported—problems throughout the world, as many cases remain concealed.

Historically, mental health issues and treatment needs were viewed as being the same for both men and women. In 1990, after the National Institutes of Health's admission that many of its studies had not included women, there was a newfound focus on women's health in general. Further investigation into the field of mental health found significant inequities in mental health and gender, prompting extensive research on the differences in mental disorders in males and females.[1] The 1990s, dubbed "The Decade of the Brain," featured many research advances in neuroscience and behavioral science. Not only were differences noted in the ways in which mental disorders affected males and females, but mental illness was also recognized as a major public health problem. The new millennium has already seen more advances in the field of mental health, with the continued introduction of novel pharmaceuticals into the marketplace, legislative advancements such as the Mental Health Parity Act,* and better understanding of the genetic basis for many mental health disorders.

Mental disorders are not uncommon. Half of all American adults experience mental illness in their lifetime; unfortunately, fewer than 50% of people with mental disorders seek professional treatment. The World Health Organization (WHO) and the National Institute of Mental Health (NIMH) report that for women worldwide, depression is now a leading cause of lost years of healthy life.[1,2] This chapter describes some of the more common mental disorders and explains how mental health is an important health issue at all stages of women's lives.

Perspectives on Mental Health

Epidemiological Data

According to the National Institute of Mental Health, an estimated 22.1% of Americans age 18 and older—about one in five adults—suffer from a diagnosable mental disorder in a given year. This figure translates to roughly 45 million people.[3]

---

*Millions of Americans with mental disorders do not have equal access to health insurance. In fact, many health plans discriminate against these people by limiting mental health and substance abuse health care through the imposition of higher co-payments and deductibles and lower annual and lifetime spending caps. The Mental Health Parity Act was passed by Congress in 1996 to eliminate annual and lifetime dollar limits for mental health care for companies with more than 50 employees.

In addition, 4 of the 10 leading causes of disability are mental disorders.[4] In the United States, mental illness accounts for more than 15% of the overall burden of disease from all causes. Data from studies conducted by the WHO, the World Bank, and Harvard University, compiled by the Global Burden of Disease study team,[5] revealed that mental illness, including suicide, ranks second in terms of burden of disease in the United States, with the leader being cardiovascular disease.

Men and women are equally likely to suffer from mental disorders; however, the prevalence of certain disorders varies by gender. In addition, men and women often experience the disorders in different ways. For example, differences have been reported in age of onset of symptoms, frequency of psychotic symptoms, course of disease progression, social adjustment, and long-term outcome.[6] It is believed that these variations in mental illness may be a result of distinct brain structures, as seen in animal studies, and the presence of different sex hormones in males and females, which cause neurons to act differently. Evidence shows that the development of brain hemispheres in males may not be similar to that in females, possibly resulting in females using their brains in different ways than males. Studies on gender patterns in the use of the brain show, for example, different areas of the brain being used by males and females when decoding words and deciphering emotion. Boys and girls are also diagnosed and treated differently by primary care physicians when they have mental health issues.[7] Table 12.1 lists disorders that show evidence of gender differences in the context of mental illness.

Gender differences exist not just in the prevalence of specific mental health disorders among women and men, but also in the way the diseases manifest themselves in the two genders.

Economic Dimensions

The economic effects of mental disorders are wide ranging and long lasting. These disorders impose a range of costs on individuals, families, and communities

Table 12.1 Gender Differences in Mental Illness

- Women have twice the rate of clinical depression.
- Women have four times the incidence of seasonal affective disorder.
- Women experience more of the depressed phase of bipolar disorder and have more rapid cycling between mania and depression.
- Women are nine times more likely to suffer from anorexia nervosa and bulimia nervosa.
- Twice as many women suffer from panic disorder.
- Women are more likely to have phobia and experience more intense symptoms.
- Borderline personality disorder and histrionic personality disorder are diagnosed in more women.
- Men are more than three times as likely to be diagnosed with antisocial personality disorders than women.
- There are greater rates of somatization in women.
- More women attempt suicide, although more men are successful at their attempts.

as a whole. Measurable components of the economic burden of mental disorders include the following elements:

- The need for mental health and social services
- Lost employment and reduced productivity
- The financial burden placed on families and caregivers
- Increased levels of crime and a greater threat to public safety
- The negative impact of premature mortality

Treatment for mental disorders is often a costly undertaking. Prescription drugs can be very expensive, especially for those individuals without adequate health insurance or insurance that does not cover pharmaceuticals. Inpatient and outpatient mental healthcare services also are very expensive and usually require ongoing follow-up. Because many people with mental disorders have difficulty holding down jobs for long periods of time, they are at increased risk for being uninsured. The cost of depression to the United States, is estimated to be $44 billion per year in terms of treatment and lost productivity, more than the costs for cardiovascular disease.[8] Costs associated with mental healthcare can create further problems in enabling access to adequate care.

Legal Dimensions

In general, people with mental disorders are not more likely to commit crimes than the general population. If they are left untreated or are undertreated, however, a correlation between mental illness and crime does exist, especially among individuals with psychotic and mood disorders. Mental illness has created an interesting element of the law, as prosecutors and judges seek to identify, through the help of experts, when an individual can be held responsible for his or her own actions and whether that person is competent to stand trial. Many people are not identified as suffering from a mental disorder during the legal process. About 16% of all inmates in state adult correctional facilities are identified as mentally ill, according to a 2001 Justice Department report.[9] The report also found that 79% of such prisoners were receiving some type of mental health therapy. About 60% of those diagnosed as mentally ill receive psychotropic medications, which include antidepressants, stimulants, sedatives, and tranquilizers. A higher percentage of female inmates than male inmates are receiving treatment for mental health. In fact, one in four female prisoners is on medication.

There are additional legal and ethical challenges centered on care and decision making for mentally ill people. The forced sterilization of mentally ill women continues to be a global concern, for example. In 1883, Sir Edward Galton, a cousin of Charles Darwin, suggested that better breeding would improve the human race. From this idea, the eugenics movement was born. **Eugenics** argued that humans could breed out the health problems in society, such as mental illness. As part of this movement, sterilization was recommended to prevent people with mental ill-

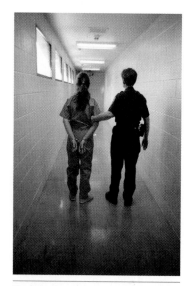

■ Data reveal that about 16% of all inmates are mentally ill.

nesses from having children who, it was believed, would also be mentally disabled or promiscuous. This philosophy gained traction around the world, and became a practice adopted by the German government under Hitler in the early 1930s. Forced sterilization was also commonly practiced in the United States on mentally ill, poor, and minority women. Most states have since passed laws banning forced sterilization of mentally ill patients, though the practice persists in some areas.

Mentally ill homeless people create a host of legal and ethical dilemmas for policymakers and program coordinators. Many of these individuals have become homeless as a result of cuts in federal and state funding to inpatient mental facilities and outpatient mental health clinics. These funding cuts continue to spur the rapid release of thousands of patients who are not capable of caring for themselves, which hampers the ability of newly diagnosed individuals to receive initial treatment. Without appropriate care and access to consistent medications and treatment, and with continued exposure to the stress of living on the street, many mentally ill homeless people experience a worsening of their mental conditions and overall health. As a result, homeless people with mental disorders have a high incidence of run-ins with the law based on their threatening behavior, substance abuse, or other disorderly conduct. The connection between the inability of many mentally ill people to access appropriate care and the incidence of criminal behavior has inspired the creation of social programs that seek to improve quality of life for the mentally ill in the United States.

Political Dimensions

The mission of the NIMH, which is part of the National Institutes of Health, is to reduce the burden of mental illness through research on the mind, brain, and behavior. NIMH also takes the lead in understanding the effects of behavior on HIV transmission and pathogenesis, and in developing effective behavioral preventive interventions. It conducts a wide range of research, research training, research capacity development, and public information outreach and dissemination programs

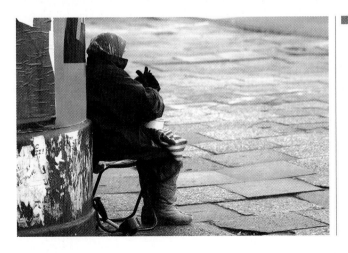

Mentally ill homeless people present a host of legal and ethical dilemmas for society.

to fulfill its mission. NIMH has identified the following areas of emphasis for its work over the next five years:

- Measure the extent of mental health disparities
- Conduct basic behavioral research on stress and coping
- Study macro-structural factors in HIV/AIDS and mental disorders
- Conduct pharmacogenetic and pharmacokinetic studies on mental disorders
- Study factors that produce health disparities in treatment responses, adherence, outcomes, and quality
- Study suicide, depression, and other severe mental illnesses in minority populations
- Identify factors that overcome health disparities related to health service delivery and use by ethnic populations
- Improve interaction with academic research initiatives, especially in the area of disparities research

These goals represent the backbone of the United States' national mental health research agenda.

Clinical Dimensions of Mental Illness

Mood Disorders

Mood disorders (also known as **affective disorders**) are conditions characterized by extreme disturbances of mood. They result from out-of-balance neurotransmitters, genetics, and environmental factors. There are two categories of mood disorders: unipolar disorder, which includes depression and dysthymia, and bipolar disorder, which includes manic depression.

Depression

Depression is a medical illness affecting the mind as well as the body that is usually triggered by stressful life events. A persistent sad mood as well as other mental and physical symptoms, which may manifest either suddenly or gradually, are characteristics of depression (Table 12.2). People with depression often feel undesirable and inadequate. They anticipate rejection and dissatisfaction from their interactions and experiences, and they blame themselves when their negative expectations are fulfilled. Depression can affect interpersonal relationships, job performance, creativity, and the ability to be a fully functional parent and partner.

Depression may coexist with other physical and mental illnesses or may be mistaken for Alzheimer's disease in the elderly. Certain medical conditions, such as thyroid disease, multiple sclerosis, and cancer, can result in depression. Depression also may arise as a response to a serious illness, a consequence of substance abuse, or a side effect of certain medications. In addition, depression frequently accompanies a number of chronic diseases, including coronary heart disease, diabetes, stroke, cancer, and HIV/AIDS.

Table 12.2	Symptoms of Depression	
Persistent sad mood	Loss of interest in pleasurable activities
Constant feelings of sadness	Sleep disturbances
Excessive crying	Appetite and weight changes
Low energy	Thoughts of death or suicide
Feelings of worthlessness or hopelessness	Physical symptoms that do not respond to treatment
Difficulty concentrating or making decisions	

Hormonal shifts during reproductive-related events and their link to mental illness have been the subject of much controversy. For example, it was previously believed that hormones were solely responsible for depression during premenstrual syndrome (PMS); however, research now shows that hormones may trigger, but are not solely responsible for, PMS-related depression. Severe depression during PMS, called premenstrual dysphoric disorder (PMDD), affects 3% to 7% of menstruating women.[10]

Postpartum depression is a type of depression that affects 10% to 15% of all new mothers. This condition is different from postpartum blues, which occurs in the first 10 days after delivery and is quite common and typically mild. Often referred to as the "baby blues," postpartum blues affects as many as 80% of new mothers and no intervention is needed. In contrast, postpartum depression begins three to six months after delivery and is more severe than postpartum blues, although less severe than postpartum psychosis. Postpartum depression is more common in women with a history of depression, marital issues, lack of social support, or a history of negative life experiences. A woman with postpartum depression may have various symptoms of depression and thoughts of hurting herself or her baby (Table 12.3). Although it often goes unnoticed and untreated, postpartum depression can greatly affect the mother and child as well as damage the relationship between the parents. It can be treated with therapy and medication.

Another hormone-related event that has been linked to mental illness is menopause. Conflicting reports have surfaced regarding whether women are at greater risk for depression during the years surrounding menopause. Some studies show that women who experience depression during the menopause years often have a history of depressive illness or have certain identifiable stressors. Certain

Table 12.3	Symptoms of Postpartum Depression	
Anxiety	Lack of interest in the baby
Feelings of hopelessness and guilt	Thoughts of suicide
Panic attacks	Thoughts of hurting self or baby
Insomnia	

events occurring around this age—for example, a change in job status, children leaving home, and the responsibility of caring for aging parents—may lead to psychological stress.

Research has shown that levels of the neurotransmitter **serotonin** are lower in people with major depression. Medications that boost levels of serotonin, called selective serotonin reuptake inhibitors (SSRIs), have proven able to relieve symptoms of depression. One study found that men's brains make 52% more serotonin than do women's brains, possibly explaining why depression can manifest differently in men and women.[11]

Genetics also play a major role in depression. Someone with a family history of depression is significantly more likely to develop depression than someone with no family history of the disease. Studies have shown that children with one depressed parent are two to three times more likely to experience depression by age 18 than are children without depressed parents. The risk doubles if both parents suffer from depression.[12]

A particular form of depression called **seasonal affective disorder (SAD)** is caused by seasonal shifts in daylight hours, which affect a person's circadian rhythm or sleep-wake cycle. SAD often affects women in their reproductive years. Its symptoms include some of the atypical symptoms of depression, such as increased appetite, lethargy, and carbohydrate cravings. Researchers believe the cause of SAD may be related to melatonin disturbances. Therapeutic doses of bright light in the morning can help to relieve this condition.

Depression is estimated to affect more than 21% of women, making it twice as common in women as in men and the most common mood disorder among women. Adolescent females have an unusually high rate of depression. Before puberty, boys are more likely than girls of the same age to be diagnosed with depression or depressive symptoms. After puberty, however, there is a significant change in the incidence numbers and girls are far more likely to be diagnosed with depression.[13] Between the ages of 30 and 44—typically the years of childbearing and childrearing—rates of depression are three times greater for women than they are

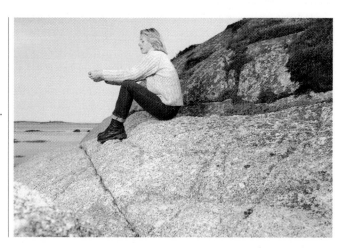

■ Therapeutic doses of bright light in the morning can help relieve depression caused by seasonal affective disorder (SAD).

for men. There also is evidence of a greater incidence of depression in the elderly, especially in women who are widowed, are in poor physical health, and have lost some or all of their independence. Medical illness and the effects of multiple medications in the elderly make it even more difficult to diagnose depression.

Researchers are examining whether the higher rates of depression in women are truly representative of a greater incidence of depression or whether the rates reflect gender-based differences in the acknowledgment of mental illness or ability to recognize symptoms. Women also have higher rates of victimization from physical abuse, sexual harassment, and rape. Acts of violence such as these tend to foster low self-esteem, a sense of helplessness, social isolation, and depression. Being a caregiver for young children, aging parents, or ill family members—roles often filled by women—also has been noted as a risk factor for depression.

Dysthymia

Dysthymia is a milder, yet more chronic, form of depression. It is diagnosed when symptoms last at least two years in adults or one year in adolescents and children. People with dysthymia exhibit a depressed mood and at least two other symptoms of depression, such as poor appetite or overeating, sleep difficulties, or low self-esteem. Dysthymia often begins in childhood or adolescence, but can occur at any age. Because it often develops at a young age, the depressed state becomes integrated within the woman's personality. It then becomes normal for a woman with dysthymia to see herself and the world from a negative perspective. The condition is comparable to depression in that it occurs at similar rates and has similar risk factors.

Manic Depression

Manic depression, also known as **bipolar disorder,** is characterized by wide mood swings that can occur within hours or days. Mood swings occur in everyone, of course, but people with bipolar disorder experience exaggerated moods that can last for weeks or even months. A person with manic depression often has periods of normal behavior, but these periods are always followed by up-and-down cycles. A manic episode is a period of abnormally euphoric or irritable mood that occurs at least once per week. During this time, a person has inflated self-esteem, unrealistic ideas about her abilities, increased energy and talkativeness, decreased need for sleep, increased sexual drive, and poor sense of judgment. Manic depression may take years to recognize and diagnose.

More than 3 million Americans have manic depression, which affects equal numbers of men and women. Gender differences are apparent in the manifestation of the disease, however, with women typically having more depressed episodes and more rapid cycling between depression and mania than do men.

Treatment

Eighty percent of people with depression respond positively to treatment. Antidepressant drugs are used to reduce sadness; they work by influencing the function of certain neurotransmitters called monoamines. Serotonin and norepinephrine,

■ Many women are turning to herbal remedies for the treatment of depression. St. John's wort (*Hypericum perforatum*) is used in the treatment of mild to moderate depression in Europe.

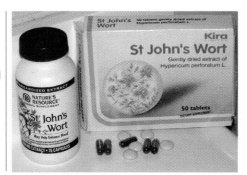

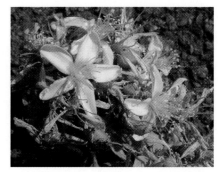

for example, are both types of monoamines. Tricyclic antidepressants (TCAs) and monoamine oxidase inhibitors (MAOIs) are types of antidepressants that affect these monoamines. These antidepressants are not always the drugs of choice, however, because of the side effects of these agents and the dietary restrictions imposed with the use of the MAOIs. SSRIs, as mentioned earlier, work better for certain people and on certain types of depression, and they have fewer side effects than both the TCAs and the MAOIs. Examples of SSRIs commonly used to treat depression include Wellbutrin, Prozac, and Paxil—three antidepressants that have become familiar household names. These prescription medications are often prescribed in combination with psychotherapy. Several of the most prescribed antidepressants have recently become available in generic formulations, making them less expensive and more accessible for many potential users.

Many women are turning to herbal remedies for the treatment of depression. St. John's wort (made from a yellow-flowering plant called *Hypericum perforatum*) is used in the treatment of mild to moderate depression in Europe; in Germany, it is used more widely than any other form of antidepressant. Although this herb has been used for centuries for medicinal purposes, the composition of St. John's wort and its mechanism of action are not well understood. Some evidence suggests that the herb may work for mild depression, but not for treating major depression of moderate severity. More studies need to be conducted to obtain conclusive results. Because the U.S. Food and Drug Administration (FDA) classifies herbal products as dietary supplements, St. John's wort can be sold without requiring studies on its dosage, safety, or effectiveness. Also, St. John's wort can interact with certain drugs, such as those used for HIV or cancer treatment, and can limit the effectiveness of these drugs. Clinical studies are under way to rigorously examine the effectiveness of such herbal treatments. Until the results of these studies become available, women should speak with their healthcare providers before taking any type of medication, including herbal remedies.

Unlike in depression, the goal of treatment of dysthymia is not to return a woman to her normal self, but rather to help her create a healthy self.[14] In addition, dysthymia responds better to long-term psychotherapy than it does to medications. Bipolar disorder is usually treated with lithium and anticonvulsants. Interpersonal therapy is typically used in conjunction with drug therapy for severe cases of mood disorders or alone for mild depression. Without treatment, mood disorders become more severe and episodes of depression become more frequent. Only one-fourth of people with depression actually seek treatment.

Anxiety Disorders

Feeling anxious or panicky is not a disorder. Some people, however, exhibit an extreme reaction to real or perceived dangers (Table 12.4) and may even mistake anxiety for a heart attack. These feelings and symptoms are the result of the fight-or-flight response, which activates the sympathetic nervous system to produce stress hormones in the adrenal glands. After a person either is removed from danger or no longer feels threatened, other hormones are produced to counteract the stress response and bring about calm. The fight-or-flight response is a normal response. In people with anxiety disorders, however, it is activated in situations in which no real danger exists and their reaction is more extreme than the reaction of the average person.

In the past, **anxiety disorders** as well as other mental disorders were defined as neuroses—conditions characterized by symptoms of anxiety or phobia, or feelings of conflict that caused difficulty in a person's life but were believed to be self-generated. The term "neurosis" is now considered obsolete, and these types of symptoms are referred to as belonging to a specific disorder.

Anxiety disorders are the most common mental health problem in the United States, affecting approximately 13% of the population. Only 25% of those affected seek treatment. Women are two to three times more likely than men to suffer from any type of anxiety disorder, and more than 30% of women experience an anxiety disorder at some time in their life.[15]

Generalized Anxiety Disorder

Generalized anxiety disorder (GAD) is characterized by chronic and exaggerated worry and tension that lasts for at least six months. It is a relatively mild condition, although it often is complicated by coexisting conditions such as depression, alcohol use, and other anxiety disorders. Symptoms of generalized anxiety disorder include the following:

- Muscle tension
- Irritability

Table 12.4 Symptoms of Anxiety Disorder

Feelings of terror and dread	Chest pain
Feelings of apprehension and uncertainty	Fainting
Nervousness	Difficulty breathing
Irritability	Sweating
Rapid heartbeat	Belief that feelings are signs of a heart attack

- Inability to relax
- Difficulty concentrating
- Fear of losing control
- Headaches
- Nausea

A woman also may constantly anticipate disaster, but she often realizes that her worry and stress are unwarranted and unnecessary. The symptoms do not interfere with daily life, but they cause unnecessary distress and discomfort.[16]

Phobias

Phobia is not just extreme fear, but irrational fear. More women are affected by phobias than are men, and women's symptoms are usually more intense than those of their male counterparts. Phobias are the most common type of anxiety disorders and encompass different types of fear. For example:

- A woman may fear a particular object or situation, a condition known as simple or specific phobia. Claustrophobia, the fear of enclosed places, is considered a simple phobia.
- Social phobia involves fear or extreme embarrassment of being in a social setting. It is twice as common in women as in men. A common social phobia is fear of public speaking or, in its limited form, performance anxiety.
- Fear of being in a situation that might provoke a panic attack or from which escape may be difficult is known as agoraphobia. This phobia often coexists with panic disorder.

Lowered self-esteem and depression often accompany phobias. Women with phobias may have problems with drugs or alcohol, which are used to ease anxiety and depression. Phobias seem to run in families and usually appear around adolescence or adulthood.

Panic Disorder

Panic disorder affects 3 to 6 million Americans and is twice as common in women as in men. This disorder is characterized by panic attacks—periods of intense fear accompanied by physical and emotional distress that may last anywhere from five to 20 minutes.[17] The panic attack often strikes without warning. Its symptoms have often been mistaken for a heart attack:

- A pounding heart
- Sweating
- Weakness
- Dizziness
- Lightheadedness
- Chest pain

- Nausea or stomach upset
- Flushes or chills
- Shortness of breath
- A fear of dying

An initial panic attack usually occurs in a person's twenties during transition periods, times of considerable stress, or crises and often sends the individual to the emergency room. Some women have an isolated attack without ever developing the disorder; nevertheless, repeated panic attacks are a definitive sign of panic disorder. After experiencing one or more attacks, many women begin to suffer from anticipatory anxiety and anticipatory attacks, awaiting an impending attack. Anticipatory attacks can result in agoraphobia—fear of the place where a panic attack previously occurred or a place that looks difficult to escape if necessary. Panic disorder is often accompanied by other conditions, including both mental disorders, such as depression, and physical ailments, such as irritable bowel syndrome.

Obsessive-Compulsive Disorder

Obsessive-compulsive disorder (OCD) affects 5 million people in the United States, with rates nearly equal for men and for women.[18] People with this type of anxiety disorder suffer from an endless cycle of disturbing thoughts, known as obsessions, and rituals, known as compulsions, intended to rid themselves of the thoughts. The rituals performed create a sense of safety and provide relief from the intrusive anxiety-causing obsessions. Common obsessions/compulsions include fear of germs or dirt, which is resolved by long periods of scrubbing hands and endless cleaning, and fear of bringing harm to someone, which is relieved by saying a certain phrase in a certain manner to prevent harm. For example, a woman may say her friend's name three times whenever she leaves the house to protect her friend from getting hurt. Other signs include the following:

- Spending significant time counting or performing repetitive tasks
- Checking appliances numerous times to confirm that they are turned off or doors to confirm that they are locked
- Having a preoccupation with symmetry and order

People with OCD are aware that their fears and behaviors are irrational, yet the obsessions and compulsions are uncontrollable without help. To warrant a diagnosis of OCD, the behaviors must take up hours of the day and significantly interfere with daily life.

Post-traumatic Stress Disorder

Post-traumatic stress disorder (PTSD) is an extremely debilitating illness that occurs after an exposure to a terrifying event such as a personal assault, a natural or human disaster, an accident, or military combat. The disorder originally was recognized in soldiers after combat, but researchers later realized that any event outside the range of normal human experiences could trigger the disorder in vulnerable people.

PTSD is estimated to affect approximately 4% of adults in the United States, although it can occur at any age. Survey results show that females' risk of developing PTSD following trauma is twice that of males. Females also are more likely to develop long-term PTSD and have higher rates of co-occurring medical and psychiatric problems with the disorder.

Symptoms of PTSD usually begin within three months of a traumatic event and include flashback episodes, nightmares, reexperiencing or reliving of the traumatic event, and emotional numbness. Women with PTSD often have difficulty sleeping, suffer from depression and anxiety, and experience irritability and outbursts of anger. Physical symptoms may include headaches, chest pain, gastrointestinal complaints, and increased alcohol or substance abuse. To be considered PTSD, symptoms must last for more than one month.

Whether a person experiences PTSD following a traumatic event is affected by an individual's response to stress, perception of the event, and social support. The following factors may increase the risk of developing the disorder:

- A personal history of mental disorders
- A family history of anxiety disorders
- Prolonged separation from parents in earlier childhood
- Abuse as a child
- Exposure to other traumatic experiences at a young age[19]

Researchers have found that people who experience PTSD have abnormal levels of hormones involved in the stress response, such as higher levels of epinephrine and norepinephrine and lower levels of cortisol. People with PTSD also have higher levels of opiates, a neurotransmitter that is produced in the body to mask pain. This increased level may be the cause of the emotional numbness seen in people with PTSD.[20]

Treatment

Most anxiety disorders are treated using a combination of therapy, antianxiety medications, and antidepressants. Treatment for phobias may include **cognitive behavioral therapy** and medications, such as certain antidepressants and beta blockers. Some people may not seek treatment if the feared object or situation is easy to avoid; however, these people often make significant decisions so as to avoid the phobic object or situation. Early treatment of panic disorder can stop the progression of disease to agoraphobia. Cognitive behavioral therapy has been shown to help 70% to 90% of people suffering from panic disorder; improvement is usually evident within six to eight weeks. Panic disorder also may be treated with antidepressants and benzodiazepines.

Many women have tried using an herbal supplement called kava to bring relief to their symptoms of anxiety. Kava (*Piper methysticum*) is a plant native to the South

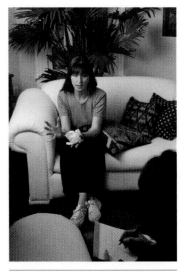

■ Professional counseling helps many people suffering from mental disorders.

Pacific that is used in a traditional beverage and has been promoted as an herbal supplement to provide relaxation; to relieve anxiety, stress, and tension; and to counter sleeplessness. Although the FDA has not determined the benefits of kava dietary supplements, the agency has advised consumers of the potential risk of severe liver injury associated with the use of this herb. Numerous reports of liver-related injuries, including hepatitis, cirrhosis, and liver failure, have surfaced in the United States and other countries.

As with other anxiety disorders, some people with obsessive-compulsive disorder may find relief with antidepressants, psychotherapy, and behavior therapy. Full-blown OCD is more difficult to treat, however. Exposure/response therapy is a type of treatment that first exposes a person to the feared object or obsessive thought/idea; the person then is prevented from carrying out the compulsion associated with the obsession. The intention is to show the person that nothing drastic will occur if the compulsive behavior is not completed.

Treatment for PTSD can include various types of therapy as well as antianxiety medications and antidepressants. Types of therapy used include cognitive behavioral therapy, group therapy, exposure/response therapy, and virtual reality.

Eating Disorders

An eating disorder is a form of mental illness characterized by a distorted body image and disordered eating behaviors. People with eating disorders often suffer from other mental disorders, such as depression, anxiety disorders, and substance abuse. Many people have eating disorder problems but do not meet the criteria for anorexia, bulimia, or binge eating disorder.

There is no single explanation for why an eating disorder evolves. Eating disorders often begin with dieting; however, before dieting, other factors have already affected a person's mindset. Women may have a biological vulnerability to eating disorders. Levels of certain neurotransmitters and hormones that affect not only one's mood, but also appetite and eating behavior, may be altered in women with eating disorders. For example, the hormone serotonin creates feelings of satiety after eating and may be present at lower levels in women with bulimia. Therefore, these individuals tend to not feel as satisfied and may binge as a result. Poor self-image, depression, anxiety, loneliness, and certain family and personal relationships may contribute to the development of an eating disorder, too. The stresses associated with adolescent and adult life also can precipitate anorexia or bulimia.[21]

Our culture, with its unrelenting idealization of thinness and "the perfect body," is also partly to blame. Consider the rise in pro–eating disorder Web sites that share information among those with eating disorders on how to better meet their disordered goals of weight loss and behavior control. Referred to as "pro-ana" for "pro-anorexia" and "pro-mia" for "pro-bulimia," the authors of these sites see them as a way to create a sense of support and community among people of like thinking. Many health professionals, however, see them as very dangerous and have mounted campaigns with Internet service providers to have the sites removed.

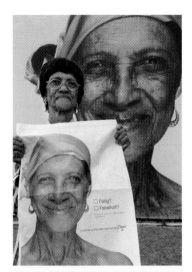

■ Dove's Campaign for Real Beauty challenges the definition of beauty by featuring women whose appearance does not fit the stereotypical definition of beauty. The ads encourage women to reconsider society's definition of beauty and the way the media shapes perceptions of beauty.

Body Image

The image of an ideal body varies over time and among cultures. The models of beauty over the last 50 years, for example, have evolved from voluptuous and curvaceous, to emaciated, to sculpted and visibly muscular. Many white Americans see the ideal as tall and thin with blonde hair and blue eyes. Blacks, in contrast, may see beauty as more flexible and incorporate attitude and style—not just shape and size—into their definition of the ideal. Although eating disorders have always been more prevalent in whites, they now are on the rise among other ethnic groups, due in part to young women acculturating to the American ideal and the newfound popularity of women of different ethnic backgrounds in the modeling and acting industries. There is an even higher risk of eating disorders for women whose occupations or hobbies emphasize beauty and thinness, such as actors, models, gymnasts, dancers, and performers in general.[22]

The *female athlete triad*—the interrelationship between disordered eating, amenorrhea, and osteoporosis—usually begins with disordered eating. Poor nutrition and intense athletic training cause weight loss and a decrease in or shutdown of estrogen production. Consequently, amenorrhea occurs. The final condition in the triad, osteoporosis, may follow if estrogen levels remain low and the woman's diet is lacking in calcium and vitamin D. Although the triad can occur in any athlete, those at greatest risk are endurance athletes such as distance swimmers and runners, and athletes in sports where slim appearance is highly valued, such as gymnasts and figure skaters.

Women who suffer from eating disorders are most likely to tie their self-esteem to their weight and their body image. As Natalie Angier in *Women—An Intimate Geography* frankly states,

> Girls, poor girls, are in the thick of our intolerance and vacillation. Girls put on body fat as they pass into adulthood . . . And then they are subject to the creed of total control, the idea that we can subdue it and discipline our bodies if we work very very hard at it . . . Dieting becomes proxy for power, not simply because girls are exposed through the media to a smothering assemblage of slender, beautiful models, but because adolescent girls today are laying down a bit of fat in an era when fat is creeping up everywhere and is everywhere despised.[23]

Angier argues that women need to help debunk the myth of an ideal body image. The idea that there is or can be a perfect body has been fostered by airbrushed models on magazine covers. The diet industry has helped to promote this idea even more by marketing items ranging from low-fat shakes for immediate weight loss to "cellulite" busters to get rid of dimpling on thighs. Instead, girls and women should encourage each other to accept themselves and their bodies while continuing to strive for accomplishment in areas other than their appearance.

Anorexia Nervosa

Anorexia nervosa is an eating disorder characterized by deprivation of food and a body weight of at least 15% below the normal weight for a person's height and age. It is classified in the American Psychiatric Association's *Diagnostic and Statistical Manual of Mental Disorders,* fourth edition (DSM-IV), as an eating disorder associated with the following factors:

- Refusal to maintain an adequate weight
- Intense fear of gaining weight
- Distorted body image
- In women, three consecutive missed periods without pregnancy (amenorrhea)

Physical symptoms of anorexia nervosa include a significant loss of weight, a refusal to eat, amenorrhea, and a denial of unusual eating behaviors or weight change. A diagnosis may be made only when a woman has become amenorrheic, meaning that she has missed three or more consecutive menstrual periods. Psychological symptoms of this eating disorder include a distorted body image, confusion of self-image, a sense of being incompetent, depression, and withdrawal from others.[24] Individuals also tend to become socially withdrawn as the disorder progresses. Researchers note that the most notable belief shared by women with anorexia is that weight, shape, or being thin is the predominant reference for establishing personal value or self-worth.[25] Other identified psychological features of the illness include the following:

- A frustration over becoming overweight
- A fear of losing control over eating
- A loss of judgment relative to the requirement of food as a basic need for the body
- An unrealistic sense of body image

Women with anorexia often display obsessive-compulsive behaviors, such as obsessing about becoming fat and, consequently, compulsively exercising or practicing odd eating rituals to avoid becoming fat. Other compulsive activities may include constant weighing, looking in the mirror, and taking body measurements. Women with anorexia also are obsessed with food and eating, and will often cook, prepare, and shop for food for others. They will eat in secret and reject food in public. Table 12.5 compares the symptoms of anorexia nervosa with those of bulimia nervosa.

Anorexia nervosa usually strikes in early to late adolescence. A general characteristic of the anorectic personality is a feeling of overall ineffectiveness as a person. The typical anorexic woman is highly critical of herself, has poor self-esteem, and believes that she is quite inadequate in most areas of personal and social functioning. She often feels powerless and unable to control many areas of her life, so she establishes power over her food intake and weight. Because of her perfectionist tendencies, the woman with anorexia believes that the ultimate sign of control is a "perfect" body. Symptoms of depression, with large mood swings, are commonly

I look in the mirror and see myself as grotesquely fat—a real blimp. My legs and arms are really fat and I can't stand what I see. I know that others say I am too thin, but I can see myself and I have to deal with this my way.

100-pound anorexic girl

Table 12.5	Symptoms of Anorexia Nervosa/Bulimia Nervosa

Symptoms of Anorexia Nervosa	**Symptoms of Bulimia Nervosa**
Loss of at least 15% of body weight	Repeated (usually secretive) episodes of bingeing and vomiting
Intense fear of weight gain	
Distorted body image (feeling fat even when too thin)	Feeling out of control during a binge
	Purging after a binge (vomiting, use of laxatives or diuretics, excessive exercise)
Absence of three consecutive menstrual periods (amenorrhea)	
	Frequent dieting
Insistence on keeping weight below a healthy minimum	Extreme concern with body weight and shape

Table 12.6	Medical Complications of Anorexia Nervosa

Dehydration	Lethargy
Reduced body fat resulting in low body temperature and the inability to stand cold	Constipation
	Organ damage and failure
Mild anemia	Loss of essential minerals, including those necessary for regulating heartbeat and keeping the bones strong
Amenorrhea	
Abdominal pain	

seen in individuals with the disorder. Various medical conditions also may arise from anorexia, as described in Table 12.6.

There has been a disturbing increase in "pro-ana" (supporting anorexia) Web sites. These sites offer their viewers tips on starving themselves, hiding their habits, and different ways to purge. Because eating disorders are often intensely private, these Web sites can offer those suffering from the disorder a sense of community and understanding. Unfortunately, the behavior they support can be life threatening.

Bulimia Nervosa

Bulimia nervosa is a disorder characterized by cyclic binge eating **(bingeing)** followed by purging. Bulimia was first identified in 1873. By the 1940s, it was considered symptomatic of anorexia nervosa—self-imposed starvation. In 1979, bulimia nervosa was first described as a separate disorder from anorexia. Prevalence rates for bulimia range from 1% to 16%, with the highest rates occurring in adolescents and young adults.[24]

Bulimia nervosa is classified in the DSM-IV as an eating disorder associated with four factors:

- Recurrent episodes of binge eating (at least two episodes per week for at least three months)

- A feeling of lack of control over eating behavior during the binge
- Regular engagement in purges
- Persistent over-concern with body shape and weight

Bulimia is a progressive disorder that usually begins with extreme hunger as a result of long periods of food deprivation from fasting or dieting and subsequent attempts at eating while still trying to control weight. Women with this eating disorder often maintain normal body weight but are extremely dissatisfied with their bodies. Some bulimics have reported that in their preadolescent years, they gained feelings of self-control and power through this self-denial. The situation progresses to out-of-control binges/purges because the artificial elimination methods have relieved the feeling of being "stuffed," and the bulimic believes it is a good way to lose weight.

Binges often occur when bulimics feel that they have passed a self-imposed limit on acceptable food intake. Consequently, they feel defeated and generally gorge until they are interrupted or the food runs out. During such binges, the caloric intake may range from 2,000 to 3,000 calories and generally lasts for less than two hours but has been reported to last as long as eight hours. The binge foods of choice are usually high-calorie, easily ingested "junk" food that requires little preparation and can be obtained while keeping the binge secret from others.

Bulimics have been known to use several modes of purging:

- Emetics
- Diuretics
- Laxatives
- Fasts
- Enemas
- Diet pills
- Chewing for hours and then spitting out the food
- Regurgitation by placing fingers or other objects down the throat
- Excessive exercise

The number of different methods of purging is a stronger index of the severity of the woman's condition than is the frequency of use of any one type.

The binge-purge cycle may occur anywhere from once or twice weekly to several times daily. The psychological components of the cycle vary from person to person, though most people with this disorder share certain similarities. The cycle begins in response to a strong emotion, either positive or negative; this can be a food craving, stress, sleeplessness, anxiety, joy, excitement, physical or emotional pain, helplessness, hopelessness, loneliness, or sadness. After the binge, some women say they initially feel relaxed and soothed, but then these feelings turn to shame, guilt, and self-hatred. The women then feel the need to purge to relieve the fear of weight gain and to regain a sense of control and purity. After the purge, bulimics may feel relieved that they have controlled their weight but guilty and negative about succumbing to the cycle again. These feelings of guilt invariably lead the bulimic to perpetuate the behavior.

Bulimia has traditionally afflicted adolescent to young adult females from middle-class backgrounds, but it affects members of other groups as well. Many women trace their cyclical behaviors to transitional points in their lives when they were changing their dependent status, such as when they were going to college or getting married. Also, in the past several decades, the media have promoted unreasonable thinness as the epitome of beauty. Many bulimic women have been socialized to attain this ideal.

The victims of bulimia often appear to be independent high achievers and are of normal weight. These young women, however, are typically perfectionist, obsessive-compulsive, depressed, intense, insecure, sensitive to rejection, anxious to please, and dependent on others. They may be socially isolated as a result of their all-consuming preoccupation with food and weight and their struggle to hide their eating behavior. Because of their strong negative self-concept, they may fear rejection. Many women with bulimia have expressed the feeling that they were deprived or lacking in affection as children, and food binges seem to fill the emotional void. The majority of women who suffer from bulimia are aware that their eating habits are abnormal, but may believe that they have the ultimate weight control secret of being able to "have their cake and eat it, too." Other factors thought to contribute to the development of bulimia include family problems, maladaptive behavior, self-identity conflicts, history of sexual abuse, and cultural overemphasis on physical appearance. In addition to the psychological problems, bulimia nervosa can cause a variety of physical problems (Table 12.7).

Binge Eating Disorder

Binge eating disorder (BED) is characterized by compulsive overeating without attempting to purge. Defining factors of BED include recurrent episodes of binge eating at least two days per week for a minimum of six months, as well as an overall sense of loss of control over the binges (Table 12.8). Women with BED also have a preoccupation with food and weight, as well as a distorted body image.

Binge eating disorder is different from non-purging bulimia nervosa, because people with non-purging bulimia binge after periods of fasting and use excessive exercise as a way to compensate for their binges. Most people who suffer from BED are obese and have a long history of weight fluctuations. Women who suffer from BED are at high risk for medical problems associated with obesity, as well as depression and anxiety due to guilt and feelings of self-disgust. Many people with BED have reported histories of major family dysfunction and childhood abuse.

Because binge eating disorder has been identified only recently, no standard treatment programs have been developed for it. Most people who have BED are treated in conventional weight-loss programs for obesity, which pay little attention to bingeing—even though 10% to 20% of the people in these programs have binge eating disorder. Most people who have the disorder accept this situation because they are more concerned about their obesity than their bingeing.

Table 12.7	Medical Consequences of Binge Eating/Purging

Medical Consequences of Binge Eating

Hypoglycemia—a sugar deficiency that may cause dizziness, headaches, fatigue, irritability, numbness, anxiety, and depression.

Neurological abnormalities.

Lethargy, inactivity, lowered metabolism.

Medical Consequences of Purging

Spontaneous regurgitation ("reverse peristalsis" after about five years of persistent vomiting).

Dental erosion on the palatal (inner) surface of the teeth as a result of the continual exposure to stomach acids in vomitus. This erosion is compounded by high sugar intake; excessive citric juices, which are taken to quench continuous thirst; and decreased saliva. Eventually erosion may lead to cavities, tooth loss, faulty bite, and gum disease.

Abscesses and sores in the mouth.

Bleeding in and tearing of the esophagus.

Choking feelings from stomach protrusion into the diaphragm—known as a hiatal hernia.

Salivary gland infection and swelling.

Hypokalemia—a deficiency of potassium because of impairment in the uptake of minerals in the alimentary canal. Hypokalemia leads to muscle fatigue, numbness, erratic heartbeat, kidney damage, and paralysis depending on the duration of the disorder.

Sodium and potassium deficiencies—mineral deficiencies that cause electrolyte imbalances, dehydration, kidney malfunction, seizures, and muscle spasm depending on the severity of the illness. Sodium deficiency leads to loss of skin elasticity, dry tongue, and low blood pressure.

Substance abuse of laxatives and diuretics, which leads to or is concurrent with abuse of and addiction to appetite suppressants, including cocaine and amphetamine/diet pills.

Constipation for laxative users; intestinal distress similar to inflammatory bowel disease for irritant (castor oil, cascara) users.

Table 12.8	Loss of Control in Binge Eating Disorder

A person must have at least three of these five criteria:

- Rapid eating
- Eating when not physically hungry
- Eating while alone
- Eating until feeling uncomfortable
- Feeling self-disgust concerning the binge

Treatment

Eating disorders are intensely secretive in most cases. Due to the nature of either not eating enough, bingeing and purging, or excessive exercise behaviors, however, friends and family members of girls affected by these disorders often have an idea that they are occurring. Many try to ignore their suspicions so as to protect the privacy of their friend or family member or out of a wish not to interfere. Women with bulimia are often able to identify themselves. In contrast, women with anorexia are often in denial about their condition and usually are brought to treatment by concerned family members. Many women enter therapy to treat an eating disorder only after being persuaded to do so by people in their lives. It thus becomes extremely important for people to confront the women in their lives when they suspect disordered eating, and to provide them with support in finding the appropriate help. As with all health interventions, sensitivity and care need to be taken when discussing eating disorders with individuals, and one needs to have an understanding of the very central and painful role the disorder may play in an individual's life.

Several approaches are used to treat eating disorders, including motivating the patient, enlisting family support, and providing nutrition counseling and psychotherapy. Behavior modification therapy and drug therapy, such as antidepressants, may be used as well. Hospitalization may be required for those patients with life-threatening complications or extreme psychological problems. If the patient's life is not in danger, treatment may be provided on an outpatient basis and may last for a year or longer.

In individual sessions of psychotherapy, the victim is encouraged to explore her attitudes about weight, food, and body image. Then, as she becomes more aware of her problems in relating to others and dealing with situational stress, the focus changes to her self-esteem, guilt, anxiety, depression, or helplessness. The issue of weight gain for people with anorexia or weight loss for those with binge eating disorder is normally not dealt with initially. Instead, constructive, nonjudgmental feedback is given to promote growth and independence. In behavior modification therapy, the focus is on eliminating self-defeating behaviors.

Other types of therapy may be used in conjunction with individual therapy. Family therapy is usually encouraged to improve overall family functioning. Group therapy may help to reduce feelings of isolation and secrecy and may be especially important for bulimics. Self-help groups are usually an adjunct to primary treatment. Through sharing of experiences, members provide mutual emotional support, exchange information, and diminish feelings of isolation.

Based on the treatment of bulimia nervosa, specific treatments for binge eating are being developed, including psychotherapy and drugs such as antidepressants and appetite suppressants. Although both treatments are reasonably effective in controlling binge eating, psychotherapy appears to have longer-lasting effects.

Treatment is often a lengthy and difficult process, with many women suffering from relapses. Most experts agree that a realistic body image concept is a precondition for recovery from an eating disorder. Treatment and prevention strategies often emphasize the importance of accepting one's body and developing positive self-esteem. Some evidence suggests that anorexia nervosa may be treated successfully, but most evaluations are not so encouraging. Although treatment is lengthy and difficult, it is necessary. Studies show that one in 10 cases of eating disorders leads to death through starvation, cardiac arrest, gastric hemorrhaging, or suicide.[26]

Other Disorders

Personality Disorders

Personality disorders are characterized by distorted and inflexible thoughts and behaviors that make it impossible for a person to live a productive life or establish fulfilling relationships. These types of disorders have created controversy in the field of psychiatry because it is often difficult to decide when the personality style of a person becomes deviant. For a woman to be diagnosed with a personality disorder, she must be experiencing long-term patterns of the distorted thoughts and behaviors and these behaviors must cause interpersonal trouble. A number of different personality disorders exist (Table 12.9), with histrionic and borderline personality disorders being the most commonly diagnosed in women.

Many people with personality disorders never enter treatment, although those who do usually seek help for depression or anxiety. Treatment can be beneficial, and it often involves long-term psychotherapy, cognitive behavioral therapy, and/or family or group therapy. Medications are frequently given in conjunction with psychotherapy to relieve symptoms of depression or anxiety. Antidepressants, antianxiety medications, and anticonvulsants are examples of such medications.

Table 12.9   Types and Symptoms of Personality Disorders

Antisocial: disrespectful of others; often in trouble with authorities

Avoidant: extremely inhibited socially; low self-esteem; intense fear of rejection

Borderline: poor self-image; unstable relationships; mood swings; impulsive behavior; extreme fear of being abandoned; self-destructive behaviors such as drug abuse, casual sex, and binge eating

Dependent: submissive; feelings of worthlessness; allows others to make important decisions; common in women who have suffered domestic abuse

Histrionic: seeks attention; acts overly emotional to attract desired attention; constantly seeks approval; is demanding and needy in relationships

Narcissistic: needs constant admiration and attention; has low self-esteem and an exaggerated sense of her own importance; constantly worried what others think of her

Obsessive-compulsive: obsessive about certain areas of life, including work; perfectionist tendencies; controlling personality

Paranoid: extremely distrustful; suspicious of others; extremely jealous, unforgiving, and quick to anger

Passive-aggressive: passively resists taking on responsibilities; consistently fails to live up to demands placed on her; often is irritable and complaining, resulting in problems in relationships

Schizoid: cannot form close relationships; has a very limited range of emotions; may lead to schizophrenia

Schizotypal: cannot form close relationships; eccentric in behavior; experiences distorted thinking and strange speech and behavior patterns; suffers from extreme social anxiety; often suspicious of others

Schizophrenia

Psychosis is a severe mental disorder characterized by loss of contact with reality and severe personality changes. **Schizophrenia,** a type of psychosis, represents an extraordinarily complex group of disorders and is the most chronic and disabling of the severe mental disorders. Many subtypes of schizophrenia exist, each of which is characterized by specific symptoms and a certain degree of disease severity. The word "schizophrenia" comes from the Greek word for "split," describing the splitting of coherent thoughts in those who suffer from the illness.

Schizophrenia afflicts about 2.5 million Americans, with men and women being affected equally. Gender differences are apparent in the development of the disease, however. Men are more likely to be affected between the ages of 16 and 25, whereas women are more likely to have a disease onset between the ages of 25 and 30. Women typically start with a milder form of the disease, experiencing more mood symptoms than psychoses. A significant proportion of women with schizophrenia experience an increase in symptoms during pregnancy and the postpartum period.

Symptoms of schizophrenia can appear either gradually over a period of years or suddenly. Women may have hallucinations and delusions, disordered thinking, and an impaired ability to manage emotions, interact with others, and think clearly. Some women have chronic suffering, whereas others experience random episodes of symptoms throughout life. Chronic sufferers often require long-term treatment and never fully recover to normal functioning. Studies show that vulnerability to schizophrenia is inherited. Researchers have identified subtle abnormalities in the structure, function, and biochemistry of brains of people with schizophrenia. They also are looking at the possibility that inappropriate neuron connections are made during fetal development but that the effects of the defect do not become apparent until puberty.

Fewer than half of people with schizophrenia get adequate treatment. New medications that cause fewer side effects have been developed over the last decade. A newly developed class of drugs, the atypical antipsychotics, are more effective than older types of drugs, but have much more severe side effects. Psychotherapy and support groups also may be helpful for some patients. Schizophrenia is a difficult disease; only one in five people recovers completely and one in 10 takes his or her own life.[27]

Dissociative Disorders

Dissociative disorders develop as an unconscious way to protect oneself from emotional traumas by detaching from a part of one's personality. These disorders occur as a response to a severe childhood trauma. The created defense appears helpful to the individual, but is actually detrimental to the process of recovery.

Several types of dissociative disorders exist, with the most common being dissociative identity disorder, also known as multiple personality disorder. Dissociative identity disorder is associated with early childhood abuse and usually has its onset in late adolescence or early adulthood. The disorder is progressive in nature and often coexists with personality disorders. Women with this disorder are unable to process

My brother had schizophrenia. He just started hearing voices when he was in his twenties. He was married, in graduate school, and he just fell apart. I took care of him, but my family was too embarrassed to deal with him. He hated the way the medication made him feel and he hated how he was when he was off the drugs, so he took his own life. I was so angry with him for doing that, at myself for not being able to prevent it, and at my family for not helping him. But now I feel that I need to do something—to educate people about mental illness, to advocate for research to get better treatment, and to help erase the stigma that goes along with mental disorders.

26-year-old woman

their thoughts, feelings, memories, and actions into a complete and single state of consciousness. Signs of dissociative identity disorder include amnesia, lack of reality, and detachment from oneself through depersonalization. People with dissociative identity disorder often hurt themselves intentionally in acts of self-mutilation. Treatment includes psychotherapy to integrate the various personalities and to resolve feelings surrounding the traumatic event.

Dissociative amnesia, another form of a dissociative disorder, is loss of memory resulting from trauma. Depending on the form of dissociative amnesia, either some or all of the experiences from various time periods are blocked out. Therapy is used to help the person adjust to the current situation rather than to resolve the past.

Suicide

In most cases, there are warning signs that a person is at risk of suicide. More than 90% of people who kill themselves have depression or another diagnosable mental or substance abuse disorder. Adverse life events like a death in the family, a relationship breakup, or financial ruin, along with other risk factors, also may make a person more likely to take his or her own life. It is important to remember, though, that suicide is not the normal response to stress. Many people have considered suicide at some point in their lives when they were depressed or experienced something very bad. Most would never act on these thoughts, and are thus not considered suicidal.

Risk factors for someone being suicidal include the following:

- Adverse life events in combination with other factors such as depression
- Prior suicide attempt
- Family history of mental disorder or substance abuse
- Family history of suicide
- Family violence, including physical or sexual abuse
- Firearms in the home
- Incarceration
- Exposure to suicidal behavior of others, including family members, peers, and even the media

Although more women than men report attempts at suicide, more men complete the act. In 1999, suicide was the eleventh leading cause of death in the United States—the eighth leading cause of death for males, and the nineteenth leading cause of death for females. For many people, an attempt at suicide is a "cry for help." In adults, the strongest risk factors for attempting suicide are depression, substance abuse, and separation or divorce. Risk factors for children and adolescents include depression, substance use, and aggressive behavior. Friends and family members of people with known depression or with one of the risk factors mentioned earlier should pay close attention to their loved ones. If they demonstrate suicidal behaviors or discuss suicidal wishes, it is important to seek professional psychiatric, social work, or medical help immediately.

Suicide has become a major problem in many developing countries and Eastern European countries. Among rural communities in China and many former Soviet bloc countries, it is currently the leading cause of death for young women.

Preventive interventions for suicide are often intensive. They typically require learning new coping skills, recognizing the underlying factors causing distress, and receiving appropriate treatment for existing mental and substance abuse disorders.

Factors Affecting Mental Health

Most mental disorders are caused by a combination of biological, psychosocial, and environmental factors. Psychosocial and environmental factors change throughout a woman's lifetime and influence the way a woman views herself, responds to stress, and interacts with others. Factors such as an increased negative concept of self or low self-esteem, or experiences such as abuse or trauma, can make a person vulnerable to mental illness.

Biological Factors

Biological factors vary among mental illnesses, but often include genetic predisposition to a disease, abnormal brain structure or function, and irregular levels or activity of neurotransmitters or hormones.

Many studies have been conducted on twins and families to determine genetic factors that create vulnerability to mental illness. Most people with mental disorders have a history of mental illness in their family, providing evidence of a genetic link. To add further evidence, limited studies on twins who were separated at birth show similar rates of mental illness among sets of twins.

Another possible biological factor in mental illness is the influence of hormones during reproductive-related events. Although studies have produced conflicting findings, it appears that a change in levels of hormones has some effect on mental well-being and may be a factor in depression during premenstrual syndrome, postpartum depression, and postpartum psychosis. Brain structure and function, as well as neurotransmitter levels, also have been studied to identify gender-related differences and differences between people with and without mental illness.

Nutrition

Several studies have looked at the impact of diet on mental health. The Food and Mood project out of the United Kingdom found that certain foods tend to increase stress levels while others help to calm the physiological effects of stress. "Food stressors" include chocolate, caffeine, sugar, and alcohol. Supporting foods include water, vegetables, fruit, and oil-rich fish. The study also found that eating regular meals and eating healthy snacks has a positive effect on mental health.

The impact of nutrition on mental health is considered secondary, however, to other, more central physiological and environmental factors.[28]

Social and Psychosocial Factors

Social and psychosocial factors change throughout a woman's lifetime and influence the way a woman views herself and interacts with others. Women with low incomes, low levels of education, and poor employment environments have higher rates of mental illness than do women of a higher socioeconomic status. These higher rates likely result from a combination of the undervalued or nonvalued roles that these women fill and the financial difficulties that accompany such roles. Women in roles not highly valued by society, such as full-time homemakers, often suffer from low self-esteem. Also, women who are trying to fill multiple roles often feel overwhelmed, which may lead to low self-esteem and, in some cases, depression. One interesting study that looked at the value of roles and self-esteem was conducted among Amish women. In Amish society, the woman's role as mother is highly valued and considered equal to the man's role as breadwinner. Results of the study showed that these women did not have low self-esteem and that there were no gender differences in the rate of depression among the Amish.[8]

Gender roles are created by the way parents view their male and female children and the values placed on different genders by society. They create stereotypes for males and females and dictate appropriate behavior for each sex. Societal constraints often present a black-and-white picture of gender—for example, seeing men as aggressive and women as passive, men as independent and women as dependent, men as stoic and women as emotional, men as strong and women as weak. Consequently, parents often interact with girls and boys differently, encouraging girls to be delicate, nurturing, nonaggressive, and sensitive to the feelings of others, and teaching boys to be assertive, aggressive, and dominant. For many women, aggression can turn inward, resulting in aggression directed at oneself and manifested as depression or another mental illness.

As children reach puberty, gender differences become even more apparent. A girl's success is often based on popularity and attractiveness, whereas a boy's success is often based on athleticism and academic achievement. Factors such as these lead many girls to base their self-esteem on their physical appearance and body weight. One study showed that women appear to attribute their successes to luck and their failures to lack of ability, whereas men attribute their successes to ability and their failures to bad luck.[8]

Research also shows that on all grade levels, girls receive less attention than boys do. Studies by the American Association of University Women revealed that girls' skills in science and mathematics lag by junior high, as does their self-esteem. Other studies have shown that girls generally make better grades than boys do, but that girls experience more internal costs—worry, anxiety, and depression—despite their academic success. As the authors of one study note, "although girls may have

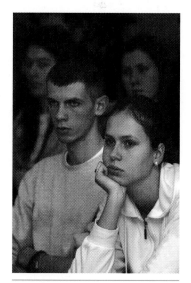

Young girls often lag behind boys in self-esteem and they are more likely to experience depression.

the edge over boys in terms of their performance in school, this edge is lost when it comes to the experience of internal distress."[29]

As girls reach the transition to puberty and become more self-critical, the rate of depression among girls increases, and the gap between the rates of depression for boys and girls expands. In addition, the different socialization of boys and girls as they age affects how women respond in relationships and handle stress, and possibly affects a woman's risk of mental illness.

Discrimination—being singled out by others based on sexual, ethnic, or physical characteristics—is another risk factor for mental illness. It can be manifested in many aspects of a woman's life, including work, marriage, and social status. Discrimination is one form of abuse, which in turn is a risk factor for mental illness. Abuse, whether physical or mental, puts women at high risk for developing mental disorders such as depression, post-traumatic stress disorder, or obsessive-compulsive disorder. Many people with mental disorders suffered from childhood abuse or traumas, and their disorders represent a response to their repressed emotions. This factor may partly account for women's increased incidence of certain mental disorders, because women are at a higher risk of being victimized through rape, abuse, and sexual harassment.

Other reasons that women suffer from mental disorders may relate to their individual personality traits. Women who are prone to pessimistic thinking, have a low self-esteem, feel they have little control over life events, and worry excessively are at higher risk for depressive and anxiety disorders. Many women also have a heightened sense of sympathy and empathy, which leaves them more vulnerable to suffering from depression after tragic events. Some experts believe that these characteristics are part of how females are conditioned versus males.

Stress

Stress is the response, be it physical, mental, or emotional, that a person displays when subjected to any type of stressor. Stressors can range from daily hassles to life-altering events, and they are experienced and perceived by people in very different ways. The changing and conflicting roles for women often create greater stress and, therefore, a higher possibility of the development of several mental health problems. Today's women face special stressors. More women are members of the paid workforce, especially those with young children. Although studies show that, on average, women who work outside the home are happier than those who do not, women still experience greater stress from having to satisfy numerous demands and fill multiple roles. For most women, responsibilities inside the home have remained the same, creating a "second shift" after a woman returns from her day job. Domestic chores, child care, and running errands sap women of their energy and cause stress that affects both their home life and their work life.

In general, people perceive, evaluate, and respond to stressors in diverse ways. Women and men may respond differently to overwhelming stress, for example. Men respond positively with physical activity, but negatively through aggression and substance abuse. In contrast, women often internalize their stress and, in doing so, abuse their self-image to produce feelings of failure and blame. Acute stress can be helpful for energizing and motivating a person, but chronic stress can overload a person and cause emotional symptoms such as edginess and distorted thinking. Chronic stress also can lead to physical symptoms such as increased heart rate and blood pressure, and lowered immune defense to common colds and other illnesses.[12]

People adopt different strategies to cope with the stress in their lives. Because stress levels change over time, individuals may adjust their coping mechanisms accordingly. Positive ways of coping with stress include relaxation techniques; supportive, positive interactions with friends and family; and exercise. People with better coping skills are less distressed overall and suffer from less pain, anxiety, depression, illnesses, and "burnout."

Stages of Life

Certain stages in a woman's life can significantly affect her emotional well-being and contribute to problems that may increase stress and lead to mental illness.

Adolescence is the age of self-doubt. Girls experience significant peer pressure while going through the physical and hormonal changes of puberty. As a girl becomes more aware of fitting into the "ideal" body image, her body changes, often adding more fat, developing wider hips, and bringing a sense of awkwardness. Teenage girls also are in the stage of forming an identity for themselves, exploring sexuality, making education and possibly career choices, establishing independence, and creating separation (which often causes conflict) from their parents. For adolescents, risk factors for mental disorders include lack of parental support, sexual abuse, low self-esteem, and weak relationships with friends or family. Some teens may not exhibit the usual signs of severe distress and may express their lack of mental wellness through substance abuse, disordered eating, behavior problems, and sexual promiscuity. Studies show that female high school students have significantly higher rates of depression, anxiety disorders, eating disorders, and adjustment disorder than their male counterparts, who have higher rates of disruptive behavior disorders.

Early adulthood brings many decisions, including those concerning career choices, relationships such as marriage or intimate partnerships, and childbearing. Reproductive events at this time in a woman's life, such as pregnancy, post-pregnancy, infertility, or the decision not to have children, may create personal stress and relationship tension. Many women also experience increased independence at this time in their lives, as well as increased financial obligations and responsibilities at work and at home.

Many women in adolescence and early adulthood begin to experiment with recreational drug use. Among women with mental health disorders, substance abuse is a common occurrence. This problem may result from these women attempting to self-medicate and cope, or from the fact that their mental disorders inhibit their reasoning skills. In addition, the prolonged use of illicit drugs can put people at higher risk for developing mental disorders. This pattern creates a "chicken or the egg" paradigm in the relationship between drug use and mental disorders.

Studies have shown that between 30% and 60% of drug abusers have mental health disorders; depression and attempted suicide are common among female substance abusers. For many of these abusers, their depressive symptoms predated their use of alcohol and other drugs. Rates of drug abuse or dependence among anorexics range from 5% to 19%; among bulimics, these rates are significantly higher, ranging from 8% to 36%.[26] These women may abuse cocaine, heroin, or methamphetamines to lose weight because these substances act as appetite suppressants. Estimates of the number of patients with bipolar disorder who also have a substance abuse problem range from 30% to 60%. In fact, substance abuse is more likely to be present with bipolar illness than with any other disorder. Individuals with bipolar disorder who abuse drugs or alcohol may have an earlier onset and worse course of illness than those who do not.

As women reach midlife, many continue to deal with career issues and financial burdens and struggle to balance their many roles of mother, wife, daughter, friend, sibling, employer, employee, and self. Women also may be dealing with stress from growing children and aging parents. The support and joy that a woman's relationships offer are often important counterbalances to the stress of managing her everyday life. As she nears late adulthood, a woman may be fortunate enough to feel satisfied with her life's accomplishments and be financially secure. If she is struggling with retirement issues, physical health, unaccomplished areas of her life, ill parents, or adult children with difficulties, however, she may feel overwhelmed by stressors that are not fully within her control.

The major mental health problems in the elderly are depression, **organic brain syndrome,** and **dementia.** A majority of the elderly people affected are women, possibly because women constitute a larger percentage of the elderly population than men. Depression is widely underdiagnosed and undertreated in the elderly population. An estimated 6% of Americans age 65 and older have a diagnosable depressive illness in any given year. Older adults in the United States are also disproportionately likely to commit suicide. Although people age 65 and older make up only 13% of the U.S. population, they accounted for 19% of all suicides in 1997.[30]

Poor physical health, limited independence, loss of privacy and freedom, and loss of one's partner or friends are contributors to stress and poor mental health in older women. Cognitive impairments in the elderly are often the result of some form of dementia, but may result from severe depression. In many cases, depression occurs concurrently with chronic medical conditions such as heart disease, diabetes, and cancer. Because of the common occurrence of depression in the elderly, many healthcare providers as well as patients and caregivers believe that depression is a normal part of aging or a normal consequence of chronic disease. Depression in older women leads to disorientation, loss of short-term memory, verbal difficulty, and inappropriate reasoning skills. Personality impairments also may result from dementia or depression or from a decrease in overall physical health.[31]

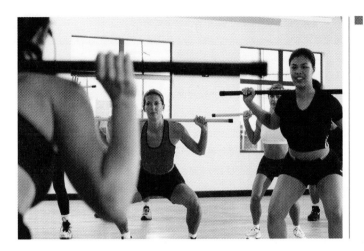

■ Women can improve their mental health by integrating physical activity into their day.

■■■■

Informed Decision Making

Good mental health is not simply the absence of mental illness. Mentally healthy people, as stated by the National Institutes of Health, are able to "...understand they are not perfect nor can they be all things to all people. They experience a full range of emotions . . . and can reach out for help if they are having difficulty with major traumas and transitions."[32]

The first step in maintaining emotional well-being is to take care of oneself. Women tend to put other people's needs before their own, creating greater stress and more illness for themselves. Women can improve their mental health by getting a good night's sleep, eating healthful foods, and integrating physical activity into their day. Women also can learn positive coping strategies to help them deal more effectively with stress. These methods of coping may better help women to handle bad moods, control their anger, and manage their stress.

The next step is to seek help. If a woman finds herself unable to cope with life's daily challenges, feels unhappy or anxious most of the time, or feels unstable mentally, she should go for treatment. Self-Assessment 12.1 can help a woman determine whether she needs to seek help.

Seeking professional help is a personal decision. To make progress, a woman must be an active and responsible participant in her treatment. Her first responsibility is to find a mental health provider whom she can trust. Psychiatrists, psychologists, and social workers are all certified and licensed practitioners who have education and training in helping people with mental health problems. When looking for a therapist, a woman should ask questions about the therapist's licensing, number of years of practice, experience treating someone with a similar medical problem, fees, types of insurance that are accepted, and methods of treatment used.

Self-Assessment 12.1

Determining One's Need to Seek Professional Help

Experiencing any of the following symptoms for several weeks may be an indication that a person needs to seek professional help.

_____ Feelings of sadness, hopelessness, or worthlessness

_____ Loss of energy and drive

_____ Behavioral changes, such as restlessness, irritability, or self-destructive behavior

_____ Physical symptoms, such as headache, nausea, backache, or unexplained pain

_____ Prolonged worry or anxiety without any identifiable cause or reason

_____ Sudden episodes of intense and overwhelming fear for no apparent reason

_____ Irrational and uncontrollable fear or panic when exposed to a particular object or situation

_____ Frequent thoughts or talk about death or suicide

Many studies have proved the benefit of combining therapy and medication. There are four basic forms of therapy:

- Traditional psychotherapy, which deals with psychosocial aspects of depression and is often referred to as "talk therapy"
- Psychodynamic psychotherapy, which deals with experiences from childhood to resolve rooted problems
- Cognitive behavioral therapy, which works to identify and correct patterns of thinking and behaviors
- Interpersonal psychotherapy, which focuses on present problems and helps with improving relationships, communication skills, and coping skills

New medications have made it easier to bring more immediate relief to people with mental disorders. Many of the new medications have fewer and less serious side effects than their predecessors. Medications for mental illness include anti-

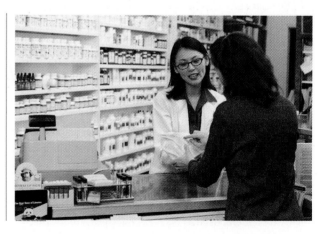

■ New medications have made it easier to bring more immediate relief to people with mental disorders.

depressants, lithium (used for bipolar disorder), antianxiety medications, and antipsychotic medications.

Another type of biomedical therapy is electroconvulsive therapy (ECT). Although much unfavorable publicity has arisen regarding ECT, research shows circumstances in which its use is medically justified. ECT is used in cases involving extreme suicide risk, psychotic agitation, or severe weight loss or physical disability. It also may be used in those people who do not respond to medications. People undergoing this type of therapy receive a muscle relaxant and general anesthesia; the application of electrical stimulation through electrodes in repeated treatments then produces a seizure in the brain. The short-term side effects of ECT include memory loss and cognitive problems. Studies show that 80% to 90% of people with severe depression improve dramatically after receiving ECT.[33]

Summary

Even with the acknowledgment of mental health as a significant issue, a stigma persists surrounding mental illness and its treatment. Viewing mental illness as a "weakness" creates a new barrier to treatment, above and beyond such existing barriers as limited access to mental health services, lack of insurance coverage, and the time involved in recovery. For people with mental disorders, the stigma leads to a

Profiles of Remarkable Women

Carola Eisenberg, M.D. (1917–)

Carola Eisenberg is a lecturer in the Department of Social Medicine at Harvard Medical School. A native of Argentina, Eisenberg first became interested in psychiatry and medicine as a teenager when she accompanied her father on a tour of Argentina's state psychiatric hospital. The conditions horrified her, prompting her to begin working at the hospital and studying to become a psychiatric social worker. She later attended medical school with an almost exclusively all-male student body.

After completing medical school in 1943 as one of only a handful of women graduates, Eisenberg came to the United States to pursue her study of child psychiatry. She accepted a fellowship at the Johns Hopkins University School of Medicine, where she later became an assistant professor of pediatrics and psychiatry. In 1968, Eisenberg became a staff psychiatrist at MIT's Student Health Service. Four years later, she became MIT's first woman Dean of Student Affairs. In 1978, she was asked to serve as Dean of Student Affairs at Harvard Medical School.

Eisenberg began working for human rights with the American Public Health Association after the sons of two friends were murdered by the military dictatorship in Argentina. She eventually met up with a number of other physician colleagues who joined together to form Physicians for Human Rights (PHR). Since its inception, PHR has grown to include approximately 5,000 health professionals. Eisenberg integrates human rights and the responsibilities of physicians into her teaching at Harvard while she continues to lecture on psychiatry.

Profiles of Remarkable Women

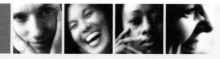

Dorothea Lynde Dix (1804–1887)

Dorothea Lynde Dix was a nurse and humanitarian who was instrumental in the reform of treatment of the mentally ill. Dix became interested in this issue when she visited a prison in Massachusetts that housed a number of mentally ill people. She saw naked prisoners in chains being kept in filthy quarters, with visible signs of harsh treatment and abuse. Dix spent the next two years researching the situation and then reported her findings to the Massachusetts legislature. Responding to her plea for humane care for the mentally ill, Massachusetts took action and moved the mentally ill people to an asylum. Dix sought change all over the United States through legislative reform, and her work prompted the establishment of 32 mental health hospitals across the United States. Dix also made an international impact, recommending reforms for prisons in Italy, France, Russia, Scotland, and Turkey.

greater loss of self-esteem and social acceptability. People with mental disorders may also fear repercussions in their careers or fear the loss of children in welfare rulings or divorce settlements. Many people have extreme views of those with mental illness and say that they would exclude them from a job or not consider them for an intimate relationship.[34, 35] Although today individuals with mental disorders face less discrimination than in the past, the harmful stereotypes associated with mental illness still affect fair access to health care, job opportunities, and general attitudes from the public. It is important for everyone to learn the signs and symptoms of mental illness so that steps can be taken to prevent and treat mental illness and maintain good emotional health.

■■■■

Topics for Discussion

1. Popular television and movie stars are often pencil thin, and young girls seek to emulate their favorite stars. What advice can an older sibling provide to a younger sister who is unhappy because she cannot achieve a size similar to her favorite star?

2. What can be done to reduce the stigma and shame that still surround mental illness?

3. How can mental health be addressed within the context of criminal rehabilitation?

4. A young woman suspects that her friend has an eating disorder. What can she do? What if her friend denies the disorder in spite of overwhelming evidence?

5. A depressed woman fears seeking treatment because she is afraid that it will affect her ability to be promoted at work. What can she do?

6. What are the ethical dilemmas with mental health?

Profiles of Remarkable Women

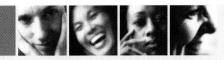

Tipper Gore (1948–)

Mary Elizabeth Aitcheson, nicknamed "Tipper" by her mother, grew up in Arlington, Virginia. Tipper met her future husband, Albert Gore, at his high school prom when she was 16, and they soon began dating. Gore headed north to study at Harvard University, and Tipper followed one year later to attend Boston University, where she majored in psychology. They were married in 1970, following Tipper's graduation, when she was just 21 and Gore was 22.

In 1975, Tipper received her master's degree in psychology from George Peabody College at Vanderbilt University in Tennessee, while she raised their first child and worked part-time as a newspaper photographer. Upon her husband's decision to run for Congress, Gore quit her job to help with his campaign and eventually moved to Washington, D.C., upon his election. As a Congressional spouse, she helped form the Congressional Wives Task Force, serving as Chair in 1978 and 1979. The task force sought to draw attention to the violence that children are exposed to through the media. She subsequently co-founded the Parents' Music Resource Center (PMRC) in 1985 to promote parental and consumer awareness of issues in popular entertainment marketed to children. Ultimately, the PMRC was successful in gaining a voluntary agreement between the Recording Industry Association of America and the National Parent Teacher Association to place consumer labels on music with violent or explicit lyrics. Those warning labels are still in use today and have served as a model for labeling efforts for television and other media. In 1987, Gore authored her first book, *Raising PG Kids in an X-Rated Society,* which detailed her efforts to seek responsibility from the entertainment industry. Gore later generated considerable controversy for her stands against sexually explicit lyrics and violent references in popular music.

A major advocate for the homeless, Gore co-founded and chaired Families for the Homeless in 1986, a nonpartisan partnership of families that raises public awareness of homeless issues. She forged a partnership with the National Mental Health Association (NMHA) to produce a major photographic exhibit entitled "Homeless in America: A Photographic Project," which toured the nation. During her husband's vice presidency, Gore shifted her focus to mental health and children's issues, supporting the Children's Health Initiative and the Mental Health Parity Act. As Mental Health Policy Advisor to President Clinton, Gore was committed to eradicating the stigma associated with mental illness. Throughout her tenure, she worked to educate Americans about the need for quality, affordable mental health care. In 1989, her son Al was hit by a car and nearly killed. It took him a year to recover from his injuries. Gore later revealed she had suffered from clinical depression and had undergone treatment for depression following the accident. She was motivated to publicly speak about her personal struggle with depression by her desire to help eliminate the stigma attached to mental illness.

7. What should you do if someone tells you they are thinking about suicide?

8. How can someone who doesn't want to be "medicated" treat depression? What are some things individuals can do to support pharmaceutical or therapy-based interventions?

■ ■ ■ ■
Web Sites

American Psychological Association: http://www.apa.org

Anxiety Disorders Association of America: http://www.adaa.org

Depression and Bipolar Support Alliance: http://www.dbsalliance.org

Depression and Related Affective Disorder Association: http://www.drada.org

National Association of Anorexia Nervosa and Associated Disorders: http://www.anad.org

National Eating Disorders Association: http://www.nationaleatingdisorders.org

National Institute of Mental Health: http://www.nimh.nih.gov

National Mental Health Information Center: http://www.mentalhealth.org

References

1. World Health Organization. (2000). *Women's Mental Health: An Evidence-Based Review*. Geneva: World Health Organization (unpublished document WHO/MSD/MHP/00.1).

2. World Health Organization. (2001). *World Health Report 2001, Mental Health: New Understanding, New Hope*.

3. Narrow, W. E. One-year prevalence of mental disorders, excluding substance use disorders, in the U.S.: NIMH ECA prospective data. Population estimates based on U.S. Census estimated residential population age 18 and over on July 1, 1998. Unpublished.

4. Murray, C. J. L., and Lopez, A. D., eds. (1996). *Summary: The Global Burden of Disease: A Comprehensive Assessment of Mortality and Disability from Diseases, Injuries, and Risk Factors in 1990 and Projected to 2020*. Cambridge, MA: Harvard University Press.

5. Murray, C. J. L., and Lopez, A. D. (2000). Progress and directions in refining the global burden of disease approach: a response to Williams. *Health Economics* 9: 69–82.

6. Lapine, J-P. (2001). Epidemiology, burden and disability in depression and anxiety disorders. *Journal of Clinical Psychology* 62(suppl 13).

7. Burt, V. K., and Hendrick, V. C. (2001). *Concise Guide to Women's Mental Health*, 2nd ed. Washington, DC: American Psychiatric Publishing.

8. Stewart, W. F., et al. (2003). Cost of lost productive work time among U.S. workers with depression. *Journal of the American Medical Association* 289(23): 3155–3144.

9. Beck, A. J., and Maruschak, L. M. (July 2001). *Mental Health Treatment in State Prisons*. Bureau of Justice Statistics. Available online at http://www.ojp.usdoj.gov/bjs/pubalp2.htm.

10. Halbreich, U., Borenstein, J., Pearlstein, T., and Kahn, L. S. (2003). The prevalence, impairment, impact, and burden of premenstrual dysphoric disorder (PMS/PMDD). *Psychoneuroendocrinology* 28(3): 1–23.

11. Nishizawa, S., Benkelfat, C., Young, S. N., et al. (1997). Differences between males and females in rates of serotonin synthesis in human brain. *Proceedings of the National Academy of Science* 94(10): 5308–5313.

12. Silberg, J., Pickles, A., Rutter, M., et al. (1999). The influence of genetic factors and life stress on depression among adolescent girls. *Archives of General Psychiatry* 56: 225–232.

13. Baron-Faust, R. (1997). *Mental Wellness for Women.* New York: William Morrow.

14. National Institute of Mental Health. (1999). *Depression: What Every Woman Should Know.* Available online at http://www.nih.nimh.gov.

15. Anxiety Disorder Association of America. (2003). *Statistics and Facts About Anxiety Disorders.* Available online at http://www.adaa.org/mediaroom/index.cfm.

16. Barlow, D. (2001) *Anxiety and Its Disorders: The Nature and Treatment of Anxiety and Panic* (second edition). New York: Guilford Press.

17. National Institute of Mental Health. (1999). *Facts About Panic Disorder.* Available online at http://www.nimh.nih.gov/publicat/panicfacts.cfm.

18. National Institute of Mental Health. (1999). *Facts About Obsessive-Compulsive Disorder.* Available online at http://www.nimh.nih.gov/publicat/ocdfacts.cfm.

19. National Center for PTSD, Department of Veteran's Affairs. (2006). What Is Post-Traumatic Stress Disorder? Available online at http://www.ncptsd.va.gov/facts/general/fs_what_is_ptsd.html.

20. Holbrook, T. L., Hoyt, D. B., Stein, M. B., et al. (2002). Gender differences in long-term posttraumatic stress disorder outcomes after major trauma: women are at higher risk of adverse outcomes than men. *Journal of Trauma* 53(5): 882–888.

21. Steiner-Adair, C., Sjostrom, L. A., Franco, D. L., et al. (2002). Primary prevention of risk factors for eating disorders in adolescent girls: learning from practice. *International Journal of Eating Disorders* 32(4): 401–411.

22. Dorian, B. J., and Garfinkel, P. E. (1999). The contributions of epidemiologic studies to the etiology and treatment of the eating disorders. *Psychiatric Annals* 29(4): 187–192.

23. Angier, N. (1999). *Woman: An Intimate Geography.* New York: Houghton Mifflin.

24. Kaye, W. H., Klump, K. L., Frank, G. K., and Strober, M. (2000) Anorexia and bulimia nervosa. *Annual Review of Medicine* 51: 299–313.

25. Blank, S., Zadik, Z., Katz, I., et al. (2002). The emergence and treatment of anorexia and bulimia nervosa. A comprehensive and practical model. *International Journal of Adolescent Medicine and Health* 14(4): 257–260.

26. Vitiello, B., and Lederhendler, I. (2000). Research on eating disorders: current status and future prospects. *Biological Psychiatry* 47(9): 777–786.

27. National Institute of Mental Health. (1999). *Schizophrenia Research at the National Institute of Mental Health.* Available online at http://www.nih.nimh.gov.

28. Lawson, W. (2003). *Eat right to fight stress. Psychology Today.* Available online at http://www.psychologytoday.com/articles/pto-2633.html.

29. Pomerantz, E., Rydell Altermatt, E., and Saxon, J. (2002). Making the grade but feeling distressed: gender differences in academic performance and internal distress. *Journal of Educational Psychology* 94(2).

30. American Association of Suicidology. (2002). *Elderly Suicide Fact Sheet.* Available online at http://www.211bigbend.org/hotlines/suicide/suicideandtheelderly.pdf.

31. Nadien, M. (1996). Aging women: issues of mental health and maltreatment. *Annals of the New York Academy of Sciences: Women & Mental Health* 789: 129–145.

32. National Institute of Mental Health. (1992). *You Are Not Alone . . . Mental Health/Mental Illness Decade of the Brain.* DHHS Publication No. (ADM) 92-1178.

33. National Institute of Mental Health. (1999). *Depression Research at the National Institute of Mental Health.* Available online at http://www.nih.nimh.gov.

34. Krisner, K. (September 2002). Eliminating the stigma of mental illness is the first stage in treatment. *Managed Healthcare Executive.* Available online at http://managedhealthcareexecutive.com/mhe/.

35. Raingruber, B. (2002). Client and provider perspectives regarding the stigma of and nonstigmatizing interventions for depression. *Archives of Psychiatric Nursing* 16(5): 201–207.

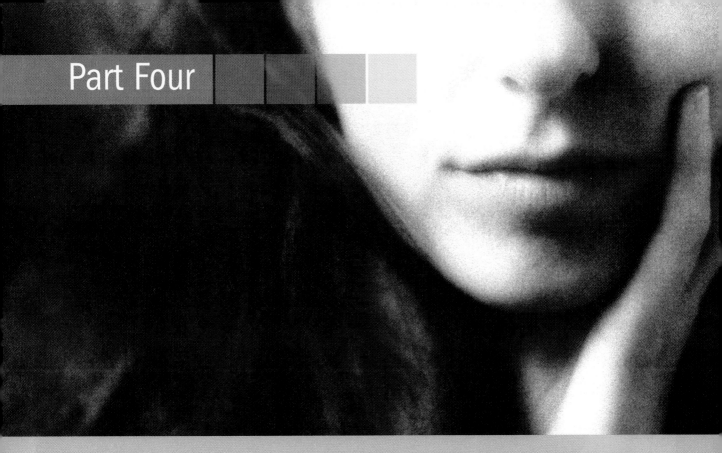

Part Four

Interpersonal and Social Dimensions of Women's Health

Chapter Thirteen

Substance Abuse

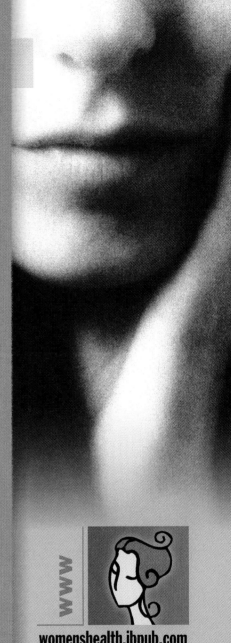

Chapter Objectives

On completion of this chapter, students should be able to discuss:

1. Substance use and abuse in women from sociocultural, legal, and economic perspectives.

2. Various dimensions of smoking.

3. The effects of smoking on a global scale.

4. Health consequences of smoking, including cardiovascular disease, cancer, other chronic diseases, and risks during pregnancy.

5. The significance of involuntary smoking from a health perspective.

6. Nicotine's role as an addictive drug and the reasons why women continue to smoke.

7. Basic strategies for quitting smoking and smoking cessation methods.

8. Epidemiological trends and various perspectives on alcohol use and abuse.

9. The physiological effects of alcohol on the body.

10. Alcoholism, the symptoms of alcoholism, and approaches to understanding alcoholism.

11. The basic treatment dimensions of alcoholism and special issues for women.

12. The mechanisms for drug entry into the body.

13. Abuse and misuse of legal and illegal drugs.

14. The risks and effects of various types of drugs.

15. The development of drug dependency and basic approaches to drug abuse treatment.

womenshealth.jbpub.com

Women's Health Online is a great source for supplementary women's health information for both students and instructors. Visit

http://womenshealth.jbpub.com to find a variety of useful tools for learning, thinking, and teaching.

Introduction

Substance abuse is defined as the overuse of, misuse of, or addiction to any chemical substance such as tobacco, alcohol, or drugs (which includes over-the-counter [OTC] and prescription medications, as well as illicit drugs). Substance abuse and substance abuse–related problems are among society's most pervasive health and social concerns. Smoking tobacco, for example, is the major preventable cause of death and disease in the United States and contributes significantly to the two leading killers in the United States, cardiovascular disease and cancer. Alcohol is associated with personal health consequences as well as alcohol-related injuries, fatalities, and crime. Over-the-counter and prescription drug abuse and misuse affect people of all ages, and are especially dangerous when combined with other medications or alcohol. Illicit drug use has profoundly affected the health of men, women, and children in the United States. Drug abuse is related to cardiac illness and death, neurological damage, fetal and infant morbidity and mortality, and infection with HIV and hepatitis.

Women are significantly affected by the entire spectrum of drug issues. An understanding of drugs, medications, dependency, and treatment issues within biological, social, and cultural contexts provides a foundation for understanding how drugs influence the quality of women's health.

Substance Use and Abuse

A **drug** is any chemical other than food that is purposely taken to affect body processes. Throughout history, people have used natural and manufactured drugs to alter their moods and serve as health aids. Opium, first cultivated in the Middle East and Asia, was used both therapeutically to induce calm and relieve pain and recreationally to induce euphoric dream states. Native Americans have used peyote,

■ Opium was used both therapeutically to induce calm and relieve pain and recreationally to induce euphoric dream states.

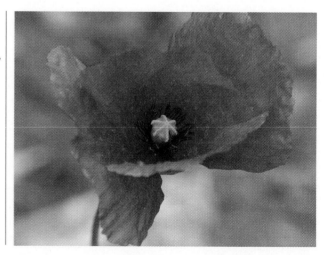

a potent hallucinogenic drug, as part of their religious practices for hundreds of years. Ancient Greek culture documented the use of many medicines, including perhaps the first hypodermic needle–like device for drug administration.

Today, drugs are consumed for legitimate health reasons, such as fighting off infections, as well as for illegal reasons, such as taking them for "fun" or pleasure. **Recreational drugs** are those drugs taken purely for fun. Although most people associate this term with illegal substances, legal substances such as alcohol, tobacco, caffeine, and many prescription drugs (such as amphetamines and tranquilizers) are also considered to be recreational drugs. All drugs, whether legal or illegal, prescribed by a doctor or purchased over-the-counter, are complex compounds that affect the body's activities.

Drugs are generally defined in terms of their legal or illegal status. The legal status of drugs, however, changes with time, customs, beliefs, and geography. In the 1920s and 1930s, for example, alcohol was illegal and marijuana was legal. Today, the reverse is true. In the early 1900s, opium, morphine, and cocaine were openly advertised and sold as "remedies" in the form of tonics, syrups, and elixirs. Coca-Cola was originally sold as both a remedy and a refreshing beverage; it contained cocaine until 1906, when the cocaine was replaced by caffeine. Today, marijuana use is tolerated in the Netherlands and in small amounts in most of Europe. Medical marijuana is legal in some countries, and a number of states in the United States have passed laws permitting marijuana use by patients with a doctor's approval. In 2005, the U.S. Supreme Court ruled that doctors can be blocked from prescribing marijuana, meaning the federal government can override state laws on patient use. Examples of illegal (illicit) drugs in the United States include marijuana, cocaine, and heroin. Despite a declared "war on drugs," drug availability continues to grow. No sector of American society is immune to illegal drugs.[1] (See Table 13.1.)

Currently legal drugs include alcohol, nicotine, caffeine, OTC drugs, and drugs obtained with a medical prescription. Prescribed medications are legal drugs that can be obtained only through the authorization of a licensed physician or dentist.

Using a drug for a purpose other than that for which it was originally intended constitutes **drug misuse.** Drug misuse includes taking more or less of a prescribed drug or using an outdated or a friend's prescribed medication. The most frequently misused OTC drugs are painkillers, sedatives, and stimulants.

Excess drug use that is inconsistent with accepted medical practice constitutes **drug abuse.** The most frequently abused prescribed medications include sleeping pills, antianxiety medications, opiates (analgesics composed of morphine or codeine), amphetamines, and steroids.

The dangers of misusing or abusing a particular drug are often associated with the drug's ability to cause addiction, or physical dependence. Many legal drugs—including barbiturates, tranquilizers, analgesics, opiates, alcohol, and tobacco—are addictive and can cause physical dependence. Besides physical dependence, drugs can create a **psychological dependence,** called habituation. Habituation is the repeated use of a drug because the user finds that each use increases pleasurable feelings or reduces feelings of anxiety, fear, or stress. Habituation becomes

| Table 13.1 | Any Illicit Drug Use in Lifetime, Past Year, and Past Month among Persons Aged 12 or Older, by Demographic Characteristics: Percentages, 2003 |

Demographic Characteristic	Time Period		
	Lifetime	Past Year	Past Month
Total	46.4	14.7	8.2
Age			
12–17	30.5	21.8	11.2
18–25	60.5	34.6	20.3
26 or older	46.1	10.3	5.6
Gender			
Male	51.2	17.2	10.0
Female	41.9	12.4	6.5
Ethnicity/Race			
Not Hispanic or Latino	47.7	14.7	8.2
White	49.2	14.9	8.3
Black or African American	44.6	15.4	8.7
American Indian or Alaska Native	62.4	18.9	12.1
Native Hawaiian or other Pacific Islander	51.0	18.5	11.1
Asian	25.6	7.1	3.8
Two or more races	60.1	20.1	12.0
Hispanic or Latino	37.0	14.7	8.0

Note: Any illicit drug includes marijuana/hashish, cocaine (including crack), heroin, hallucinogens, inhalants, or any prescription-type psychotherapeutic used nonmedically.

Source: SAMHSA, Office of Applied Studies, National Survey on Drug Use and Health. (2003).

detrimental when the person becomes so consumed by the need for the drugged state of consciousness that all energies are directed to compulsive drug-seeking behavior.

Drugs can enter the body through several modalities:

- *Oral administration.* Taking a drug in capsule, tablet, or liquid form in the mouth and swallowing it is the most common way of consuming a drug. Drugs taken orally do not reach the bloodstream as quickly as those taken by other means.

- *Through the lungs.* The user sniffs a powder, such as cocaine, inhales gases, aerosol sprays, or fumes from solvents or other compounds that evaporate

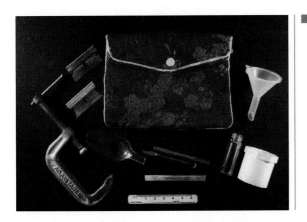

There are several ways that drugs can enter the body.

quickly, or smokes a substance. Inhaling drugs can produce serious, even fatal consequences.

- *Use of a syringe.* Drugs may be injected subcutaneously (under the skin), intramuscularly (into the muscle tissue), or intravenously (directly into a vein). An intravenous injection results in the drug getting into the bloodstream immediately. Intramuscular and subcutaneous injections are slower in action.

Several factors influence the effects of a drug:

- Each person responds differently to different drugs at different times and in different settings. A drug may intensify a woman's underlying emotional state at the time that it is taken. For example, a woman who is feeling depressed may feel more depressed.

- Generalized physical conditions such as a cold, pregnancy, or menstruation may make the body more vulnerable to the effects of a drug.

- Genetic differences among individuals may account for varying drug responses.

- Mindset has been shown to play a role in drug effects. Someone who snorts cocaine to enhance sexual pleasure may feel more stimulated simply because that is what she expects to happen.

- Social setting may influence drug effects. Drug effects at a noisy, crowded party are different from the effects produced at an intimate, subdued event.

Tolerance is the body's ability to withstand the effects of a drug. Continued use of certain drugs results in increased tolerance and decreased responsiveness, so increasingly larger doses become necessary to achieve a constant effect. Larger doses increase the risk of toxicity—the level at which a drug becomes poisonous to the body. Toxicity may result in either temporary or permanent, minor or major, body damage or death.

The use of several drugs at once is known as polyabuse. The average user who enters treatment is on five different drugs. The more drugs used, the greater the chance of side effects, complications, and possible life-threatening situations.

Sociocultural Dimensions of Women and Drug Use

The path toward drug abuse is believed to be complex, yet patterned, for women. The typical pattern begins with a breakdown of protective factors, such as family or environment, and results in an increase in fears, anxieties, phobias, and failed relationships. Studies indicate that several factors increase the likelihood of drug abuse in women:

- Significant life stresses, such as divorce, loneliness, and dissatisfaction with a career[1]
- Sexual abuse and physical abuse, beginning before the age of 11 and occurring repeatedly[2]
- Issues such as low self-esteem, self-deprecation, anxiety, and conflict

Society's double standard for women prevails in drug use. A harsher stigma has always been placed on the addicted woman than on the addicted man. The greater social sanctions against addiction in women make some women less willing to seek help and their friends and families less willing to recognize the addiction and intervene.

Females also have a higher rate of substance abuse co-occurring with other psychiatric disorders, such as depression, anxiety, post-traumatic stress disorder, eating disorders, and borderline personality disorder.

Legal Dimensions of Substance Abuse

Criminalizing drug use disproportionately affects people of color. For example, while African Americans constitute 14% of marijuana users in general, they account for nearly one-third of all marijuana arrests. Hispanic and African American drug offenders both have a greater chance of being sentenced to prison than white drug offenders (40% and 20% greater, respectively). African Americans also receive longer prison terms for drug offenses than whites do, serving nearly as much time in prison for a drug offense as whites do for a violent offense.[3]

According to the U.S. Surgeon General's Office, since 1980 the number of women in prison has increased at nearly double the rate for men. There are now nearly seven times as many women in state and federal prisons as in 1980; in particular, the number of women incarcerated for drug offenses has risen 888% since 1980, and minority women (African American and Hispanic) represent a disproportionate share of this increase. For example, in New York, minority women accounted for 91% of prison sentences for drugs, although they make up only 32% of the state's population.[4] Minority women are also least likely to receive effective drug treatment. Once arrested, many addicts are incarcerated where their addiction is either left untreated or worsens due to the widespread (albeit underground) availability of drugs in many prisons.

In addition to the legal status of the drugs themselves, some unique legal considerations are associated with drug use among women. Of particular concern is drug use during pregnancy. Pregnant drug users are at increased risk for miscarriage, ectopic pregnancy, stillbirth, low weight gain, anemia, hypertension, low-birthweight babies, and other medical problems. HIV infection, a possible consequence of intravenous drug use, is another risk among pregnant drug users. Approximately 4% of pregnant women between the ages of 15 and 44 reported being current users of illicit drugs in 2001; this number represents roughly half the rate found among nonpregnant women in the same age group (8.3%). The rates of drug use among pregnant (15.1%) and nonpregnant (14.1%) women age 15 to 17 were nearly equal.[1]

A number of states are now dealing with prenatal substance abuse through their legal systems. Some states require healthcare professionals to report prenatal drug exposure; others have amended their child welfare laws to include prenatal substance abuse, using this as evidence of child abuse to end or diminish parental rights. This approach shifts the focus to punishment and away from the urgent need to provide appropriate drug treatment programs for women. Only a few states have viewed drug use by pregnant women as a sign of the need for treatment, forcing pregnant users into inpatient treatment programs. According to the Women's Law Project, punitive reproductive health policies have an especially negative effect on low-income women and women of color. About 80% of pregnant women charged with crimes for drug abuse are women of color, and drug testing of newborns is implemented almost exclusively by public hospitals that predominantly serve low-income women.[5] Such policies may have the effect of discouraging women from seeking needed prenatal care or drug treatment.[6] The threat of criminal punishment fosters a climate of fear and mistrust between doctors and patients, potentially causing harm to the health of both women and their future children.

Economic Dimensions of Substance Abuse

According to the Office of National Drug Control Policy, drugs lead to 52,000 deaths and cost $110 billion per year in the United States.[7] The effects of drug use can be considered on both an individual and societal level. Individual effects include:

- Physiological changes
- Mental dependence
- Conflicts in relationships

Societal costs include:

- Burden of drug-related crime
- Creation of treatment facilities
- Loss of individual productivity
- Care for children of drug-dependent parents
- The policing of illicit drug availability
- Treatment of medical complications resulting from inappropriate drug use

The United States spends about $40 billion per year on the "war on drugs." While the federal government spends more than $18 billion, state and local governments spend at least another $20 billion trying to stem the drug tide.[8, 9] Around the world, illicit drugs are one of the most lucrative exports for many countries.

The economic and social forces that come into play between drug users and drug sellers are significant. Across the board, drug use is more prevalent among people of lower socioeconomic status. Use of certain drugs, such as crack cocaine, is much more common among poorer people than among affluent people. These drugs tend to be relatively affordable on a per-dose basis. Most often drugs are exchanged for money, but frequently they are exchanged for sex. This practice is most common among poor female drug users, with crack addiction being a prevalent precursor to such behavior. Exchanging drugs for sex puts women at heightened risk for acquiring a sexually transmitted disease, such as HIV infection, and for becoming a target for sexual violence.

Tobacco use and abuse have their own economic dimensions. Today, the price of a pack of cigarettes averages more than $2, with many states piling on hefty additional taxes. As a result, a pack-a-day smoker may spend close to $1,000 annually to fund her habit. In November 1998, 46 states and the tobacco industry settled the states' Medicaid lawsuits for recovery of their tobacco-related healthcare costs. The tobacco industry committed to pay the states roughly $206 billion over the next 25 years. As part of the settlement, additional payments of $5 billion were to be made to 14 states to compensate them for potential harm to their tobacco-producing communities. Four states (Mississippi, Texas, Florida, and Minnesota) settled their tobacco lawsuits separately for a total of $40 billion to be paid over the next 25 years. The money from these settlements was initially meant to be used for state health programs and antismoking campaigns. As states run into budget crises, however, much of the tobacco settlement money is being devoted to other programs.

Tobacco

Cigarette smoking is a major preventable cause of premature morbidity and mortality in the United States today. Tobacco causes more death and suffering than any other human-made material. Half of all Americans who smoke will die of a smoking-related disease. Surpassing breast cancer in 1987, lung cancer has become the leading cause of cancer death among U.S. women. Roughly 90% of all lung cancer deaths and 30% of all cancer deaths are attributable to smoking.[10] Clearly, the health consequences of smoking are devastating to women's health.

Smoking is a complex addictive behavior, but smokers are not the only individuals affected by their tobacco use. Involuntary smokers—the nonsmoking spouses, partners, co-workers, children, and even pets of smokers who inhale either the exhaled smoke from smokers or the wafts from their cigarettes—experience significant smoking-related morbidity and mortality as well.

Epidemiological Trends and Issues

Tobacco was one of the New World "discoveries" of Spanish explorers 450 years ago, although archaeological and historical evidence suggests that the use of tobacco by women antedated European consumption of the products. Tobacco became an accepted component of early colonial life, and New England colonial women reputedly smoked while performing routine domestic duties. Through the next century, tobacco was also snuffed (inhaled), dipped, and chewed.

Cigarette smoking gradually increased in popularity. Technological "improvements" to cigarettes enhanced the ease of inhalation and modified their flavor and aroma. The 1920s were a critical period of change for women, characterized by radically altered social and cultural patterns. During this period, the tobacco industry began its portrayal of smoking as a form of rebellion, romance, and emancipation for women. Women began to smoke openly in public settings, and female cigarette smoking prevalence rates rose from 2% in 1930 to 34% in 1965.

Today, about one in four women younger than age 25 and one in five women in general in the United States smoke cigarettes. Smoking rates among adults have declined by nearly half since 1965.[11,12] The decline does not seem to affect all groups of women equally, however. Current smoking rates vary based on education and race/ethnicity (see Figure 13.1 and Table 13.2).

Among adults in the United States, American Indian/Alaska Natives have the highest prevalence of tobacco use. Asian Americans and Hispanic women have the lowest prevalence. Among African Americans, Asian Americans, Pacific Islanders, Hispanics, American Indians/Alaska Natives, and whites, a higher percentage of men than women are cigarette smokers.

Among high school girls, smoking rates recently peaked in the mid-1990s but have since dropped rather dramatically. More than half of all high school students have tried smoking, establishing a pattern for becoming smokers as adults. As with adults, rates of current cigarette smoking varied among high school students by race/ethnicity (see Figure 13.2). In addition, about 15% of high school students in the United States reported smoking cigars, with males being two times more likely to do so than females.[13,14]

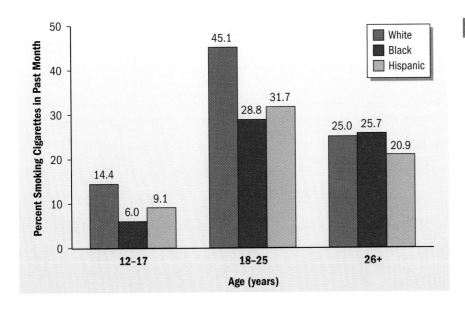

Figure 13.1

Current cigarette use, by race/ethnicity and age, 2004.

Table 13.2 Percentage of Persons Aged ≥18 Years Who Were Current Smokers,* by Sex and Selected Characteristics—National Health Interview Survey, United States, 2004

Characteristic	Men	Women	Total
Race/Ethnicity			
White, non-Hispanic	24.1	20.4	**22.2**
Black, non-Hispanic	23.9	17.2	**20.2**
Hispanic	18.9	10.9	**15.0**
American Indian/ Alaska Native	37.3	28.5	**33.4**
Asian[†]	17.8	4.8	**11.3**
Education[‡]			
<8 years	23.5	10.5	**16.7**
9–11 years	38.3	29.8	**34.0**
12 years (no diploma)	29.9	21.9	**25.5**
GED[§] diploma	42.1	36.6	**39.6**
High school graduate	27.2	21.2	**24.0**
Associate degree	24.6	18.0	**20.9**
Some college	24.6	20.3	**22.2**
Undergraduate degree	13.5	10.1	**11.7**
Graduate degree	7.9	8.1	**8.0**
Age Group (years)			
18–24	25.6	21.5	**23.6**
24–44	26.3	21.4	**23.8**
45–64	25.0	19.8	**22.4**
≥65	9.8	8.1	**8.8**
Total	**23.4**	**18.5**	**20.9**

*Persons who reported smoking ≥100 cigarettes during their lifetime and at the time of interview reported smoking every day or some days.
[†]Does not include Native Hawaiians or other Pacific Islanders.
[‡]Persons aged ≥25 years.
[§]General Educational Development.

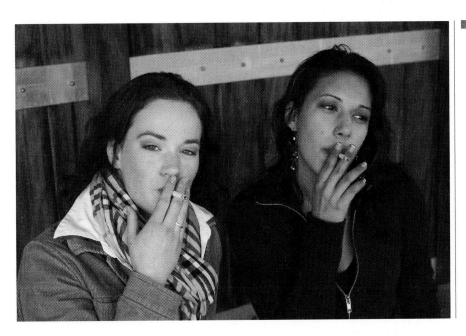

■ Females are beginning to smoke at younger ages, increasing their risk for suffering from smoke-related deaths.

Other tobacco products, such as chew or dip, are popular in certain geographic regions and among athletes. Many young athletes falsely consider the nonsmoking form of tobacco to be safer and less likely to negatively affect their athletic performance.

Societal Costs of Smoking

The human costs are the greatest toll associated with smoking. Annual tobacco-related deaths exceed the number of deaths from alcohol, cocaine, heroin, homicide,

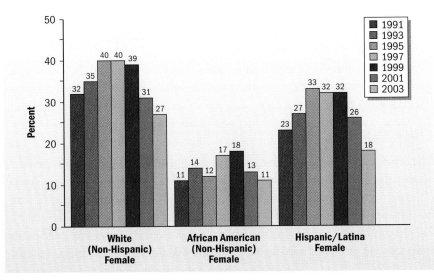

*Smoked cigarettes on one or more of the 30 days preceding the survey.

Figure 13.2

Current* cigarette smoking among female high school students, by race/ethnicity, 1991–2003.

Source: American Cancer Society, Surveillance Research. (2004). Youth Risk Behavior Surveillance System. *Morbidity and Mortality Weekly Report* 53 (23): 499–502.

suicide, car accidents, fire, and AIDS combined. Each year, approximately 435,000 deaths in the United States are attributed to cigarette smoking.[15,16] Passive smoking, or involuntary smoking, causes thousands of deaths each year as well. Smoking causes more than $150 billion per year in health-related costs, such as mortality-related productivity costs and medical expenditures for both adults and newborns.[16]

Smokers pay a human cost before dying as well. The smoking-related diseases of cancer, emphysema, and cardiovascular disease exact a toll measured in terms of suffering and disability. The estimates of costs are probably low, considering the costs for burn care from smoking-related fires and medical care costs associated with diseases from secondhand smoke, and are difficult to measure.

Legal Dimensions of Tobacco Use

All 50 states and the District of Columbia have placed some sort of restriction on smoking in certain places. The laws range from restrictions in designated areas to sweeping prohibitions in all public places and workplaces. Examples of recent smoking legislation include the following:[17A]

- **Taxes.** All 50 states and the District of Columbia impose a cigarette excise tax. Rhode Island has the highest tax at $2.46 per pack and South Carolina has the lowest at $0.07 per pack. The national average for state cigarette excise taxes is $0.90 per pack.

- **Youth Access.** All 50 states and the District of Columbia prohibit the sale of tobacco products to minors. Age restrictions vary by state; in most states, tobacco sales to youths younger than 18 are banned. Alabama, Alaska, and Utah prohibit sales to minors younger than age 19. Eighteen states and the District of Columbia require a photo ID from purchasers who appear to be younger than 18. Penalties for purchasing tobacco vary by state as well. Eight states may suspend a minor's driver's license; 14 states require attendance of a smoking education/cessation program; and 25 states order minors to pay a fine and perform community service.

- **Tobacco Product Vending Machine Sales.** Forty-six states and the District of Columbia have restrictions on where vending machines can be placed. A number of states prohibit tobacco vending machines everywhere except for bars and taverns; some states include restrictions on machines in workplaces. Two states, Idaho and Vermont, prohibit tobacco vending machines altogether.

Advertising is clearly effective in perpetuating and promoting specific products to selected groups. Cigarette advertising is especially effective in increasing cigarette consumption by recruiting new smokers, enticing former smokers to relapse, making it more difficult for current smokers to quit cigarettes, and acting as an external cue or reminder to smoke. In the past, tobacco companies have targeted specific audiences and promoted specific brands with a calculated strategic effort. Minority communities and young women have been aggressively singled out, for example. Several brands are specifically targeted to the African American community and are heavily advertised in African American–oriented media. Other advertising and promotional campaigns have sought to introduce "feminine" cigarettes, which are slim or "ultra-slim" and characterized by decorative borders and sophisticated designer packaging.

Cigarette manufacturers have responded to legal restrictions by increasing their advertising budgets. In 1998, the year that national advertising restrictions took effect, the combined marketing budget of the four largest cigarette manufacturers was $6.7 billion. By 2003, it had increased to more than $15 billion. These extra funds have been invested in new and innovative promotional campaigns.[17B]

Smoking and Women Worldwide

Around the world, nearly one-third of all adults (approximately 1.1 billion people) are estimated to be smokers. This high prevalence makes involuntary inhalation of tobacco smoke almost unavoidable throughout much of the world. Because tobacco smoking has primarily been a custom and addiction of men, women and children represent the majority of the world's passive or involuntary smokers.

The World Health Organization (WHO) estimates that approximately 700 million, or almost half, of the world's children are exposed to environmental tobacco smoke (ETS). Because the home is a predominant location for smoking, women and children are exposed to tobacco smoke most often as they carry out the tasks and pastimes of their daily lives—doing chores at home, eating, entertaining, and even sleeping. The exposures at home may be compounded for many women and children by additional exposures at work and school.[18]

Tobacco companies are savvy in the ways they lure new smokers, particularly women. According to WHO, many tobacco companies cleverly link the emancipation of women in the developing world with smoking, similar to methods that

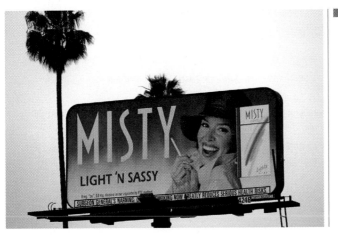

▣ Tobacco companies are savvy in the ways they lure new smokers, particularly women.

were used in Western countries decades ago. According to the Institute for Global Tobacco Control, governments in developing countries may be less aware of the harmful effects of tobacco use on women and children and are preoccupied with other health issues; they mostly see tobacco as a problem confined to men. If no dramatic changes in prevention and cessation occur, the prevalence of smoking among women in developed and developing countries could rise to 20% by 2025.[18] To counter this trend, international non-governmental organizations are banding together to address smoking as a global health crisis, especially among women. Specific research and programs are being initiated across the globe to halt women's initiation of smoking and to address the harmful effects of exposure to ETS.

Health Consequences for Women Who Smoke

Tobacco use is the single most important preventable cause of death and disease in the United States (see Table 13.3). Almost half of all smokers between the ages of 35 and 69 die prematurely. Health risks to smokers depend not only on their smoking status, but also on specific smoking behaviors and the duration of such behaviors. Morbidity and mortality rates vary directly with the amount smoked, the depth of cigarette inhalation, the "tar" and nicotine content of cigarettes, and the duration of smoking. Inhalation patterns and puffing behavior determine exposure to carbon monoxide and other toxic compounds. Mortality rates also vary inversely with initiation of smoking—in other words, the earlier a woman begins to smoke, the shorter her life. On average, women who smoke will lose 14.5 years of life from smoking.

Symptoms of smoking-related illness usually take years to develop, although irritation symptoms such as watery eyes, nasal irritation, squinting, and coughing develop fairly soon after a woman starts smoking. Smoking affects not only the smoker, but also others in the smoker's environment, including unborn babies (Figure 13.3). In addition, smoking causes premature signs of aging including wrinkles, blotchy skin, and discolored teeth.

Table 13.3   **Women's Health Consequences of Smoking**
Increased risk for cancer—lungs, larynx, oral cavity, esophagus, kidneys, and cervix
Increased risk for chronic obstructive pulmonary disease (COPD)—chronic bronchitis, emphysema
Increased risk for cardiovascular disease—myocardial infarction, chronic ischemic heart disease, arteriosclerotic vascular disease, subarachnoid hemorrhage, malignant hypertension
Complications of pregnancy and infant health—increased risk for low-birthweight babies, fetal growth retardation, preterm babies, ectopic pregnancy, spontaneous abortion, fetal death, SIDS, and neonatal death
Other risks—osteoporosis, urinary incontinence, decreased fertility, earlier menopause, peptic ulcer disease, and migraine headaches

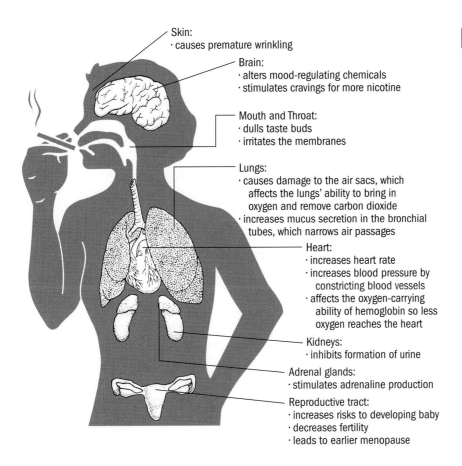

Figure 13.3

Physiological effects of cigarette smoking.

Skin:
· causes premature wrinkling

Brain:
· alters mood-regulating chemicals
· stimulates cravings for more nicotine

Mouth and Throat:
· dulls taste buds
· irritates the membranes

Lungs:
· causes damage to the air sacs, which affects the lungs' ability to bring in oxygen and remove carbon dioxide
· increases mucus secretion in the bronchial tubes, which narrows air passages

Heart:
· increases heart rate
· increases blood pressure by constricting blood vessels
· affects the oxygen-carrying ability of hemoglobin so less oxygen reaches the heart

Kidneys:
· inhibits formation of urine

Adrenal glands:
· stimulates adrenaline production

Reproductive tract:
· increases risks to developing baby
· decreases fertility
· leads to earlier menopause

Cardiovascular Disease

Cigarette smoking accounts for more than 50,000 deaths in women per year. Coronary heart disease is the major cause of death among both men and women in the United States. Cigarette smoking doubles a woman's risk of myocardial infarction (heart attack) and doubles to quadruples her risk of sudden cardiac death. The use of oral contraceptives by women smokers, especially women older than age 35, increases the risk of myocardial infarction, stroke, and blood clots. Oral contraceptive users over the age of 35 who smoke are advised to stop smoking or change their method of contraception. Young and middle-age women who smoke have substantially higher rates of both fatal and nonfatal stroke than nonsmokers. Each year, more than 8,800 deaths from stroke and 40,000 deaths from coronary heart disease are attributed to smoking in women (see Figure 13.4).[19] Smoking is also a major risk factor for arteriosclerosis and peripheral vascular disease.

Like cigarettes, cigars increase a person's risk of developing cardiovascular disease. Heavy smoking of cigars, especially for people who inhale, increases risk of coronary heart disease and chronic obstructive pulmonary disease.

Figure 13.4

U.S. male and female deaths attributable to cigarette smoking.

Source: Centers for Disease Control and Prevention. (2005). *Morbidity and Mortality Weekly Report* 54 (25): 625–628.

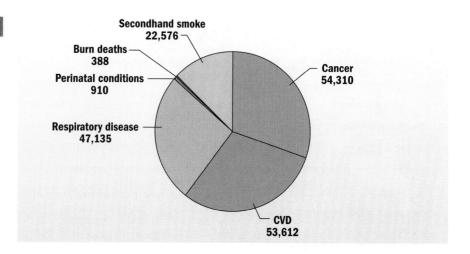

Cancer

Cigarette smoking has been shown to be a major risk factor for cancers throughout the body. More than 150,000 cancer deaths in the United States are associated with smoking each year, with 50,000 of these deaths occurring in women.[19] Smoking is associated with an increased risk of at least 15 types of cancer, including cancer of the lung, larynx, pharynx, mouth, esophagus, kidney, pancreas, and bladder in women (see Figure 13.5). Cigarette smoking and possibly exposure to passive smoke increase a woman's risk of cervical cancer as well.

Lung cancer death rates for women have increased by 400% over the past 30 years, and lung cancer is now the leading cause of cancer-related deaths among women.[18] Smoking accounts for more than 80% of lung cancer deaths in women.

Cigar smoking, like cigarette smoking, is associated with cancer of the lung, oral cavity, and esophagus.

Other Health Consequences

Cigarette smoking severely damages the respiratory system. About 8.6 million people will suffer smoking-related chronic conditions of the respiratory system. **Chronic obstructive pulmonary disease (COPD),** also known as **chronic lower respiratory disease (CLRD)** or **chronic obstructive lung disease (COLD),** is characterized by permanent airflow obstruction and extended periods of disability and restricted activity. COPD encompasses many conditions, including emphysema and chronic bronchitis, which usually occur together:

- With **emphysema,** the limitation of airflow results from irreversible disease changes in the lung tissue after years of assault on the lung tissue. The air sacs in the lungs are destroyed, which compromises the lungs' ability to bring in oxygen and remove carbon dioxide from the body. As a result, breathing becomes labored, and increased demand is placed on the heart.

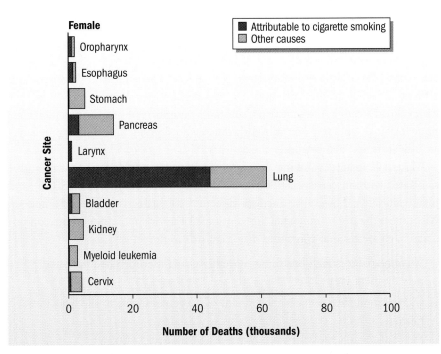

Female

Legend: ■ Attributable to cigarette smoking □ Other causes

Cancer Site (y-axis): Oropharynx, Esophagus, Stomach, Pancreas, Larynx, Lung, Bladder, Kidney, Myeloid leukemia, Cervix

Number of Deaths (thousands) (x-axis): 0, 20, 40, 60, 80, 100

Figure 13.5

Annual number of cancer deaths* attributable to smoking in females, by site—United States, 1995–1999.

Source: U.S. Department of Health and Human services. (2004). *The Health Consequences of Smoking: A Report of the Surgeon General.* Atlanta, GA: U.S. Department of Health and Human Services, Centers for Disease Control and Prevention, National Center for Chronic Disease Prevention and Health Promotion, Office of Smoking and Health.

*Among women 35 and older

- **Chronic bronchitis** is characterized by constant inflammation of the bronchial tubes. The inflammation thickens the walls of the bronchi, and the production of mucus increases, resulting in a constricting or narrowing of the air passages.

Cigarette smoking is the major risk factor for developing COPD, with 80% of all COPD deaths in women in the United States being attributed to smoking.[10] In 2002, 51% of all COPD deaths were in women. Females who smoke also are 10.5 times more likely to die from emphysema or chronic bronchitis than are nonsmokers.

Women who smoke face an increased risk of osteoporosis and early menopause, with smokers reaching spontaneous menopause one to two years earlier than non-smoking women. The age differences in menopause appear to be smoking-dose dependent. Women smokers also appear to have prematurely wrinkled skin and facial aging, and they often look older than their stated age.[20] One study also indicated that a significant relationship exists between premature gray hair and smoking.[21] Another correlation has been established between smoking and fertility, suggesting that women who smoke experience more fertility problems than do nonsmoking women. Smokers also appear to have more frequent episodes of back pain than nonsmokers, especially women who have been diagnosed with adolescent idiopathic scoliosis (sideways curve of the spine that results in an S shape of the back and is diagnosed during the teenage years).[22]

Cigarette smoking also can worsen the symptoms or complications of allergies, asthma, and existing disorders of the pulmonary and circulatory system.

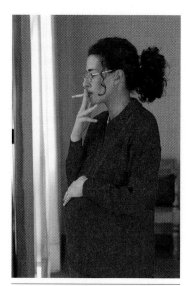

■ Smoking presents many risks to a woman and her unborn child.

Smoking and Pregnancy

Quitting smoking may be one of the most significant things a pregnant woman can do to optimize the well-being of her baby. Smoking is believed to be associated with 17% to 30% of low-birthweight babies, 14% of preterm deliveries, and 10% of all infant deaths. Although the prevalence of smoking during pregnancy has declined steadily in recent years, substantial numbers of pregnant women continue to smoke, and only one-third of women who stop smoking during pregnancy are still abstinent one year after the delivery.[23]

Maternal cigarette smoking during pregnancy also retards fetal growth and is associated with miscarriage, stillbirth, sudden infant death syndrome (SIDS), and infant mortality. These risks increase directly with increasing doses of smoking. Nicotine and carbon monoxide are considered the two most important components in cigarettes that constitute major hazards to the fetus.

- Nicotine reduces fetal breathing movements and uterine blood flow, and increases fetal heart rate.
- Carbon monoxide reduces the amount of oxygen available to the fetus by as much as 25%.

One large study showed that prenatal smoking could affect an infant's lung function two months before the baby was born by altering the structure of the baby's lungs and airways.

Maternal prenatal smoking is not the only detrimental smoking source for infants. Studies suggest that paternal smoking may present a risk for babies as well. Women can continue to transmit smoking effects via breast milk after the baby is born.

Involuntary Smoking

Involuntary smoking, also known as "passive smoking" or environmental tobacco smoke (ETS), occurs when nonsmokers breathe air contaminated by smokers. Involuntary smoking is not benign—it causes increased morbidity and mortality in healthy nonsmokers, young infants and children, and possibly even the family pet. Each year, as many as 35,000 to 40,000 deaths from heart disease, 3,000 deaths from lung cancer, and 150,000 to 300,000 lower respiratory infections in infants are estimated to occur due to ETS exposure.[13]

ETS is of special concern for babies and young children, for whom the major source of smoke exposure is the home. Involuntary smoking increases a child's risk of low birthweight; sudden infant death syndrome (SIDS); acute lower respiratory tract infections, such as bronchitis and pneumonia; induction and exacerbation of asthma; chronic respiratory symptoms; and middle-ear infections. In adults, ETS increases the risk of lung cancer, heart disease, and nasal sinus cancer. It also has been suggested that a link exists between ETS exposure and the following conditions:

- Spontaneous abortion
- Adverse effects on cognition and behavior
- Exacerbation of cystic fibrosis
- Decreased pulmonary function in adults
- Cervical cancer

For adults living in households where no one smokes, the workplace is the greatest source of exposure to ETS. The separation of smokers and nonsmokers within the same airspace may reduce, but does not eliminate, the exposure of nonsmokers to ETS. In one study, bartenders in San Francisco showed significant improvement in their respiratory symptoms after the new California laws requiring smoke-free bars went into effect; this improvement was seen within six weeks of the new laws.[24] As noted earlier, legislation in many states has mandated that many workplaces follow a nonsmoking policy. In 1986, only 3% of the United States' workforce was in a smoke-free environment. Nearly 70% of the U.S. workforce currently works under a smoke-free policy.[25]

Smoking as an Addiction

Although tobacco smoke contains literally thousands of compounds, the most significant from a health perspective are nicotine, tar, and carbon monoxide.

- **Nicotine** is the addictive element in cigarettes. It has several effects on the body, including increasing blood pressure, increasing heart rate, and negating hunger.
- Tar is a thick, sticky, dark fluid produced when tobacco is burned. It actually consists of hundreds of compounds, many of which are **carcinogenic** (capable of promoting growth of cancerous cells) in their own right. Through inhalation, tar settles and accumulates throughout the oral cavity and pulmonary system. The combination of tar and smoke further compromises the cardiopulmonary system.
- Carbon monoxide is another deadly by-product of cigarettes. This gas interferes with the ability of the blood to carry oxygen, impairs normal functioning of the nervous system, and contributes to degradation of the cardiopulmonary system.

Smoking addiction is defined as dependence on tobacco such that stopping smoking results in withdrawal symptoms. Smoking is clearly an addictive behavior, and, as noted above, nicotine is the addictive pharmacological component. Self-Assessment 13.1 provides an opportunity to assess whether an individual is addicted to cigarette smoking (or to another drug).

Smoking cessation results in withdrawal, an adverse reaction characterized by unpleasant symptoms and an intense psychological and physiological demand for nicotine. Symptoms of withdrawal usually include the following:

- Cigarette craving
- Irritability

It's Your Health

Strategies to Quit Cigarettes Gradually

Wait 15 minutes after the initial urge for a cigarette. This delay gives a feeling of control, and sometimes the urge will simply go away.

When an urge for a cigarette presents, use a distraction such as drinking water, making a phone call, taking a short walk, or brushing teeth.

Avoid the places where the smoking habit has thrived—a favorite chair, lingering after a meal, a coffee break.

Establish nonsmoking hours and gradually extend them.

Buy cigarettes only by the pack and never buy the same brand twice in a row.

Try to buy cigarette brands with successively lower levels of tar and nicotine.

Make it harder to get your cigarettes. Keep them in a locked drawer or with a friend.

Declare former smoking areas to be nonsmoking areas, such as the car, house, and office.

Don't empty ashtrays.

Collect cigarette butts and take a deep breath of the collection every day as a reminder of how dirty and smelly the smoking habit is.

Keep a daily record to document and reinforce progress with quitting.

Self-Assessment 13.1

Are You Addicted to Cigarettes?

Carefully read and answer each of the following questions honestly.

1. Have you ever failed in an attempt to give up cigarettes? yes no
2. Have you ever failed in an attempt to cut back on cigarettes? yes no
3. Have you ever failed in an attempt to switch to a lower-tar and lower-nicotine cigarette? yes no
4. When you have not smoked a cigarette for a while, do you feel any withdrawal symptoms, such as an urge for a cigarette, irritability, anxiety, difficulty concentrating, or drowsiness? yes no
5. Have you developed any smoking-related side effects, such as a morning cough or a hoarse voice, yet continue to smoke? yes no

If you answered "yes" to any of these questions, you are probably hooked on cigarettes and have an addiction to tobacco. It is time to quit cigarettes, and seek help from your healthcare provider if necessary.

- Restlessness
- Anxiety
- Difficulty in concentrating
- Headache
- Drowsiness
- Varied gastrointestinal disturbances such as diarrhea and constipation

The wide range of withdrawal symptoms that occur with cigarette smoking cessation, both physical and psychological, show considerable variability in their duration and intensity. For heavy smokers, withdrawal symptoms may occur within two hours of the last cigarette. The peak period of physiological symptoms from smoking cessation is usually 24 to 48 hours into abstinence, but many smokers report "craving" cigarettes for as long as a year. Withdrawal symptoms include depression, feelings of frustration and anger, irritability, troubled sleep, difficulty in concentrating, restlessness, headache, tiredness, and increased appetite.

Why Women Smoke

Women often initiate cigarette smoking in adolescence in the context of social interactions with peers. Adolescents are more likely to be smokers if their parents, older siblings, or peers smoke. Many smokers report that their primary reason for smoking is to give them something to do in social situations and/or to "fill time." Smoking dependence in females appears to be controlled less by the actual nicotine and more by the social situations in which smoking occurs. (See **It's Your Health** on page 531.)

Nicotine may have several different effects, sometimes acting as a relaxant and at other times functioning as a stimulant. This compound in itself reinforces and strengthens the desire to smoke. It also may facilitate short-term memory, help in performing certain tasks, reduce anxiety, negate hunger symptoms, temporarily relieve feelings of depression, and increase pain tolerance.

Fear of unwanted weight gain is a reason that many women have cited for not quitting smoking. Even many pregnant women who smoke indicate that their reason for doing so is to avoid weight gain. Smokers do tend to weigh less than nonsmokers. There is no scientific consensus yet regarding the physiological or biochemical mechanism that is responsible for this relationship between weight regulation and smoking behavior. Some evidence indicates that nicotine elevates the body's basal metabolic rate (BMR). Studies show that women gain an average of 5 pounds upon quitting smoking, but exercise combined with a smoking cessation program can decrease this weight gain and increase rates of abstinence from smoking.[26]

Women's concerns about weight gain and the maintenance of their smoking behavior sadly reflect their willingness to risk long-term detrimental—and potentially catastrophic—consequences in exchange for dealing with body image and weight-control issues. Teenage girls, in particular, often believe that smoking helps them control their weight, and this belief dissuades many from quitting this behavior. Health professionals, educators, mothers, and other female role models must strike a balance between recognizing that girls have concerns about their weight, while trying to refocus them on healthy behaviors, self-esteem, and safer coping strategies.

Quitting Smoking

Quitting smoking is the most significant personal behavior that one can undertake to improve one's health. Although the recovery from smoking takes time, cessation of smoking results in a gradual decrease in cancer and cardiovascular disease risk. For example, after 10 to 20 years of cessation, lung cancer rates for former smokers approach the rates of lifetime nonsmokers. Unfortunately, no such relationship exists between smoking cessation and lower risk of COPD. With cessation of smoking, the rate of functional pulmonary loss declines, but the previously lost function cannot be regained. Overall, however, timely cigarette smoking cessation is the best prevention of symptomatic pulmonary disease.

Quitting smoking is not an easy process. The woman who wants to quit smoking on her own has two options:

- Gradual reduction is a process of not only gently tapering the number of daily cigarettes smoked, but also cutting back on the relative amount of tar and nicotine by changing brands to those with lower and lower levels of these substances. Many strategies can be used in the process of gradual reduction, all of which serve to modify traditional smoking behavior and reinforce progress toward total cessation.

- Going "cold turkey" means making a decisive, sudden break from cigarettes. Some people find that they are able to go cold turkey if they do it one day at a time. They promise themselves to be smoke free for 24 hours; at the end of

It's Your Health

Common Rationalizations of Women Smokers

It can't be as bad as they say.

The government wouldn't let them sell cigarettes if they were that harmful.

My aunt lived to be 80 and she smoked.

We all have to die sometime.

I have so much stress in my life.

I really need cigarettes to make things better.

I DON'T want to gain weight.

It is okay if I smoke because I eat well and exercise every day.

I only smoke at work, not at home.

I only smoke low-tar cigarettes.

I am too busy to eat, and smoking helps me to control my hunger.

I had smoked for years before I became pregnant with my first child. I quit smoking while I was pregnant, but as life became more stressful, I started again—just having a cigarette after a bad day or if my friends were over. Gradually, I began to smoke more and more. Four years later, my daughter told me that my mouth smelled bad, like I "lit a fire in it." I knew then that I had to quit this disgusting habit. Although I don't smoke anymore, I still want one after lunch, when I have a drink, just at certain times of the day. I will always be addicted.

32-year-old woman

that day, they reaffirm their commitment to another smoke-free day. It may take several weeks or months for a former heavy smoker to become confident about the newly acquired nonsmoking status.

Smoking cessation programs have evolved since 1964, when the first Surgeon General's Report on Smoking and Health was published. Intervention strategies for smoking cessation now include a variety of treatment modalities. They may be individualized or group based, formal or informal in design. Multicomponent, behaviorally oriented programs seem to elicit the most favorable results for short-term and long-term cigarette cessation. These programs often incorporate several treatment modalities, including aversive conditioning, contracting, self-control, stimulus control, group support, and cessation maintenance. Pharmacological agents, such as nicotine gum and transdermal nicotine patches, are often used with multicomponent treatment programs as well. Although not all studies have produced consistent results, a number of investigations have shown that use of nicotine gum, in conjunction with sessions of counseling to deal with psychological issues, can help some people stop smoking. Transdermal nicotine patches are proving to be a more effective alternative than the gums. Other forms of treatment for smoking cessation that are available by prescription include nasal sprays, lozenges, and a special inhaler. Although the option has not yet been proven effective by scientific studies, some people find hypnosis or acupuncture to be helpful in their quest to stop smoking. Research efforts to develop a vaccine for the prevention and treatment of tobacco addiction are currently under way.

Alcohol

Pure **alcohol** is a colorless liquid obtained by fermentation of a sugar-containing liquid. Ethyl alcohol (ethanol) is the type of alcohol found in alcoholic beverages. The amount of alcohol varies from beverage to beverage (Table 13.4). Nearly the same amount of alcohol is present in a 12-oz bottle or can of beer (4% alcohol), 5 oz of table wine (10% alcohol), and 1.25 oz of distilled spirits (40% alcohol). The National Institute on Alcohol Abuse and Alcoholism recommends that individuals who choose to drink and are not specifically at risk for alcohol-related problems

Table 13.4   Alcohol Content in Beverages

Serving Size	Beverage	Alcohol by Volume (%)
12 oz	Light beer	2.4
12 oz	Beer	4.0
5 oz	Wine	10.0
1.25 oz	Vodka (80 proof)	40.0
	Whiskey (86 proof)	43.0

Each contains approximately 0.5 oz of alcohol.

should not exceed the one to two drinks per day limit recommended by the U.S. dietary guidelines.

Blood Alcohol Concentration

Blood alcohol concentration (BAC) is a physiological indicator used by clinicians and law enforcement officials to determine whether a person is legally "drunk." BAC is expressed in terms of the percentage of alcohol in the blood. A BAC of 0.10 (which is technically 0.10%) indicates the presence of approximately one part of alcohol per 1,000 parts of other blood components. As seen in Table 13.5, a BAC of 0.10 results in significant compromise of mental and psychomotor capabilities. In all 50 states, driving with a BAC of 0.08 or higher is illegal. The punishment for violating this limit, as well as the number and kind of other laws related to driving while intoxicated, vary from state to state.

Many factors affect BAC and an individual's response to alcohol. For example, BAC is increased when greater amounts of alcohol are consumed at a faster rate and are consumed without food. Stronger drinks, smaller body size, older age, and being Asian or Native American also lead to increased BAC levels when drinking. In Asians and Native Americans, the metabolic process is unable to break down alcohol as quickly as the corresponding mechanism in whites. In addition to higher BACs, many Asians and Native Americans experience effects such as nausea, headaches, and flushing of the skin when they drink.

With regular alcohol consumption, more and more alcohol is required to achieve the same desired psychological effect, although motor coordination and judgment are impaired at the same level. After several years of drinking, some individuals

Table 13.5 Blood Alcohol Concentrations

BAC	Effects
0.02–0.04	No overt effects; feelings of muscle relaxation and slight mood elevation
0.05–0.06	Relaxation and warmth; slight decrease in reaction time and slight decrease in fine muscle coordination
0.08–0.10	Balance, speech, vision, and hearing slightly impaired; euphoric feelings; increased loss of motor coordination
0.11–0.12	Difficulty with coordination and balance; distinct impairment of mental facilities and judgment
0.14–0.15	Major impairment of mental and physical control; slurred speech, blurred vision, and lack of motor skill
0.20	Loss of motor control; substantial mental disorientation
0.30	Severe intoxication with minimum conscious control of mind and body

Greater levels lead to unconsciousness, coma, and death from respiratory failure.

Source: Substance Abuse and Mental Health Services Administration.

develop "reverse tolerance" and actually become intoxicated after drinking only a small amount of alcohol.

Epidemiological Trends and Issues

Although alcohol consumption is generally considered a personal and private issue, its effects permeate all sectors and dimensions of society. Alcohol has been a constant component of American life since colonial days. Attempts to control, restrict, or abolish alcohol in the United States have all met with failure. In 1919, the 18th Amendment to the Constitution was ratified in an attempt to stop the rapid growth of alcohol addiction. During the Prohibition era, illegal sales of bootlegged beverages and prescription "medications" prevailed as people sought ways around the ban. Prohibition was officially repealed in 1933 by the ratification of the 21st Amendment.

During the nineteenth and early twentieth centuries, most people who opposed alcohol consumption believed that alcoholics were morally weak. Today, there is a greater awareness of the highly complex nature of alcoholism. The public admissions of alcoholism by prominent women such as Betty Ford, Drew Barrymore, Elizabeth Taylor, and Mary Tyler Moore have reinforced the fact that alcoholism is a personal and pervasive health problem that affects women from all walks of life.

According to the U.S. Department of Health and Human Services, 44% of females age 12 and older report current (past-month) alcohol use; 56% of women age 18 to 25 report current drinking; and 18% of girls aged 12 to 17 report alcohol use.[27] Sixty-two percent of white women age 18 to 44 currently drink compared with 40% of black women, 40% of Hispanic women, and 31% of Asian/Pacific Islander women.[28] Although black women are less likely than white women to drink, if they drink, they are more likely to drink heavily. Nearly 4% of black women are heavy drinkers, compared with 2.8% of white women age 18 to 44.[29] In general, women not only are less likely to drink than men, but they also generally drink less and are less likely to become alcohol dependent.[30]

Cultural factors influence the prevalence of alcoholism because the perception of drunken behavior as deviant depends on the culture in which it occurs. It has been suggested that when drinking is a part of family rituals or ceremonies and when there is great disapproval of public drunkenness, there is a corresponding lower prevalence of heavy drinking. Gender-based social norms often contribute to alcohol consumption patterns. For example, in some cultures, men are drinkers while women generally abstain.

Alcohol consumption rates also vary by region and by level of education. Alcohol use is higher in the Northeast (55.5%), Midwest (53.7%), and West (50.8%) than in the South (45.1%); the rate of alcohol use is also higher in large metropolitan areas (52%) as compared with small metropolitan and nonmetropolitan areas (49.7% and 43.7%, respectively).[27] Higher levels of education are associated with greater prevalence of current use of alcohol. Individuals with higher levels of education tend to be moderate drinkers more so than those who are less educated; 67.6% college graduates and 36.4% of adults with less than a high school degree are current drinkers.[27]

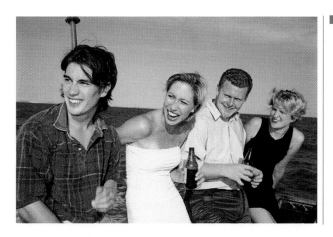

■ Alcohol is an accepted and often traditional part of many social events.

Psychosocial Dimensions of Alcohol Use and Alcoholism

Social phenomena contribute to alcohol consumption by women and influence their access to recovery services. Society's double standard for women certainly prevails where alcoholism is concerned. The popular media and folklore portray a male drunk as comical and lovable, but a drunken woman as loose, weak, and immoral. This double standard extends into the treatment arena. The greater social sanctions applied to alcoholism in women make some women less willing to seek help and others less willing to recognize that they need help. Because alcoholic women violate the stereotype of feminine behavior, they often distress their families and friends and even the health professionals who might support them.

Depression has been found to be associated with alcohol consumption and has been suggested as a factor in the alcohol drinking behavior of women. As in the age-old question of "which came first, the chicken or the egg?", it is difficult to establish whether alcohol is a symptom of depression or a consequence of it.

Victimization is another factor associated with alcohol-related problems. In one large study, researchers found that women who reported being sexually abused in childhood were more likely to experience alcohol-related problems as adults. Physical abuse as an adult is also a factor that may increase a woman's risk for alcohol abuse or dependence.[31] The relationship between victimization and alcohol may be confounded by the fact that victimization often leads to depression, which in turn is associated with alcohol use.

Although the literature includes few studies on alcohol and drug use among lesbians, it has been suggested that lesbians consume more alcohol for longer periods and are more likely than heterosexual women to use alcohol in combination with other drugs.[32] Lesbian women may be at greater risk of alcohol problems because of the social disapproval directed at their sexual orientation.

Societal Costs of Alcohol Use and Alcoholism

With more than 113 million Americans reporting current use of alcohol and 12 million calling themselves heavy drinkers, the economic, social, and personal costs of alcohol-related crimes, accidents, illnesses, and deaths are profound. It has been estimated that the cost of alcohol abuse and alcoholism in the United States is $148 billion, including $19 billion for healthcare expenditures.[33] Almost 70% of the costs of alcohol abuse are related to lost productivity—45% to alcohol-related illness and 21.2% due to premature death. In addition, underage drinking costs Americans more than $58 billion per year.[34]

The costs to society from alcohol cannot be measured just in terms of dollars; the human costs of drinking are incalculable. Alcohol contributes to significant morbidity and mortality among Americans (Table 13.6). Approximately 100,000 people die each year in the United States as a result of alcohol. Its use is associated with more than 45% of all motor vehicle crash fatalities, roughly one-third of all homicides and suicides, and 22% of all fatal boating accidents.[35] Alcohol contributes to several often-fatal illnesses, most notably liver disease, cancer, and cardiovascular disease. The death rate among women alcoholics is higher than that among male alcoholics because women alcoholics have an increased risk for suicide, alcohol-related accidents, cirrhosis, and hepatitis.[36]

Legal Issues of Alcohol Use and Alcoholism

There are many legal issues related to drinking. During the Prohibition era, alcohol was illegal in the United States. Although a constitutional amendment made it legal again, both states and the federal government have since enacted several laws that limit its use. Nationally, alcohol use is limited to people older than age 21. In most other countries, no such age limit exists. In many Muslim countries, such as Saudi Arabia, however, alcohol use remains illegal.

In addition to setting age limits on alcohol use, states have enacted other laws governing drinking and driving, drunk and disorderly behavior, purchase of alcohol for a minor, and driving with an open container of alcohol; all of these laws limit how and when individuals can consume alcohol. Most of the penalties associ-

---

Table 13.6   Complications from Chronic Alcohol Consumption

Cancer:
  Cancer of the liver, larynx, esophagus, stomach, colon, breast, and skin (malignant melanoma)

Cardiovascular effects:
  Hypertension, stroke, and cardiovascular disease

Organ damage:
  Brain, stomach, colon, pancreas, and kidneys

Diabetes

Fetal alcohol syndrome

Impotency and infertility

Diminished immunity

Sleep disturbances

ated with alcohol abuse or misuse involve misdemeanor charges or fines, but some—for example, drunk driving violations—entail mandatory jail time in many states.

Effects of Alcohol

Alcohol functions as a central nervous system depressant that effectively impairs all major body systems. When consumed in small quantities, it has a mild, relaxing effect. Consumption of larger quantities results in compromised sensory motor coordination, judgment, emotional control, and reasoning capabilities. As seen in Figure 13.6, because alcohol circulates throughout the body, nearly all bodily functions can be affected by increased alcohol consumption. It usually takes about 15 minutes for alcohol to reach the bloodstream, and the peak effect occurs in one hour. Once in the bloodstream, alcohol is quickly carried to the liver, heart, and brain.

The liver is the organ most vulnerable to alcohol because it metabolizes alcohol. Heavy drinking may lead to alcoholic hepatitis, which is characterized by inflammation and destruction of liver cells, and **cirrhosis,** which produces progressive scarring of liver tissue. Approximately 10% to 35% of heavy drinkers develop alcoholic hepatitis and 10% to 20% develop cirrhosis.[37] Compared with men, women develop

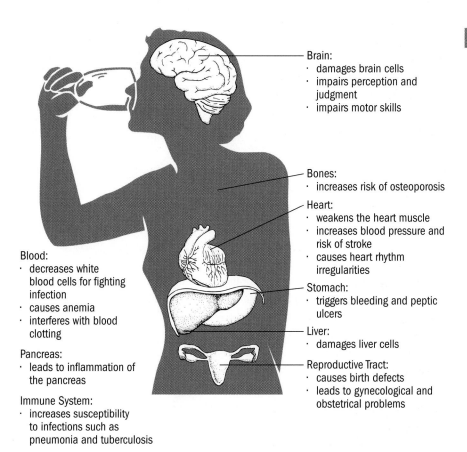

Blood:
· decreases white
  blood cells for fighting
  infection
· causes anemia
· interferes with blood
  clotting

Pancreas:
· leads to inflammation of
  the pancreas

Immune System:
· increases susceptibility
  to infections such as
  pneumonia and tuberculosis

Brain:
· damages brain cells
· impairs perception and
  judgment
· impairs motor skills

Bones:
· increases risk of osteoporosis

Heart:
· weakens the heart muscle
· increases blood pressure and
  risk of stroke
· causes heart rhythm
  irregularities

Stomach:
· triggers bleeding and peptic
  ulcers

Liver:
· damages liver cells

Reproductive Tract:
· causes birth defects
· leads to gynecological and
  obstetrical problems

Figure 13.6

Physiological effects of alcohol.

alcohol-induced liver disease over a shorter period of time and after consuming less alcohol.[38]

Chronic heavy alcohol consumption is also associated with cardiovascular damage. Consuming one or two alcoholic drinks per day appears to lower the death rate from coronary heart disease; however, heavier drinking increases the risk of alcohol-associated heart muscle disease. In response to the evidence that one or two drinks per day may prevent heart attacks and stroke, researchers are investigating the effects of light alcohol consumption on the liver. Alcohol also is associated with various cancers, although there is still controversy surrounding the association between alcohol and breast cancer (Chapter 10).

Perhaps the most dramatic effects of alcohol are on the brain and behavior. As a central nervous system depressant, alcohol alters the activity of brain neurons, resulting in impaired sensory, motor, and cognitive function. Moderate amounts of alcohol also have disturbing effects on perception, judgment, and psychomotor skills. Alcohol's anesthetic effect may cause diminished perception of pain and temperature, possibly leading to serious injury or exposure to extreme temperatures. Although drinking may decrease judgment, increase interest, and reduce inhibitions in sex, it also impairs a man's ability to achieve or maintain an erection and a woman's ability to achieve orgasm. Additional drinking results in a progressive reduction in behavioral activity, which may lead to sleep, general anesthesia, coma, and even death.

Alcohol is particularly dangerous when combined with other drugs, such as depressants and antianxiety medications. Of the 100 most frequently prescribed drugs, more than half contain at least one ingredient that interacts adversely with alcohol. Combining alcohol with drugs may produce an effect greater than that expected with either substance taken alone (Table 13.7). Acetaminophen (brand name Tylenol) can be especially toxic to the liver when taken in combination with many drinks, in rare cases leading to acute hepatic failure.

Heavy alcohol consumption typically leads to several nutritional problems for the chronic user. Because alcohol dulls the senses of taste and smell, heavy drinkers often skip meals and develop nutritional deficiencies. Alcohol consumption also has been associated with osteoporosis due to alcohol's ability to block the absorption of calcium. Chronic consumption disrupts normal digestive processes, resulting in gastritis (inflammation of the stomach lining), stomach ulcers, and intestinal lesions, which interfere with the metabolism of vitamins and minerals. In addition, alcoholism has been associated with thiamine (vitamin B_1) deficiency, which is believed to play a critical role in diseases of the nervous, digestive, muscular, and cardiovascular systems.

Physiologically, women appear to have less body water than men of similar body weight and produce lower levels of alcohol dehydrogenase, the enzyme responsible for ethanol metabolism. As a result, women absorb about 30% more alcohol than men do into the bloodstream before it can be metabolized in the liver.[39] The alcohol reaches women's brains and other organs more quickly, resulting in more rapid intoxication than in men as well as more organ-specific ethanol toxicity. For a woman of average

Table 13.7   Alcohol and Drug Interactions

Type of Drug	Examples	Possible Effects
Analgesics (narcotic)	codeine, Demerol, Percodan	Increased CNS depression possibly leading to respiratory arrest and death
Analgesics (nonnarcotic)	aspirin, acetaminophen, ibuprofen	Gastric irritation and bleeding Increased susceptibility to liver damage
Antidepressants	Tofranil, tricyclics (Elavil)	Increased CNS depression, decreased alertness
Antianxiety drugs	Valium, Librium	Increased CNS depression, decreased alertness
Antihistamines	Actifed, Dimetapp, cold medications (prescribed and over-the-counter)	Increased drowsiness
Antibiotics	penicillin, erythromycin	Nausea, vomiting, headache Some antibiotics are rendered less effective
CNS* stimulants	caffeine, Dexedrine, Ritalin	Somewhat counter depressant effect of alcohol but do not influence level of intoxication
Diuretics	Lasix, Diuril, Hydromox	Reduction in blood pressure with possible lightheadedness
Psychotropics	Tindal, Mellaril, Thorazine	Increased CNS depression possibly leading to respiratory arrest
Sedatives	Dalmane, Nembutal, Quaalude	Increased CNS depression possibly leading to respiratory arrest and death
Tranquilizers	Valium, Miltown, Librium	Increased CNS depression, decreased alertness and judgment

*CNS: Central nervous system.

size, one drink has the same effect as two drinks have on the average-sized man. Women alcoholics also are more likely to suffer liver damage than men.

Hormone levels play a role in alcohol metabolism. Studies have indicated that both the menstrual cycle and the use of oral contraceptives influence blood alcohol levels. The rate of alcohol metabolism and peak BAC attained with a standard dose of alcohol may vary depending on estrogen levels. Moderate alcohol consumption may increase estrogen levels in postmenopausal women taking oral contraceptives and hormone replacement therapy.[40] These variances may help explain why some women have difficulty predicting their response to alcohol and their feelings of loss of control over their responses.

Alcohol can have a detrimental influence on reproductive health and pregnancy. Although alcohol crosses the placental barrier, its effects on the developing fetus vary because of differences in the degree and timing of exposure, genetic differences in maternal metabolism of alcohol, maternal nutritional status, and possible interaction with other drug compounds. Women who are alcoholics or who drink heavily during pregnancy have a higher rate of spontaneous abortion. A direct effect of alcohol in pregnant women is fetal alcohol syndrome (FAS). This syndrome is distinguished by specific physical and mental abnormalities in infants born to mothers who drank alcohol during pregnancy (see Chapter 6). FAS has the following symptoms:

- Small body size and weight
- Slower than normal development and failure to catch up
- Skeletal deformities
- Facial abnormalities
- Organ deformities
- Central nervous system handicaps[41]

Alcohol consumption may inhibit the release of oxytocin and prolactin, two hormones that are important for initiation and maintenance of lactation. It also may alter the composition of a woman's breast milk and impair the infant's suckling behavior.[42]

Alcohol plays an indirect role in many unwanted pregnancies and sexually transmitted diseases (STDs). Because of impaired judgment and reasoning from intoxication, contraception may be forgotten or ignored, judgment may be distorted, and danger may not be perceived. In addition to unwanted pregnancies and STDs, alcohol is often a factor in acquaintance rape cases and incidents of pressured sex.

Chronic heavy drinking also may be associated with menstrual disorders, infertility, and possibly early menopause.

Alcoholism

Alcoholism has officially been recognized as a disease for more than 25 years. The traditional definition of an alcoholic is a person whose consumption of alcohol interferes with a major aspect of her life. Alcoholism has since been redefined as a primary, chronic disease with genetic, psychological, and environmental factors influencing its development and manifestations. Alcohol has a generational cyclic effect. Children of alcoholics are more likely to suffer abuse, to have psychological or emotional problems, to become alcoholics, and to marry alcoholics. A large national study reported that approximately one in four U.S. children is exposed at some time before age 18 to alcoholism and/or alcohol abuse.[43]

Chronic alcohol abuse usually manifests itself as one of the following patterns:

- Daily intake of large amounts of alcohol
- Regular heavy drinking on weekends
- Periods of sobriety between binges of daily heavy drinking that may last for weeks or months

Alcoholism generally appears between ages 20 and 40, but can present in childhood or early adolescence. Alcohol becomes a problem when an individual is no longer able to control when and how much drinking takes place. Clinical diagnosis of alcoholism is based on the presence of at least three of the following symptoms, persisting for a month or more or occurring repeatedly over a longer period of time:

- Alcohol taken in large amounts (5 or more drinks per day)
- Persistent desire to quit drinking or one or more unsuccessful attempts to cut down or quit alcohol
- Considerable time spent obtaining, using, or recovering from alcohol
- Continued drinking despite social, psychological, or physical symptoms such as ulcers that are caused or worsened by alcohol
- Withdrawal symptoms, such as physical trembling, sweating, high blood pressure, delusions, and hallucinations, when alcohol intake is curbed
- The avoidance or relief of withdrawal symptoms by drinking
- Desire or need for a drink to start the day
- Denial of an alcohol problem
- Sleep problems
- Attempts to control drinking by changing brands or going on the wagon
- Depression and paranoia
- Failure to recall what happened during a drinking episode
- Dramatic mood swings
- Participation in behaviors or activities while drinking that are regretted afterward
- The experience of the following symptoms after drinking: headaches, nausea, stomach pain, heartburn, gas, fatigue, weakness, muscle cramps, irregular or rapid heart rate

I used to think that I couldn't be an alcoholic. I had a good job and I drank only wine. I certainly don't look like an alcoholic, whatever that look is. It took a long time for me to admit that I really was dependent on that wine. I needed it every day just to dull the world.
30-year-old woman

Risk Factors for Alcoholism

As mentioned earlier, family history of alcohol problems, early initiation of drinking, and victimization are all factors that may increase a woman's risk for alcohol abuse or alcoholism. Studies on identical twins as compared with fraternal twins, for example, show that identical twins are more likely to have similar rates of alcohol dependence, abuse, and heavy consumption, suggesting a genetic component to alcoholism.[44] There is also a significant association between alcoholism in people who were adopted and their biological parents, further reinforcing this hypothesis.[38] A large nationwide survey showed that more than 40% of persons who initiated drinking before age 15 were considered alcohol dependent at some point in their lives.[45] Women who were sexually, verbally, or physically abused also reported more alcohol-related problems.

Many psychiatrists believe that alcohol abuse is a symptom of a personality disorder and that drinking alcohol is the person's way of seeking relief from stress. The act and the effects of drinking reinforce drinking behavior, and the cycle of abuse begins. Traits associated with alcoholism, such as history of antisocial behavior, high levels of depression, and low self-esteem, have been identified.

Treatment Dimensions of Alcoholism

The most difficult and significant step for an alcoholic is admitting to an alcohol problem. Often well-intended friends or family members, out of fear, embarrassment, loyalty, or hope, shield the alcoholic from the truth. Confrontation—either personal or via an accident or drunk-driving conviction—that makes the individual acknowledge the alcohol problem is often a turning point in seeking assistance (Self-Assessment 13.2). Recovery from alcoholism is enhanced when the person has a strong emotional support system, including concerned family, friends, and employer.

Alcoholism is a complex problem, and each case must be treated with sensitivity and recognition of its unique situation and contributing factors. Standard treatment programs focus on the relief of physiological dependence but do not eliminate the underlying disease. Individual personality, psychological factors, and sociocultural factors must be addressed to help the alcoholic regain control of her life. Alcohol treatment programs often follow three steps in the treatment of alcoholism:

1. Managing acute intoxication episodes
2. Correcting chronic health problems associated with alcoholism
3. Changing long-term behavior

The most successful treatment modalities combine different approaches and provide ongoing support for people who are learning to live without alcohol. Many alcohol treatment facilities assist clients in overcoming their physical addiction to alcohol and helping them deal with their withdrawal symptoms (Table 13.8) through detoxification programs. Detoxification programs are generally available in medical or psychiatric hospitals. Psychological addiction is usually addressed immediately after the detoxification process is completed. Programs such as Alcoholics Anonymous (AA), which is entirely run by volunteers who are recovering alcoholics, provide support for people trying to maintain their abstinence from alcohol. Studies conducted by Alcoholics Anonymous show that the average length of sobriety for its members is more than eight years; 50% of members have been sober for more than five years, 24% for between one and five years, and 26% for less than one year. Since the organization began in 1935, Alcoholics Anonymous has supported more than 100,000 groups and had over 2 million members in 150 countries.[46] AA meetings can now be found in towns and cities across the country almost every day of the week.

Women alcoholics who enter treatment programs have special needs. Their treatment programs must be culturally sensitive and incorporate issues such as age, socioeconomic status, drug use, and sexual orientation into their format. Strategies that have been proposed for assisting women in addressing their alcohol problems include use of culturally appropriate, nonstigmatized language; development of supportive case management; implementation of a mentoring or buddy system; expansion of childcare services; and creation of a multimedia campaign that educates women.

Self-Assessment 13.2

National Council on Alcoholism Self-Test: Do You Have a Drinking Problem?

1. Do you occasionally drink heavily after a disappointment or a quarrel, or when your parents give you a hard time?   yes   no

2. When you have trouble or feel pressured at school, do you always drink more heavily than usual?   yes   no

3. Have you noticed that you are able to handle more liquor than you did when you were first drinking?   yes   no

4. Did you ever wake up on "the morning after" and discover that you could not remember the evening before, even though your friends tell you that you did not pass out?   yes   no

5. When drinking with other people, do you try to have a few extra drinks that others DON'T notice?   yes   no

6. Are there certain occasions when you feel uncomfortable if alcohol is not available?   yes   no

7. Have you recently noticed that when you begin drinking you are in more of a hurry to get the first drink than you used to be?   yes   no

8. Do you sometimes feel a little guilty about your drinking?   yes   no

9. Are you secretly irritated when your family or friends discuss your drinking?   yes   no

10. Have you recently noticed an increase in the frequency of your memory blackouts?   yes   no

11. Do you often find that you wish to continue drinking after your friends say that they have had enough?   yes   no

12. Do you usually have a reason for the occasions that you drink heavily?   yes   no

13. When you are sober, do you often regret things you did or said while drinking?   yes   no

14. Have you tried switching brands or following different plans for controlling your drinking?   yes   no

15. Have you often failed to keep the promises you've made to yourself about controlling or cutting down on your drinking?   yes   no

16. Have you ever tried to control your drinking by changing jobs or moving to a new location?   yes   no

17. Do you try to avoid family or close friends while you are drinking?   yes   no

18. Are you having an increasing number of financial and academic problems?   yes   no

19. Do more people seem to be treating you unfairly without good reason?   yes   no

20. Do you eat very little or irregularly when you are drinking?   yes   no

21. Do you sometimes have the shakes in the morning and find that it helps to have a little drink?   yes   no

22. Have you recently noticed that you cannot drink as much as you once did?   yes   no

23. Do you sometimes stay drunk for several days at a time?   yes   no

24. Do you sometimes feel very depressed and wonder whether life is worth living?   yes   no

25. Sometimes after periods of drinking, do you see or hear things that aren't there?   yes   no

26. Do you get terribly frightened after you have been drinking heavily?   yes   no

Those who answer "yes" to two or three of these questions may wish to evaluate their drinking in these areas. "Yes" answers to several of these questions indicate the following stages of alcoholism:

Questions 1–8: Early Stage: Drinking is a regular part of your life.

Questions 9–21: Middle Stage: You are having trouble controlling when, where, and how much you drink.

Questions 22–26: Beginning of the Final Stage: You no longer can control your desire to drink.

Source: National Council on Alcoholism and Drug Dependence, Inc. (http://www.ncadd.org).

Table 13.8	Alcohol Withdrawal Symptoms	
Irritability	Dry mouth
Agitation	Elevated blood pressure
Depression	Headache
Lack of concentration	Anxiety
Body tremors	Puffy, blotchy skin
Nausea and vomiting	Fitful sleep with nightmares
Generalized weakness, achiness	Brief hallucinations
Sweating	Delirium tremens (DTs)
Fever	

Drugs

No drug use is benign. At a minimum, all psychoactive drugs affect the central nervous system. Many habitual drug users end up in the emergency room as a result of overdosing, accident, or injury related to the drug use (see Table 13.9). In addition to the direct physiological effects and risks of drug use, additional risks may be associated with the administration of drugs to the body. For example, the process of using needles to inject drugs presents serious risks beyond those of using drugs. Many diseases, including hepatitis and HIV, can be transmitted from one person to another via contaminated injection equipment. The effects and risks of drugs are summarized in Table 13.10.

Epidemiological Trends and Issues

According to the National Survey on Drug Use and Health, more than 51 million women ages 12 and older reported using an illicit drug at some point in their lives. This represented an increase from 34.7% in 2000 to 41.9% in 2003. The rate of current illicit drug use was 6.1% for females and 10.6% for girls age 12 to 17.[27]

Drug overuse and misuse are particular problems among older women. Although they are generally not users of illicit drugs, older women are likely to be consumers of high levels of medications. Elderly women represent 11% of the general population, but they receive more than 25% of all written prescriptions.[29] Medications such as sedatives, hypnotics, antianxiety drugs, antihypertensive drugs, vitamins, analgesics, diuretics, laxatives, and tranquilizers are prescribed for elderly women at a rate that is 2.5 times the prescription rate for elderly men. Women are diagnosed with anxiety and depression disorders more often than men are, so they are prescribed drugs more often to treat these disorders. Gender differences in weight, body composition, gastric emptying time, cerebral blood flow, and use of hormones in contraception and hormone replacement therapy can influence the effect these drugs have in women.

Table 13.9	Number of Female Emergency Department Drug Mentions, 2000–2002		
Drug Type	2000	2001	2002
Alcohol in combination	80,948	85,328	79,957
Cocaine	59,314	65,713	69,852
Heroin	30,146	30,023	31,173
Marijuana	33,334	37,781	41,707
Methamphetamine	4,841	6,680	6,565
MDMA (ecstasy)	2,011	2,331	1,987
LSD	948	820	112
PCP	1,720	1,683	2,738
Total mentions	513,271	538,166	553,874

Source: Substance Abuse and Mental Health Services Administration. (2004). Emergency Department Trends from the Drug Abuse Warning Network.

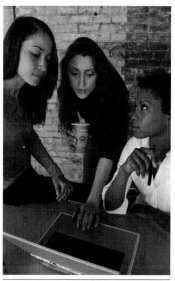

■ There is no particular stereotype of a drug-dependent woman.

Although many use prescribed medication appropriately, some older women develop a dependency on sleeping pills, muscle relaxants such as Valium, or diet pills. In the 1950s and 1960s, a high percentage of middle-class women were prescribed these medicines, which were widely viewed as acceptable coping tools. Today, many of these women continue to see the use of these drugs as an acceptable way to dull emotions, anxiety, or stress caused by the demands of everyday life.

Stimulants

Stimulants affect the central nervous system and increase heart rate, blood pressure, strength of heart contractions, blood glucose level, and overall muscle tension. Collectively, these effects place additional stress on the body.

Caffeine, one of the most widely used stimulants in the world, is found in many different sources. It has a variety of effects:

- Relief of drowsiness
- Help in the performance of repetitive tasks
- Improved mental capacity for work
- Increased basal metabolic rate

In addition, caffeine has been shown to trigger anxiety, insomnia, irregular heartbeat, faster breathing, upset stomach and bowels, dizziness, and headaches. Women who drink a lot of caffeine and then suddenly stop their consumption may experience headaches, irritability, and fatigue.

Table 13.10 Summary of Effects and Risks of Drugs

Cocaine and Crack

Names	"Coke," "snow," "lady," "rock," "blow"
Physiological effects	Speed up physical and mental processes; create sense of heightened energy and confidence
Health effects	Headaches, exhaustion, shaking, blurred vision, nausea, seizures, loss of appetite, loss of sexual desire, impotence, impaired judgment, hyperactivity, babbling, paranoia, violence
Long-term risks	Nasal damage (if snorted); lung damage (if smoked); hepatitis and HIV (if injected); damage to heart and blood vessels; chest pain; heart attack; disruptions in cardiac rhythm; stroke; damage to liver
Special risks to women	Increased danger of miscarriage and physical and mental impairment of the fetus; increased risk of congenital malformations, fetal deaths, and SIDS

Amphetamines

Names	Benzedrine ("bennies"), dextroamphetamine (Dexedrine, "dex"), methamphetamine (Methedrine, "meth," "crank"), Desoxyn ("copilots"), methylphenidate (Ritalin), pemoline (Cylert), phenmetrazine (Preludin), "black beauties"
Physiological effects	Speed up physical and mental processes; lessen fatigue; boost energy; sense of excitement
Health effects	Loss of appetite; blurred vision; headache and dizziness; sweating; sleeplessness; trembling; anxiety and paranoia; delusions and hallucinations
Long-term risks	Cardiovascular damage—hypertension, stroke, heart failure; malnutrition, vitamin deficiencies; skin disorders; ulcers; sleeplessness; fever; brain damage; depression; violent behavior; fatal overdose
Special risks to women	Not yet determined

Barbiturates

Names	Pentobarbital (Nembutal, "yellow jackets"), secobarbital (Seconal, "reds"), thiopental (Pentothal), amobarbital (Amytal, "blues," "downers"), phenobarbital (Luminal, "phennies"), methaqualone ("love drug," Quaalude, "ludes," "Q"), sopor ("Sopors")
Physiological effects	Mild intoxication, drowsiness, lethargy, decreased alertness
Health effects	Drowsiness, poor coordination, slurred speech, impaired judgment, hangover, confusion, irritability; cold skin; depressed respirations; rapid heart rate
Long-term risks	Disrupted sleep; impaired vision; increased risk of fatal overdose with increased use
Special risks to women	Risk of birth defects and subsequent behavioral problems if used during pregnancy

Antianxiety Drugs

Names	Benzodiazepines: chlordiazepoxide (Librium), diazepam (Valium), oxazepam (Serax), flurazepam (Dalmane); dicarbamates: meprobamate (Equanil, Miltown)
Physiological effect	Slows down central nervous system
Health effects	Slurred speech, drowsiness, stupor
Long-term risks	Physical and psychological dependence; possible fatal overdose; withdrawal can lead to coma, psychosis, and death
Special risks to women	Menstrual irregularities and failure to ovulate have been reported

Table 13.10 Summary of Effects and Risks of Drugs (continued)

Marijuana and Hashish

Names	Marijuana ("pot," "grass," "Mary Jane"), hashish ("hash")
Physiological effects	Relaxes the mind and body; heightens perceptions
Health effects	Increased heart rate; dry mouth and throat; impaired perceptions and reactions; lethargy; nausea; disorientation, possible hallucinations, heightened anxiety
Long-term risks	Psychological dependence; impaired thinking, perception, memory, and coordination; increased heart rate and hypertension; compromised immunity
Special risks to women	Prenatal use may lead to fetal effects, including small head, poor growth, lower birthweight

Psychedelics

Names	LSD ("acid"), mescaline, PCP ("angel dust," "peace pill")
Physiological effects	Alters perceptions and produces hallucinations
Health effects	Increased heart rate, hypertension, fever, headache, nausea, sweating, and trembling; delusions and unpredictable violence
Long-term risks	Possible flashbacks, psychological dependence; stupor, coma, convulsions, heart and lung failure; brain damage
Special risks to women	Effects on fetus unknown

Inhalants

Names	Depends on specific product
Physiological effects	Temporary feelings of well-being; giddiness; hallucinations
Health effects	Nausea, sneezing, coughing, nosebleeds, loss of appetite, decreased heart and breathing rates; impaired judgment; loss of consciousness
Long-term risks	Hepatitis, liver and kidney failure; respiratory impairment; blood abnormalities; possible suffocation
Special risks to women	Not yet determined

Opiates/Synthetic Narcotics

Names	Opium, morphine, codeine; heroin ("horse," "junk," "smack," "downtown"); methadone (Dolophine, "meth," "dollies"); hydromorphone (Dilaudid, "little D"); oxycodone (Percodan, "perkies"); meperidine (Demerol, "demies"); propoxyphene (Darvon)
Physiological effects	Relaxation of the central nervous system; pain relief; temporary sense of well-being
Health effects	Nausea and vomiting; restlessness; reduced respirations; lethargy; weight loss; slurred speech; mood swings; sweating
Long-term risks	Physical dependence; malnutrition; compromised immunity; hepatitis; HIV; skin lesions; fatal overdose
Special risks to women	Higher risk for preterm labor, intrauterine growth retardation, and preeclampsia

Cocaine is a popular stimulant drug that is ingested by approximately 1.5 million Americans, with an estimated 682,000 people being considered frequent users (using cocaine on 51 or more days during the past year).[47] The immediate effects of cocaine last 5 to 15 minutes because the drug is rapidly metabolized by the liver. With repeated use, the brain becomes tolerant to cocaine, and users need more of it to get high.

Crack is a smokable mixture of cocaine and baking soda. Because it sets off rapid ups and downs, this drug produces a powerful chemical and psychological dependence. Crack users often need another "hit" within minutes of the previous one. Smoking cocaine in its "freebase" form also delivers a concentrated high that can disappear within seconds.

Cocaine and crack are dangerous for both pregnant women and their unborn babies, causing miscarriages, premature labor, low-birthweight babies, and babies with small head circumferences. Women who use cocaine while pregnant are more likely to miscarry in the first three months of pregnancy than other groups of women are, including those who do not use drugs and those who use heroin or narcotics. Infants born to cocaine and crack users suffer major complications, including drug withdrawal and permanent disabilities. Because cocaine affects blood pressure, it can deprive the fetal brain of oxygen or cause brain vessels to burst, so that the fetus experiences the prenatal equivalent of a stroke, resulting in permanent physical and mental damage. In addition, cocaine babies have higher-than-normal rates of respiratory and kidney problems. Visual problems, low birthweight, seizures, depression, lack of coordination, and developmental retardation are common among cocaine babies as well.

Amphetamines are manufactured chemicals sold under a variety of names. Generally found in pill form, they may also be ground and sniffed or made into a solution for injection. Amphetamines were once widely prescribed for weight control because they suppress the appetite and stimulate the central nervous system. A serious side effect of these drugs is the strain placed on the cardiovascular system, which can lead to severe cardiovascular damage. Use of methamphetamine, a form of amphetamine often referred to as "meth," "crank," or "ice," has skyrocketed in recent years as the drug has become cheaper and more widely available.

Anabolic steroids are synthetic derivatives of the male hormone testosterone. These powerful compounds are legitimately prescribed for treatment of burns and injuries, but athletes and others who want to appear muscular and athletic have increasingly illegally misused them. Women who take anabolic steroids risk development of a deepened voice, breast reduction, enlargement of the clitoris, changes in or cessation of the menstrual cycle, and growth of facial hair. Other potential effects include an increased risk of heart disease or stroke, liver tumors and jaundice, acne, bad breath, aching joints, and increased aggression. Both men and women run a risk of HIV transmission when needles are shared for steroid injection. Anabolic steroid users can become increasingly aggressive and paranoid. Studies have shown steroids to be addictive substances that create the same problems with dependence and withdrawal as cocaine.

Depressants and Antianxiety Drugs

Drugs that relax the central nervous system are called depressants, sedatives, or hypnotics. The most widely used depressant is alcohol. Depressants have a synergistic effect when they are mixed together. As the user builds up tolerance, the likelihood of a potentially fatal overdose increases.

Barbiturates are depressants that are used medically for inducing relaxation and sleep, relieving tension, and treating seizures. They may also be administered intravenously as a general anesthetic. Low doses of barbiturates produce mild intoxication and euphoria and decrease alertness and muscle coordination. With a higher dose, the person may suffer slurred speech, decreased respiration, cold skin, weak and rapid heartbeat, and unconsciousness. Side effects of these drugs include drowsiness, impaired judgment and performance, and a hangover that may last for hours or days. Regular barbiturate use leads to physical dependence. Barbiturate addicts tend to be sleepy, confused, or irritable.

Barbiturates also present problems in pregnancy. These drugs easily cross the placenta and can cause birth defects and behavioral problems. Babies born to mothers who abused sedatives during pregnancy may be physically dependent on the drugs and are more prone to respiratory problems, feeding difficulties, disturbed sleep, sweating, irritability, and fever.

Barbiturate withdrawal is a time-consuming process and medically difficult to manage. Withdrawal symptoms include anxiety, insomnia, delirium, and convulsions. Systemic dependence is so critical that occasionally an abrupt ending of barbiturate use leads to death.

Antianxiety drugs, such as benzodiazepines, are primarily prescribed to treat tension and muscular strain. The most commonly used benzodiazepines are alprazolam (Xanax) and diazepam (Valium). Benzodiazepines are relatively fast-acting medications, creating effects in less than an hour. Drowsiness and loss of coordination are the most common side effects. When used in combination with other substances, such as alcohol, benzodiazepines can cause serious and possibly life-threatening complications. When taken with benzodiazepines, medications such as anesthetics, antihistamines, sedatives, muscle relaxants, and some prescription painkillers may increase central nervous system depression. Similar to the barbiturates, high doses of these drugs result in slurred speech, drowsiness, and stupor. Physiological and physical dependence on antianxiety drugs may occur within two to four weeks. Withdrawal symptoms from antianxiety drugs may include coma, psychosis, and death.

Cannabis (Marijuana)

Cannabis, known as marijuana, "pot," or "weed," consists of a mixture of crushed leaves and flower buds of the *Cannabis sativa* plant; this drug is usually ingested by smoking. **Hashish** also is an extract of cannabis, but is two to 10 times as concentrated as marijuana. Tetrahydrocannabinol (THC) is the primary psychoactive ingredient in both drugs.

It's Your Health

Indications of Drug Use

Abrupt change in attitude, including a lack of interest in previously enjoyed activities

Frequent vague and withdrawn moods

Sudden decline in work or school performance

Sudden resistance to discipline or criticism

Secret telephone calls and meetings with a demand for greater personal privacy

Increased frustration levels

Decreased tolerance for others

Change in eating and sleeping habits

Sudden weight loss

Evidence of drug use

Frequent borrowing of money

Stealing

Disregard for personal appearance

Impaired relationships with family and friends

Disregard for deadlines, curfews, or other regulations

Unusual temper flare-ups

New friends, especially known drug dealers, and strong allegiance to these friends

Source: National Institute on Drug Abuse (NIDA), National Institutes of Health.

When taken in low to moderate doses, the effects of marijuana are similar to the effects of alcohol and some tranquilizers. In contrast to alcohol, however, marijuana at low doses does not dull sensation, but rather may cause slight alterations in perception. Its immediate physical effects include an increased heart rate, bloodshot eyes, and dry mouth and throat. High doses diminish the ability to perceive and react and cause sensory distortion. Hashish users may experience vivid hallucinations and LSD-like psychedelic reactions, and some people experience acute panic attacks.

Chronic use of marijuana has been shown to suppress ovulation and alter hormone levels in women. Frequent use of this drug during pregnancy may result in lower-birthweight infants and appears to be associated with impaired verbal, perceptual, and memory skills, as well as difficulties with decision making and sustained attention in children.[1] Studies show conflicting results regarding smoking marijuana and its relationship to cancer. Frequent marijuana use has been linked to cancer of the head and neck as well as bladder cancer.

Marijuana for medical use has been a subject of controversy for many years. The drug has been studied for its possible analgesic effect; its potential for reducing spasms and spasticity produced by multiple sclerosis and partial spinal cord injury; its use for chemotherapy-related nausea and vomiting; its ability to lower intraocular pressure to treat glaucoma; and its work as an appetite stimulant for wasting syndrome due to HIV infection, anorexia, and cancer.[48] Some believe that evidence for the prescription of marijuana remains inadequate and that other medications produce similar results without the side effects. Many others believe that marijuana is useful and find ways to obtain the drug for medical purposes.

Psychedelics and Hallucinogens

Hallucinogenic drugs create changes in perceptions and thoughts. A common feature of a hallucinogenic experience is the suspension of normal psychic mechanisms that integrate the self with the environment. Some of the more common effects induced by hallucinogenic drugs include changes in mood, sensation, perception, and relations. These drugs produce tolerance to the **psychedelic** effects, but do not create physical dependence or produce symptoms of withdrawal, even after long-term use. As with most psychoactive drugs, however, there is a danger of psychological dependence.

Peyote and lysergic acid diethylamide (LSD) are both hallucinogens. Mescaline is the active ingredient in peyote, a spineless cactus with a small crown, or button, that is dried and then swallowed. From earliest recorded time, natives in northern Mexico and the southwestern United States have used peyote as a part of traditional religious rites. LSD ("acid") also is ingested orally and produces hallucinations, including bright colors and altered perceptions of reality.[49] The hallucinogenic experience, or "trip," is characterized by slight increases in body temperature, heart rate, and blood rate; sweating; chills; and sometimes headaches and nausea. A "bad trip" may result in an acute anxiety reaction that may trigger panic, depression, confusion, fear of insanity, and distorted thoughts and perceptions. Although this drug does not produce physical dependence, evidence of psychological dependence has been found. The most common delayed reaction of LSD is a "flashback," in which individuals reexperience the perceptual and emotional changes originally produced by the drug.

Narcotics

Narcotics include the opiates—opium and its derivatives, morphine, codeine, and heroin—and some other non-opiate synthetic drugs. All narcotics have sleep-inducing and pain-relieving properties. They may be used medically for pain relief, but they have a high potential for abuse. Narcotics relax the user and, when injected, may produce an immediate rush. They also may result in restlessness, nausea, and vomiting. With large doses, the skin becomes moist, cold, and bluish, and the pupils become smaller. Respiration slows, and the user become unresponsive. Death is possible. Over time, opiate users may develop heart infections, skin abscesses, and congested lungs. Infections from unsterile equipment increase the risk of hepatitis, tetanus, and HIV infection. Heroin use among young women has increased in recent years as availability of the drug has spread from urban to suburban environments. Among students surveyed, roughly 1.5% of eighth graders, tenth graders, and twelfth graders reported using heroin at least once during their lifetimes. More than 14% of eighth graders, 18% of tenth graders, and 30% of twelfth graders reported that heroin was "fairly easy" or "very easy" to obtain.[50]

Although narcotics such as heroin affect a woman's ability to conceive, many addicts still can become pregnant. Use of heroin during pregnancy is believed to affect the developing brain of the fetus and possibly cause behavioral abnormalities in childhood. A baby of a heroin addict is born an addict as well and often suffers severe withdrawal symptoms after birth.

Inhalants

Inhalants are chemicals that produce vapors with psychoactive effects and are predominantly abused by pre-adolescents and young adults. Many products that are used

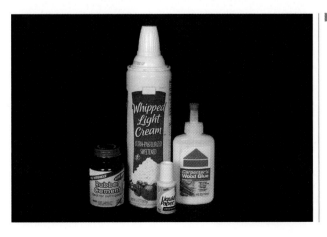

■ Many products that are used as inhalants are not meant for inhalation and are extremely dangerous.

in this way are not meant for inhalation, such as solvents, aerosols, cleaning fluids, and petroleum products. Most inhalants produce the same effects as anesthetics—namely, they slow down bodily functions. At low doses, users may feel slightly stimulated; at higher doses, they may feel less inhibited. Regular use of inhalants leads to tolerance, so the user needs increasingly higher doses to attain the desired effects. Inhalants may cause serious medical complications, such as hepatitis with liver failure, kidney failure, respiratory impairment, destruction of bone marrow and skeletal muscles, blood abnormalities, and irregular heartbeat. Because many inhalants are widely available household products, inhalants are often tried by young people or those who cannot afford or have access to more illicit drugs.

Designer Drugs

Designer drugs are produced in chemical laboratories and then sold illegally. Such synthetic narcotics are particularly dangerous because they are more powerful than those derived from natural substances. The risk of brain damage or fatal overdose from ingestion is correspondingly higher.

MDMA (3,4-methylenedioxymethamphetamine), commonly known as "ecstasy," is an example of a designer drug. It is somewhat related to mescaline and amphetamines. It has been identified as one of the "club drugs" that include GHB, Rohypnol, Ketamine, and methamphetamine. Ecstasy use is dramatically increasing among young women. In the United States, the drug has been associated with a predominantly white, middle-class population. Immediate effects of the drug include a feeling of warmth and openness. Delayed responses, usually within a day, include insomnia, muscle aches, fatigue, and difficulty concentrating. Chronic use of MDMA has been shown to cause brain damage in humans; the extent of damage is directly correlated with the extent of MDMA use. Heavy users also have significant impairments in visual and verbal memory.[51, 52]

Prescription Drugs

The three classes of prescription drugs most commonly abused are opioids prescribed for pain, which include morphine, codeine, and oxycodone (e.g., OxyContin, Percodan, Percocet); central nervous system depressants for anxiety and sleep disorders such as barbiturates and benzodiazepines (e.g., Valium, Librium, and Xanax); and stimulants for sleep disorders and attention-deficit hyperactivity disorder (e.g., Dexedrine and Ritalin). Any of these medications, when used improperly, can lead to serious health consequences and even death. Prescription drug use and abuse are on the rise in the United States, especially among older adults, adolescents, and women. In 2003, more than 6.3 million Americans reported currently using prescription drugs for nonmedical purposes (see Figure 13.7).[53]

Drug Dependency

Drug dependency refers to the attachment—physical or psychological (or both)—that a person may develop to a drug. *Physical dependence* occurs when phys-

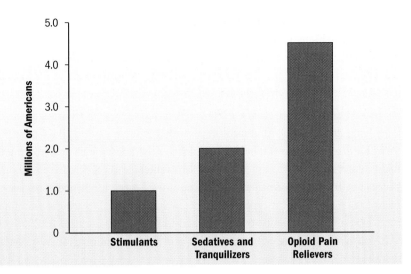

Figure 13.7

More than 6.3 million Americans reported current use of prescription drugs for nonmedical purposes in 2003.

Source: Office of Applied Studies, Substance Abuse and Mental Health Services Administration. (2004). *National Survey on Drug Use and Health.*

iological changes in the body's cells cause an overpowering, constant need for a drug. If the drug is not taken, the user develops withdrawal symptoms, such as intense anxiety, extreme nausea, and deep craving for the drug. Tranquilizers, painkillers, barbiturates, and narcotics may produce physical dependence. *Psychological dependence,* also referred to as habituation, results in a strong craving for a drug because it produces pleasurable feelings or relieves stress or anxiety. Physical and psychological dependence do not always coexist. For example, marijuana and LSD may not create physical dependence, but their continued use has been demonstrated to cause psychological dependence.

Cross-tolerance, or cross-addiction, often presents with drug dependency. In this condition, a state of physical dependence exists in which psychological need for one psychoactive substance leads to dependence on similar substances.

Treatment Dimensions of Drug Dependency

There are three basic approaches to drug-abuse treatment: detoxification, therapeutic communities, and outpatient drug-free programs. Different forms of intervention may help different people and be applicable to different dependencies.

- *Detoxification* is the supervised withdrawal from drug dependence, either with or without medication, in a hospital or outpatient setting.

- *Therapeutic communities* are highly structured, drug-free environments in which abusers live under strict rules while participating in group and individual therapy.

- *Outpatient drug-free programs* are available through community and treatment facilities. Self-help programs include Narcotics Anonymous (NA) and Pills Anonymous (PA), which follow the philosophy of Alcoholics Anonymous. In these programs, users admit to their helplessness and put their faith in a "higher power." Many people do not recognize their own drug problems, and require intervention by friends and family before they will seek treatment (see Self-Assessment 13.3).

Drug dependency treatment programs must address the spectrum of physical and psychosocial issues that confront the addict. These challenges are especially difficult for female addicts, who experience an array of concerns such as contraception, pregnancy, motherhood, childrearing, and health problems in addition to the underlying drug dependency. Evidence suggests that women are less likely to seek treatment for drug abuse, and they respond differently than men to drug treatment. Female addicts often are caregivers and are reluctant to seek care for themselves because of the needs of others. In addition, they more often need specialty treatment than males.[54] These types of services include prenatal treatment, mental health services, domestic violence counseling, and childcare assistance. In 2000, 60% of U.S. substance abuse treatment facilities provided special programs or services for women.[55]

Psychosocial and behavioral treatment programs that emphasize increased self-esteem and choosing positive life options may be more successful with certain women. Unfortunately, few programs focus on the special needs of women or acknowledge the barriers that women must overcome to obtain treatment. These

Self-Assessment 13.3

Do I Have a Drug Problem?

Carefully read and honestly respond to the following statements:

1. Sometimes I am preoccupied with getting and taking a drug.   yes   no

2. Sometimes I don't go to an important event at school or work, or a social or recreational event, so that I can get or take a drug instead.   yes   no

3. I continue to use a drug despite the fact that it makes things with my family or friends worse, or it interferes with school or work activities.   yes   no

4. I have developed a specific physical or mental condition from my drug use (example, irritated nose from cocaine).   yes   no

5. I have repeatedly tried to cut down or eliminate my use of a drug.   yes   no

6. I am sometimes unable to fulfill my obligations (to family, friends, work, or school) because of my drug use.   yes   no

7. I feel specific symptoms when I cut back or eliminate the drug.   yes   no

8. I sometimes take another drug to relieve withdrawal symptoms.   yes   no

9. I sometimes use the drug in larger doses or over a longer period than recommended.   yes   no

10. I need to take more of the drug now than I did before to get the same effect.   yes   no

If you answered "yes" to any of these statements, it is important to seek help now with your drug problem.

barriers may include, but are not limited to, lack of day care for children, lack of safe drug-free housing, fear of losing their children, financial and legal difficulties, lack of transportation, and health problems requiring services beyond drug treatment. In addition, treatment needs of women should be evaluated with the realization that women do not constitute a homogenous group, but rather run the gamut of pregnant women, adolescent users, older women, single professionals, and housewives, to name but a few subgroups.[32]

Informed Decision Making

The use of drugs, alcohol, or tobacco is a personal responsibility issue. Personal responsibilities include:

- Understanding the breadth of impact that use of a particular substance can have on a person's physical and psychological well-being;

- Being aware of how the substance affects personal behaviors and the assessment of reality; and

- Being able to ascertain and acknowledge that a problem with substance abuse may be present.

Recognizing the warning signs of substance dependence or addiction and seeking early treatment intervention are signs of initial success in addressing the issue. Maintaining abstinence after treating the problem is an ongoing process.

Tobacco

Informed consumers are aware of the multidimensional and interdependent issues of smoking and realize that this problem has no immediate or simple solution. If a woman is a smoker, the single most significant step she can take to improve her chances of well-being is to quit smoking. Regardless of the difficulty—and breaking any addictive behavior is undeniably difficult—there are no excuses or rationalizations that suffice or compare to the devastating consequences of smoking.

The avoidance of involuntary smoking is not as simple as it sounds. Although legislation now restricts smoking in many areas, smoking still occurs in many restaurants, bars, smoking lounges, and places of employment. Also, children are subjected to smoking in their own homes, cars, and even in the womb before birth. Nonsmokers' desire for a "smoke-free" environment presents a potential threat to smokers, who feel that their rights to smoke are violated. Is it possible for both nonsmokers and smokers to coexist in "separate but equal" environments? This question and others are currently being considered in legal and legislative debates. The challenge for nonsmokers is to assert their right to a smoke-free environment in a nonviolent but assertive manner. Much of the resistance by smokers is defensive, as they are reminded of their own need to quit and their fear of failure and frustration with the process.

Women often do not consider tobacco to be a drug. In reality, tobacco can decrease the effects of certain medications such as acetaminophen, antidepressants, and insulin taken for diabetes. Smoking also increases the risk of heart and blood vessel disease when taking oral contraceptives. Tobacco should be identified as a drug when healthcare providers inquire about medications or drug use.

Alcohol

If a woman chooses to drink, several suggestions can help provide her with a framework for decision making and skills development for responsible and safe drinking behavior. For those with a propensity toward excessive drinking, it is important to set a limit and stick to it. A limit of one or two drinks per day may be a reasonable amount for some; only drinking during social activities and only drinking on weekends are other possible limits. The development of alternatives to drinking is a critical task to avoid turning to alcohol when upset or depressed. Alcohol neither "fixes" a problem nor provides an "escape." When drinking becomes the primary focus of an activity, a significant risk for serious long-term alcohol problems arises.

Communication skills are an important component of responsible drinking. Learning to say, "No, thank you, I have had enough to drink," is an important step in exercising personal power and control over drinking behavior. Pacing alcohol consumption is important as well. Bingeing Friday night on a week's worth of alcohol is not the same as moderately paced drinking throughout the week. Also, recognize that alcoholic beverages are not good or wise thirst quenchers, as alcohol leads to dehydration. A glass of water or juice can effectively quench one's thirst and is better than having an alcoholic drink. Food should be consumed before drinking, so it is a good idea to eat something before going to a party or meeting someone for a drink.

Helping others to drink in moderation is also a personal responsibility issue. It is not wise to push drinks or refill empty glasses quickly. Food helps to slow the absorption of alcohol and should be encouraged first, particularly if guests have not eaten for a while. Nonalcoholic beverages should always be available as well. Perhaps the most important responsibilities are never to serve alcohol to a guest who seems intoxicated and never to permit an intoxicated person to operate a vehicle. Assuming responsibility includes making contingency plans for intoxication. The early identification of designated drivers helps ensure safe transportation home for guests. If intoxication occurs despite efforts to prevent it, assume responsibility for the health and safety of guests by providing transportation home or overnight accommodations. Stay with the person if he or she is vomiting. If the person is lying down, turn his or her head to the side and protect the person from swallowing the vomit. Monitor the breathing status. If there are any signs of unconsciousness or respiratory problems, seek immediate medical attention. Remember that the only thing that sobers a drunk person is time. (See Table 13.11.)

Table 13.11 How Do You Handle an Intoxicated Person? Dos and Don'ts

DO demonstrate concern for the person's welfare. Talk in a calm, nonjudgmental voice to reassure him or her.

DO find out what the person was drinking, how much, over what time period, and if the alcohol was consumed with any other drugs or medicines.

DO explain what you intend to do, speaking in a clear, firm, reassuring manner.

DO arrange for someone to stay with a person who is vomiting.

DO encourage the intoxicated person to lie down and sleep, making sure to lie on his or her side. This positioning prevents accidental death by choking should he or she begin to vomit. Be sure to check the person every 30 minutes for the first two hours and then every hour to make sure the person is responsive and breathing. If the individual does not respond, call for emergency assistance (e.g., 911). Remember, a person's blood alcohol concentration (BAC) level may continue to rise depending on how much the individual has had to drink and how recently he or she consumed the alcohol.

DO call for help if the person becomes uncontrollable or you sense an impending medical emergency.

DON'T attempt to constrain the person.

DON'T keep the person awake.

DON'T give the person any medication, even aspirin. Aspirin may irritate the stomach lining.

DON'T give the person food, coffee, tea, or other liquids. He or she is at risk for choking.

DON'T induce vomiting.

DON'T give the person a cold shower.

DON'T assume that every intoxicated person who passes out will sleep it off. Check his or her breathing at regular intervals.

DON'T let a drunk person operate a car, motorcycle, or bicycle.

DON'T leave him or her alone.

Life-Threatening Situations

Unconsciousness

Respiratory difficulties (weak breathing, cessation of breathing, or a person with bluish or pale-colored skin)

Increased, decreased, or irregular pulse (severe circulatory problems are indicated by an irregular pulse or a pulse above 100 or below 60 beats per minute)

Vomiting while semiconscious or unconscious

Source: Reprinted by the permission of Julie Barnes, coordinator, Substance Abuse Services, University of Northern Iowa.

Drugs

Understanding the short- and long-term negative effects that drugs can have, while also developing personal strengths and self-confidence, is the foundation that enables a woman to resist drugs effectively. Knowing how to cope with stress in a healthy way can minimize the likelihood that a woman will turn to drugs as a coping mechanism. The enhancement of self-esteem is another significant personal strength that provides a foundation for drug avoidance.

Early identification and treatment offer hope to the person who is using drugs. Unfortunately, many people either fail or refuse to see the signals that a person is using drugs. Knowing what to do when someone has a drug problem is another dimension of personal responsibility. Many treatment and counseling centers offer free telephone services that provide advice on assessing the situation and helpful resources for action. Confronting the substance abuser is sometimes best handled by a group of loved ones and in the presence of a trained counselor. Outlining how the abuse has affected each person in the abuser's life and how much each person cares about the abuser helps to balance the information. It is unrealistic to expect the abuser to quit without assistance. Although offering support is beneficial, the abuser needs to know that treatment and therapy are necessary.

Informed decision making is also an essential responsibility with prescribed and OTC medication use. Many women have little or no idea why they take certain prescribed medications, or they have multiple and vague reasons for using complex OTC medications. Drugs, whether prescribed or self-medicated, can have powerful adverse reactions with other drugs, certain foods, alcohol, tobacco, and caffeine. Older women are often subject to dangerous and possibly fatal drug interactions due to the numerous medications and supplements they are taking. Because many of the most serious effects of drugs are often wrongly attributed to "being depressed" or "growing old," women should know about possible adverse drug reactions and side effects so such events can be recognized and reported. They should also know which foods and other drugs interact with the medications being taken and whether specific dietary recommendations have been identified for the medications.

Co-dependency

The concept of co-dependency is important for many women who become embroiled within the chaos of another person's life. The term "co-dependent" is used to describe a person obsessed, tormented, or dominated by the behavior of others. Growing out of the older notion of "co-alcoholic," a term once applied to the wives of heavy drinkers, the premise of co-dependency is that everyone in an alcoholic's family is diseased. Consciously or unconsciously, and to their lifelong detriment, co-dependents interact with the drinker and "enable" this person to drink. Co-dependents often feel helpless, miserable, hopeless, and angry as they accept the victim role. A woman may be co-dependent in a relationship with a lover, spouse, parent, child, or friend. A co-dependent typically feels responsible for the behavior and mood of the other.

The co-dependent must learn how to separate her own life from that of the addicted person's. The recovery from co-dependence is similar to recovery from alcohol dependence in that only the co-dependent can take the necessary steps toward her own recovery. A co-dependent must learn not to try to control someone else's life and to stop playing the victim role. Many co-dependents have received useful support and encouragement from various programs, such as the Twelve-Step Program of Al-Anon, a support group for family and friends of alcoholics.

Profiles of Remarkable Women

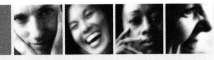

Betty Ford (1918–)

Elizabeth Ann (Betty) Bloomer was born in Chicago and raised in Grand Rapids, Michigan. Bloomer studied dance with Martha Graham in New York City before returning to Grand Rapids at the age of 24. In Grand Rapids, she worked as a fashion coordinator and formed her own dance group, working with handicapped children to teach them the value of rhythm and movement.

In 1948, Bloomer married Gerald R. Ford, two weeks before he was elected to the U.S. Congress. The couple lived in Alexandria, Virginia, for most of the 25 years of Ford's Congressional career. Betty Ford dedicated much of her time to the extracurricular activities of her four children, and also spent time with the Congressional Wives Club, the 81st Congress Club, and the National Federation of Republican Women. Just as the Fords were planning to retire from Congress in 1973, Gerald Ford was selected to serve as Vice President of the United States. Eighteen months later, following Richard Nixon's resignation, he was sworn in as President of the United States.

Betty Ford directed her efforts as First Lady toward handicapped children and women's issues. She was very involved with the passage of and attempts to ratify the Equal Rights Amendment. In 1974, while First Lady, she was diagnosed with breast cancer. She used this event as a springboard to become an honest and vocal advocate for increased awareness about breast cancer and other women's health issues. By openly discussing her ordeal with breast cancer, Ford helped millions of troubled women throughout the United States to understand their illness and take personal responsibility for their bodies. Ford later served as co-chairman for the Susan G. Komen Foundation for Breast Cancer, founded in 1982 by Komen's sister, Nancy Brinker. She was awarded the first Boehm porcelain "Peace Rose" by the Komen Foundation for her prominent role in support of breast cancer research and education, and was even further honored by the award being renamed "The Betty Ford Award." Each year, Ford presents this award to a new recipient for his or her role in the fight against breast cancer.

In 1982, Ford co-founded the Betty Ford Center in Rancho Mirage, California, which offers treatment programs to assist women, men, and their families in starting the process of recovery from alcoholism and other drug dependencies. In 1987, Ford published a book, *Betty: A Glad Awakening,* which recounted her own recovery from chemical dependency in 1978. Once again, she helped millions of people by taking a candid approach to a traditionally stigmatized illness. Ford continues to be an active and outspoken advocate for improved awareness, education, and treatment for alcohol and drug addiction. Today, the Betty Ford Center is regarded as the premier substance abuse treatment facility in the nation.

Betty Ford has been honored many times by many prestigious groups for her public service and outstanding humanitarian contributions. She continues to serve as Chairman of the Board of Directors of the Betty Ford Center and is very involved with handicapped children, the arts, breast cancer issues, arthritis, AIDS, and other issues of significance to women.

Summary

Despite the overwhelming evidence of the detrimental effects of tobacco, alcohol, and drugs, many women continue to abuse them and risk further harm to themselves, their children, and others in their environment. Eliminating smoking is a cornerstone of the improvement of women's health in the United States. Smoking cessation is a significant positive change that a woman can make toward improving her health status. Women also must exercise caution and wisdom with alcohol and legal

Profiles of Remarkable Women

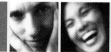

Drew Barrymore (1975–)

Drew Barrymore was born into an acting family; her kin include the legendary actors Lionel, John, and Ethel Barrymore. Drew Barrymore began her career at the age of just 11 months, appearing in a Puppy Choice dog food commercial. She got her first movie role at the age of two, playing a boy in *Suddenly Love.* At age five, she appeared in *Altered States,* and she was turned into a household name when she starred in the blockbuster *E.T.: The Extraterrestrial.* She continued her appearance in films, including Stephen King adaptations *Firestarter* (1984) and *Cat's Eye* (1985).

Soon after, Barrymore tried alcohol for the first time at age nine and marijuana at age 10. She then turned to cocaine, stirred controversy with her near-nude appearances in *Far from Home,* and was forced into ASAP Family Treatment Center, a drug rehabilitation clinic. Following rehab, Barrymore published a memoir entitled *Little Girl Lost* and made a comeback in Hollywood in the early 1990s.

Barrymore's persistence and energy have helped her recover from the difficulties of growing up in front of the camera and in the public eye, and have shaped her into a strong and determined woman. She has not only appeared in numerous successful movies, but has also produced her own films, including *Never Been Kissed, Charlie's Angels,* and a remake of *Donnie Darko.* A dedicated philanthropist, Barrymore often donates her time and resources to a number of charities. She is actively involved in volunteering for and supporting animal rights issues and anti-fur campaigns, urging young people to vote, and advocating for children's rights.

drug use. Knowing the consequences of drinking alcohol, being "alcohol wise," and assuming personal responsibility are the first steps in controlling alcohol use. Reducing the kinds and amounts of drugs taken—recreational drugs, prescribed medications, OTC medications, and substances such as caffeine—should also be an important health goal.

■ ■ ■ ■

Topics for Discussion

1. Should pregnant women be permitted to drink alcohol, use drugs, or smoke? Should states intervene in cases of maternal substance use?

2. Is it a sign of personal weakness or strength for a woman to admit that she has a problem with alcohol or drugs?

3. What should a woman do or say when she knows her friend has a problem with drugs or alcohol, but the friend does not think that she has a problem?

4. Can smokers' rights and nonsmokers' rights both be protected at the same time?

5. How can young girls be educated to resist peer pressure and advertising pressure to initiate cigarette smoking?

6. List all chemicals and substances that you use to change your state of consciousness, such as caffeine, tobacco, alcohol, prescription drugs, over-the-counter drugs, and illegal drugs. Try to give up one or more of these substances for a period of time, and replace it with a healthy behavior such as exercise. Keep a record of how you feel and any changes that you notice in your health or behavior.

7. Should natural substances and over-the-counter medicines be regulated in the same way that prescription drugs are?

8. Is it better to put drug addicts in jail or to send them to mandatory drug treatment programs?

9. Is there any validity to the arguments to legalize marijuana? What about other illicit drugs? Discuss the pros and cons of a change in policy in this area.

Web Sites

Alcoholics Anonymous: http://www.alcoholics-anonymous.org

Health and Human Services Drug and Alcohol Information: http://www.health.org

Recovery Services: http://www.soberrecovery.com

Substance Abuse and Mental Health Services Administration: http://www.samhsa.gov

Surgeon General's Guide to Quitting Smoking: http://www.surgeongeneral.gov/tobacco/consquits.htm

References

1. Substance Abuse and Mental Health Services Administration, U.S. Department of Health and Human Services. (2002). *2001 National Household Survey on Drug Abuse.*

2. National Center on Addiction and Substance Abuse, Columbia University. (2003). *The Formative Years: Pathways to Substance Abuse Among Girls and Young Women Ages 8–22* (PDF).

3. The Sentencing Project. (2005). *Briefing: The Federal Prison Population: A Statistical Analysis.*

4. Mauer, M., Potler, C., and Wolf, R. (1999). Gender and justice: women, drugs, and sentencing policy. *The Sentencing Project.*

5. Center for Women Policy Studies. (2001). *Women, Pregnancy and Substance Abuse.*

6. Poland, M. C., et al. (1993). Punishing pregnant drug users: enhancing the flight from care. *Drug and Alcohol Dependence* 31.

7. Office of National Drug Control Policy. (2003). *Drug Fact Sheet.* Published by the U.S. Department of State. Available online: http://usinfo.state.gov/products/pubs/archive/drugfacts/.

8. Office of National Drug Control Policy. (2000). National Drug Control Strategy FY2001 Budget Summary, page 2.

9. Drucker, E. (January/February 1998). Drug prohibition and public health. *Public Health Reports 114.* U.S. Public Health Service.

10. U.S. Department of Health and Human Services. (2004). *The Health Consequences of Smoking: A Report of the Surgeon General.* Atlanta, GA: US DHHS, CDC, NCCDPHP, Office of Smoking and Health.

11. National Center for Health Statistics. (2003). *Health, United States, 2003 with Chartbook on Trends in the Health of Americans.* Hyattsville, MD: Public Health Service.

12. Centers for Disease Control and Prevention. (2004). Cigarette smoking among adults—United States, 2002. *Morbidity and Mortality Weekly Report* 53(20): 427–431.

13. American Cancer Society. (2005). *Cancer Facts and Figures, 2005.*

14. Centers for Disease Control and Prevention. (2003). Youth risk behavior surveillance—United States. *Morbidity and Mortality Weekly Report* 53(SS-2).

15. Mokdad, A. H., Marks, J. S., Stroup, D. F., and Gerberding, J. L. (2004). Actual causes of death in the United States, 2000. *Journal of the American Medical Association* 291(10): 1238–1245.

16. Centers for Disease Control and Prevention. (2002). Annual smoking-attributable mortality, years of potential life lost, and economic costs—United States, 1995–1999. *Morbidity and Mortality Weekly Report* 51: 300–303.

17A. American Lung Association. (2005). State Legislated Action on Tobacco Issues (Overview). Available online at http://slati.lungusa.org/StateLegislate Action.asp.

17B. Alexander, W. (2006). *The New Face of Cigarette Advertising: Cigarette Marketing Strategies Emerging After the MSA.* UNC-Chapel Hill, Chapel Hill, North Carolina.

18. Samet, J., and Yoon, S. Y., eds. (2001). *Women and the Tobacco Epidemic: Challenges for the 21st Century.* World Health Organization.

19. Centers for Disease Control and Prevention. (2005). Annual smoking-attributable mortality, years of potential life lost, and productivity losses—United States, 1997-2001. *Morbidity and Mortality Weekly Report* 54(25): 625–628.

20. Matikainen, T. (2001). Aromatic hydrocarbon receptor-driven Bax gene expression is required for premature ovarian failure caused by biohazardous environmental chemicals. *Nature Genetics* 28: 355–360.

21. Mosley, S. G., and Gibbs, A. O. C. (1996). Premature grey hair and hair loss

among smokers: a new opportunity for health education? *British Medical Journal* 313: 8.

22. Scott, S. C., et al. (1999). The association between cigarette smoking and back pain in adults. *Spine* 24(11): 1090–1098.

23. *Women and Smoking.* (2001). Report of the Surgeon General.

24. Eisner, M. D., Smith, A. K., and Blanc, P. D. (1998). Bartenders' respiratory health after establishment of smoke-free bars and taverns. *Journal of the American Medical Association* 280: 1909–1914.

25. Ong, M. K., and Glantz, S. A. (2004). Cardiovascular health and economic effects of smoke-free workplaces. *American Journal of Medicine* 117(1): 32–38.

26. Marcus, B. H., et al. (1999). The efficacy of exercise as an aid for smoking cessation in women. *Archives of Internal Medicine* 159: 1229–1234.

27. Substance Abuse and Mental Health Services Administration. (2005). *Results from the 2004 National Survey on Drug Use and Health: National Findings.* NS-DUH- Series H-28, DHHS Publication No. SMA 05-4062. Rockville, MD: Office of Applied Studies.

28. *Alcohol Use Among Adults: United States, 1997–98.* Advance Data No. 324. PHS 2001–1250.

29. National Center for Health Statistics. (1999). *Health, United States, 1999, with Health and Aging Chartbook.* Hyattsville, MD: National Center for Health Statistics.

30. Su, S. S., Larison, C., Ghadialy, R., et al. (1997). *Substance Use Among Women in the U.S. SAMHSA Analytic Series A-3.* Rockville, MD: Substance Abuse and Mental Health Services Administration.

31. Miller, B. A. (1998). Partner violence experiences and women's drug use: exploring the connections. In: Wetherington, C. L., and Roman, A. B. (eds.) *Drug Addiction Research and the Health of Women.* Rockville, MD: National Institute on Drug Abuse, 407–416.

32. Wetherington, C. L., and Roman, A. B. (1998). *Drug Addiction Research and the Health of Women: Executive Summary.* Rockville, MD: National Institute on Drug Abuse, NIH Publication no. 98-4289.

33. National Institute on Alcohol Abuse and Alcoholism. Drinking in the U.S.: main findings from the 1992 National Longitudinal Alcohol Epidemiologic Survey (NLAES). *U.S. Alcohol Epidemiologic Data Reference Manual, vol. 6, ed. 1.* Bethesda, MD: National Institute on Alcohol Abuse and Alcoholism.

34. Levy, D. T., Stewart, K., and Wilbur, P. M. (1999). *Costs of Underage Drinking.* Pacific Institute. Written for the U.S. Department of Justice, Office of Juvenile Justice and Delinquency Prevention.

35. National Institute on Alcohol Abuse and Alcoholism. (1997). *9th Special Report to the U.S. Congress on Alcohol and Health from the Secretary of Health and*

Human Services. Rockville, MD: National Institute on Alcohol Abuse and Alcoholism, NIH Publication no. 97-4017.

36. *Journal of the American Medical Association* news release. (March 12, 1996).

37. National Institute on Alcohol Abuse and Alcoholism. (1998). *Alcohol Alert No. 42: Alcohol and the Liver.* Rockville, MD: National Institute on Alcohol Abuse and Alcoholism.

38. National Institute on Alcohol Abuse and Alcoholism. (1999). *Alcohol Alert No. 46: Are Women More Vulnerable to Alcohol's Effects?* Rockville, MD: National Institute on Alcohol Abuse and Alcoholism.

39. Taylor, J. L., Dolhert, N., Friedman, L., et al. (1996). Alcohol elimination and simulator performance of women and men aviators: a preliminary report. *Aviation, Space, and Environmental Medicine* 67(5) 407–413.

40. Longnecker, M. P., and Tseng, M. (1998). Alcohol and postmenopausal women. *Alcohol Health and Research* 22(3): 185–189.

41. Abel, E., and Sokol, R., for National Institute on Alcohol Abuse and Alcoholism—Missouri Department of Health, State Center for Health Statistics. (1992). A revised conservative estimate of the incidence of FAS and its economic impact. *Alcoholism: Clinical and Experimental Research* 15(3).

42. Heil, S. H., and Subramanian, M. G. (1998). Alcohol and the hormonal control of lactation. *Alcohol Health and Research* 22(3): 178–184.

43. Ellis, D. A., Zucker, R. A., and Fitzgerald, H. E. (1997). The role of family influences in development and risk. *Alcohol Health and Research World* 21(3): 218–225.

44. Prescott, C. A., Aggen, S. H., and Kendler, K. S. (1999). Sex differences in the sources of genetic liability to alcohol abuse and dependence in a population-based sample of U.S. twins. *Alcoholism: Clinical and Experimental Research* 23(7): 1136–1144.

45. Grant, B. F., and Dawson, D. A. (1997). Age at onset of alcohol use and its association with DSM-IV alcohol abuse and dependence. Results from the National Longitudinal Alcohol Epidemiologic Survey. *Journal of Substance Abuse* 9: 106–110.

46. Alcoholics Anonymous. (2004). *Alcoholics Anonymous 2004 Membership Survey.*

47. Office of Applied Studies, Substance Abuse and Mental Health Services Administration, U.S. Department of Health and Human Services. (2002). *The NHSDA Report: Substance Abuse or Dependence.*

48. National Institute on Drug Abuse. (1997). *Workshop on Medical Utility of Marijuana: Report to the Director of NIH by the Ad Hoc Group of Experts.* Bethesda, MD: National Institutes of Health.

49. National Institute on Drug Abuse. (2002). *Facts About Drugs Parents Need to Know.*

50. National Institute on Drug Abuse and University of Michigan. (2004). *Monitoring the Future 2004 Data from In-School Surveys of 8th- 10th-, and 12th-Grade Students.*

51. McCann, U. S., Mertl, M., Eligulashvili, V., and Ricaurte, G. A. (1999). Cognitive performance in (+/−) 3,4-methylenedioxymethamphetamine (MDMA, "ecstasy") users: a controlled study. *Psychopharmacology* 143: 417–425.

52. Bolla, K. I., McCann, U. D., and Ricaurte, G. A. (1998). Memory impairment in abstinent MDMA ("ecstasy") users. *Neurology* 51: 1532–1537.

53. National Institute of Drug Abuse. (2005). *Prescription Drugs: Abuse and Addiction.* NIDA Research Report. NIH Publication Number 05-4881.

54. Office of Applied Studies, Substance Abuse and Mental Health Services Administration. (2002). *National and State Estimates of the Drug Abuse Treatment Gap: 2000 National Household Survey on Drug Abuse* (NHSDA Series H-14, DHHS Publication no. SMA 02-3640). Rockville, MD: Substance Abuse and Mental Health Services Administration.

55. Office of Applied Studies, Substance Abuse and Mental Health Services Administration. (2002). *The DASIS Report: Facilities Offering Special Programs or Services for Women.* Based on the Drug and Alcohol Services Information System (DASIS), the primary source of national data on substance abuse treatment.

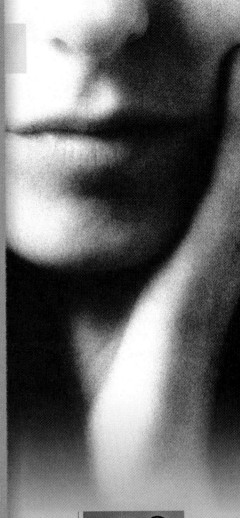

Chapter Fourteen

Violence, Abuse, and Harassment

Chapter Objectives

On completion of this chapter, the student should be able to discuss:

1. The different forms of violence.

2. Violence from a sociocultural, historical, and economic perspective.

3. The influence of poverty, alcohol and drugs, and the media on violence.

4. Violence as a global issue.

5. Types of family and intimate violence.

6. The definition of stalking and actions a woman can take to protect herself.

7. Forms of battering, including physical, sexual, property, psychological, and social violence.

8. Violence in lesbian relationships.

9. Concerns with battering during pregnancy.

10. Battering in women with disabilities.

11. Concepts and issues of child abuse.

12. Concepts and issues of elder abuse.

13. Differences between stranger and intimate rape.

14. Effects of rape on physical health, mental health, sexual intimacy, and relationships.

15. Prevalence of violence toward women by strangers.

16. Sexual harassment as a form of social control and its effects on women in the workplace.

17. Strategies for effective communication to deal with intimate violence and sexual harassment.

womenshealth.jbpub.com

Women's Health Online is a great source for supplementary women's health information for both students and instructors. Visit

http://womenshealth.jbpub.com

to find a variety of useful tools for learning, thinking, and teaching.

Introduction

Violence takes place throughout modern society, and it occurs in many forms. In its broadest sense, *violence* refers to the unjust use of force and power. This definition implies much more than physical forms of violence and includes social norms, values, and political and economic policies. In 2002, the World Health Organization (WHO) compiled the first comprehensive summary of the problem of violence on a global scale in *The World Report on Violence and Health*.[1] The typology in the *World Report* classifies violence into three categories according to who commits the violent act: self-directed violence, interpersonal violence, and collective violence.

Self-directed violence includes suicidal behavior and **self-mutilation** (see **It's Your Health**). Suicide is discussed in further detail in Chapter 12.

Interpersonal violence includes family/partner violence toward a child, partner, or elder and community violence toward an acquaintance or a stranger. Family and intimate violence—including stalking, domestic battering, child abuse, elder abuse, and rape in many cases—are major facets of the violence epidemic. Although most intimate violence qualifies as a crime, historical and cultural traditions to a large extent have condoned violence within the family setting. Violence by strangers—such as robbery, carjackings, aggravated assault, rape, and homicide—affects women as either the victims of the crime itself or the victims of the situation through loss of a partner or family member. Sexual harassment must be considered a form of violence as well, because it also involves an unjust use of power.

Collective violence is an act of violence by people as a group in an effort to achieve social, political, or economic objectives. It can take a variety of forms, including armed conflicts; genocide, repression, and other human rights abuses; terrorism; and organized violent crime. Many acts of violence toward women evolve as a result of women's subordinate status in society. Forms of abuse affecting women as a group in certain populations include female genital mutilation, female infanticide, trafficking of women and girls for sexual exploitation, and acts of rape during war. These acts of abuse have traditionally been associated with countries other than the United States; recent evidence shows that these offenses against women occur worldwide.

Violence often has mental and physical consequences for its victims, including long-term disability or death. Each year, more than 1.6 million people worldwide lose their lives to violence. Indeed, violence is among the leading causes of death for people age 15 to 44 years old.[1] Women are disproportionately victims of violence throughout the world. It is estimated that more than 2.5 million females experience some form of violence each year. Nearly two out of three of those females have been attacked by a family member or an acquaintance.[2]

This chapter provides an overview of violence, focusing on interpersonal violence and the issues that contribute to violence and victimization. Informed decision-making criteria for women are reviewed as well.

Perspectives on Violence, Abuse, and Harassment

Sociocultural Issues

Cultural differences in values, attitudes, and behavioral norms across ethnic and racial groups must be considered in any examination of violence. Unfortunately, data are scarce in this area. Overall, it has proved difficult to assess attitudes toward rape and other violent crimes. Some studies indicate that the public tends to blame victims of rape, rather than those who commit the violent act. In some cases, people believe the violence was justified.

Cultural attitudes about violence toward women may be based on societal acceptance of male dominance. In many cultures, both men and women believe that a man has the right to control his wife's and daughters' behaviors and that a disobedient woman should be punished. By legitimizing these acts of violence, cultures perpetuate violence against women. Women are particularly vulnerable to abuse by their partners in societies where there are marked inequalities between men and women, rigid gender roles, weak sanctions against violent behavior, and cultural norms that support a man's right to sex regardless of a woman's feelings. Studies around the world have identified a list of events that seem to "trigger" violence in intimate relationships, as seen in Table 14.1.[3]

Society's tolerance of rape between intimate partners, especially married partners, is an important dimension of violence. Many people believe that marriage affords men the right to have sex with their wives at any time. In these settings, if the wife refuses, the husband can force her to have sex or punish her through violent means. "Blaming the victim" is a key concept in relationship violence from a women's health perspective. Women who feel they are at fault or that they

> *I feel like it was my fault that I was raped. I had a little too much to drink and I went back to my apartment with him. I wanted to kiss him, but I didn't want to have sex. When he started forcing me to do more than kiss, I asked him to stop. But he wouldn't listen. I probably shouldn't have invited him back with me and I feel guilty for leading him on.*
>
> **19-year-old college sophomore**

Table 14.1   Events Commonly Cited as an Abuser's Rationale for Violence Toward Women

- Not obeying one's husband or partner
- Talking back to one's husband or partner
- Not having food ready on time
- Failing to care adequately for the children or the home
- Questioning one's husband or partner about money or girlfriends
- Going somewhere without permission
- Refusing one's husband or partner sex
- Expressing suspicions of infidelity

Source: Heise, L., Ellsberg, M., and Gottenmoeller, M. (December 1999). Ending violence against women. *Population Reports, Series L, No. 11.* Baltimore, MD: Johns Hopkins University School of Public Health, Population Information Program. Reprinted with permission.

"deserved" punishment may not report a rape. Certain factors, including a woman's style of dress, her relationship with the assailant, evidence of resistance, presence of alcohol or drugs, and location of the incident, may affect a third party's attitude toward the rape and contribute to his or her belief that the rape may actually be "excusable" or "understandable."

Cultural differences in reporting of rape may lead to further insight regarding society's view of rape and differing views among people of different racial and ethnic backgrounds. One large national survey found that American Indian/Alaska Native women were significantly more likely to report rape and physical assault than were women of other backgrounds. Asian/Pacific Islander women were least likely to report rape victimization. Hispanic women were less likely to report rape victimization than were non-Hispanic women in regard to non-intimates; however, in a more recent survey, Hispanic women were significantly more likely than non-Hispanic women to report that they were raped by a current or former intimate partner at some time in their lifetime (Figure 14.1).[4] The explanation for these differences is unclear. More research is needed to determine whether the reporting of incidents of violence is based on the existence of less violence in certain racial and ethnic groups or on social, demographic, and environmental factors that keep a woman from reporting an incident.[5]

Historical Trends

Historically, it has been socially acceptable for a husband to physically discipline his wife. In England, husbands were not punished for murdering their wives until the nineteenth century. The United States followed English law and allowed physical discipline of wives by their husbands until U.S. courts criminalized wife beating in the twentieth century.[6]

Rape also has been documented in American history since the arrival of the Europeans. Spanish explorers used female Native American captives for sexual services and raped Native American women whose tribes they conquered. Native

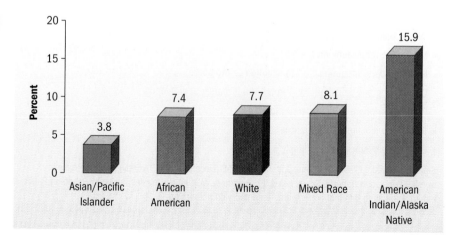

Figure 14.1

Percentage of women reporting rape in their lifetime by race/ethnicity of victim.

Source: Tjaden, P., and Thoennes, N. (2000). *Extent, Nature, and Consequences of Intimate Partner Violence.* Washington, DC: National Institute of Justice, Office of Justice Programs, U.S. Department of Justice.

American cultures, however, prohibited rape, and it had rarely occurred until the arrival of the explorers. Fears of brutal rapes by Native American men were found to be unsubstantiated during colonial-era "Indian" wars. Indeed, English women who had been held captive reported no such treatment.[7]

In seventeenth-century New England in particular, female servants were at high risk of rape and sexual harassment. During that era, an estimated one-third of rape victims were female servants, even though that group represented only 10% of the total population.[7] Later, in the South, where slave labor was increasingly used instead of indentured servants, African female servants found themselves victimized by white owners and overseers who viewed them as property—available for service of their sexual needs. Some historians assert that rape was used to dominate female slaves in a system that otherwise treated them as equals to male slaves.[8]

Poverty Influences

Poverty has been identified as an extremely important factor in many aspects of violence. Low income and joblessness contribute substantially to family violence. The relationship between violence, poverty, and joblessness may be a result of feelings of inadequacy and low self-esteem brought on by unemployment, stress associated with financial instability, and/or an inability to provide for one's family. Often, these emotions turn to frustration and anger, and eventually lead to fighting within the household. In turn, displaced anger can result in violence toward one's partner or children. Unemployed individuals also spend significantly more time in the home, allowing ample opportunities for tensions to rise.

The feminization of poverty refers to the fact that women and children are overwhelmingly the victims of poverty. Women often remain trapped in abusive relationships because of their financial dependence on the abuser. Studies show that women living in households with the lowest annual household income are victimized nearly seven times more than women living in households with the highest income.[9] Living in circumstances of stress and poverty can also lead some women to become perpetrators of violence against their children, spouses, or family members.

Alcohol and Drug Influences

Substance use and abuse consistently have been found to be associated with all forms of relationship violence. It is unclear whether a direct cause-and-effect relationship exists between the use of drugs or alcohol and violence or whether this situation involves two overlapping social epidemics. Violence in a home may cause depression and lack of self-esteem, possibly leading to an increased use of alcohol abuse. Conversely, conflicts in interpersonal relationships may arise as a consequence of substance use and abuse and lead to violent behavior.

Data from the National Crime Victim Survey highlight the strong association between interpersonal violence and substance use. Among victims able to tell whether there was substance use by the perpetrator, 75% reported alcohol or other drug use by the offender at the time of the crime.[10] American Indians, who are

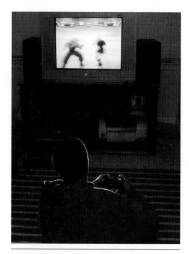

▓ Gaming violence has been shown to influence children and adolescents.

victimized at rates twice as high as the national average, are more likely to experience violence by an offender of a different race. Alcohol can play a significant role in violence, especially among certain groups. For example, 62% of American Indian victims report an offender who was under the influence of alcohol, compared to 42% for the national average.[11]

Media Influences

Media access through television, movies, video and computer games, and the Internet is a major influence in the lives of Americans, especially children and adolescents. Media can be a powerful tool for positive learning and entertainment, but can also pose a threat to emotional and physical safety.

The influence of the media in American culture remains a hotly debated topic among policymakers, educators, and prevention professionals. A number of studies have found that violence and sex on television and in other media constitute an important and unrecognized influence on children and adolescent health and behavior. In addition, unwanted exposure to sexual pictures and sexual solicitations on the Internet create safety concerns for today's parents. According to the Youth Internet Safety Survey conducted by the U.S. Department of Justice, one in five children (10 to 17 years old) receives unwanted sexual solicitations online.[12] The Internet has made it easier for pedophiles to gain access to pornographic collections as well as to solicit children online. Child pornography has devastating effects on children, both on those who are exploited in the actual pictures and on those who view it. To counter this problem, the National Center for Missing and Exploited Children, in partnership with the Federal Bureau of Investigation, Bureau of Customs Immigration Enforcement, U.S. Secret Service, U.S. Postal Inspection Service, and state and local law enforcement in Internet Crimes Against Children Task Forces, operates the national CyberTipline and the national Child Pornography Tipline. These tiplines allow people to report suspicious behavior to a reliable source that can follow up on a possible danger.

Costs of Victimization

The cost of crime is great, with crime victims experiencing a number of losses relating to the crime. The financial burden to the victim includes healthcare costs for treating any physical and mental injuries, as well as lost wages for missed workdays. Other costs may include stolen property in burglaries and expenses for repairing or replacing damaged property. There are costs that impose a burden on society as well, such as police services, fire services, and state victims' services. In the United States, all levels of government combined spent $147 billion for police protections, corrections, and judicial and legal activities in 1999.[13] Victims of violent crime and their families received $370 million in compensation benefits in 2001, an increase of $52 million over the benefits distributed in 2000. This compensation was mainly for medical expenses, lost wages, and mental health counseling.[14]

But the cost burden of violence includes much more than just financial losses. Intangible losses, such as long-term pain and suffering and reduced quality of life, are much more difficult to quantify. Studies show a significant relationship between intimate partner violence and chronic pain, depression, low self-esteem, and substance abuse. Victims of violence also may experience higher rates of attempted suicide and heart disease.[15] All of these findings lead to even higher direct medical costs and consequently more losses for the victim. In a study measuring the cost of human life conducted by the U.S. Department of Justice, it was found that the intangible loss of quality of life exceeds the tangible losses for victims of all crimes, with the exception of arson cases from which there are no injuries.[16]

Legal Dimensions

The number of violent crimes by intimate partners against females has significantly decreased over the past decade. This decrease has been attributed to the Violence Against Women Act (VAWA) of 1994, which was reauthorized in 2000 and again in 2005 to continue existing programs and increase funding. Important aspects of VAWA include these provisions:

- Making it a crime to cross state lines to continue to abuse a spouse or partner
- Creating tough new penalties for sex offenders
- Prohibiting anyone facing a restraining order for domestic abuse from possessing a firearm
- Providing a substantial commitment of federal resources for police, prosecutors, and prevention service initiatives in cases involving sexual violence or domestic abuse
- Requiring sexual offenders to pay restitution to their victims
- Requiring states to pay for rape examinations
- Providing funds for federal victim-witness counselors
- Extending rape shield laws to protect crime victims from abusive inquiries into their private conduct
- Requiring that released offenders report to local enforcement authorities

Global Issues

Violence is a global issue. According to a 2000 UNICEF study, 20% to 50% of the female population of the world will become victims of domestic violence at some point in their lives.[17] Partner violence accounts for a significant number of deaths among women; studies from a range of countries show that 40% to 70% of female murder victims were killed by a husband or a boyfriend, often during an ongoing abusive relationship. In many countries, deaths are concealed as accidents. For example, it is suspected that many deaths of women in India that are recorded as "accidental burns" were actually murders where women were doused with kerosene and set on fire.[1]

I cannot describe how I felt when it was over. I was wondering if it would have been better if I had died. I was humiliated, angry, hurt, and so violated. He had been someone I had trusted—I thought that he was a friend. Looking back, though, there were clues to his violent nature. I had ignored them. It was a mistake for which I paid dearly.

18-year-old student

In some countries, nearly one in four women reports sexual violence by an intimate partner and as many as one-third of adolescent girls report forced sexual initiation. Tens of thousands of women each year are subjected to sexual violence in healthcare settings, including sexual harassment by providers, genital mutilation, forced gynecological exams, and obligatory inspections of virginity. Rape is also used as a documented weapon of war. For example, during the Bosnia–Herzegovina conflict, estimates of the number of women raped by soldiers range from 10,000 to 60,000.[1]

Worldwide data on child abuse are scarce; nevertheless, it is estimated that 57,000 homicides occurred among children younger than 15 years of age worldwide in 2000. Nonfatal child abuse also occurs in virtually every country. In a study conducted in the Republic of Korea, for example, 67% of parents admitted whipping children to discipline them and 45% reported hitting, kicking, or beating their children. In Ethiopia, 21% of urban schoolchildren and 64% of rural schoolchildren reported bruises or swelling from parental punishment.[1]

In Southeast Asia, hundreds of thousands of children are involved in the sex trade, and poverty in those countries continually drives more boys and girls into this arena. Although the demand is driven mostly by local clients, sex tourism continues to grow and fuel the market in countries such as Thailand, Cambodia, and Vietnam. In Cambodia, almost all of the girls in prostitution are the main providers for their families. Children as young as age 12 from poor families are sold by parents or agents into the sex trade.

Elder abuse also occurs on a global scale. In some countries, rapid socioeconomic change weakens family networks that once supported older generations. For example, countries of the former Soviet Union have a growing number of elderly who are left to fend for themselves, resulting in numerous cases of elder neglect. Theft of agricultural products and livestock has been identified as a type of abuse endured by older people in rural areas of the Caribbean.

Family and Intimate Violence

Family and intimate violence refers to violence between individuals in a significant relationship; it can be directed toward former or current spouses or partners, dates, elders, and children.

Violence against women is primarily intimate violence. In the United States, one out of every four women will experience violence by an intimate partner at some point during her lifetime. Family and intimate violence includes many forms of mental and physical crime, as well as threatening with injury (see Self-Assessment 14.1).

Stalking

Stalking, as defined by the National Institute of Justice, is a "course of conduct directed at a specific person that involves:

Recognizing a Potentially Abusive Partner

1. Did the person grow up in a violent family? Was he or she abused as a child?
2. Is the person jealous of your friendships and does he or she try to control the time you spend with other people?
3. Does the person lose his or her temper frequently and overreact to minor problems and frustrations?
4. Does the person abuse alcohol or drugs?
5. Does the person control the finances and make all the decisions within the household?
6. If male, does he have a distorted concept of manhood? Does he have traditional ideas about women's roles versus men's roles?
7. Do you fear the person when he or she is angry?
8. Has the person used physical or psychological coercion to pressure you for sex? Has he or she ever physically assaulted you?

If you answer "yes" to one or more of these questions, you may be at risk of abuse. Talk to your healthcare professional about ways to prevent abuse before it happens.

- Repeated visual or physical proximity (with "repeated" meaning on two or more occasions);
- Nonconsensual communication;
- Verbal, written, or implied threats; or
- A combination thereof that would cause fear in a reasonable person."[18]

A large survey in the United States found that stalkers frequently were a current or former spouse, cohabiting partner, or date at some point in the stalked women's lives.[3] The same survey found a strong association between stalking and other forms of violence in intimate relationships. Eighty-one percent of women stalked by a current husband, former husband, or cohabiting partner were physically assaulted by that partner; 31% also were sexually abused by that partner.[4]

Although every stalking case is different, a stalker's behavior typically becomes more and more threatening, serious, and violent. The behavior may begin with making harassing calls, watching or following someone, sending unwanted mail, or making verbal threats. The stalking activity generally escalates from what initially may be bothersome and annoying, to the level of obsessive, dangerous, violent, and potentially fatal acts. Some stalkers may not have a violent motive, but still may cause harm if jealousy or anger is involved.

States have passed laws to prevent stalking and punish those who engage in acts of stalking. The first anti-stalking law was passed in California in 1990 in response to several high-profile cases in which the perpetrators stalked and eventually killed their victims. In each case, the victim had notified the police of the stalker's threatening behavior, yet the police were unable to do anything legally unless the stalker acted on the threats. The California law gave law enforcement officers the right to intervene in stalking cases before the stalker acted on his or her threats. Since then, all states have passed similar laws. Restraining or protection orders can be issued to protect citizens against stalking situations. A woman who believes she is being stalked should take action, as outlined in Table 14.2.

Another form of stalking, called **cyberstalking,** is defined as threatening behavior or unwanted advances directed at another using the Internet and other forms of online communications. Victims are targeted through chat rooms, e-mail, and message boards. The stalker may send obscene, threatening, or improper messages; a barrage of unwanted e-mails; or electronic viruses. Online stalking often turns into offline stalking, bringing a real threat of physical harm to the victim. Law enforcement agencies estimate that cyberstalking is a factor in 20% to 40% of all stalking cases. Although current state laws encompass any type of unwanted communication with the victim, many states are now further protecting their residents from cyberstalking by specifically including electronic transmission of communication.

Domestic Violence

Domestic violence, also referred to as **battering,** occurs when a person subjects a current or former romantic partner to forceful physical, social, and psychological

Table 14.2   Guidelines for Women Who Are Being Stalked
These guidelines provide practical information for a woman who believes she is being stalked, but is not in imminent danger. The guidelines do not guarantee her safety, but rather they should reduce her risk of harm.

- Record each incident of stalking with great detail. This record can be used as evidence against the perpetrator if necessary.
- Let family and friends know about the stalker. This protects not only the victim but also those close to the victim.
- Be extremely alert when away from home; carry a whistle to alert others nearby or a cellular phone to report suspicious behavior or to contact someone for help if necessary.
- Seek protection, restraining, or stay-away orders.
- Inquire about the state's stalking laws because each state's laws differ, and see how they apply to this specific case.
- Note any illegal acts by the stalker, such as entering the residence without permission, destroying property, and so on. By reporting these acts to the police, the acts are not only documented for future evidence but may also require that the stalker be incarcerated or ordered to stay away from the woman.
- Create a safety plan. Keep a list of important numbers, such as law enforcement, legal representation, and safe places. Victims may want to keep important items and extra money in one place to grab in a rush if necessary.
- Other preventive measures include changing the locks on doors; adding extra outside light around the residence; maintaining an unlisted phone number; varying regular routes; staying in public places when out of the house; and informing neighbors so that they can alert someone if they see something suspicious.

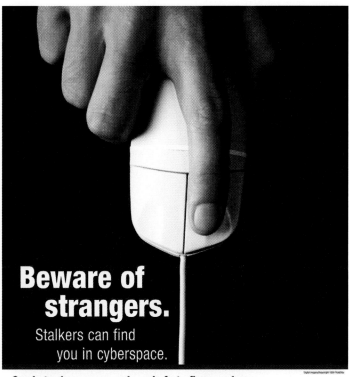

Beware of strangers.

Stalkers can find you in cyberspace.

One in twelve women and one in forty-five men has been stalked at some time in their life. Protect yourself.

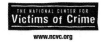

The Internet provides many perpetrators with opportunities to stalk. Reprinted with permission from the National Center for Victims of Crime.

behavior so as to coerce her, without regard to her rights. Battering includes five types of interpersonal violence: physical, sexual, property, psychological, and social. Physical violence includes slapping, choking, punching, kicking, pushing, and using objects as weapons. Forced sexual activity constitutes sexual violence. Property violence denotes threatened or actual destruction of property. Psychological and social forms of violence include threats of harm, physical isolation of the woman, extreme jealousy, mental degradation, and threats of harm to children, pets, or other loved ones.

Battering of women is a major health problem. It occurs in families of all racial, economic, educational, and religious backgrounds. Although the reasons for violence are not always clear, some causes of domestic violence, and violence in general, have been identified (see Table 14.3). Battering tends to be a pattern of violence rather than a one-time occurrence. During the six months following an episode of domestic violence, 32% of women are victimized again. Nearly half of the men who beat their wives do so at least three times per year.[19] Violence in a home often involves more than the adult couple. Each year, an estimated 3.3 million children are exposed to violence against their mothers or other female caretakers by family

Table 14.3	Causes of Violence

Root Causes of Domestic Violence

- Power and control
- Growing up in a cycle of violence and abuse
- Distorted concept of manhood

Root Causes of Violence

- Poverty and unemployment
- Underemployment and economic disequilibrium
- Lack of housing and displacement
- Circumstances of racism and injustice
- Alcohol and substance abuse
- Hopelessness and despair

Source: Office of Women's Health Report. (1997). *Domestic Violence Facts.* Department of Health and Human Services.

members.[20] Research suggests that almost all of these children are aware of the violence in their homes; even if they do not see it, they hear the screams and see the bruises, broken bones, and abrasions sustained by their mothers.[21] In homes in which partner abuse occurs, it is estimated that children are 1,500 times more likely to be abused than children in homes where no abuse is present.[22]

Domestic violence is thought to be more prevalent among immigrant women than among U.S. citizens. Immigrants from certain cultures condone the use of violence from a man toward his wife or other women in the family. Women from these cultures may not have access to legal and social services, as well as extended family or other support networks. Immigrant women also may not feel that they are protected by the U.S. legal system or may feel that they are unable to seek help from authorities if their immigrant status is unstable.[23–25] Studies involving Latina, South Asian, and Korean immigrants demonstrated that 30% to 50% of these women have been sexually or physically victimized by a male intimate partner.[26]

Although battering of women occurs at all socioeconomic levels of society, the rate of intimate violence against women generally decreases as household income levels increase (Figure 14.2).[27] Spousal abuse perhaps appears more frequently under economically disadvantaged conditions because educated, middle-class, and affluent women tend to have more resources with which to avoid or leave violent relationships. For example, affluent women may seek confidential professional help and not use residential shelters.

Regardless of socioeconomic status, battering is a major cause of injury to women in the United States (Table 14.4). Relationship violence can and often does lead to death. In recent years, the mortality rate from relationship violence has been high: an intimate killed about 33% of female murder victims. In the United States, more

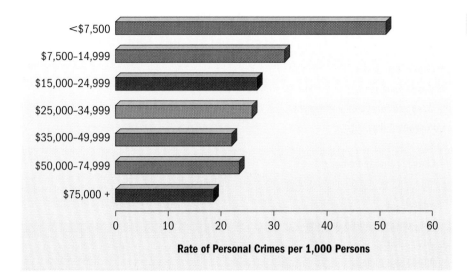

Figure 14.2

Victimization rates for persons age 12 and older, by annual family income victims.

Source: Greenfield, L., (2005). *Criminal Victimization in the United States, 2003 Statistical Tables. National Crime Victimization Survey* (NCJ 207 811). Washington, DC: U.S. Department of Justice.

than three women are murdered every day by an intimate partner.[28] Battering is often underdiagnosed during medical visits because both the patient and her healthcare provider may be reluctant to initiate or discuss the topic. In a recent study, 92% to 98% of women did not discuss their experiences of abuse with their healthcare providers.[29] Although most states have mandatory reporting requirements for child abuse or elder abuse, only a small number of states have a corresponding requirement for healthcare providers to report battering of women.

Battering in Same-Sex Relationships

Although research on domestic violence has increased considerably in the last two and a half decades, only recently has attention been given to the problem of partner abuse among homosexual couples. Research in this area is especially difficult. In 2001, there were 5,046 reported incidents of domestic violence affecting lesbian, gay, bisexual, or transgender victims in the United States; 43% of these victims identified themselves as female.[30] In terms of race/ethnicity, 27% of the victims were white, 15% Hispanic, 10% African American, and 3% Asian/Pacific Islander.

Lesbian victims of partner abuse are doubly stigmatized—first because of their victimization and second because of their sexual orientation. Many lesbians perceive battering as a heterosexual phenomenon and therefore may not recognize the patterns of abuse within their own relationships.[31] Additionally, fewer protective measures from the legal system are available to lesbians. Such victims of domestic violence often find it difficult to seek assistance from the courts and police when their relationships are not recognized in many states' legislatures. Most battering-related services are designed for heterosexual female victims and heterosexual male offenders, making it difficult for lesbians to find support. This lack of services is believed to be a major contributor to the lack of recognition of lesbian, bisexual, and gay domestic violence.

Table 14.4   Health Outcomes of Violence Against Women—
Partner Abuse, Sexual Assault, Child Sexual Abuse

Nonfatal Outcomes

Physical Conditions

- Injury and functional impairment
- Permanent disability
- Severe obesity
- Chronic pain syndrome
- Irritable bowel syndrome and other gastrointestinal disorders

Mental Health

- Post-traumatic stress disorder
- Depression
- Anxiety disorders
- Eating disorders
- Sexual dysfunction
- Low self-esteem
- Substance abuse

Negative Health Behaviors

- Smoking, alcohol and drug abuse
- Sexual risk-taking
- Physical inactivity
- Overeating

Reproductive Health

- Unwanted pregnancy
- Sexually transmitted diseases/HIV
- Gynecological disorders, including pelvic inflammatory disorder
- Pregnancy complications, including low birthweight and miscarriage

Fatal Outcomes

- Homicide
- Suicide
- Maternal mortality
- AIDS-related death

Source: Heise, L., Ellsberg, M., and Gottenmoeller, M. (December 1999). Ending violence against women. *Population Reports, Series L, No. 11*. Baltimore, MD: Johns Hopkins University School of Public Health, Population Information Program. Reprinted with permission.

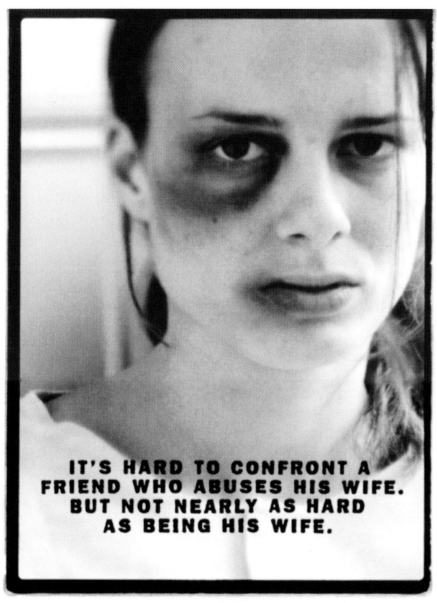

At least one out of every three murdered women is killed by her husband or boyfriend. Reprinted with permission from the Family Violence Prevention Fund.

IT'S HARD TO CONFRONT A FRIEND WHO ABUSES HIS WIFE. BUT NOT NEARLY AS HARD AS BEING HIS WIFE.

So you know your friend is an abuser. Do you ignore it or bring it up? Ignoring it is easy. Bringing it up is awkward. You could lose a friend. But maybe bringing it up is the only way to really be a friend. Telling him you know, telling him it's wrong, telling him it's a punishable crime, could be doing him a big favor. Maybe he needs someone to talk to. Maybe he needs someone to say, "No, it's not OK." But more important than his feelings, his wife's well-being, her very life may be in your hands. We can give you some information that may help. Call us at 1-800-END ABUSE.

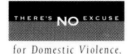

THERE'S **NO** EXCUSE for Domestic Violence.

Family Violence Prevention Fund

Battering During Pregnancy

Women are not immune to battering during pregnancy. Each year, as many as 324,000 pregnant women experience intimate partner violence.[32] Battering during pregnancy has numerous consequences. Women who are battered may be less likely to seek prenatal care and gain sufficient weight. They also may be more likely to engage in harmful behaviors such as smoking or alcohol use. Battering during pregnancy is linked to an increased risk of miscarriage, premature labor, fetal distress, and low birthweight. Blunt abdominal trauma can lead to fetal death or low birthweight by provoking preterm delivery. Excessive stress and anxiety for the mother also may cause adverse effects.[3] To date, only limited research regarding violence during pregnancy has been conducted. More research is needed to identify additional issues that may precipitate battering of pregnant women.

Battering in Women with Disabilities

Violence and abuse are significant problems for people with disabilities. Women with disabilities experienced abuse as often as women without disabilites, at a rate of 52%. One study found that women with disabilities and women without disabilities were equally likely to report experiencing physical, sexual, or emotional abuse at some point in their lives. Women with disabilities, however, were more likely to report multiple perpetrators, longer duration of abuse and more intense experiences of abuse.[33]

Disabled women are most commonly abused by an intimate partner, followed by a family member, a personal care attendant, a stranger, or a healthcare provider. The abuse often begins subtly, as the abuser tries to determine how much violence will remain unnoticed. Abuse may take the form of psychological, physical, or financial abuse, or it may involve neglect by withholding care, medication, or mobility devices.

Many people with disabilities are especially vulnerable to victimization because of their real or perceived inability to fight or flee, or to tell anyone about the abuse. Many battered women's shelters may be inaccessible or lack attendant care or per-

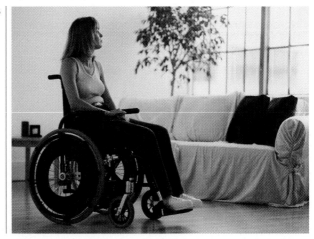

▦ Women with disabilities face unique challenges with violence.

sonnel who are trained in working with specific conditions. A woman therefore may find herself trapped in an abusive situation. Consequently, healthcare practitioners need to find ways to conduct at least part of their visit with a woman with disabilities in private. This opportunity allows a woman to answer questions and confide in her practitioner without a caretaker or family member being present.[34]

Child Abuse

As defined by the amended 1996 Child Abuse Prevention and Treatment Act, **child abuse and neglect** includes any act or the failure to act on the part of a parent or caretaker that presents an imminent risk of serious harm or actually results in serious physical or emotional harm, sexual abuse, exploitation, or death of a child. A child is defined as a person younger than age 18, except in sexual abuse cases, in which the age is specified by the child protection laws of the child's state of residence. Included in the definition of child abuse and neglect is the withholding of medically indicated treatment that in a professional's medical judgment would be effective in improving or curing a life-threatening condition. The four major types of maltreatment of children include physical abuse, child neglect (failure to provide for a child's basic needs including physical, education, or emotional needs), sexual abuse, and emotional abuse.

In the United States, an estimated 906,000 children were victims of abuse and neglect in 2003 (roughly 50% boys and 50% girls). More than 80% of these children were maltreated by one or both parents, most commonly the female parent; women represented nearly 60% of all perpetrators of such violence. The abuser's gender differed by type of maltreatment: neglect and medical neglect were most often attributed to female perpetrators, whereas sexual abuse was most often attributed to male perpetrators. The median age of perpetrators was 31 years for women and 34 years for men.[35]

Approximately 60% of the maltreated children suffered neglect, including medical neglect; nearly 20% suffered physical abuse; approximately 10% were sexually abused; and 5% were emotionally maltreated. Many children suffer more than one type of maltreatment. Studies show that an estimated 1,500 children died as a result of child abuse or neglect; only a small percentage of these child fatalities occurred in foster care. More than half of all victims were white, one-fourth were African American, and one-tenth were Hispanic; however, rates of victimization were highest among Pacific Islander, American Indian/Alaska Native, and African American children (see Figure 14.3). Reasons for child abuse and neglect as reported by state agencies included substance abuse by one or both of the parents, poverty or other economic strain, parental capacity and skill, and other incidents involving domestic abuse.

In a survey by the National Center on Child Abuse Prevention Research, 85% of states reported substance abuse as a major problem in families with suspected child maltreatment.[36] Research also suggests that although children from all socioeconomic levels suffer from abuse and neglect, children from families with annual incomes of

Figure 14.3

Frequency of victimization of U.S. children by race/ethnicity, 2003.

Source: U.S. Department of Health and Human Services, Administration on Children, Youth and Families. (2005). *Child Maltreatment 2003*. Washington, DC: U.S. Government Printing Office.

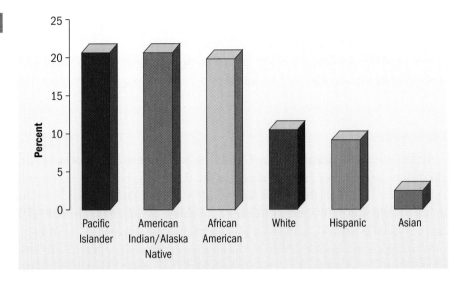

less than $15,000 were more than 25 times as likely to suffer maltreatment than were children from families with annual incomes of $30,000 or more.[37] There are a number of problems associated with poverty that may contribute to child maltreatment: more transient residence, poorer education, and higher rates of substance abuse and emotional disorders. Moreover, families at the lower socioeconomic levels have less adequate social support systems to assist parents in their child care responsibilities.

Almost without exception, abusive parents were themselves abused or neglected as children. This underscores the resulting cycle of abuse: Battered children often grow up to become battering adults. Child abuse is frequently a symptom of family violence. One large study revealed that women who had both witnessed violence between their parents and been victims of parental abuse themselves were twice as likely to abuse their partner or children than were women who had been exposed to only one or the other type of violence. Women appeared to be most strongly influenced by their mother's behavior. With every witnessed incident in which the woman's mother had attacked her father, there was an increased likelihood that the woman would

- Abuse her child;
- Abuse her partner; or
- Become the victim of her current partner.[38]

Several psychological traits have been associated with child abusers:

- Immaturity and dependency
- A sense of personal incompetence
- Difficulty in seeking pleasure and finding satisfaction as an adult
- Social isolation
- A reluctance to admit the problem and seek help

- Fear of spoiling children
- A strong belief in the value of punishment
- Unreasonable and age-inappropriate expectations of children
- Low personal self-esteem

Any combination of these traits results in an inability to cope and problem-solve effectively when a problem or crisis evolves. In such cases, the outcome may ultimately be abuse.

The most largely victimized age group is the youngest (0 to 3 years of age), with victimization decreasing with age (see Figure 14.4). A history of child abuse can lead to behavioral and psychological problems, relationship problems, low self-esteem, depression, suicidal behavior, alcohol and substance abuse, sexual dysfunction, and sexual risk-taking later in life.[3]

Elder Abuse

As the number of people older than age 60 has rapidly grown, so has the number of abuse cases involving elderly victims.[39] **Elder abuse** is a serious problem for women because they generally live longer than men. In most cases, elders become increasingly dependent on others for their care as they get older. Even after accounting for their larger share of the aging population, women still accounted for two-thirds of all elder abuse reports.[40] There are three major situations for abuse of the elderly:

- Domestic abuse (maltreatment by someone who has a relationship with the victim)
- Institutional abuse (maltreatment by staff in a residential facility)
- Self-neglect (failure to care for oneself)

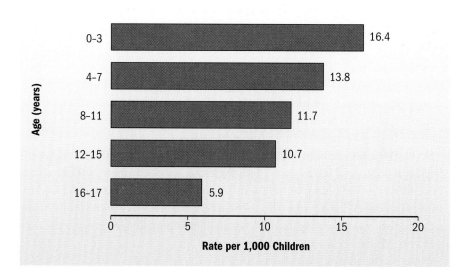

Figure 14.4

Victimization rates by age group, 2003.

Source: U.S. Department of Health and Human Services, Administration on Children, Youth and Families. (2005). *Child Maltreatment 2003*. Washington, DC: U.S. Government Printing Office.

Within these situations, the National Center on Elder Abuse defines seven types of elder abuse:

- *Physical elder abuse* is defined as the use of physical force that results in bodily injury, physical pain, or impairment.
- *Sexual elder abuse* is defined as nonconsensual sexual contact of any kind with an elderly person.
- *Emotional or psychological elder abuse* is the infliction of anguish, pain, or distress through verbal or nonverbal acts.
- *Financial or material exploitation* occurs when an elder's funds, property, or assets are misused or misappropriated by another.
- *Neglect* refers to the refusal or failure of a caretaker to perform his or her obligations or duties to an elderly person. Neglect can be active, when the failure or refusal to acknowledge an obligation is intentional, or passive, when the failure is unintentional.
- *Self-neglect* is the failure to provide oneself with adequate food, water, clothing, shelter, safety, personal hygiene, and medication, thereby threatening the elderly person's own health or safety.
- *Abandonment,* also known as "granny dumping," occurs when an elderly person is deserted by an individual who has physical custody of the elder or by a person who has assumed responsibility for providing care to the elder.

Elder abuse has been discovered in people of all racial, ethnic, and economic backgrounds in the United States. In general, elders who are unable to care for themselves are more likely to suffer abuse. Researchers have found that in 90% of substantiated cases, perpetrators of elder abuse were family members, with two-thirds being adult children or spouses. Men were more likely to be perpetrators of abuse in cases of abandonment, physical abuse, emotional abuse, and financial and material exploitation. Women were slightly more likely to be perpetrators in cases of neglect. In self-neglect cases, approximately two-thirds of elders were female, 75 or older, and white.[39]

In one survey conducted in the United States, 36% of nursing-home staff reported having witnessed at least one incident of physical abuse of an elderly patient in the previous year, 10% admitted having committed at least one act of physical abuse themselves, and 40% said that they had psychologically abused patients.[40] Abusive acts within institutions include physically restraining patients, depriving them of dignity and choice over daily affairs, and providing insufficient care (allowing them to develop pressure sores, for example).

Several factors have been identified that contribute to a high stress level for relatives of a dependent older person and, therefore, may contribute to elder abuse. These factors include caregiver stress, impairment of the dependent elder, and resentment of dependency, especially as the level of dependency increases. In many cases of abuse, caregivers are unprepared, unable, or unwilling to provide the necessary care. Elder abuse is also related to emotional problems, such as alcohol or drug use by the abuser, social isolation of the abuser and the abused, and lack of

My granddaughter and her boyfriend always take money from me. The other day, when I asked them to leave my house, they pushed me. They're always yelling at me and telling me how much they hate caring for me. My daughter who lives with me pretends she doesn't see it. But who can I tell? If I report them, I'll end up in a nursing home all alone.

82-year-old woman

community support. It has also been hypothesized that the abuser may be repeating a cycle of violence, similar to the cycle identified in cases of child abuse and neglect. That is, the abuser of an elderly parent may have been abused by the parent in childhood, or the abuser may have witnessed the same type of elder abuse by the parent against the abuser's grandparent.

Rape and Sexual Assault

Rape and sexual assault are violent crimes of aggression. Rape is defined as an event occurring without consent, involving the use of force or the threat of force to sexually penetrate the victim's vagina, mouth, or rectum.[4] Sexual assault often refers to forced sexual contact, but this term is frequently used as an all-encompassing descriptor for any type of unwanted sexual advances as well. A large survey conducted by the National Institute of Justice and the Centers for Disease Control and Prevention found that one of six women and one of 33 men in the United States has been the victim of attempted or completed rape as a child or an adult.[4] Determining an accurate estimate of the number of women raped per year is quite difficult given the significant underreporting of the crime. In 2004, there were 204,370 reported victims of rape, attempted rape, or sexual assault in the United States. Of these individuals, 95,420 were victims of sexual assault, 43,440 were victims of attempted rape, and 65,510 were victims of completed rape.[41] Nine out of every 10 rape victims were female.[41]

Rape may occur among strangers or intimates. Acquaintance rape, or **date rape,** is defined as rape in which the victim and the rapist were previously known to each other and may have interacted in some socially appropriate manner. In 2004, 67% of rape victims knew their assailant. Approximately 47% were raped by a friend or acquaintance, 17% by an intimate, and 3% by another relative; 31% of victims were raped by a stranger; and in 2% of the cases, the relationship could not be identified (see Figure 14.5).[41] Rape by a co-worker, teacher, professor, a husband's friend, or boss—anyone the individual knows—is considered acquaintance rape.

Many victims of rape are children and adolescents; about 44% of rape victims are younger than age 18 and about 15% are younger than age 12.[41] Although physical abuse and neglect account for the greatest portion of child abuse incidents, child sexual abuse is another tragic dimension of child abuse in general. Of the substantiated child abuse cases in 2000, 10% comprised sexual abuse cases.[42] It is difficult to determine the incidence rate of sexual abuse among children. One recent report found that 13% of girls and 3.4% of boys had been sexually abused.[43] In reported cases, three-fourths of adolescent sexual assault victims knew their attackers—21.1% were family members and 32.5% were acquaintances or friends.[43] Males are reported to be the abusers in most sexual abuse cases involving children.

In many cases of date or acquaintance rape, the rape has been facilitated by the use of drugs to render the victim unconscious or incapacitated. Flunitrazepam, commonly known as Rohypnol, is one type of "date rape drug." This drug is ten times as strong as Valium and is tasteless and odorless. It dissolves in liquid, takes effect

My stepfather started fondling me when I was 6. It evolved into sex by the time I was 12. I think my mother knew, but she had so many other problems to deal with. I had three younger sisters and I was so afraid for them. He said that he wouldn't touch them if I wouldn't tell "the secret." I was trapped. Eventually I found out that he was telling them the same thing. I have been in therapy for a year. I am still so hurt and so angry. The feelings and memories just won't go away.

21-year-old woman

Figure 14.5

Perpetrator relationship to victim in cases of sexual assault/rape.

Source: Catalano, S.M. (2005). *Criminal Victimization, 2004*. Washington, DC: Bureau of Justice Statistics, U.S. Department of Justice.

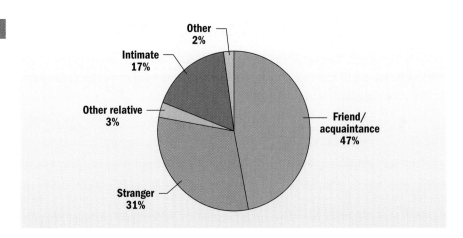

quickly, and produces memory loss for as long as eight hours. Rohypnol is especially popular on high school, college campuses, and as well as nightclubs. Many women have been raped after consuming a drink with the drug dissolved in it. The use of the drug is extremely dangerous and can cause death. Gamma hydroxybutyrate (GHB) and gamma butyrolactone (GBL) are found in liquid form and have also been associated with sexual assault. Abuse of GHB and GBL can lead to coma and seizures. Ketamine, used as a tranquilizer in cats, is another common date rape drug that is snorted. It is referred to as "special K" and can cause death.

Rape also can happen in a marriage, during a legal separation, or after a divorce. Rape in marriage is often called spousal rape or marital rape. Historically, husbands had unlimited sexual access to their wives and, therefore, rape within marriage was not recognized as a crime. In 1993, marital rape became a crime in all 50 states. Many states provide exemptions for certain situations, such as mental or physical impairment of a woman rendering her unable to consent, that protect husbands from being prosecuted for rape. One study found that nearly 14% of women who had been married were the victims of at least one attempted or completed rape by their husbands or ex-husbands.[44]

In addition, rape can occur between people of the same sex. The National Violence Against Women Survey found that 10.8% of women rape or sexual assault victims were assaulted by a female.[4] Results of one study of sexual coercion within gay and lesbian relationships indicated that 50% of the lesbians who had experienced sexual coercion reported unwanted penetration, and 32% reported unwanted fondling.[45]

Rape is often characterized as not being a "clear-cut" crime such as murder. Societal pressures and norms have reinforced beliefs that rape is sometimes justifiable, depending on the circumstances. For various reasons, most rapes go unreported. In fact, an estimated 58% of rapes are never reported to the police.[41] These unreported rapes may be perceived as a threat to public safety, because if the rapists are not dealt with in the criminal justice system, their violent behavior may con-

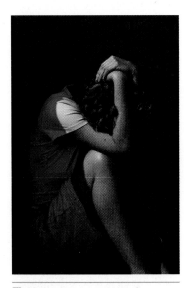

■ Most rapes go unreported.

It's Your Health

Information About "Date Rape Drugs"

Rohypnol (roofies, ruffies, roach, R2, rophies, la roche, rib, mind eraser, the forget pill, the date rape drug)

- **Characteristics:** small white pill (often has "ROCHE" on one side for Hoffmann-La Roche, its manufacturer, and a circled "1" or "2" on one side); can be swallowed as a pill, dissolved in a drink, or snorted; tasteless and odorless
- **Effects:** may feel dizzy, disoriented, nauseated, sleepy, extremely relaxed, or drunk; can cause difficulty speaking or moving, unconsciousness, and loss of memory; effects may last from two to eight hours.

Gamma Hydroxybutyrate (GHB, liquid ecstasy, easy lay, liquid X, energy drink, somatomax, scoop, Georgia Home Boy, grievous bodily harm, goop)

- **Characteristics:** white powdered material or liquid form
- **Effects:** may feel drowsy, dizzy, or nauseated; may cause unconsciousness, seizures, severe respiratory depression, and coma

Ketamine (special K, vitamin K, cat tranquilizer, k)

- **Characteristics:** white powdered material, similar to cocaine; can be snorted, smoked with marijuana, or dissolved in beverages
- **Effects:** short-acting hallucinatory effects; can affect the senses, judgment, and coordination for 18 to 24 hours

Ways to Protect Yourself

- Don't leave a beverage unattended or accept a drink from an open container.
- Don't drink from someone else's drink.
- Don't drink any beverage with a funny taste, odor, residue, color, or consistency.
- Go to parties with trusted friends; watch out for each other and leave together.

tinue. The underreporting of rape is due to a number of factors, including the pattern of "blaming the victim." Many women fear unwanted publicity from making a formal complaint, and others distrust hospital and law enforcement agencies. Reasons for women not reporting rape include feelings of shame or guilt, fear that they would not be believed, and fear of reprisal or punishment if the rapist is an acquaintance or employer.

Around the world, countless women in prisons and jails are at risk of rape and other forms of sexual violence. Reporting procedures in prisons are often ineffectual, and complaints are routinely ignored. To make matters worse, punishment for the crime is rare and some inmates face retaliation from the offender if a report is made.

Reducing Risk of Rape/Sexual Assault

Risk reduction for rape entails taking actions—by both women and society as a whole—to eliminate the inappropriate use of physical and sexual force. These

It's Your Health

Reducing the Risk of Date Rape

Be wary of a relationship that is operating along classic stereotypes of dominant male and submissive, passive female. The dominance in ordinary activities may extend to the sexual arena.

Be wary when a date tries to control behavior or pressures others in any way.

Be explicit with communication. Don't say "no" in a way that could be interpreted in any way as a "maybe" or "yes."

Avoid ambiguous messages with both verbal and nonverbal behavior. Saying "no" and permitting heavy petting implies confusion or ambiguity.

First dates with an unknown companion may be safer in a group.

Avoid remote or isolated spots where help is not available.

Limit alcohol and illegal drug use.

It's Your Health

Myths and Facts About Rape

Myth: Rape only occurs in the "bad part of town," not in nice neighborhoods.

Fact: Six out of 10 sexual assaults take place at the victim's own home or at the home of a friend, neighbor, or relative.

Myth: Rape occurs only late at night, in the dark.

Fact: Forty-three percent of rapes occur between 6 P.M. and midnight; 24% of rapes occur between midnight and 6 A.M.; and the other 33% take place between 6 A.M. and 6 P.M.

Myth: If a person pays for a date, he or she has the right to expect something back, such as sex.

Fact: No one ever owes anyone sex.

Myth: If a person returns to his or her date's apartment or house, the date has the right to expect sex.

Fact: Consent for sexual contact is not defined by one's willingness to enter someone else's home or inviting someone into his or her home, including a date.

Myth: People who commit rapes are unable to control their sexual urges.

Fact: Rapists are not driven by uncontrollable sexual urges, but rather by the need to feel powerful and in control. Forcing someone to engage in sexual intercourse against her or his will is an act of violence and aggression. Sex is the weapon used to humiliate and control the victim.

Myth: Rapists are always strangers to the victim.

Fact: Approximately 66% of rape victims know their assailant.

Myth: All rapists are African American men who rape white women.

Fact: In approximately 88% of rapes, the victim and the offender are members of the same race. Whites tend to rape whites; blacks tend to rape blacks.

Myth: All rapists are men.

Fact: Although men commit 99% of forcible rapes, women do commit rape and other sexual assault offenses. In 2000, 300 women were serving time for rape and 900 more for other sexual assaults in the United States.

Myth: Only promiscuous women or women wearing provocative clothing are victims of rape.

Fact: Neither provocative dress nor promiscuous behavior is an invitation for unwanted sexual activity. Forcing someone to engage in nonconsensual sexual activity is sexual assault, regardless of the way the person dresses or acts.

Myth: All rape victims are women.

Fact: In 2001, one in every 10 rape victims was male.

Myth: Women who are raped were asking for it.

Fact: No one deserves to be raped. A victim should never be blamed for the actions of the perpetrator.

Sources: National Crime Victimization Survey, 1999; National Crime Victimization Survey, 2000; Sex Offenses and Offenders. Bureau of Justice Statistics, U.S. Department of Justice, February 1997.

strategies include measures to reduce one's susceptibility to physical assault. This does not mean that women are "at fault" if communication attempts fail and a rape subsequently occurs; it does mean that women owe it to themselves to communicate explicitly their intent, or lack thereof, in sexual matters.

An important concept in reducing the risk of rape, particularly date and marital rape, is formalized preparation and training. Four critical components should be included in any risk reduction program for rape:

1. Discussion and understanding of the facts of rape and dispelling the myths of rape

2. Skills training in developing honest and direct communication about dating and sexual needs and desires

3. Practical interventions (combination of audiovisual presentations, group discussions, and role playing)

4. Preparation for what to do when rape occurs, with an emphasis on early support and counseling

These measures are valuable in improving a woman's self-esteem and self-confidence as well as for providing practical rape intervention strategies and a heightened awareness of local supportive resources and services.

Response to Rape/Sexual Assault

In the event that rape or sexual assault occurs, a woman's first concern should be finding safety and calling the police. The police will assist the victim in seeking medical attention, which is important for treating any physical injuries, testing for sexually transmitted diseases (STDs) and HIV/AIDS, and collecting medical evidence for prosecution. It is important to report the assault to the police immediately; the decision about whether to prosecute the offender can be made later. A woman also should contact her local rape crisis center to inquire about counseling and support.

Reactions to and recovery from rape show considerable variability among individuals. Victims of rape often suffer from mental health problems, gynecological issues, negative health behaviors, chronic health conditions, and even fatal outcomes. Rape also may lead to unwanted pregnancies and STDs, including HIV/AIDS. Being tested immediately after the incident for STDs may help a woman prevent long-term consequences from disease. Post-exposure prophylactics, including antibiotics, emergency contraceptive pills, hepatitis B vaccination, and antiretroviral drugs, can be administered.

A common psychological reaction to violent encounters, such as rape, is post-traumatic stress disorder (PTSD; see Chapter 12). At some point during their lifetimes, 31% of all rape victims develop PTSD; rape victims are 6.2 times more likely to develop PTSD than nonvictims.[46] See Chapter 12 for more information on PTSD.

Rape trauma syndrome is another condition associated with rape victims. It is usually described as having two phases. The first phase, or acute phase, includes the immediate emotions following the event. These emotions can vary and include, but are not limited to, shock, anger, numbness, guilt, disbelief, embarrassment, shame, feelings of being unclean, anxiety, denial, fear, self-blame, or restlessness. This phase is often characterized by significant disruption in a woman's life. The second phase of rape trauma syndrome includes attempts at reorganizing one's life and lifestyle, and learning to cope again. Victims may decide to change schools, jobs, or routes to school or work in an attempt to remove reminders of the event from their daily lives. Overwhelming feelings often develop that the victim may not directly link to the rape. Often the rape is repressed and not acknowledged (sometimes for years), but the feelings do not disappear. Depression, guilt, and loss of self-esteem are common reactions during this phase. Other psychological problems include suicide attempts, eating disorders, substance abuse, social phobia, and other anxiety disorders. Major depressive episodes are three times more prevalent among rape victims than among nonvictims. Rape victims are 4.1 times more likely to have contemplated suicide and 13 times more likely to have attempted suicide.[46] Being a victim of rape can also have a significant negative impact on a woman's sexual health and intimacy. Mediating factors that may influence how a woman reacts to a rape experience include individual coping and reaction patterns, demographic variables, characteristics of the assault, historical variables, and social supports.

Violence by Strangers

Although relatives or acquaintances of the victim commit most violent offenses, the number of crimes committed by strangers is increasing. These crimes include such acts as carjacking, robbery, murder, gang violence, sexual assault, and rape. Victimization rates of men exceed those of women in all types of violent crimes, except rape and sexual assault. In general, women are more likely to be victimized by an intimate than by a stranger, except in cases of robberies. Strangers also commit roughly two-thirds of the aggravated assaults against females.[41]

Another aspect of stranger violence is the concept of hate crimes, crimes that "manifest evidence of prejudice based on race, religion, sexual orientation, or ethnicity." In 2004, 9,021 hate crime incidents were reported to U.S. law enforcement. More than half of these crimes were motivated by race; religious bias accounted for 16%; sexual orientation for 16%; ethnicity for 13%; and disability for 0.8%.[47]

Although stranger victimization cannot always be avoided, people can take a number of measures to protect themselves. When alone, women should avoid isolated areas and carry a whistle or cellular phone, if possible, in case of emergency. Flashy jewelry and large sums of money should be worn or carried using discretion when visiting high-crime areas. Women who are aware of their surroundings and use common sense can greatly reduce their risk of victimization; this does not mean, however, that women who are victimized are at fault. The circumstances and characteristics of each violent crime and each victim are unique, and it is not practical or realistic to imagine that these strategies alone could prevent all types of violence. Prevention is just the best—albeit limited—tool currently available to women.

Sexual Harassment

Although **sexual harassment** can occur in any setting, it has been most commonly reported in the workplace. The stereotype of sexual harassment, as in many forms of violence, involves a male harasser and a female victim. In reality, sexual harassment recognizes no gender boundaries—the victim and the harasser may even be the same sex. Three types of harassment have been defined:

- *Gender harassment* constitutes behavior that conveys a degrading or hostile attitude toward women.
- *Unwanted sexual attention or advances* include behaviors such as staring, commenting, touching, or repeated requests for dates or sexual favors.
- *Sexual coercion*, also referred to as quid pro quo (defined as an "equal" exchange or substitution), is the use of threats or bribery to obtain sexual favors.

The offensive conduct may interfere with a woman's ability to perform her regular duties at work and often creates an intimidating or hostile working environment. Women who are at the greatest risk for sexual harassment are those in careers traditionally considered to be male occupations. Sexual harassment can be initiated by anyone, but it is more likely to be used by someone with more power or authority than the recipient. In addition to suffering physical and emotional victimization, the threat of economic vulnerability often leaves the victim with the feeling that she has few real options in the situation.

Sexual harassment is often trivialized and not recognized as a violation of rights or personal dignity. Excuses are often encountered with such behavior, but these excuses serve to perpetuate power disparity and further dehumanize women. As with other forms of sexual victimization, harassment operates as an instrument of social control.

Sexual harassment on the job can appear in many forms, and its ramifications can be devastating. A common situation involves a boss or supervisor who requires sexual services from an employee as a condition for keeping a job or getting a promotion. Less blatant forms of workplace sexual harassment include being subjected to obscenities or being made the target of sexual jokes and innuendoes. Personal humiliation and degradation are outcomes of workplace sexual harassment, and the financial consequences of not complying with sexual coercion on the job may be devastating. Many victims, especially if they are supporting families, cannot afford to be unemployed. Also, many find it difficult to seek other work while they are employed. If they are fired for refusing to be victimized, unemployment compensation is not always available. When it is available, the amount usually represents just a fraction of the person's regular salary. Thus, a person who quits or is fired as a result of sexual harassment faces the prospect of severe financial difficulties.

It's Your Health

Common Excuses for Sexual Harassment

"Sexual harassment is a trivial distraction from the real work."
Sexual harassment can have long-term emotional impact on the victim. The emotional and economic impact of sexual harassment is not trivial in nature or form.

"I didn't mean any harm. I was just having fun."
Sexual harassment is similar to poking someone with a stick. The fun is one-sided and unfair.

"She should take it as a compliment that we like her when we say things like that."
Unwanted and unsolicited sexual advances and innuendoes, particularly from others in positions of power, can be frightening. The victim can hardly feel "complimented" when she feels threatened and put down.

"She just wanted to make trouble here with a complaint."
Women are caught between the proverbial rock and a hard place. If they accept the harassment, they perpetuate the behavior and risk further, and perhaps worse, harassment. If they file a complaint, they are labeled as troublemakers, with no guarantees that the situation will be corrected. Filing a complaint may also place a woman's job security or career in jeopardy.

Employers are becoming increasingly more sensitive to this issue, perhaps motivated in part by a number of court decisions that have awarded large payments to victims. It is an employer's responsibility to maintain a workplace that is free of sexual harassment by educating employees about which behaviors constitute harassment and taking appropriate measures if these behaviors occur.[48] The U.S. Department of Labor Employment and Training Administration can provide training guidelines for the workplace.

A new report from the American Association of University Women found that nearly two-thirds of college students have encountered some type of sexual harassment while at college. More than half of female students have been subjected to sexual comments and jokes, and about 35% have experienced physical harassment by being touched or grabbed in a sexual manner. Students who are lesbian, gay, bisexual, or transgender are more than twice as likely to be harassed as heterosexual students. Only 7% of students reported the harassment. Many students actually admit to sexually harassing other students; the reason more than half gave for the harassment was "I thought it was funny."[49]

Victims of sexual harassment may experience a range of adverse emotional and physical effects, including anger, humiliation, shame, embarrassment, nervousness, irritability, and lack of motivation. Guilt is another common feeling, as if the victim has done something wrong to encourage the harassment. The sense of alienation and helplessness reported by many victims of sexual harassment is similar to that experienced by many rape victims. Sexual harassment victims may also experience psychosomatic effects, including headaches, stomach ailments, back and neck pain, and a variety of other stress-related ailments.

Dealing Effectively with Harassment

A number of options are available to the individual who experiences sexual harassment. First, the victim should recognize that criminal charges can be filed against the perpetrator. If the coercion falls short of attempted rape or assault, it is often wise to confront the person responsible for the harassment. The confrontation should be stated in clear terms, and the specific behaviors should be identified as sexual harassment. The victim should make it clear that the behavior is unwelcome and will not be tolerated and that, if it continues, charges will be filed through appropriate channels. Some victims carefully document what has occurred and provide a written confrontation rather than undertake a verbal discussion. Others may choose to seek out the assistance of their human resources department if the sexual harassment occurs within a work setting.

If the behavior does not stop, the next step is to discuss it with the supervisor of the person responsible for the harassment. It is often helpful to talk to other employees—many times there is more than one victim. Discussing the matter with other employees provides peer support and pressure for the behavior to stop. Official complaints can be filed with local or state Human Rights Commissions or Fair Employment Practice Agencies.

A guy I worked with would always come up behind me and start rubbing my shoulders. When I asked him to stop, he told me that I needed to relax, that he was just trying to help by giving me a massage. I didn't know who to tell, but it made me really uncomfortable, especially because he continued to do it even after I asked him to stop. Eventually, I went to our Human Resources department and it turned out that another co-worker had just reported him for making lewd comments to her. Within a week, he was fired. Although I felt bad at first for turning him in, it just made me too uncomfortable and nervous to work with him. I think I did the right thing.

26-year-old computer programmer

If legal action is necessary, lawsuits can be filed in federal courts under the Civil Rights Act. They can also be filed under city or state laws prohibiting employment discrimination. One lawsuit can be filed in a number of jurisdictions. A person who has been the victim of sexual harassment is more likely to receive a favorable court ruling if attempts were made to resolve the problem within the organization before taking the issue to court.

Informed Decision Making

Knowing the facts about violence can lead to a certain level of paranoia and anger, both unhealthy conditions. Identifying the factors that contribute to violence and working to eliminate them are much more constructive reactions to potential or perceived threats of violence. For example, although miscommunication is clearly not the only or major cause of rape, it is often a factor. Misinterpretation of communication is frequently cited as a reason for the high prevalence of date rape and courtship violence. Women and men need to communicate more effectively, both in terms of their feelings and in explicitly stating their needs in the relationship, each person's responsibility within the family, and personal preferences and wishes regarding sexual behavior.

Many people still believe that men should be aggressive and that women should be passive, compliant, and pleasing to others. When people—whether male or female—buy into these stereotypes, it sets the stage for problems. Men and women may act the way they think that they are "supposed to act" and expect their partners to act the way they are "supposed to act" in return. For example, women who have been socialized to be passive may not think that they have a right to express their opinions openly and freely. Men who have been socialized to live up to a "macho" image may think that they need to "score" with women or control women to be "real" men. They may expect women to go along with their need to prove themselves or believe that a woman means "yes" when she says "no."

To address these stereotypes, a woman must take several steps:

- Recognize the inherent limitations in any stereotype
- Be open in discussing values with respect to relationships and sexuality
- Decide for herself and be explicit about when she will or will not have sex
- Understand that coercion and violence are never acceptable or deserved within a relationship
- Avoid situations where inebriation by one or both parties makes open and clear communication difficult

Many women find it difficult to talk openly about relationships and sexuality. Instead of using clear communication, they rely on assumptions, hints, innuendoes, and considerable hope that their partner understands. Unfortunately, such telepathic communication is highly unreliable. Expectations and values about relationships

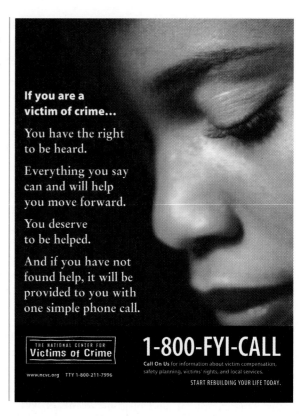

■ Reaching out for help can be the most important step. Reprinted with permission from the National Center for Victims of Crime.

and sexuality should be explicitly expressed. Communication is bidirectional: In a relationship, each person must carefully listen to the other person and confirm what has or has not been said.

Finally, "no" means "no."

Sources of Help

Women in dysfunctional relationships first need to identify and acknowledge the presence of the problem. Denial, avoidance, and protection of the dysfunctional partner often prevent or delay such acknowledgment, particularly for women who may have grown up in a dysfunctional family situation.

Professional assistance is needed in the form of counseling and support when the problem has been identified. Most communities have services and facilities to support female victims of violence, including local crisis hotlines. Hotline counselors can provide callers with phone numbers of facilities that provide counseling, supportive services, and emergency shelter. Shelters provide physical safety, psychological counseling, and referral services. Many local organizations have been organized by women who have been battered themselves and recognize the need for sensitive and protected outreach services. Support groups provide the opportunity for women to share common concerns, fears, and information. For many women, the most im-

Profiles of Remarkable Women

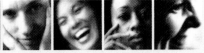

Byllye Yvonne Avery (1940–)

Byllye Y. Avery, founder of the National Black Women's Health Project (now called the Black Women's Health Imperative), has been a women's healthcare activist for 20 years. After receiving her B.A. in psychology from Talladega College and her master's degree in education focusing on special education from the University of Florida, Avery taught special education to emotionally disturbed students and consulted on learning disabilities in public schools and universities throughout the southeastern United States.

In 1976, Avery co-founded the Gainesville Women's Health Center. In 1978, she co-founded Birthplace, an alternative birthing center in Gainesville, Florida. Avery moved to Atlanta in 1981 to begin the National Black Women's Health Project (NBWHP), a nonprofit organization committed to defining, promoting, and maintaining the physical, mental, and emotional well-being of black women. A dreamer, "visionary," and grassroots realist, Avery has combined activism and social responsibility in developing a national forum for the exploration of health issues of black women, the gathering and documenting of the black women's health experiences in America, and the provision of a supportive atmosphere for black women.

In addition, Avery has become involved in the health of women on an international level. In 1986, she undertook health awareness and advocacy programs for Caribbean women in Barbados through the University of the West Indies. She also worked with the Belize Rural Women's Association to organize multiethnic women so as to establish health priorities. In 1988, Avery spent time in Kenya and was instrumental in the formation of self-help groups there. She organized and established a health agenda for African Brazilian women in Sao Paulo through the Geledes Black Women's Institute and participated in the Kellogg International Leadership Program in southern Africa, Latin America, and the United States from 1989 to 1994. Avery also served as a consultant with the Ford Foundation, Office for West Africa, in 1996 and participated in discussions to form self-help groups with the Development Exchange Center.

For two years, Avery served as a visiting fellow at the Harvard University School of Public Health. She has also served on the Advisory Committee on Research on Women's Health at the National Institutes of Health and the Women's Cancer Advisory Board at the Dana Farber Cancer Center in Boston. She has been a board member of the National Women's Health Network, the New World Foundation, the Boston Women's Health Collective, the Global Fund for Women, and the International Women's Health Coalition.

Avery has been involved in numerous film projects including *It's Up to Us,* a PBS documentary; *On Becoming a Woman: Mothers and Daughters Talking Together;* and *On Becoming a Cameroonian Woman: Mothers and Daughters Talking Together.* Avery authored a book in 1998, entitled *An Altar of Words,* which examines words such as "activism," "belonging," "empowerment," "imagination," "pride," and "wisdom" through intimate meditations.

portant step in taking control of a violent situation is admitting there is a problem and reaching out for help.

■■■■

Summary

Violence is harmful to individuals, families, and society. Women bear a disproportionate burden as victims of violence. Violence affects women not only as the actual victims of crimes, but also as the wives, girlfriends, mothers, and daughters of male victims or male perpetrators, and as the perpetrators themselves. Many women are left alone to raise children; girls are raised without fathers; and some women lose their sons. These women, as well as women as victims of violence, are all at risk of psychological reactions, such as a general loss of self-esteem, depression, anxiety disorders, and suicide. Children in battering households may experience illness, emotional problems, increased fears, increased risk of abuse, injuries, and death. They also may learn to accept abusive behavior as a role model. In addition, battering leads to high societal costs, such as increased crime; legal, medical, and counseling costs; and an overall decrease in quality of life. Efforts are urgently needed to address and reduce the full spectrum of violence against women.

Topics for Discussion

1. How does style of dress serve as a form of nonverbal communication? How can this communication be interpreted or misinterpreted?

2. How do sociocultural values and attitudes contribute to the continuing victimization of women?

3. What can a woman do to reduce her risk of assault?

4. What should a woman do if she believes that a friend is in an abusive relationship?

5. Do cultural practices and rituals that involve body modifications qualify as self-mutilation? What are some examples of these practices?

6. What are some steps that may be involved during a rape exam? What evidence may be collected to help in making a case against a rapist?

Web Sites

Children's Defense Fund: http://www.childrensdefense.org

Family Violence Prevention Fund: http://www.endabuse.org

National Center on Elder Abuse: http://www.elderabusecenter.org

National Center for Missing and Exploited Children: http://www.missingkids.com

National Committee for the Prevention of Elder Abuse:
http://www.preventelderabuse.org

NYC Gay and Lesbian Anti-Violence Project: http://www.avp.org

Rape, Abuse and Incest National Network (RAINN): http://www.rainn.org

Self-Abuse Finally Ends (SAFE): http://www.selfinjury.com

U.S. Department of Justice, Office on Violence Against Women:
http://www.usdoj.gov/ovw

References

1. World Health Organization. (2002). *World Report on Violence and Health: Summary.* Geneva: World Health Organization.

2. Office of Women's Health Report. (1997). *Domestic Violence Facts.* Department of Health and Human Services.

3. Population Information Program, Johns Hopkins University School of Public Health. (1999). Ending violence against women. *Population Reports* Series L, no. 11, vol. XXVII, no. 4.

4. Tjaden, P., and Thoennes, N. (2000). *Extent, Nature, and Consequences of Intimate Partner Violence: Findings from the National Violence Against Women Survey.* Washington, DC: National Institute of Justice, Office of Justice Programs, U.S. Department of Justice.

5. Tjaden, P., and Thoennes, N. (1998). *Prevalence, Incidence, and Consequences of Violence Against Women: Findings from the National Violence Against Women Survey.* Washington, DC: National Institute of Justice, Office of Justice Programs, U.S. Department of Justice.

6. Attorney General's Family Violence Task Force. (1989). *Domestic Violence: A Model Protocol for Police Response.* Harrisburg, PA: Attorney General's Family Violence Task Force.

7. D'Emilio, J., and Freedman, E. B. (1988). *Intimate Matters.* New York: Harper and Row.

8. Davis, A. Y. (1983). *Women, Race, and Class.* New York: Vintage Books.

9. Rennison, C. M., and Welchans, S. (2000). *Intimate Partner Violence. Bureau of Justice Statistics.* Washington, DC: U.S. Department of Justice.

10. Greenfield, L. (ed.). (1998). *Alcohol and Crime: An Analysis of National Data on the Prevalence of Alcohol Involvement in Crime.* Prepared for The Assistant Attorney General's National Symposium on Alcohol and Crime. Washington, DC: U.S. Department of Justice.

11. Bureau of Justice Statistics. (2004). *American Indians and Crime, 1992–2002.* Washington, DC: U.S. Department of Justice.

12. Finkelhor, D., Mitchell, K. J., and Wolak, J. (2000). *Online Victimization: A Report on the Nation's Youth.* National Center for Missing and Exploited Children.

13. Gifford, S. (2002). *Justice Expenditure and Employment in the United States, 1999.* Washington, DC: Bureau of Justice Statistics, U.S. Department of Justice.

14. National Association of Crime Victim Compensation Boards. (2002). Compensation at record heights! *Crime Victim Compensation Quarterly* 3: 1.

15. National Center for Injury Prevention and Control. (2002). *CDC Injury Research Agenda.* Atlanta, GA: Centers for Disease Control and Prevention.

16. U.S. Department of Justice. (1994). *The Cost of Crimes to Victims: Crime Data Brief.* Washington, DC: Office of Justice Programs.

17. Kapoor, S. (2000). *Domestic Violence Against Women and Girls.* UNICEF: Innocenti Research Centre.

18. Greenfield, L., et al. (1998). *Violence by Intimates: Analysis of Data on Crimes by Current or Former Spouses, Boyfriends, and Girlfriends. Bureau of Justice Statistics Factbook.* Washington, DC: U.S. Department of Justice.

19. American Medical Association. (1994). *Diagnostic and Treatment Guidelines on Domestic Violence.* SEC:9-677:3M:9/94.

20. American Psychological Association. (1996). *Violence and the Family: Report of the American Psychological Association.* Presidential Task Force on Violence and the Family.

21. Family Violence Prevention Fund. (July 2003). *The Effects of Domestic Violence on Children.* Available online at http://www.endabuse.org.

22. Bureau of Justice Assistance. (1993). *Family Violence: Interventions for the Justice System.* Washington, DC: U.S. Department of Justice.

23. Anderson, A. (1993). License to abuse: the impact of conditional status on female immigrants. *Yale Law Journal* 102: 1401.

24. Orloff, L. E., et al. (1995). With no place to turn: improving advocacy for battered immigrant women. *Family Law Quarterly* 29(2): 313.

25. Erez, E., and Hartley, C. C. (2003). Battered immigrant women and the legal system: a therapeutic jurisprudence perspective. *Western Criminology Review* 4(2).

26. Raj, A., and Silverman, J. (2002). Violence against immigrant women: the roles of culture, context, and legal immigrant status on intimate partner violence. *Violence Against Women* 8(3).

27. Greenfield, L. (2005). *Criminal Victimization in the United States, 2003 Statistical Tables. National Crime Victimization Survey* (NCJ 207811). Washington, DC: U.S. Department of Justice.

28. Bureau of Justice Statistics Crime Data Brief. (February 2003). *Intimate Partner Violence, 1993–2001.*

29. Wijma, B. (2003). Gynecologists could help identify sexual, physical, and emotional abuse. *Lancet* 361: 2107–2113.

30. Baaum, R., and Moore, K. (2002). *Lesbian, Gay, Bisexual, and Transgender Domestic Violence in 2001.* New York: National Coalition of Anti-violence Programs.

31. National Coalition of Anti-violence Programs. (1998). *Annual Report on Lesbian, Gay, Bisexual, and Transgender Domestic Violence.* Washington, DC: Violence Against Women Office, Office of Justice Programs, U.S. Department of Justice.

32. Gazmararian, J. A., et al. (2000). Violence and reproductive health: current knowledge and future research directions. *Maternal and Child Health Journal* 4(2): 79–84.

33. Nosek, M. A., Hughes, R. B., Taylor, H. B., and Howland, C. A. (2004). Violence against women with disabilities: the role of physicians in filling the treatment gap. In: S. L. Welner and F. Haseltine (eds.), *Welner's Guide to Care of Women with Disabilities.* Philadelphia: Lippincott, Williams, and Wilkins, 333–345.

34. Weiner, S. (1999). *A Provider's Guide for the Care of Women with Physical Disabilities and Chronic Medical Conditions.* North Carolina Office on Disability and Health.

35. U.S. Department of Health and Human Services, Administration on Children, Youth and Families. (2005). *Child Maltreatment 2003.* Washington, DC: U.S. Government Printing Office.

36. National Center on Child Abuse Prevention Research. (2001). *Current Trends in Child Abuse Prevention, Reporting, and Fatalities: The 1999 Fifty State Survey.* Chicago: Prevent Child Abuse America.

37. U.S. Department of Health and Human Services, National Center on Child Abuse and Neglect. (1996). *Third National Incidence Study of Child Abuse and Neglect: Final Report* (NIS-3). Washington, DC: U.S. Government Printing Office.

38. Heyman, R. E., and Slep, A. M. S. (2002). Do child abuse and interparental violence lead to adulthood family violence? *Journal of Marriage and Family* 64: 864–870.

39. National Center on Elder Abuse. (1998). *The National Elder Abuse Incidence Study: Final Report.* National Center on Elder Abuse at the American Public Human Services Association in Collaboration with Westat.

40. Toshia, T., and Kuzmeskus, L. M. (1999). *Types of Elder Abuse in Domestic Settings—Elder Abuse Information Series,* no. 1. Grant No. 90-am-0660, May 1996. Updated by National Center on Elder Abuse, May 1999.

41. Catalano, S. M. (2005). *Criminal Victimization, 2004.* Washington, DC: Bureau of Justice Statistics, U.S. Department of Justice.

42. Snyder, H. (2000). *Sexual Assault of Young Children as Reported to Law Enforcement: Victim, Incident, and Offender Characteristics.* Washington, DC: Bureau of Justice Statistics, U.S. Department of Justice.

43. National Institute of Justice. (2003). *Youth Victimization: Prevalance and Implications.* Washington, DC: U.S. Department of Justice.

44. Russell, D. (1990). *Rape in Marriage.* Bloomington, IN: Indiana University Press.

45. Waldner-Haugrud, L. K., and Vanden Gratch, L. (1997). Sexual coercion in gay/lesbian relationships: descriptives and gender differences. *Violence and Victims* 12(1): 87–98.

46. Kilpatrick, D. G., Edmunds, C. N., and Seymour, A. K. (1992). *Rape in America: A Report to the Nation.* Arlington, VA: National Victim Center.

47. U.S. Department of Justice. (2004). *Hate Crime Statistics, 2004: Uniform Crime Reports.* Washington, DC: Federal Bureau of Investigation, Criminal Justice Information Services Division.

48. O'Hare, E. A., and O'Donohue, W. (1998). Sexual harassment: identifying risk factors. *Archives of Sexual Behavior* 27(6): 561–580.

49. American Association of University Women. (2006). *Drawing the Line: Sexual Harassment on Campus.*

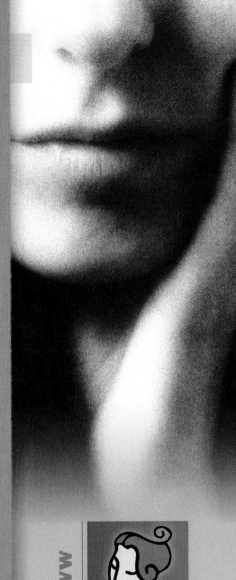

Chapter Fifteen

Women in the Workforce

Chapter Objectives

On completion of this chapter, the student should be able to discuss:

1. Historical trends related to women in the workforce.

2. Occupational trends of women.

3. Work issues for special populations.

4. Work-related barriers specific to low-income women and women on welfare.

5. The wage gap between the two genders and the concepts of the "glass ceiling" and the "sticky floor."

6. The connection between work, family, and personal life.

7. The lack of basic benefits and family-friendly work policies for a significant number of women.

8. The effects of housework, child care, elder care, and the work environment on a woman's general well-being.

9. Work-related stress and the comparison of mental well-being of employed women versus nonworking women.

10. Musculoskeletal injuries in the workplace and ways to protect against these injuries.

11. Chemical, biological, and physical hazards in the workplace and their effects on women's reproductive health.

12. Global dimensions of women in the workforce.

13. Ways for employers and employees to increase productivity and satisfaction.

womenshealth.jbpub.com

Women's Health Online is a great source for supplementary women's health information for both students and instructors. Visit

http://womenshealth.jbpub.com

to find a variety of useful tools for learning, thinking, and teaching.

Introduction

Over the past several decades, numerous women have joined the workforce. In 1900, women made up roughly one-fifth (18.3%) of the labor force with 5.3 million women working. These numbers rose to 29.6% of the labor force in 1950 (18.4 million women) and increased even more to 46.6% of the labor force in 2001 (66 million women).[1–3] Women are still not reaching the highest echelons of the work world in great numbers. In 2005, only two *Fortune* 500 companies had female CEOs and only 10% had women holding at least one-fourth of their officer positions.

The rising number of women in the workforce has highlighted many new issues, including pay differentials between genders, the balancing of work and family, health and safety in the workplace, and the struggle for many women between choosing a career and choosing to stay home. On average, full-time women employees with the same job responsibilities who are performing at equal levels as their male counterparts now earn $0.80 for every $1 earned by men.[4] These inequities have yet to be solved by awareness campaigns or legislation. Women also typically shoulder more of the burden of family and household responsibilities than men do, often working at their paying jobs and then taking on a "second shift" of responsibilities when they return home. Some women who choose to stay home feel conflicted by their choice, as do some women who choose to pursue a career and leave their child with a surrogate provider.

As women have increased their presence in the workforce, general health and safety issues have arisen. Workstations, tools, and protective equipment have traditionally been designed for men and therefore may compromise the health and safety of women. Health hazards from biological, chemical, and disease-causing agents are significant in many predominantly female occupations, including the textile, laundry, and meat industries; health care; and food preparation. Additionally, physically intense activities or exposure to certain substances while on the job can harm working women who are pregnant.

■ While women make up half of the workforce, they continue to earn less than their male counterparts for the same responsibilities.

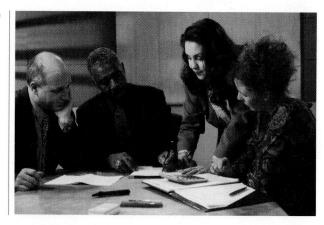

In this chapter, gender differences in the workplace, the balancing of work and family, and occupational safety issues are discussed. In addition, the chapter presents strategies for decreasing job stress and increasing workplace satisfaction.

Trends and Issues

Historical Issues

In colonial times, all members of the family worked together as an economic unit. Although the majority of women's paid jobs outside the home appeared to be extensions of their household duties—making clothing, cleaning house, teaching, or cooking—women also worked as blacksmiths, silversmiths, shopkeepers, and operators of grist mills. When their husbands were off at sea or at war, women continued to operate the family businesses until the husbands returned; other women accompanied troops to war and served as nurses and cooks. Some women even became spies or posed as men and entered battle.

The Industrial Revolution brought women into the factories, providing many with new skills, educational opportunities, and social outlets. Many European women immigrated to the United States to work as indentured servants, with hopes of a more promising future. Workplace violence, sexual harassment, and unfair pay were issues for a number of these women, who were often physically and sexually abused on the job, and deprived of personal freedom and financial compensation. Because many women's positions were viewed as temporary, working women typically earned enough wages to help make ends meet, but not enough to make a comfortable living.

In the mid-1800s, Charlotte Woodward campaigned to change laws to give women rights to their earnings, as opposed to the custom of husbands having ownership of their wives' money. The New York Married Women's Property Act, which was passed in 1848, represented a major step for women's rights; by 1860, other states had passed similar laws.[5] It was not until 1974, however, that Congress passed the Equal Credit Opportunity Act, which made it unlawful for creditors to discriminate against women on the basis of sex or marital status, thereby enabling women in the United States to establish their own credit lines.

Women continued to find opportunities to earn wages, with many working to build professional careers as lawyers, journalists, physicians, and teachers. Wyoming was the first state to provide equal pay for female teachers under a law passed in 1869, followed soon thereafter by California.[5] Although exceptions did arise, most women continued to work in occupations traditionally associated with women—for example, nursing, clerical work, and domestic servant positions.

When World War II began, the types of jobs available to women increased dramatically. "Rosie the Riveter" became the symbol for women workers in the U.S. defense industries. More than 6 million women, from all backgrounds and from all over the country, worked at industrial jobs that challenged traditional notions of women's capabilities and ensured American productivity that helped win the war. During the war years, women became streetcar conductors, taxicab drivers, machine operators, business managers, and railroad workers. They unloaded freight, worked

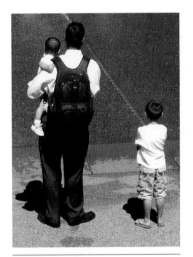

Men and women are redefining traditional roles and responsibilities for their families.

in lumber mills and steel mills, and made munitions. In essence, women occupied almost every aspect of industry. This trend led to a rise in salaries and an overall commitment by women to their jobs, though many women lost their new positions when the men returned from war.

In the post–World War II era, the number of women in the workforce has continued to grow. Today, women are more likely than men to attend college, a major change from 30 years ago. The desegregation of college majors has led more women into fields such as architecture, business, and the sciences.[6] Many women are postponing childbearing and marriage, having smaller families, and, in turn, focusing on building their careers and developing themselves as individuals before taking on the roles of wife and mother. Women have opened up numerous opportunities for themselves by attending college, fighting for equal rights in the workplace, and breaking barriers in many occupations traditionally associated with men. Despite all of the advances, however, gender discrimination in jobs persists.

Occupation Trends of Women

The realities of women in the workforce can be better understood by looking at the rates of participation in the workforce according to age and educational level, the professions in which women are concentrated, and the percentage of women-owned businesses. Such statistics begin to paint a more complete picture of women's opportunities and persistent hurdles, and they show how solving the dilemma of child care would affect many women's ability to work (Table 15.1).

Of the 108 million women age 16 and older in the United States, approximately 60% are in the labor force either working or looking for work.[3] Women age 35 to 44 represent the highest percentage of working women (Figure 15.1).[7] This may

Table 15.1   Employment Status of Women with Children, 2004 (in millions)

	Employed		Unemployed	
	Total	Percent	Total	Percent
Women, age 16 and over	64,412	55.9%	3,789	5.6%
With children younger than 18 years old	24,413	66.6%	1,501	5.8%
With children 6 to 17 years old, none younger	15,006	73.7%	776	4.9%
With children younger than 6 years old	9,407	57.8%	724	7.1%
With children younger than 3 years old	4,983	52.9%	417	7.7%
With no children younger than 18 years old	40,000	50.9%	2,289	5.4%

Source: U.S. Department of Labor. (February 2004). *Women in the Workforce: A Databook.* p. 15.

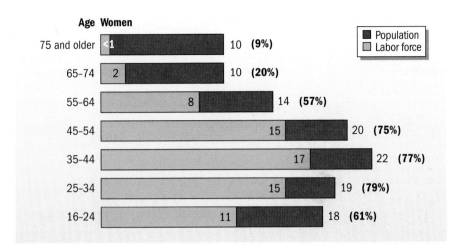

Figure 15.1

Labor force participation rates for women by age, 2002.

Source: U.S. Department of Labor, Bureau of Labor Statistics.

be partly due to the fact that women are more likely to participate in the workforce as their children get older. More than three-fourths of women age 25 years and older who are employed are college graduates. Most working women (75%) are employed full time (Table 15.2). In addition, nearly 50% of multiple jobholders are women.[8]

While women work in all industries and contribute in multiple ways to the economy, their participation is often concentrated in certain sectors. The majority of employed women work in technical, sales, and administrative support occupations (Table 15.3). Nearly one of every five employed women works as a teacher (excluding post-secondary positions), secretary, manager or administrator, or cashier.[9]

Table 15.2 Employment Status of Women, Aged 25–64, by Educational Attainment, 2004

	Participation Rate	Unemployment Rate
Total	68.5%	4.4%
Less than high school	43.6%	10.4%
High school graduate, no college	65.1%	4.9%
Some college or associate's degree	72.6%	4.2%
College graduates, total	77.5%	2.7%
Bachelor degree	75.7%	2.9%
Master's degree	81.0%	2.4%
Professional degree	80.7%	2.3%
Doctoral degree	84.9%	1.8%

Source: U.S. Department of Labor. (February, 2004). *Women in the Workforce: A Databook.* p. 22.

Table 15.3	Employed Women by Occupational Group, 2004 (numbers in thousands)

Occupation	Percentage of Total That Are Women
Healthcare practitioner and technical support	73.2%
Sales and office	63.9%
Managerial and professional specialty	50.3%
Arts, design, and entertainment	47%
Life, physical, and social science	43%
Farming, forestry, and fishing	20.6%
Architecture and engineering	13.8%
Construction and extraction	2.5%

Source: U.S. Department of Labor. (2004). *Women in the Labor Force.* Bureau of Labor Statistics.

According to the U.S. Census Bureau's Survey of Business Owners and Self-Employed Persons, women own 26% of all nonfarm businesses, totaling nearly 5.5 million businesses.[10] (Women-owned businesses are defined as privately held firms in which women own 51% or more of the firm.) More than half of such firms were in the services industry, particularly business services and personal services. Women cite a variety of reasons for starting their own businesses:

■ By breaking the barriers of traditionally male-dominated fields, women have created greater opportunities for themselves in the workplace.

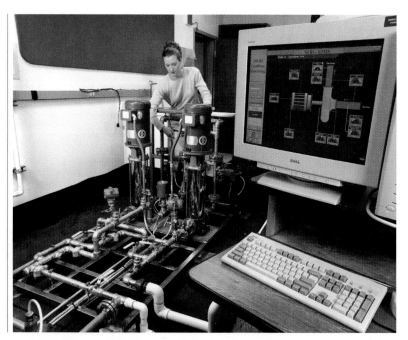

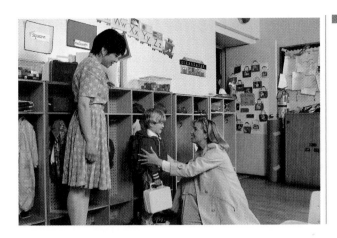

Childcare remains a major challenge for working parents.

- Flexibility
- Independence
- Outlet for creativity
- Relief from sexual harassment in the workplace
- An exit from poverty[10]

In recent years, the number of women in the workforce who have young children has significantly increased. Today, 59% of mothers with infants (younger than age 1), 65% of mothers with children younger than age 6, and 78% of mothers with children ages 6 to 17 are in the workforce.[11,12] The number of dual-earner families also has increased. Before World War II, less than 10% of the workforce was from a dual-earner family. Today, more than 42% are dual-earner families. In nearly 75% of dual-earner families, both partners work full time.[13] What is surprising is that many two-parent families with young children are having difficulty making ends meet. Fifty percent of young children are members of families with incomes less than $40,000; 25% are in families making less than $20,000.[14]

Special Populations

Women with Disabilities in the Workplace

Women with disabilities confront many barriers in the workplace:

- Lack of job opportunities or appropriate jobs
- Inaccessible work environments
- Lower wages than people without disabilities
- Discouragement by family and friends
- Fear of losing health insurance or Medicaid
- Little or no accessible parking or public transportation nearby

In addition, once a job has been secured and other barriers worked through, there still may be a need for adaptations to workstations, special work arrangements or hours, handrails or ramps, or communication access for hearing or visually impaired individuals. The severity of a woman's disability has the greatest influence on her employment status. According to the National Institute of Disability and Rehabilitation Research, only 24.7% of women with a severe disability have a job, as compared with 68.4% of women with a nonsevere disability (74.5% of women with no disability had jobs).[15] Women with disabilities are employed in a variety of occupations, including the service industry, managerial and professional occupations, and middle management positions. In terms of pay, women with disabilities earn, on average, less than women with no disabilities. Women with disabilities that directly affect their work are more likely to live below the poverty level than those people without work disabilities. Approximately 40% of women with a severe work disability are living in poverty.[15]

Older Women

Women have increasingly been participating in the part-time labor force during the traditional years of retirement. This trend is largely attributable to the fact that individuals are living longer and healthier lives and/or finding their retirement savings are not adequate to make ends meet. Older women may have special health needs as members of the workforce, including the need for easy or disabled access to a work site, close proximity to restrooms, and seats with supportive backs or armrests to assist in getting up and down. Employers should be aware of the special needs of older workers, as they provide a valuable and often highly educated supplement to the workforce.

Socioeconomic Issues

Although many women face the difficult task of finding and keeping a job that is rewarding both mentally and financially, low-income women—particularly welfare recipients—face even greater obstacles. For these women, the consequences of not finding employment or the inability to maintain a job can have devastating

◼ Older workers have unique needs in their workplace environments.

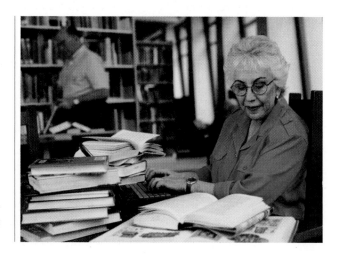

consequences. Welfare recipients and low-wage workers are disproportionately women and minorities with family responsibilities. Women heads of household represent a high percentage of this group. Welfare-to-work programs that were supported by the dramatic welfare reform passed in 1996 have helped many of these women move from welfare into paid employment. Most of these individuals work in service industries characterized by low hourly wages (averaging about $7 per hour), however, and are at significant risk for layoffs or work-hour reduction in a down economy.

Work opportunities for low-income women or women on welfare are often limited because many persons in this situation lack education, training, transportation, or child care. Many jobs available to low-income women or women on welfare either are available at odd hours (such as evening or night hours) or have shifting schedules. Both situations make transportation and childcare options even more difficult. Low-income women who live in rural areas with little or no public transportation often have trouble getting to and from job training centers, let alone to jobs. Other women are caught between taking a job to put food on the table and leaving young children at home alone because of lack of child care. For many women, even when they are able to find transportation and child care, their low wages are eaten up by the costs for those transportation and childcare services.

Low-wage jobs often provide few or no benefits, such as healthcare coverage, paid sick leave, or paid family leave. Furthermore, because the positions do not require advanced skills, employers are typically quick to replace a woman who may have to miss work because her child is sick.[16] A recent study reported that women who left welfare to work were less likely than other working women to have jobs that offered paid sick days, family leave, or flexible job schedules, even though they were more likely to have children with chronic health problems.[17]

Equal Pay for Equal Work

A great challenge for working women has been the battle of receiving equal pay for performing equal work. Men in the same jobs as women often earn more than women with the same education and years of experience.

In 2004, women who worked full time, regardless of age, race, or educational attainment, earned a median weekly salary of $573 compared with $713 for men—that is, they earned approximately three-fourths of what men make (Table 15.4).[4] This income level represented an increase from 1998 earnings for both genders. Earning differences between genders varied by demographic features, with the greatest contrast arising between men and women ages 55 to 64. The narrowest gap between earnings was among workers 20 to 24 years old; in this demographic group, women earned 94% of what men earned (Figure 15.2).[4] As a result of these differences, the average 25-year-old woman who works full time, year-round, until retiring at age 65 will earn $523,000 less over her lifetime than the average working man.[18] To elucidate this point even further, men with a professional degree have average annual incomes of more than $70,000, while women with the same degree average $40,000 per year. In other words,

I have a high school degree and a few college-level courses, but I can't get a job that pays enough to cover child care and bills. I'm now living with my mom, and she basically takes care of my kids. But I want to make it on my own! How can I afford to go back to school and take care of my kids at the same time? If I don't go to school, how can I get a job to make enough money to support us? I feel like I'm stuck in a situation that I'll never get out of.

26-year-old woman with two children under the age of 5

Table 15.4   Women's and Men's Median Weekly Earnings by Selected Characteristics, 2004

Characteristic Age	Women ($)	Men ($)
Total, 16 years and older	573	713
16 to 19	293	318
20 to 24	391	417
25 to 34	561	639
45 to 54	625	857
55 to 64	615	843
65 and older	478	641
Race/Ethnicity		
White	584	732
Black	505	569
Hispanic	419	480
Asian	613	802
Educational Attainment		
Less than a high school diploma	344	446
High school graduate, no college	488	645
Some college or associate degree	577	761
College graduates	860	1143

Source: Bureau of Labor Statistics. (2005). *Highlights of Women's Earnings in 2004*. U.S. Department of Labor.

Figure 15.2

Women's median weekly earnings as a percentage of men's, by age, 2004.

Source: Bureau of Labor Statistics. (2005). *Highlights of Women's Earnings in 2004*. U.S. Department of Labor.

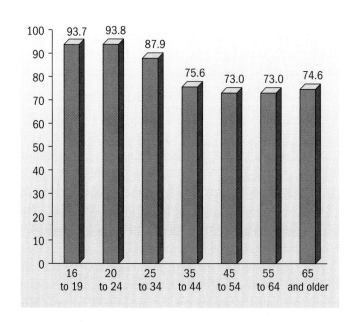

these women work Monday through Friday to earn what a man in a comparable position has earned by noon on Wednesday.[19]

The pay gap is closing in some fields, but not in others and not quickly enough. For example, in comparison to men in the same occupation, on a weekly average:

- Women lawyers make almost $500 less
- Women bartenders make about $70 less
- Women engineers make about $150 less
- Women doctors make nearly $500 less
- Women registered nurses make about $100 less
- Women professors make nearly $300 less[3]

Not only do women make less money than men in virtually every profession, but women are clustered in low-paying professions.[19] In 2004, women earned 80.3% of what men earned.[20] Less than 2% of all working women earn more than $75,000 per year.[21] Many women are worried about the "sticky floor"—employment practices that keep full-time, working women right at the poverty threshold level. One-fourth of women who work full time do not earn enough to move their families above the federal poverty threshold. At the other extreme, women continue to fight against the "glass ceiling" phenomenon—employment practices that effectively keep working women out of top-ranking positions. For example, according to a 2002 report, women held only 15% of corporate officer positions in the *Fortune* 500 companies, and there were only six women chief executive officers in all *Fortune* 500 firms. Changes are occurring, although the rate of change is slow.

Besides lower wages, a grim reality for working women is the lack of paid sick or family leave, childcare benefits, flexibility of schedule associated with employment, and employer-provided health insurance, pension plans, or retirement benefits. According to a survey conducted by the AFL-CIO:

- 54% of women reported no paid leave to care for a baby or an ill family member.
- 74% say their employers do not offer childcare benefits.
- 34% have no flexibility or control over their schedule.[22]

In addition, two-thirds of the approximately 60 million women working outside of the home in the United States do not have pension plans; those who do receive half the benefits enjoyed by their male counterparts.[19]

Although gender discrepancies in income are often thought of as a woman's issue, it is clearly a family issue. With more women in the workforce, more families are depending on dual incomes. In the AFL-CIO's 1997 Ask a Working Woman Survey, almost two-thirds of working women and more than half of married women said that they provided half or more of their family's incomes.[23] In 1970, women maintained 5.6 million families in the United States, meaning that there was no other provider in the household; in 2000, women maintained 13 million (18%) of the 71 million families in the country. Women maintained 14% of white families, 47% of black families, and 24% of Hispanic-origin families. Given the large number of women who are the sole providers for their families and work in low-paying jobs, it comes as no surprise that 27% of all families maintained by women were below the poverty level in 1998.[19]

Race/Ethnicity Issues

In general, women occupy proportionally more of the lower-paying jobs than men do, and they receive fewer benefits and less flexibility in their working conditions than men do. Minorities—and especially minority women—are even more likely to be in these less desirable positions. While white workers of either gender earned more than their black and Hispanic counterparts, white women's average weekly earnings ($584) were 14% higher than black women's ($505) and 28% higher than those of Hispanic women ($419).[4]

In 1999, women were one-third more likely than men to be among the working poor, and African American and Hispanic women were two to three times more likely than white women to be members of the working poor group.[24] Less than 2% of white women, 1% of African American women, and 1% of Hispanic women earn more than $75,000 per year; meanwhile, 70% of white women, 73% of African American women, and 82% of Hispanic women earn less than $25,000 per year.[21] Recent studies have shown, however, that minorities are moving most rapidly from welfare to work programs. In fact, African American women have had a steeper decline in welfare participation than white participants over the same period.

Achieving Equal Pay

One key factor for women who are seeking to help themselves is education. Completing high school is the first step in increasing one's potential income. The median income for women increased by 33% for those with a high school degree, and another 25% for those with an associate's degree.[19]

To achieve fair compensation for their work, women should learn what fair and equitable pay is for their position and experience, be aware of the laws that prohibit pay discrimination against women, and support efforts to bring "pay equity" to their workplaces. Employees should encourage their employers to implement a pay equity policy, along with a way of creating a grading system to categorize jobs based on education, skills, and experience. Pay rates should be adjusted so that jobs of equal value are paid equally.

Balancing Work and Family Life

Thirty-four percent of women say that the biggest problem facing women today is combining family and work.[25] Women continually juggle many tasks in an effort to perform well at work, run a household, provide a loving home for their children, spend quality time with their partners, and provide care for their elders. Women who have multiple roles, as mother and provider for example, have a lower incidence of depression and other mental health problems than women who have only one role; however, in many cases, having multiple roles can contribute to strain and stress.

The role of mother is often a woman's principal source of stress; she may enjoy this role and be committed to it, but nevertheless may feel strained by it. Her stress may be exacerbated by society's normative expectation of "good mothering," which does not usually encompass full-time employment.[26,27] Although being in the workforce increases a woman's opportunities for obtaining resources, power, social identity, positive self-esteem, and involvement with others, involvement in paid employment may also be a source of stress. The benefits of work are contingent on the woman's working conditions, her marital status, her stability in her job, and her ability to handle many roles at once. The more demanding and difficult the job and the less supportive the workplace, the greater the negative spillover from one's work life to one's personal life.

Working mothers often feel the stresses of work significantly more than working fathers do. Mothers, for example, often must juggle the multiple responsibilities of maintaining high job performance and being the primary caregiver for children. Single mothers frequently carry this double burden, resulting in them being even more stressed than married working women. Although men are performing more household responsibilities than they did 20 years ago, women continue to spend more time than men doing housework on top of increasing their workloads outside the home. This trend has led to an increase in the work–family life conflict experienced by these parents. One study showed that women spend 30.8 hours per week doing paid work and 25.6 hours on family care. By comparison, men spend 39.7 hours per week doing paid labor and 14.3 hours on family care or housework.[28] Housework and family care tend to be more unbalancing to a person's sense of well-being because the tasks are thought to be more repetitive, dirtier, menial, unending, and relatively inflexible. Even when men do housework, it is often work that can be scheduled, such as lawn maintenance or repairs. In contrast, women are often responsible for cleaning, cooking, and caring for children—duties that cannot be postponed.[26] Married men are more likely to have partners who are willing to take care of tasks at home, making men's lives more balanced. On the other hand, men in general do not adjust their time in response to their wives' employment status.[29]

Besides doing more housework, mothers spend more time on average with their children than fathers do. Mothers spend an average of 3.2 hours per workday with their children, whereas fathers spend an average of 2.3 hours with their offspring. Seventy percent of parents feel that they do not have enough time to spend with their children. In fact, both parents have less time for themselves than they did 20 years ago; fathers have 1.2 hours during the workday, whereas mothers have 0.9 hour.[13] Couples also have less time together. Nearly 46% of married women or women living with someone work different schedules than their partners do.[22]

One in five working parents is a member of the "sandwich generation," meaning that the individual is caring for both children and elderly relatives. More than one-third of those with elder responsibilities—men and women alike—reduced

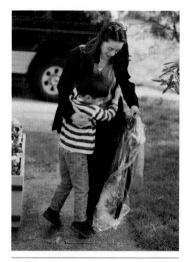

Many women who have entered the workforce continue to work on household chores and child care when they return home from work.

their work hours or took time off to provide the necessary care.[13] Fifty-four percent of Americans say they will probably be responsible for the care of an elderly parent or other relative in the next 10 years. Women account for 70% of the unpaid people caring for the elderly; they also constitute the majority of paid workers, including nurses, nurse's aides, and home healthcare workers.[25]

Child Care

Childcare facilities, relatives, and nannies have become a necessity for working families with children. More than three-fourths of preschool-age children with employed mothers are regularly cared for by someone other than their parents. Thirty-two percent of children attend daycare centers, and 16% are cared for by family members. A babysitter or nanny regularly cares for 6% of children in the child's home. Families with children between the ages of three and five say that child care is their third greatest expense after housing and food.[25] The cost of full-day child care can range from $4,000 to $20,000 per year per child. In addition to the high costs, nine out of 10 Americans describe finding quality child care as "difficult."[25,30] One study showed that 40% of rooms for infants in childcare centers actually jeopardize the health, safety, or development of children. Only 11 states require childcare providers to have any early childhood training prior to minding children in their homes.[31]

Child care does not always ease the stress for working women. In fact, 52% of women say that childcare problems affect their ability to perform well at work.[25] Eighty percent of employers reported that childcare problems force employees to lose work time. In addition, only 9% of sampled workers with children in daycare facilities report feeling "very successful" in balancing work and family.[32]

The Current Situation

Working Mother magazine rates the 100 best companies for working mothers every year, based on various measures of flexibility within the workplace, such as flextime, telecommuting, and job sharing. Companies also are rated on their propensity to listen to employees by surveying them on work–life topics and, in response to the survey results, adding features such as lactation rooms. The top-rated companies do not just offer policies, but market them as well.[33] *Ms.* magazine has reported, however, that some of these companies officially offer flextime to employees but do not necessarily practice what they preach. In many organizations, workers in low-wage jobs are half as likely as managers and professionals to have flextime; low-wage workers are also more likely to lose a day's pay when they must stay home to care for a sick child.[34]

Within many companies, only 20% of employees have access to childcare information and referral services; 25% are provided with access to eldercare information and referral services. Only 12% of employees with children younger than age six have childcare services on or near their work site that are operated or sponsored by their employers, and these facilities are usually located at headquarters where managers and executives work.[14,29] Even those lower-paid employees who have access to referrals or nearby childcare facilities usually find the fees too high for their earnings. Many of the company-operated daycare centers are open only during regular business hours, such as 8 A.M. to 6 P.M.; however, 32% of employees with young children have unpredictable or erratic work schedules, and these are the employees who are most likely to earn less than $25,000 per year.[14,22]

The Future

Many women suffer from job- and family-related stress, but do not feel they have any options that would relieve that stress. Some women aspire to the "superwoman" ideal—for example, being a high-powered executive while keeping a clean house, preparing home-cooked meals, spending quality time with her children, and being a loving and supportive wife. Women need to find their individual balance of work and family responsibilities and make changes if they are dissatisfied with their situation. For women with partners, open communication about the sharing of responsibilities can help couples to establish a good balance within their home. In situations where both partners work, sharing of chores is essential to minimize stress and maximize quality family time.

For single women, it is important to find balance between work and home responsibilities, too. This may mean reviewing policies at work that allow for job sharing or flextime, or advocating for these options if they are not provided by one's employer. Women without these options need the power and support of other women, employers, and politicians to fight for them. Women who own businesses should set examples for pay equity, fair workplaces, supportive work environments, and family-friendly policies.

Health and Safety in the Workplace

Women's work-related stress has been linked to factors such as lack of supportive workplace policies, unfair pay, concerns for quality child care, inflexible scheduling, and lack of support and help at home. In times of economic upheaval, concerns over downsizing and layoffs create even added pressures. Other stressors revolve around lack of control at work, such as high workload demands, unreasonable deadlines, role ambiguity and conflict, repetitive and boring work, and strained relationships with co-workers or supervisors.[35] The stress from this type of work often produces little job satisfaction and a poor sense of well-being. The following jobs are associated with high stress because of the need to respond to others' demands and timetables with little control over events:

- Secretaries
- Waitresses
- Middle managers
- Police officers

- Editors
- Medical interns[36]

Long-term exposure to job stress can lead to higher levels of depression, anxiety, and other mental illnesses. In one survey, 60% of employed women cited stress as their number one problem at work.[37] As jobs become more demanding and less rewarding, employees often feel more stressed by the end of the workday and have less time and energy for their families. Twenty-five percent of employees reported feeling stressed often or very often over the past three months, and 25% described feeling emotionally drained often or very often. More than one-fourth of employees are not in as good a mood as they would like for their families; 28% of people feel they have no energy for their families or other important people upon returning from work. This in turn creates a negative sense of well-being and results in negativity that affects a person's performance at work.[13]

A person's work setting can create physical stress as well, because of noise, lack of privacy, poor lighting or ventilation, poor temperature control, or inadequate sanitary facilities. Physical stress on the body is a consequence of many different occupations. Jobs that require being on one's feet for long hours can result in leg pain, swelling, and varicose veins; secretarial and computer-related jobs are often accompanied by neck and back aches and eye strain; and women on production lines suffer from musculoskeletal injuries resulting from repetitive motions. These types of difficulties are not restricted to gender, yet certain factors make women more susceptible to this type of injury. Typical designs of equipment and workstations accommodate the larger-on-average size of males as compared with females. For example, higher workstations and chairs that cannot be adjusted to the correct height for women promote poor posture, excessive reach, and strain on the neck, back, shoulders, and arms.

■ Long-term exposure to work-related stress can lead to higher levels of depression, anxiety, and other illnesses.

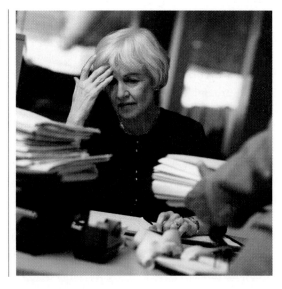

Hand tools that are designed for larger hands may create unnecessary pain, stressed muscles, and calluses. Protective equipment and clothing that are too large have a greater likelihood of slipping off, getting caught in equipment, or creating gaps for harmful agents to seep through, thereby compromising a woman's safety.

Musculoskeletal injuries, also referred to as ergonomic injuries, disproportionately affect female workers. Although women account for only 33% of the people injured at work in the United States, they constitute 64% of **repetitive motion injuries,** which include the following conditions:

- **Carpal tunnel syndrome**—a condition that occurs when tendons in the wrist become inflamed after being aggravated
- **Tendonitis**—inflammation caused by friction from overuse of tendons
- Muscle strains from overexertion

Repetitive motions can result in the compression of nerves, which, in many jobs, will occur in the nerves from the neck to the hand. Nerve injuries that result from repetitive motions may cause various symptoms, as shown in Self-Assessment 15.1. Repetitive motion injuries account for more than half of all work time lost due to injuries and illness among women (Table 15.5).[38,39]

Women in lower-wage occupations and occupations employing large numbers of women are at significant risk of musculoskeletal disorders. Examples of these occupations include nursing aides, cashiers, maids, nurses, and assemblers (Table 15.6). Many of these jobs employ a large number of minorities, such as Hispanic, Southeast Asian, and African American women. Back injuries are common among employees who need to lift large items or even people. Safe lifting can be accomplished with the correct lifting technique and awareness regarding the amount of weight being lifted.

It's Your Health

Tips for Lifting Loads Safely

- Test the weight of the load before lifting. If too heavy or awkward, enlist a co-worker to help or use a cart or dolly.
- Figure out where you need to move the load and how you are going to get to your destination before you lift.
- Lift with your legs shoulder-width apart and bend at your knees and hips, not your waist.
- Lift with tightened stomach muscles and using your leg muscles to reduce strain on your back.
- Hold the load close to your body at waist height.
- Avoid twisting during the lift; pivot your body or move your feet if necessary.
- Stretch and strengthen your back and stomach with exercises if lifting is part of your daily occupation.

Self-Assessment 15.1

Symptoms of Repetitive Strain Injuries

- Do you have numbness and/or tingling in your hand that often feels worse when you lift your hand over your head?
- Do you often experience wrist weakness?
- Do you have numbness or tingling in the inside of your arm or into your fingers?
- Do you often feel numbness or tingling in multiple fingers and does your hand often "fall asleep" at night? Do you frequently drop objects?
- Do you have achiness, stiffness, tightness, or a burning sensation in your fingers, forearm, elbow, or shoulder?
- Do you experience muscle tightness at the side of your neck?

If you are experiencing one or more of these symptoms, you may have an overuse injury. Women should speak to their healthcare provider about preventing, reducing, and/or treating these types of disorders.

Table 15.5	Ergonomic Injuries Among Women	

Description of Injury	Number of Lost-Worktime Injuries to Women	Percentage of All Workers Injured
Carpal tunnel syndrome	18,740	68%
Tendonitis	8,965	62%
Injured due to repetitive motion	43,671	64%
Due to repetitive typing or keyboard entry	10,890	89%
Due to repetitive placing/grasping	14,223	64%
Due to repetitive use of tools	4,682	46%

Source: Bureau of Labor Statistics. (2000). *Lost-Worktime Injuries and Illnesses, 2000.*

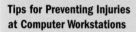

It's Your Health

Tips for Preventing Injuries at Computer Workstations

- Reduce repetitive motions by alternating tasks throughout the day.

- Take frequent breaks, and stretch during the breaks if possible.

- Avoid bending or twisting your neck, or twisting your trunk.

- Keep shoulders relaxed and arms close by sides when working.

- Maintain good posture by keeping back and neck erect with shoulders relaxed.

- Keep your feet supported on the floor or on a footrest to reduce pressure on the lower back.

- Position your computer monitor so that it is centered directly in front of you and your neck is in a neutral or straight position when viewing it.

- Reduce glare on your screen by tilting the monitor, reducing overhead lights, and avoiding direct glare from windows.

- Rest your eyes every 30 minutes by looking away from the screen and focusing on various objects around the room or outside.

Computer-related injuries have become a significant concern in the workplace because of the widespread use of computers in many occupations (Self-Assessment 15.2). Prolonged use of a computer keyboard or mouse, as well as sitting at a computer working intensively without stretching, can lead to frequent muscle aches and nerve pain in the hands, arms, shoulders, neck, and back. Another common complaint of computer workers is visual discomfort, which is accompanied by eyestrain and headaches. Being aware of these risks and correcting improper posture and techniques can help prevent discomfort and injury.

Table 15.6	Jobs with the Most Musculoskeletal Disorders for Women		

Occupation	Number of Women with Lost-Worktime Injuries	Median Hourly Wage	Median Annual Pay
Nursing aides, orderlies, attendants	41,022	$8.89	$18,491
Registered nurses	10,718	21.56	44,845
Cashiers	8,551	6.95	14,456
Assemblers	6,926	10.32	21,053
Maids and housemen	6,739	7.41	16,190
Miscellaneous machine operators	6,634	NA	NA
Laborers (except construction)	5,574	9.04	18,803
Licensed practical nurses	5,232	14.15	29,432
Sales workers, other commodities	5,079	8.02	16,361
Freight, stock, and material handlers	4,530	9.04	18,810

Sources: Bureau of Labor Statistics. (2000). *Lost-Worktime Injuries and Illnesses, 2000,* and *National Occupational Employment and Wage Estimates, 2000.*

Computer Workstation Evaluation Checklist

Posture

- Are your hands, wrists, and forearms straight, in-line, and roughly parallel to the floor?
- Is your head level or bent slightly forward and balanced?
- Is your head in line with your torso?
- Are your elbows close to your body and bent at 90 to 120 degrees?
- Are your feet fully supported by the floor or a footrest?
- Is your back fully supported when sitting vertical or leaning back slightly?
- Are your shoulders relaxed?
- Thighs and hips should be supported by a well-padded chair.
- Knees should be at the same height as the hips with the feet slightly forward.

Keyboard/Mouse

- Is your keyboard directly in front of you at a distance that allows your elbows to stay close to your body with your forearms approximately parallel with the floor?
- If you have limited desk room, do you use a keyboard tray to ensure adequate positioning?
- Is your keyboard in a position that lets you avoid reaching with the arms, leaning forward with the torso, and using extreme elbow angles?
- Can you reduce awkward wrist angles by lowering or raising the keyboard or chair to achieve a neutral wrist posture?

Seating

- Does your backrest support your lower back (lumbar area)?
- Does your seat width and depth accommodate your body? Is the seat pan not too long?
- Does the seat front not press against the back of your knees and lower legs?
- Is the seat cushioning rounded with a waterfall front devoid of sharp edges?
- If there are armrests, do they support both forearms while your complete computer tasks?

Lighting

- Does your office have well-distributed diffuse lights that reduce glare on the computer screen?
- Does your office use light, matte colors and finishes on walls and ceilings to better reflect indirect lighting and reduce dark shadows and contrast?

Computer Screen

- Is your computer display screen at right angles to windows and light sources?
- Is the monitor clean and free of dust?
- Is the top of the screen at or below eye level?

Work Techniques

- Are your computer tasks organized in such a way that allow you to vary tasks with other work activities or take micro-breaks and recovery pauses?

If you answered "No" to one or more of these questions, you are putting yourself at risk of injury. Use the checklist guidelines to improve your workplace health and avoid injuries.

Source: Adapted from the U.S. Department of Labor's Office of Safety and Health Administration's eTool, Computer Workstation Evaluation. (http://www.osha.gov/SLTC/etools/compuCterworkstations/checklist.html)

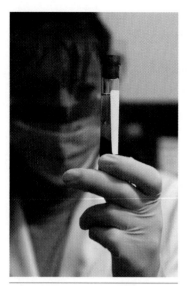

■ Healthcare workers face unique workplace hazards.

Other physical hazards of significance are the dangers posed by exposure to certain chemical, biological, and physical toxins, many of which are suspected carcinogens, allergens, or agents that cause respiratory illness. Occupational exposures occur in many of the industries that employ large numbers of women and minorities:[37]

- Meat industry: exposure to suspected carcinogenic fumes
- Laundry/dry-cleaning industry: exposure to carcinogenic solvents that increase risk of kidney, cervical, bladder, skin, and liver cancer
- Textile industry: exposure to dust that causes a variety of lung diseases
- Metal-working industry: exposure to various carcinogens that increase the risk of lung cancer
- Agriculture: exposure to pesticides and herbicides that may lead to a possible increased risk of non-Hodgkin's lymphoma and lung cancer
- Healthcare industry: exposure to numerous toxic and allergenic substances, infectious diseases, and radiation
- Service industry: exposure to excessive cigarette smoke in bars or restaurants

Healthcare workers face additional hazards, including needlestick injuries and latex allergies. Approximately 600,000 to 800,000 needlestick injuries occur annually in healthcare settings, mostly involving nurses (more than 90% of whom are women). Needlestick injuries can cause serious infections from bloodborne pathogens, such as hepatitis B, hepatitis C, and HIV, creating both physical and emotional threats to workers. In addition, 8% to 12% of healthcare workers who have frequent latex exposure develop sensitivity to this material. Symptoms can be as mild as contact dermatitis or as severe as **anaphylactic shock** (severe and possibly fatal allergic response to foreign substance, characterized by difficulty breathing and low blood pressure). The hazard from latex use is recognized in many different industries, including people in the latex-manufacturing industry, police, food handlers, and sanitation engineers.[39] Pregnant women also appear to have a higher sensitivity to latex than does the general population.[40]

The causes of most reproductive health problems are still unknown, but certain harmful substances have been identified as having reproductive effects in pregnant women. Approximately 75% of all women of reproductive age are in the workforce, and more than half of all children born in the United States are born to working mothers. Women can be exposed to many different types of health hazards at work during pregnancy. Hazards from environmental pollutants in the workplace can cause one or more effects, depending on when the woman is exposed (see Tables 15.7 and 15.8). For example, substances may cause fetal damage, such as birth defects, low birthweight, developmental disorders, miscarriages or stillbirths, infertility, menstrual cycle effects, and even childhood cancer. Other possible hazards to pregnant women include prolonged standing, lifting, and long work hours.[41]

Table 15.7 Chemical and Physical Agents That Are Reproductive Hazards for Women in the Workplace

Agent	Observed Effects	Potentially Exposed Workers
Cancer treatment drugs (e.g., methotrexate)	Infertility, miscarriage, birth defects, low birthweight	Healthcare workers, pharmacists
Certain ethylene glycol ethers	Miscarriage	Electronics and semiconductor workers
Carbon disulfide	Menstrual cycle changes	Viscose rayon workers
Lead	Infertility, miscarriage, low birthweight, developmental disorders	Battery makers, solderers, welders, radiator repairers, bridge repainters, firing range workers, home remodelers
Ionizing radiation (e.g., X rays and gamma rays)	Infertility, miscarriage, birth defects, low birthweight, developmental disorders, childhood cancers	Healthcare workers, dental personnel, atomic workers
Strenuous physical labor (e.g., prolonged standing, heavy lifting)	Miscarriage late in pregnancy, premature delivery	Many types of workers

Source: National Institute for Occupational Safety and Health. (1999). *The Effects of Workplace Hazards on Female Reproductive Health.* Department of Health and Human Services: Publication No. 99–104.

Table 15.8 Disease-Causing Agents That Are Reproductive Hazards for Women in the Workplace

Agent	Observed Effects	Potentially Exposed Workers	Preventive Measures
Cytomegalovirus (CMV)	Birth defects, low birthweight, developmental disorders	Healthcare workers, workers in contact with infants and children	Good hygienic practices such as handwashing
Hepatitis B virus	Low birthweight	Healthcare workers	Vaccination
Human immunodeficiency virus (HIV)	Low birthweight, childhood cancer	Healthcare workers	Practice universal precautions
Human parvovirus B19	Miscarriage	Healthcare workers, workers in contact with infants and children	Good hygienic practices such as handwashing
Rubella (German measles)	Birth defects, low birthweight	Healthcare workers, workers in contact with infants and children	Vaccination before pregnancy if no prior immunity
Toxoplasmosis	Miscarriage, birth defects, developmental disorders	Animal care workers, veterinarians	Good hygienic practices such as handwashing
Varicella-zoster virus (chickenpox)	Birth defects, low birthweight	Healthcare workers, workers in contact with infants and children	Vaccination before pregnancy if no prior immunity

Source: National Institute for Occupational Safety and Health. (1999). *The Effects of Workplace Hazards on Female Reproductive Health.* Department of Health and Human Services: Publication No. 99–104.

Other Health Concerns

Many women work in the informal work sector, employed in jobs that are seasonal (like agriculture) or domestic (like housecleaning). Because many of these jobs employ women who may not have official work permits or are "paid under the table" (meaning that the women do not receive benefits or declare taxes), significant additional risks are associated with them. Injuries that occur during migrant crop picking, for example, often go untreated as the workers have few resources and are afraid of drawing the attention of authorities. Additionally, women who do odd jobs around the home, such as cleaning houses or painting, often do not have health coverage or disability coverage should an injury occur.

Hazardous work environments put many youths at risk of serious injuries. Young workers have been killed on construction sites, during robberies while tending retail establishments, and while working on farms. Common nonfatal injuries incurred by young workers include sprains and strains, burns, cuts, and bruises. Homicide was the leading cause of death among youths in retail trade, accounting for nearly two-thirds of the youth fatalities in the industry. Most of these homicides were the result of robberies.[42]

Pregnant and lactating women may face additional stresses as they cope with sickness caused during pregnancy, co-workers' responses to pregnancy, and the time and privacy needs of nursing or pumping breast milk. Sexual harassment in the workplace is also a major form of stress (see Chapter 14).

Global Dimensions

Across the globe, women are becoming increasingly more active in the workforce. Approximately 70% of women in developed countries and 60% of women in developing countries are engaged in paid employment. Worldwide, more women are participating in and completing their education, resulting in better job opportunities and consequently better status in their families and society. Although much progress has been made, however, millions of women remain unprotected by labor laws and poorly compensated for their work. They are not treated as equals and often experience discrimination and significant pay differences.

The proportion of informal work done by women has increased dramatically over the last decade. In some countries of sub-Saharan Africa, for example, nearly 90% of the female labor force is in the informal economy. This informal—and often invisible—work accounts for a significant amount of output, including the production of handmade goods, services such as laundry and sewing, and vast amounts of child care. In developing countries, a great effort has been made to quantify the amount of informal work women do. By recognizing the role of the informal workforce, of which women represent the majority, the groups are helping to legitimize the work they do and help women gain access to key financial resources that could assist them in getting ahead. Examples of such efforts include microlending programs, where women are loaned small sums of money to further their businesses without the need for collateral and with reasonably low interest rates.

The rate of payback from these women-focused micro-lending programs has been higher than that observed with any other formal credit program that has been measured. Once women gain access to these loans, they have the ability to create sustainable and profitable business opportunities for themselves and their families. By having greater access to capital, women can better protect themselves from the significant workplace health hazards that present themselves in many formal and informal work environments. In addition, the money that women make from their work enterprises is overwhelmingly reinvested into the health and well-being of their families.

In terms of work and families, government policies around the world vary. It is interesting that the United States—one of the richest countries in the world—does not guarantee women any paid family leave, unlike many other countries. Worldwide, 128 countries mandate some sort of paid family leave. For example,

- In Germany, a new mother receives 14 weeks of leave at full pay.

- In Italy, a new mother receives 20 weeks of leave at full pay.

- In Canada, new mothers have the right to take a full year off from work at 60% pay.

- In Norway, new mothers can take one year off from work at 80% pay.

Informed Decision Making

Working women, with and without children, experience significant stress that affects their health, relationships, work productivity, and young children. Supportive companies produce workers who are less stressed, feel more successful in the balancing of work and family, are more satisfied with both their work and home lives, and are more loyal and committed to their employers.[25]

There are solutions. First, employers should help employees prepare to better balance parenthood and work life by offering services related to family planning,

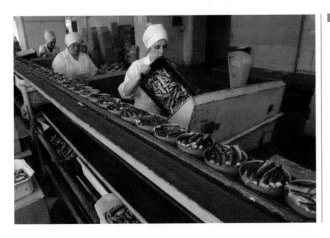

Women are becoming increasingly more active in workplaces across the globe.

I just had my second child, and I have six months off to care for him. My two-year-old goes to day care at my firm's on-site child-care center. When I return to work, I'll work part time so I get to spend time with my children. The women of my firm have said that there's no problem with taking advantage of flextime and taking off six months to care for my newborn. I hope they're right! I feel very fortunate to be part of a firm that takes such good care of its employees.

30-year-old lawyer

preconception health care and counseling, and parenting classes. Second, the Family and Medical Leave Act (FMLA) could be expanded to help families in crisis. The FMLA of 1993 provides 12 weeks of unpaid, job-guaranteed leave for employees who need to care for newborns or a seriously ill relative, or to recover from a serious illness of their own. This benefit is available to employees who have worked at least 1,250 hours over the past year for employers with 50 or more employees. Currently, the act covers only 57% of the country's private workforce.[34] Workers in entry-level, low-paying jobs are less likely to be offered a paid maternity leave than are managers and are less likely to get the time off after having a baby. Although the FMLA was originally envisioned as dealing with a women's issue, 42% of those who have requested family and medical leave since its passage are men.

Employers can also ease new mothers' return to the workplace by providing breastfeeding support through lactation assistance programs and private breastfeeding rooms. Only 10% of working mothers continue nursing for six months following birth, compared with 24% of at-home mothers. Thirty-seven percent of employers currently provide opportunities for women who are nursing to continue to do so; this provision cuts down on absenteeism and healthcare costs for both mothers and infants.[14]

In addition, employers need to help employees find affordable quality child care and elder care, develop childcare programs, or offer employee assistance for childcare facilities. Childcare assistance programs need to include more flexibility, by allowing for the needs of employees who work night and weekend shifts (Figure 15.3). Flexible work schedules, job-sharing programs, and prorated benefits for part-time and temporary employees also need to be enforced—two-thirds of part-time workers and three-fifths of temporary workers are women.[19] Many employers have established flexible work policies and are promoting the idea of a family-friendly workplace. Unfortunately, the people who need the extra support are the people who are often the least likely to receive it.

Women also need to be aware of their rights in the workplace. Discrimination should not be tolerated, and actions can be taken if a woman suspects she is being treated unfairly because of her gender, race, age, religion, pregnancy, sexual orientation, or disabilities.

Summary

The workplace has emerged as the modern-day "community" for many people. It provides a social life, a support system, and opportunities for volunteering, and it affects people's moods and their values.

- Women are particpating in all jobs and careers today, but inequities in pay and advancement persist.

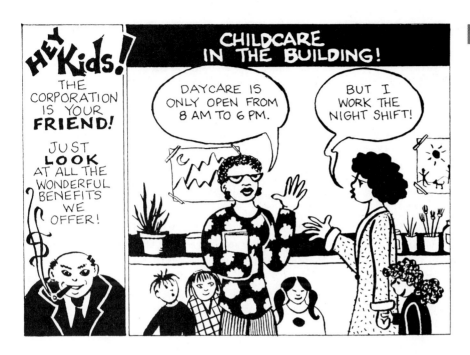

Figure 15.3

Childcare programs need to be developed with more flexibility to allow for night and weekend shifts.

Source: © Jennifer Camper.

- Women still shoulder the majority of the burden of children and home life, even when working.
- Women benefit greatly from quality, affordable, and accessible child care, enabling them to have choices about labor force participation.
- The stress of work and family, and the attempt to "do it all," is not an insignificant women's health issue.

Employers must continue to make an effort to create a more supportive and rewarding work environment. By promoting a healthy work–life balance, employers benefit, as do employees. At the same time, women should strive to find such a balance in their lives, by setting priorities, discussing options with their employers and partners, and advocating for fairness and support in the workplace.

As both genders become accustomed to a more equitable sharing of responsibilities inside and outside the home, women will be afforded a more balanced existence between work and family. As Arlie Hochschild so aptly states, "Up until now, the woman married to the 'new man' has been one of the lucky few. But as the government and society shape a new gender strategy, as the young learn from example, many more women and men will be able to enjoy the leisurely bodily rhythms and freer laughter that arise when family life is family life and not a second shift."[43]

Profiles of Remarkable Women

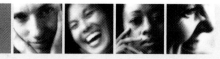

Patricia Ireland (1945–)

Patricia Ireland began her career by working as a flight attendant for Pan American World Airlines from 1967 to 1975. Upon being told that her medical benefits didn't apply to her husband even though wives of male employees were covered, Ireland sued her employer and won—a victory that marked the beginning of her activism. Ireland received her law degree from the University of Miami Law School in 1975, then worked as a partner in a major Miami law firm. She served as legal counsel to Dade County and Florida National Organization for Women (NOW) for seven years. From 1987 to 1991, Ireland served as executive vice president and treasurer of the national NOW organization.

In 1991, Ireland became president of NOW, the largest, most visible, and most successful feminist organization in the United States. Her major contributions included organizing NOW activists to defend women's access to abortion, elect a record number of women to political office, work more closely in coalitions with other social justice and civil rights groups, and champion international feminist issues.

Ireland developed NOW's Project Stand Up for Women; in 1992, she led NOW in organizing a crowd of 750,000 for the organization's March for Women's Lives. In the same year, she initiated the "Elect Women for a Change" campaign. This campaign provided feminist candidates with experienced organizers who trained and deployed volunteers to staff phone banks, distribute leaflets and posters, organize fundraisers, and get people to the polls.

As part of NOW's work with the Up and Out of Poverty Now! coalition, Ireland delivered testimony and organized lobby days, news briefings, and protests on behalf of poor women. She served on the board of the Rainbow/PUSH Coalition and, in 1993, was a co-convener and keynote speaker for the thirtieth anniversary march on Washington commemorating the legacy of Dr. Martin Luther King, Jr. She has put forth significant efforts on behalf of lesbian and gay rights, including serving as a speaker and major organizer for the 1993 March on Washington for Gay, Lesbian, and Bi Civil Rights.

Ireland was the prime architect of NOW's Global Feminist Program. In 1992, she brought together women from more than 45 countries to participate in the Global Feminist Conference. Although no longer president of NOW, Ireland continues to champion many international feminist issues.

Topics for Discussion

1. What questions should a woman ask before taking a job to ensure that she will receive all of the benefits that she may need?

2. Discuss how the cycle of poverty creates additional barriers to employment opportunities for women.

3. What strategies could women use in the workplace to determine whether chemical, biological, or physical hazards are present?

4. What are some possible strategies for women to use in finding balance in their professional, educational, and personal lives?

5. What are some possible strategies for women to use when seeking greater equity opportunities in specific workplaces?

Profiles of Remarkable Women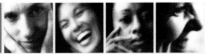

Alice Hamilton (1869–1970)

Alice Hamilton was a physician, social reformer, and professor of industrial medicine who is best known for her research on toxic substances in the workplace. Hamilton graduated from the University of Michigan Medical School in 1893. She then continued her education in Germany, where she studied bacteriology and pathology at the Universities of Leipzig and Munich. Neither university had allowed female students before, so Hamilton was permitted to attend lectures on the condition that she make herself inconspicuous to male students and professors. She then returned to the United States to study at Johns Hopkins University.

After her time at Johns Hopkins, Hamilton began teaching pathology as a professor at the Women's Medical College of Northwestern University in Chicago. It was there that she met Jane Addams and other reformers who encouraged her to find a way to apply her scientific knowledge to social problems. She immediately began to work to benefit the health of women and their families by providing a well-baby clinic for residents in the neighborhood. During the typhoid fever epidemic that struck Chicago in 1902, Hamilton made a connection between improper sewage disposal and the role of flies in transmitting typhoid fever. Living among poor working-class families, Hamilton saw firsthand the pain and suffering brought on by work-related diseases and injuries such as lead palsy and carbon monoxide gassing. She realized that these health problems were caused by unsafe working conditions and noxious chemicals; at the same time, she also saw that the industries in the United States denied responsibility for the illnesses and that states had no worker's compensation laws.

In 1908, Hamilton was named to the Illinois Commission of Occupational Diseases; in 1911, she was appointed to the U.S. Bureau of Labor as a special investigator. The Illinois Commission of Occupational Diseases was the first such commission in the world. As a result of its findings, several worker's compensation laws were passed in Illinois. Hamilton began researching occupational toxic disorders, first with the support of the State of Illinois and later from the Federal Bureau of Labor Statistics. She became a pioneer in the United States in the fields of occupational epidemiology and industrial hygiene through her investigations of lead poisoning among bathtub enamellers. Her incredible findings led to sweeping reforms that called for the reduction of occupational exposure to lead. Hamilton continued to study poisons affecting workers in the lead, munitions, and copper industries throughout the United States, traveling the country and touring mines and factories, smelters, and forges. Other Hamilton-led studies that helped influence the study of occupational health included investigations of carbon monoxide in steelworkers, mercury poisoning in hatters, and "dead fingers" syndrome among laborers using jackhammers.

In 1919, Hamilton was appointed assistant professor of industrial medicine at Harvard Medical School. The first woman faculty member of Harvard University, she remained the only woman teaching there for many years. All of her students were male because females were not admitted to the school until after World War II. Harvard set three requirements for Hamilton related to her status as a woman: She was not allowed to use the Faculty Club, she had no access to football tickets, and she was not allowed to march in commencement processions. After 1925, she served as a member of the faculty of the Harvard School of Public Health, where she continued to promote safety in the workplace as well as turn occupational health into a respected field in academia.

While at Harvard, Hamilton served two terms on the Health Committee of the League of Nations. In 1935, she retired from the university and accepted a position as consultant to the U.S. Division of Labor Standards. From 1944 to 1949, she served as president of the National Consumers' League. Hamilton's published works include *Industrial Poisons in the United States* (1925), *Industrial Toxicology* (1934), and *Exploring the Dangerous Trades* (1943). She received many honorary degrees, distinctions, and awards, including a listing in *Men of Science* in 1944 and the Lasker Award of the U.S. Public Health Association in 1947.

■■■■

Web Sites

American Federation of Labor—Congress of Industrial Organizations:
http://www.aflcio.org

Business and Professional Women/USA: http://www.bpwusa.org

Institute for Women's Policy Research: http://www.iwpr.org

National Institute for Occupational Safety and Health—Women: http://www.cdc.gov/niosh/topics/women/

National Organization for Women: http://www.now.org

U.S. Department of Labor: http://www.dol.gov

U.S. Department of Labor—Bureau of Labor Statistics: http://www.bls.gov

■■■■

References

1. U.S. Bureau of the Census. (1976). *The Statistical History of the United States—From Colonial Times to the Present.* U.S. Department of Commerce.

2. U.S. Department of Labor. (1989). *Handbook of Labor Statistics.* Bulletin 2340. Bureau of Labor Statistics.

3. U.S. Department of Labor. (2002). *Employment and Earnings.* Bureau of Labor Statistics.

4. U.S. Department of Labor. (2005). *Highlights of Women's Earnings in 2004.* Report 987. Bureau of Labor Statistics.

5. Mofford, J. H. (1996). Women in the workplace. *Women's History Magazine.*

6. Parcel, T. L. (1999). Work and family in the 21st century: it's about time. *Work and Occupations* 26(2): 264–274.

7. U.S. Department of Labor. (2000). *Employment and Earnings.* Bureau of Labor Statistics.

8. Business and Professional Women/USA. (2003). *101 Facts on the Status of Working Women.*

9. U.S. Department of Labor. (2002). *Facts on Working Women.* Women's Bureau.

10. Center for Policy Alternatives. (1999). Women and the economy—entrepreneurship. *Women's Economic Leadership Summit Report.*

11. Bachu, A., and O'Connell, M. (2000). *Fertility of American Women* (Current Population Reports P20-526). Washington, DC: U.S. Census Bureau.

12. Unpublished data from the U.S. Bureau of Labor Statistics (March 2000).

13. Tarmann, A., and Population Reference Bureau. (November 2003). *Is America Settling Down?*

14. Shore, R. (1998). *Ahead of the Curve: Why America's Leading Employers Are Addressing the Needs of New and Expectant Parents.* New York: Families and Work Institute.

15. Jans, L., and Stoddard, S. (1999). *Chartbook on Women and Disability in the United States.* An InfoUse Report. Washington, DC: U.S. National Institute on Disability and Rehabilitation Research, 18.

16. National Partnership for Women and Families. (1999). *Detours on the Road to Employment: Obstacles Facing Low-Income Women.*

17. Heymann, S. J., and Earle, A. (1999). Impact of welfare reform on parents' ability to care for their children's health. *American Journal of Public Health* 89: 502–505.

18. Institute for Women's Policy Research. (1998). *The Male–Female Wage Gap: Lifetime Earning Losses.*

19. Center for Policy Alternatives. (1999). Women and the economy—economic self-sufficiency. *Women's Economic Leadership Summit Report.*

20. U.S. Department of Labor, Bureau of Labor Statistics. (2004). *Overview of BLS Statistics on Wages, Earnings, and Benefits.*

21. AFL-CIO. (1999). *It's High Time—Past Time—for Women of Color to Earn Equal Pay.* AFL-CIO Working Women's Department.

22. AFL-CIO. (2000). *Ask a Working Woman Survey.* AFL-CIO Working Women's Department.

23. AFL-CIO. (1997). *Ask a Working Woman Survey.* AFL-CIO Working Women's Department.

24. AFL-CIO. (2003). *Fact Sheet: Equal Pay for Women of Color.* AFL-CIO Working Women's Department.

25. Center for Policy Alternatives. (1999). Women and the economy—family and work. *Women's Economic Leadership Summit Report.*

26. Milkie, M. A., and Petola, P. (1999). Playing all the roles: gender and the work–family balancing act. *Journal of Marriage and the Family* 61: 476–490.

27. Barnett, R. C., and Baruch, G. K. (1987). Social roles, gender and psychological distress. In Barnett, R. C., Biener, L., and Baruch, G. K. (eds.). *Gender and Stress.* New York: Free Press.

28. Robinson, J. P., and Godbey, G. (1997). *Time for Life.* University Park: Pennsylvania State University Press.

29. Shelton, B. A., and John, D. (1996). The division of household labor. *Annual Review of Sociology* 22: 299–322.

30. Schulman, K. (2000). *Issue Brief: The High Cost of Child Care Puts Quality Care Out of Reach for Many Families.* Washington, DC: Children's Defense Fund.

31. Children's Defense Fund. (1998). *Facts About Childcare in America.*

32. Hochschild, A. R. (1997). *The Time Bind.* New York: Holt.

33. Cartwright, C. (2002). 100 best companies for working mothers. *Working Mother.*

34. Holcomb, B. (2000). Friendly for whose family? *Ms.* X(3): 40–45.

35. Allen, K. M., and Phillips, J. M. (1997). *Women's Health Across the Lifespan: A Comprehensive Perspective.* Philadelphia, PA: Lippincott-Raven.

36. American Psychological Association. (1997). *Psychology at Work: Get the Facts.*

37. Centers for Disease Control and Prevention. (2001). *Women's Safety and Health Issues at Work.* National Institute of Occupational Safety and Health.

38. U.S. Department of Labor. (2000). *Lost-Worktime Injuries and Illnesses.* Bureau of Labor Statistics.

39. AFL-CIO. (2003). *Women Workers Need OSHA's Ergonomic Standards.* Department of Occupational Safety and Health.

40. Cheng, L., and Lee, D. (1999). Review of latex allergy. *Journal of the American Board of Family Practitioners* 12(4): 285–292.

41. National Institute for Occupational Safety and Health. (1999). *The Effects of Workplace Hazards on Female Reproductive Health.* Department of Health and Human Services: Publication No. 99-104.

42. Windau, J., Sygnatur, E., and Toscano, G. (1999). *Work Injuries of Young Workers.* Monthly Labor Review, OSHA.

43. Hochshild, A. (1989). *The Second Shift.* New York: Avon Books.

A

Abortion   The spontaneous or induced expulsion of an embryo or fetus before it is viable or can survive on its own.

Abruptio placentae   A complication of pregnancy in which the placenta separates prematurely from the wall of the uterus.

Abstinence   In terms of sex, the practice of refraining from sexual activity.

Acute disease   A disease that begins and ends quickly. Examples include pneumonia and localized infection.

Adenocarcinoma   A cancer that originates from cells of the endocrine glands.

Adenomyosis   A benign condition caused by the development of tumors on the walls of the uterus, which can bleed and cause pain during menstruation.

Adjuvant therapy   Methods such as chemotherapy and radiation therapy that enhance the effectiveness of surgery in cancer treatment.

Aerobic bacteria   Bacteria that are oxygen dependent.

Aerobic exercise   Any physical activity in which the amount of oxygen taken into the body is slightly more than, or equal to, the amount of oxygen used by the body.

Afterbirth   The placenta and amniotic sac that are expelled from the womb after a baby is delivered.

Alcohol   A colorless liquid obtained by fermentation of a sugar-containing liquid. Ethyl alcohol (ethanol) is the type of alcohol found in alcoholic beverages.

Alcoholic   A person whose experiences interfere with normal life activities due to regular and continuous drinking of alcohol.

Alcoholism   Traditionally, the disease of an alcoholic, who is a person whose consumption of alcohol interferes with a major aspect of her life. Alcoholism has since been redefined as a primary, chronic disease with genetic, psychological, and environmental factors influencing its development and manifestations.

Allopathic school   A school that teaches a system of medical practice making use of all measures proved of value in treatment of disease (i.e., conventional medicine exclusive of homeopathic practices).

Alzheimer's disease   An irreversible, progressive brain disorder that occurs gradually and results in memory loss, behavior and personality changes, and a decline in cognitive abilities.

Amenorrhea   Absence of the menstrual period in a woman by age 16 (primary amenorrhea) or absence of the menstrual period for three to six consecutive months in a woman who has had regular periods since the onset of menstruation (secondary amenorrhea). It is often caused by stress, acute weight loss, or excessive strenuous exercise.

Amniocentesis   Procedure between the sixteenth and twentieth week of pregnancy intended to detect fetal defects. The amniotic sac is punctured with a needle and syringe, and amniotic fluid is obtained for analysis.

Amnion   The innermost membrane of the amniotic sac, which contains the amniotic fluid.

Amniotic fluid   Watery fluid that surrounds a developing embryo and fetus in the uterus.

Amphetamines   Synthetic stimulants that increase energy and alertness, produce euphoria, and suppress appetite. Excessive use can cause headaches, irritability, dizziness, insomnia, panic, confusion, and delirium.

Anabolic steroids   Synthetic derivatives of the male hormone testosterone usually taken to increase muscle mass. Their use often results in serious physiological and psychological side effects.

Anaerobic bacteria   Bacteria that are intolerant of oxygen.

Analgesic   Medication that relieves pain without inducing loss of consciousness.

Anaphylactic shock   A severe and sometimes fatal allergic reaction to a foreign substance that causes symptoms such as weakness, shortness of breath, and falling blood pressure.

Androgens   Any steroid hormone (hormone made in the outer layer of the adrenal gland) that increases the development and growth of male physical qualities. Testosterone is an androgen that stimulates the growth of male characteristics.

Androgyny   A blending of typical male and female qualities in an individual.

Aneurysm   A type of weakened blood vessel that can cause a stroke. This ballooning of a weakened region of a blood vessel may result from several factors, including a congenital defect, chronic blood pressure, or an injury to the brain. If left untreated, the aneurysm continues to weaken until it ruptures and bleeds in the brain.

Angina pectoris   Chest pain resulting from insufficient supply of blood (oxygen) to the heart muscle.

Anorexia nervosa   An eating disorder characterized by self-starvation, excessive weight loss, and a host of other physiological and psychological illnesses.

Antihistamine   A medication used to reduce the effects of histamine, a substance found in body tissues that plays a role in allergic reactions.

Antioxidants   Substances that prevent cells called "free radicals" from harming the body's tissues. Antioxidants are present in many fruits and vegetables. They work to neutralize free radicals and protect genes from damage, possibly decreasing the risk of cancer and heart disease, and delaying the effects of aging.

Anxiety disorders   Group of conditions that share extreme or pathological anxiety as the principal disturbance of mood. Anxiety disorders include panic disorder, agoraphobia, generalized anxiety disorder, specific phobia, social phobia, obsessive-compulsive disorder, acute stress disorder, and post-traumatic stress disorder. Anxiety disorders are the most common mental disorder in the U.S. and affect a significant number of people worldwide.

Aorta   The great artery arising from the left ventricle of the heart; the largest artery.

Aortic valve   A valve located between the left ventricle and the aorta.

Arrhythmias   Erratic heartbeats.

Arteries   Vessels in the body that supply oxygenated blood to the tissues.

Arterioles   Small arteries.

Arteriosclerosis   Any arterial disease that leads to thickening and hardening of the arterial walls, slowing the flow of blood.

Arthritis   Inflammation of the joints. Arthritis encompasses more than 100 diseases and conditions that affect joints, the surrounding tissues, and other connective tissues.

Artificial insemination   Introduction of semen into the uterus or oviduct by other than natural means close to the time of ovulation. It is most often used when the infertility problem is male related.

Assisted reproductive technology (ART)   Any treatment or procedure that involves the handling of human eggs and sperm with the purpose of helping a woman become pregnant.

Asymptomatic viral shedding   Most often associated with herpes simplex virus infections. Viral shedding is when active herpes virus, present in the nerve cells of an infected person, moves along the nerves to the surface of the skin. Shedding often occurs without any symptoms (asymptomatic) but may still be infectious, meaning that it can be passed onto others.

Atherosclerosis   A type of arteriosclerosis characterized by deposits of fatty substances or plaques on inner walls of arteries that narrow blood vessels.

Athletic amenorrhea   The cessation of regular menstrual periods due to excessive exercising.

Atrial fibrillation   A disorder in which the heart's two small upper chambers (the atria) quiver instead of beating effectively. Because blood is not pumped completely out of them, it may pool and clot. If a piece of a blood clot in the atria leaves the heart and becomes lodged in an artery in the brain, a stroke results.

Atrium   The left or right upper blood-receiving chamber of the heart.

Autoimmune disease   A disease caused by autoantibodies or lymphocytes that attack normal components of the body—molecules, cells, or tissues—of the organism producing them. It is more common among women than men.

Azoospermia   A complete absence of sperm in the semen and often the cause of male infertility.

B

Bacteria   Single-celled organisms that multiply and cause disease by forcing the body to release poisons and germ-fighting antibodies. Unlike viral infections, bacterial infections usually can be treated by antibiotics.

Bacterial vaginosis   An inflammation of the vagina, caused by an overgrowth of the normal bacteria found in the vagina and resulting in an imbalance; the most common cause of vaginitis, this infection is sometimes, but not always, sexually transmitted.

Balloon angioplasty   A procedure used to open narrowed or blocked coronary arteries. A small, hollow tube called a catheter is inserted into an artery near the blockage. A balloon near the end of the catheter is then inflated, which helps to widen the vessel and allows blood to flow. A wire mesh stent is usually placed at the site of narrowing to keep the artery open.

Barbiturate   A class of sedatives that have a depressant effect on the central nervous system.

Bariatric surgery   Gastrointestinal surgery for obesity that alters the digestive process. The operation promotes weight loss by closing off parts of the stomach to make it smaller.

Barrier contraception   A method of birth control that provides a physical or chemical barrier to prevent sperm from fertilizing eggs. All barrier methods (except plain condoms) are used with spermicide, a chemical that breaks down the cell walls of sperm. Most barrier methods are used inside the vagina to cover the cervix and prevent sperm from entering the uterus. Male condoms are protective sheaths that enclose the penis during intercourse and ejaculation.

Bartholin's glands   Two small glands located just inside the vaginal opening that help lubricate the vagina.

Basal cell carcinoma   A nonmelanoma skin cancer that begins in the basal cells of the epidermis (outer layer of skin). It usually develops in areas exposed to the sun, such as the head and neck.

Basal metabolic rate (BMR)   The amount of energy needed to maintain essential body functions under resting conditions, usually expressed in terms of calories per hour per kilogram of body weight.

Battering   Repeatedly subjecting a person to forceful and coercive physical, social, and/or psychological behavior.

Beneficiary   In terms of insurance, an individual who is eligible to receive benefits under an insurance policy.

Benign tumor   A noncancerous growth that does not spread to other parts of the body.

Bicuspid valve   A valve that separates the left atrium and the left ventricle of the heart; also known as the mitral valve.

Bilateral salpingo-oophorectomy   Surgical excision of the fallopian tube and the ovary.

Bile   Fluid produced by the liver and stored in the gallbladder that plays a key role in the digestion of fats.

Binge eating disorder (BED)   An eating disorder characterized by lack of control over eating and overeating in secret. Victims do not force themselves to vomit, however, as in bulimia nervosa.

Bingeing   The consumption of large amounts of food that is characteristic of bulimia nervosa.

Biomedical research   Studies relating to the activities and applications of science to clinical medicine.

Cervical cap   A contraceptive device made of latex and individually customized to fit snugly over the cervix.

Cervical dysplasia   Abnormal changes in the cells of the cervix. This benign condition is considered precancerous and can develop into cancer if left untreated.

Cervicitis   An inflammation of the cervix.

Cervix   The small end of the uterus extending into the vagina.

Cesarean delivery   The surgical procedure in which an infant is delivered through an incision made in the abdominal wall and uterus.

Chemotherapy   The treatment of disease with anticancer drugs or chemicals.

Child abuse and neglect   Physical or mental injury, sexual abuse or exploitation, negligent treatment, or maltreatment of a child by a person who is responsible for the child's welfare, under circumstances that indicate that the child's health or welfare is harmed or threatened.

Chlamydia   A sexually transmitted disease (STD) that is caused by the bacterium *Chlamydia trachomatis*. Most people are asymptomatic and therefore are not aware of their infections. If left untreated, chlamydia can cause serious damage to a woman's reproductive system. Chlamydia is the most frequently reported infectious disease in the United States.

Chloasma   Darkening of skin pigment on the upper lip, under the eyes, and on the forehead—commonly linked to pregnancy or taking oral contraceptives.

Cholesterol   One of the steroids or fatlike chemical substances manufactured by the body and also consumed in foods of animal origin. It is essential for the manufacture and maintenance of cells, sex hormones, and nerves throughout the body.

Chorion   Outer membrane of the amniotic sac that expands around the fetus as it grows.

Chorionic villus sampling   A procedure performed to detect fetal abnormalities in which samples of chorionic villi are removed and examined.

Chromosomes   The structures in the nucleus of each cell composed of DNA and protein that contain the genes that provide information for the transmission of inherited characteristics.

Chronic bronchitis   Constant inflammation of the bronchial tubes. The inflammation thickens the walls of the bronchi, and the production of mucus increases, resulting in a constricting or narrowing of the air passages.

Chronic disease   A disease that lasts longer than several weeks, often for the length of a person's life; it may be ongoing or progress slowly. Examples include diabetes, heart disease, and lupus.

Chronic obstructive pulmonary disease (COPD; also known as chronic lower respiratory disease [CLRD] or chronic obstructive lung disease [COLD])   A disease characterized by permanent airflow obstruction and extended periods of disability and restricted activity.

Cirrhosis   Alcohol-induced liver disease.

Climacteric Physiological changes that occur during the transition period from fertility to infertility in both sexes.

Clinical trial A research study designed to answer specific questions about new vaccines, new therapies, or new ways of using known treatments. Clinical trials are used to determine whether drugs or treatments are both safe and effective.

Clitoridectomy The removal of the clitoris; also known as female genital mutilation or female circumcision.

Clitoris A highly sensitive structure of the female external genitalia, the only purpose of which is sexual pleasure.

Co-dependent A person in a continuing relationship with a chemically dependent person whose actions enable the addiction to continue.

Cognitive behavioral therapy A short-term treatment, usually lasting several months, that teaches people to identify and change patterns of thinking that cause them to perceive certain situations or objects as dangerous.

Coitus Technical term for penile-vaginal intercourse.

Colonoscopy An examination of the colon using a flexible, lighted instrument called a colonoscope.

Colostomy A surgically created opening from the outside of the body into the colon that provides a new path for waste material to leave the body after part of the colon has been removed.

Colostrum Early milk, or milk produced during the pregnancy and for three to five days after birth. Colostrum is yellowish in color, thicker than milk, and rich with protective antibodies and protein.

Colposcope A lighted magnifying instrument used to examine the vagina and cervix.

Colposcopy A procedure in which a colposcope is used to examine the vagina and cervix.

Complex carbohydrates One of the main sources of fuel for the muscles. Complex carbohydrates are found in breads and cereals, pasta, rice, and vegetables such as potatoes and corn.

Conception Formation of a viable zygote by the union of the male sperm and the female ovum; fertilization.

Conceptus The products of conception or fertilization, including the fertilized egg and its enclosing membranes.

Condom A barrier contraception method consisting of a sheath, preferably latex, that covers the penis during intercourse. It prevents pregnancy by collecting the semen in the receptacle tip.

Congenital heart disease A heart condition present when a baby is born. It may include many different conditions, most of which can be surgically corrected.

Congestive heart failure (CHF) A condition in which the heart loses its ability to contract properly or sufficiently to meet the demands placed on it.

Conization   The surgical removal of a cone-shaped piece of tissue intended to determine whether abnormal cells have invaded tissue beneath surface cells or to treat a precancerous lesion. Also called cone biopsy.

Contraception   Intentional prevention of conception or impregnation through the use of various devices, agents, drugs, sexual practices, or surgical procedures.

Contraceptive sponge   A contraceptive device that acts both as a cervical barrier by absorbing ejaculated sperm and as a source of spermicide. It is available without fitting or prescription.

Contraindication   A medical condition that renders a course of treatment inadvisable or unsafe that might otherwise be recommended.

Co-payment   A type of cost sharing whereby the enrollee or covered person pays a specified flat amount per unit of service or unit of time, and the healthcare insurer pays the remainder of the cost.

Coronary artery bypass surgery   A type of surgery that creates a "bypass" around the blocked part of the coronary artery to restore the blood supply to the heart muscle.

Corpus luteum   A yellowish body that forms on the ovary at the site of the ruptured follicle where the egg has been released. It secretes progesterone to help prepare the body for pregnancy.

Corset   A close-fitting undergarment or an outer garment, worn to support and shape the waistline, hips, and breasts.

C-reactive protein   A protein produced by the liver during periods of inflammation that is detectable in blood in various disease conditions. The C-reactive protein blood test is used as an indicator of acute inflammation.

Crack   A highly addictive smokeable form of cocaine; also known as "rock."

Cryosurgery   Surgical procedure that freezes and destroys abnormal tissues.

Cryotherapy   Freezing of an infected area.

Cunnilingus   Oral stimulation of the clitoris or vulva.

Cyberstalking   Threatening behavior or unwanted advances directed at another person using the Internet and other forms of online communications.

Cystic fibrosis   An abnormality of the respiratory system and the sweat and mucous glands. Cystic fibrosis is the most common genetic disorder among whites in the United States.

Cystic mastitis   The most common breast disorder in women, resulting in tender and lumpy breast tissues. Also known as fibrocystic breast disease.

Cyst   An abnormal growth of cells consisting of a thin-walled sac filled with fluid.

Cystitis   Inflammation of the bladder.

Cytomegalovirus (CMV)   A viral infection that causes mild flu-like symptoms in adults but that can cause small birth size, brain damage, developmental problems, enlarged liver, hearing and vision impairment, and other malformations in newborns. Babies with CMV are infected in utero, although only 10% of those so infected have symptoms.

Pregnant women often acquire CMV from young infected children with few or no symptoms. CMV is the most common prenatal infection today and it is an opportunistic infection of HIV/AIDS.

D

Date rape   Rape in which the victim and the rapist were previously known to each other and may have interacted in some socially appropriate manner. Also known as "acquaintance rape."

Delirium tremens (DTs)   A condition induced by alcohol withdrawal and characterized by excessive trembling, sweating, anxiety, and hallucinations.

Dementia   Cognitive decline, often occurring in old age. This mental deterioration and decline in intellectual functioning is severe enough to interfere with routine daily activities.

Depression   A mental condition in which a person feels extremely sad, worthless, and hopeless. In more severe cases, the person may experience thoughts of suicide. Types of depression include clinical depression, bipolar depression, seasonal affective disorder (SAD), dysthymia, and postpartum depression.

Diabetes mellitus   A disease characterized by abnormal glucose production or metabolism. A person with diabetes has either a deficiency of insulin (the hormone produced by the pancreas needed to convert glucose to energy) or a decreased ability to use insulin. As a result, glucose builds up in the bloodstream and, without treatment, may damage organs and contribute to heart disease.

Diaphragm   A latex, dome-shaped cap inserted over the cervix to prevent conception.

Diastolic   The second reading of blood pressure that represents the amount of pressure the blood exerts against the wall of the artery when the heart rests between beats.

Diethylstilbestrol (DES)   A synthetic estrogen originally prescribed to prevent miscarriages. DES caused malformations of the reproductive organs in some women who were exposed to the drug during fetal development.

Digital rectal examination   An examination intended to detect colorectal cancer in which the physician inserts a lubricated gloved finger into the rectum to feel for abnormal areas.

Dilation and curettage (D&C)   A minor surgical procedure in which the cervix is expanded enough (dilated) to permit the cervical canal and uterine lining to be scraped with a spoon-shaped instrument called a curette.

Dissociative disorders   Disorders that develop as an unconscious way to protect oneself from emotional traumas by detaching from a part of one's personality. These disorders occur as a response to a severe childhood trauma.

Diuretic   Drug that expedites the elimination of fluid from the body.

Dizygotic twins   Two offspring developed from two eggs released from the ovary and fertilized at the same time. They may be the same or opposite sex, and may differ physically and in genetic traits. Also called fraternal twins.

Domestic violence   Subjecting a spouse, partner, or family member to any forceful physical, social, and psychological behavior so as to coerce that person, without regard to his or her rights. Also known as battering.

Double-contrast barium enema   A type of X-ray procedure in which a mixture containing barium is inserted into the rectum. The barium mixture outlines the lower part of the bowel, enabling any blockages or abnormalities in the lining of the bowel to be identified.

Down syndrome   A congenital condition characterized by various degrees of mental retardation and abnormal development. It is caused by the presence of an extra chromosome, usually number 21 or 22.

Drug   Any chemical other than food that is purposely taken to affect body processes.

Drug abuse   The excessive use of a drug that has dangerous side effects.

Drug dependency   The attachment—physiological or psychological (or both)—that a person may develop to a drug. Physical dependence occurs when physiological changes in the body's cells cause an overpowering, constant need for a drug.

Drug misuse   The use of a drug for a purpose other than its original intent.

Dysmenorrhea   Pain or discomfort just prior to or during menstruation.

Dyspareunia   Painful intercourse, which can stem from physical or psychological causes.

Dysplasia   Abnormal cells that are not cancer. It is classified as mild, moderate, or severe.

Dysplastic nevi   Atypical moles.

Dysthymia   A form of depression that is milder and less disabling than major depression, but more chronic in nature.

E

Eclampsia   A life-threatening condition during pregnancy that causes convulsions and may lead to coma and death of the mother and baby. Eclampsia progresses from preeclampsia.

Ectoparasitic infections   Infections caused by tiny parasites that reside on the skin and survive on human blood and tissue. Infections include scabies and pubic lice ("crabs"). Parasites cause itching and may cause bumps or a rash, but are easily treated with a topical cream.

Ectopic pregnancy   The implantation of a fertilized egg outside the uterus.

Edema   An abnormal accumulation of fluid in body parts or tissues that results in swelling.

Effacement   The thinning of the cervix before delivery.

Egg donation   A type of assisted reproductive technology used when a woman is unable to produce eggs or has a genetic disorder that will be passed on to her child. Egg donors must be willing to dedicate an enormous amount of time to this effort because of the amount of drug treatment and monitoring that they must undergo.

Elder abuse   The injury, maltreatment, or neglect of an older person from a physical, psychological, or material perspective.

Electrocardiograph (ECG)   A device used to record the electric activity of the heart so as to diagnose heart problems.

Electrocautery   Electrical burning of an infected area.

Electrodessication   Tissue destruction by heat.

Embolism   A condition in which an embolus (clot) traveling in the bloodstream becomes lodged in a blood vessel.

Embolus   A clot circulating in the bloodstream that becomes lodged in a blood vessel.

Embryo   An organism in its early stage of development in humans. The embryonic period lasts from the second to the eighth week of pregnancy.

Embryo transfer   A fertility procedure in which the sperm of the infertile woman's partner are placed in another woman's uterus during ovulation. The fertilized egg is removed a few days later and transferred to the uterus of the infertile woman.

Emotional or psychological elder abuse   The infliction of mental or emotional anguish of an older person through such means as humiliation, intimidation, or threats.

Emphysema   The limitation of airflow as the result of irreversible disease changes in the lung tissue after years of assault on that tissue. The air sacs in the lungs are destroyed, and the lungs are compromised in bringing oxygen and removing carbon dioxide from the body. As a result, breathing becomes compromised, and increased demand is placed on the heart.

Endometrial hyperplasia   An overgrowth of the lining of the uterus (endometrium) resulting from lack of ovulation. Failure to ovulate leads to too much estrogen and not enough progesterone being produced by the body. When this occurs, the endometrium builds up but is not shed during the menstrual cycle.

Endometriosis   A benign condition in which tissue that looks like endometrial tissue grows in abnormal places outside the uterus.

Endometrium   The tissue that lines the inside of the uterine walls.

Environmental tobacco smoke (ETS)   Smoke resulting from others who are smoking cigarettes. Also referred to as passive or secondhand smoke.

Enzyme linked immunosorbent assay (ELISA)   Laboratory test used to detect antibodies produced in response to HIV infection. If HIV antibodies are found with this test, it is repeated. If antibodies are found on a second ELISA test, a Western Blot test is performed.

Epidemiology   The study of patterns of disease in the population; epidemiology is concerned with the frequency and type of a disease in groups of people and the factors that influence the distribution of the disease.

Epidural anesthesia   A type of anesthetic used during delivery that is injected through a catheter placed in a space beside the spinal cord. Epidurals are the most common choice of anesthesia made by pregnant women and allow the mother to be awake for the birth.

Episiotomy An incision in the mother's perineum that enlarges the opening of the vagina to provide more room for the infant during delivery and to help prevent tearing of the vaginal tissues.

Epstein-Barr virus One of the eight known types of human herpes viruses; causes mononucleosis.

Erythrocytes Red blood cells. Erythrocytes carry oxygen and carbon dioxide.

Estrogen A class of hormones that produce female secondary sex characteristics and affect the menstrual cycle.

Eugenics The study of or belief in the possibility of improving the qualities of the human species or a human population by such means as discouraging reproduction by persons having genetic defects or presumed to have inheritable undesirable traits, or encouraging reproduction by those presumed to have positive traits.

F

Fallopian tubes Tubes or ducts that allow for the passage of ova from the ovary to the uterus.

Familial adenomatous polyposis (FAP) A condition in which polyps are inherited and affect the gastrointestinal tract. Individuals with FAP develop hundreds to thousands of polyps throughout the colon at a young age.

Family and intimate violence Forms of violence that include child abuse, incest, courtship violence, date rape, battering, marital rape, and elder abuse.

Fat A lipid with one, two, or three fatty acids, responsible for multiple body functions.

Fat-soluble vitamins Vitamins absorbed with the aid of fats in the diet or bile from the liver, through the intestinal membrane and stored in the body.

Fecal occult blood testing A simple procedure of smearing a small sample of stool on a slide containing a chemical that changes color in the presence of hemoglobin. Developing tumors cause minor bleeding, which results in the presence of occult blood (small amounts of blood in the stool).

Fecundity The physical ability of a woman to have a child. Women with impaired fecundity include those who find it physically difficult or medically inadvisable to conceive or deliver a child.

Fee for service A traditional method of healthcare payment in which physicians and other providers receive payment that does not exceed their billed charges for each unit of service rendered.

Fellatio Oral stimulation of the penis or scrotum.

Female athlete triad The interrelationship between disordered eating, amenorrhea, and osteoporosis. Beginning with disordered eating, the combination of poor nutrition and intense athletic training causes weight loss and a decrease in or shutdown of estrogen production. Consequently, amenorrhea occurs. The final condition in the triad, osteoporosis, may follow if estrogen levels remain low and the woman's diet continues to lack calcium and vitamin D.

Female condom   A form of barrier contraception that lines the entire vagina, preventing the penis and semen from coming in direct physical contact with the vagina.

Female genital mutilation   Any of three types of genital mutilation: removal of the prepuce and/or the tip of the clitoris; removal of the entire clitoris (both prepuce and glans) and the adjacent labia; or removal of the clitoris, the adjacent labia (majora and minora), and the joining of the scraped sides of the vulva across the vagina. Often referred to as female circumcision or female genital cutting.

Feminism   The policy, practice, or advocacy of political, economic, and social equality for women. It is the principle that women should have rights equal to those of men.

Fertility   The state of being fertile; capable of producing offspring.

Fertility awareness methods   Several methods, including the calendar or rhythm method, the basal body temperature method, and the cervical mucus method, that can help a woman determine her most fertile time. These methods can be used to prevent pregnancy or to help a woman become pregnant.

Fertilization   The union of an ovum and a sperm.

Fetal alcohol syndrome (FAS)   Alcohol-related defects among infants due to prenatal maternal alcohol consumption. They are usually characterized by growth retardation, facial malformations, and central nervous system dysfunctions including mental retardation.

Fetal distress   Signs of distress in the fetus such as slowing of heart rate or acid in the blood.

Fetus   The unborn baby in the uterus from the eighth week of gestation until birth.

Fiber   Plant parts that cannot be digested in the human digestive tract. High-fiber diets protect against certain cancers and heart disease.

Fibroadenoma   A nonmalignant form of breast tumor.

Fibrocystic breast disease   The most common breast disorder in women, resulting in tender and lumpy breast tissues. Also known as cystic mastitis.

Fibroid   A benign uterine tumor composed of muscular and fibrous tissue.

Flexibility   The range of motion permitted by joints.

Folate   A B vitamin found in foods such as chickpeas, spinach, strawberries, kidney beans, and citrus fruits and juices.

Folic acid   A form of folate used to fortify grain-based foods, such as bread, flour, rice, pasta, and cereal. It is vital for cell growth and function and for the development of a healthy neural tube in fetuses.

Follicle stimulating hormone (FSH)   A pituitary hormone secreted by a female during the secretory phase of the menstrual cycle. It stimulates the development of ovarian follicles.

Food insecurity   Lack of access to nutritionally balanced and safe foods or having limited access to nutritious and affordable food.

Forceps Surgical instruments used for grasping. Obstetric forceps may be used to extract a baby from the birth canal during delivery.

Formulary A list of drug products that a payer has identified as part of a given health insurance product's covered benefits.

Fornication Voluntary sexual intercourse between persons not married to each other.

G

Galactosemia Inherited disease characterized by lack of enzyme needed for processing galactose (sugar in milk products); can cause mental retardation if not treated promptly.

Gamete intrafallopian transfer (GIFT) A procedure for treating infertility that involves placing sperm and egg cells into the fallopian tubes.

Gangrene Localized tissue death due to inadequate blood supply or bacterial invasion.

Gastritis Inflammation of the stomach lining.

Gender The economic, social, and cultural attributes and opportunities associated with being male or female.

Gender dysphoria The overall psychological term used to describe the negative or conflicting feelings about one's sex or gender roles.

Gender identity How one psychologically perceives oneself as either male or female.

Gender roles The public expression of one's gender identity, as well as the cultural expectations of male and female behaviors.

Generalized anxiety disorder (GAD) An anxiety disorder that causes an ongoing, general feeling of intense worry and fear, often for no apparent reason.

Generic drug The chemical equivalent of a brand-name drug that is available once the brand-name drug goes off patent. Generic drugs are typically less expensive than their brand-name counterparts.

Genetic phenotype The observable traits or characteristics of an organism—for example, hair color, weight, or the presence or absence of a disease.

Gestational diabetes A form of the disease that develops in 2% to 5% of all pregnancies, but usually disappears when the pregnancy is over.

Glycemic index A measure of how fast glucose enters the bloodstream after a carbohydrate is eaten and thus how quickly the carbohydrate increases a person's blood sugar.

Gonadotropin-releasing hormone (GnRH) Hormone responsible for reproductive hormone control; stimulates release of follicle stimulating hormone at the beginning of the menstrual cycle.

Gonadotropins Pituitary hormones that stimulate activity in the testes or ovaries.

Gonorrhea A sexually transmitted bacterial infection that can cause dangerous complications leading to infertility, ectopic pregnancy, or persistent pain in the pelvic area; it can even spread to the bloodstream and cause arthritis or life-threatening heart or brain infections.

Group B streptococcus (GBS)   A type of bacterium that can cause illness in newborn babies and pregnant women. Pregnant women with GBS do not necessarily infect their babies; however, babies who develop signs and symptoms are at risk of sepsis, pneumonia, meningitis, long-term disabilities such as hearing or vision loss, and death. Obstetricians can test women for GBS and prevent disease by administering antibiotics intravenously during labor.

H

Hallucinogenic drugs   Drugs that create changes in perceptions and thoughts. A common feature of a hallucinogenic experience is that the drug suspends normal psychic mechanisms that integrate the self with the environment.

Hashish   An extract of cannabis that is 2 to 10 times as concentrated as marijuana.

Hate crime   A crime in which the defendant intentionally selects a victim or, in the case of a property crime, the property that is the object of the crime because of the actual or perceived race, color, national origin, ethnicity, gender, disability, or sexual orientation of the person.

HDL cholesterol   A type of lipoprotein in the blood that carries cholesterol and fats out of the body. Often referred to as "good" cholesterol.

Heart attack   Death of a certain portion of the heart.

Hemoglobin   The iron-containing protein in the red blood cell that carries oxygen from the lungs to the cells and carbon dioxide away from the cells to the lungs. It is also responsible for the red color of blood.

Hemorrhagic stroke   A condition in which blood vessels leading to and within the brain rupture, causing the brain to no longer receive blood and oxygen.

Hepatitis   Inflammation and destruction of liver cells.

Hepatoma   A cancer that originates from liver cells.

Herpes simplex virus (HSV)   Virus that causes skin eruptions.

Heterosexuality   Sexual orientation to persons of the opposite sex, and/or sexual activity with another of the opposite sex.

High-density lipoprotein (HDL)   A type of lipoprotein in the blood that carries cholesterol and fats out of the body. It is often referred to as the "good" cholesterol.

Histoplasmosis   Infection caused by breathing in airborne spores of fungus; the disease primarily affects the lungs, but occasionally affects other organs. Histoplasmosis is an opportunistic infection of AIDS.

HIV (human immunodeficiency virus)   A virus that attacks and damages the white blood cells in the body's immune system that are needed to fight off infection; eventually causes AIDS (Acquired Immune Deficiency Syndrome) when so many white blood cells have been destroyed that the immune system can no longer fight off illness.

Homeostasis   A constant environment within the body.

Homocysteine An essential amino acid found in the blood. Increased levels of homocysteine can harm the artery lining and increase risk for coronary artery disease.

Homologous Refers to parts that resemble one another or originate from the same tissue, such as the external genitals, gonads, and some of the internal structures of males and females.

Homophobia Irrational fears of homosexuality, the fear of the possibility of homosexuality in oneself, or self-loathing toward one's own homosexuality.

Homosexual A person whose primary social, emotional, and sexual orientation is toward members of the same sex.

Honor killings The killing of a woman who has a (sexual) contact with a man outside the frame of marriage, even when she has been a victim of rape. It is intended to maintain and protect the honor of the family. Offenders are often younger than age 18 and are sometimes treated as heroes in their communities. Such killings have been reported in Pakistan, Jordan, Yemen, Lebanon, Egypt, the Gaza Strip, and the West Bank.

Host uterus A procedure in which the sperm from a man and the egg from a woman are combined in a laboratory. The fertilized egg is then implanted into the uterus of a second woman, who agrees to bear the child that is not genetically related to her.

Hot flash An uncomfortable sensation of menopause consisting of internally generated heat beginning in the chest and moving to the neck and head or spreading throughout the body. Also known as hot flushes.

Human chorionic gonadotropin (hCG) A hormone produced by the chorionic villi in a pregnant woman.

Human genome The DNA contained in an organism or a cell, which includes both the chromosomes within the nucleus and the DNA in mitochondria.

Human papillomavirus (HPV) A virus that causes genital warts. In women, some strains are known to cause cervical cancer.

Hunger The painful or uneasy feeling caused by the continuous and involuntary lack of food.

Hymen Tissue that partially covers the vaginal opening.

Hyperglycemia High blood sugar levels, whereby a person may become very ill. Early signs of hyperglycemia include high blood sugar, high levels of sugar in the urine, frequent urination, and increased thirst.

Hyperplasia A precancerous condition characterized by an increase in the number of normal cells.

Hypertension A blood pressure that remains elevated above what is considered a safe level. Also known as high blood pressure.

Hyperthyroidism Thyroid disease resulting from an overactive thyroid, most commonly caused by Graves' disease.

Hypoactive sexual desire disorder (HSDD)   A persistent lack of interest in or desire for sex. This disorder often reflects relationship problems, but may be caused by other physical or personal difficulties.

Hypoglycemia   Low blood sugar levels that can cause a person to become nervous, shaky, and confused and can result in the person passing out.

Hypothyroidism   Thyroid disease resulting from an underactive thyroid; most commonly caused by Hashimoto's disease.

Hysterectomy   The surgical removal of the uterus, resulting in surgically induced menopause.

Hysteroscopy   A procedure used to view the inside of the uterus through a telescope-like device called a hysteroscope.

I

Iatrogenic   Induced in a patient by a medical treatment or procedure. Used to refer to an infection or other complication of treatment.

Immune system   The body's natural defense system, which works to protect the body from pathogens.

Implantation   The embedding of the fertilized ovum in the uterine lining six to seven days after fertilization.

In vitro fertilization (IVF)   A procedure for treating infertility that involves removing the ova from a woman's ovary. The ova and the sperm (from the woman's partner) are placed in a medium; if fertilization occurs, the conceptus is injected into the woman's uterus.

Incidence   The number of new cases of a disease or condition in a given period of time.

Indemnity health insurance   A form of health insurance in which a person prepays a premium in exchange for a specific amount of monetary coverage in the event of illnesses or accidents. If an illness or accident occurs, the enrollee or the care provider submits a claim to the insurance organization. The insurance organization then reimburses the party for all or, in most cases, a percentage of the incurred costs.

Inferior vena cava   The major vein that carries oxygen-poor blood into the right atrium of the heart.

Infertility   The inability to conceive a child.

Infibulation   The removal of the clitoris, the labia majora and labia minora, and the joining of the scraped sides of the vulva across the vagina, where they are secured with thorns or sewn with catgut or thread. A small opening is kept to allow passage of urine and menstrual blood. An infibulated woman must be cut open to allow intercourse on her wedding night and is closed again afterwards to secure fidelity to the husband. Infibulation is the most extreme form of female genital mutilation.

Inhalants   Chemicals that produce vapors with psychoactive effects and are predominantly abused by pre-adolescents and young adults.

Insulin-dependent diabetes mellitus (IDDM) A type of diabetes that often appears in childhood or adolescence. It is considered an autoimmune disease because the immune system attacks and destroys the insulin-producing beta cells in the pancreas, so that the pancreas produces little or no insulin. Also called type 1 diabetes or juvenile diabetes.

Intersexuality The sexual physiology of an individual in which the person is born with sex chromosomes, external genitalia, or internal reproductive organs that are not considered "standard" as male or female.

Intracytoplasmic sperm injection (ICSI) A procedure for treating infertility that involves the injection of a single sperm directly into a mature egg.

Intrauterine device (IUD) A small, flexible, plastic T-shaped device that contains either copper or the hormone progesterone and is inserted into the uterus by a clinician to prevent pregnancy. The IUD can be left in place for 1 to 10 years, depending on the type of device.

Intrauterine growth retardation Poor fetal growth for a given duration of pregnancy.

Involuntary smoking A situation in which nonsmokers have to breathe air contaminated by smokers. Also known as passive smoking or environmental tobacco smoke (ETS).

Iron A mineral that is needed to make hemoglobin (a compound in the blood).

Ischemic stroke A condition in which blood vessels leading to and within the brain become blocked, causing the brain to no longer receive blood and oxygen.

Isoflavone A phytoestrogen that is present in soybeans and soy-based products.

J

Jaundice A condition in which accumulation of pigments in the blood produces a yellowing of the skin and eyes.

K

Kegel exercises Exercises that help strengthen the vaginal and pelvic floor muscles to help prepare the muscles for delivery; aid in a speedy recovery from delivery; help prevent or treat urinary incontinence; and help prevent or treat the loss of pelvic support.

L

Labia majora The outer lips of the vagina.

Labia minora The inner lips of the vulva, one on each side of the vaginal opening.

Lactation The production and secretion of milk by the mammary glands.

Lactational amenorrhea method (LAM) A contraceptive method used by breastfeeding women that is effective only if all three of the following criteria are met: menstrual periods have not yet returned; the mother is fully breastfeeding; and the baby is younger than six months old.

Lamaze   A method of childbirth preparation in which the expectant mother is prepared psychologically and physically through breathing exercises and concentration to control pain during childbirth while maintaining consciousness.

Laparoscopy   Examination of a woman's abdominal cavity to view the ovaries, fallopian tubes, and other structures.

LDL cholesterol   A type of lipoprotein that contains cholesterol and triglycerides and is considered harmful because it promotes fatty deposits on the inner lining of arteries. Also called "bad" cholesterol.

Left atrium   One of the two upper chambers of the heart. It receives blood with oxygen from the lungs.

Left ventricle   One of the two lower chambers of the heart. It pumps blood from the heart to the body tissues.

Lesbian   A woman whose sexual orientation is to women; a female homosexual.

Leukemia   A cancer that originates within the blood and blood-producing organs.

Leukocytes   White blood cells. Leukocytes act as scavengers to rid the blood and body of bacteria and waste. Several types of white blood cells exist, each of which has its own role in fighting bacterial, viral, fungal, and parasitic infections.

Life expectancy   The number of years a person born at a given point in time is expected to live from birth.

Lipoprotein   A compound found in the bloodstream containing a core of lipids with a shell of protein, phospholipid, and cholesterol.

Lobectomy   Removal of the lobe of a lung.

Long-term care   Custodial care provided over a prolonged or indefinite period of time, required because of a person's disability or aging. Skilled nursing facilities, or nursing homes, are the most common types of long-term care facilities.

Low-density lipoprotein (LDL)   A type of lipoprotein that contains cholesterol and triglycerides and is considered harmful because it promotes fatty deposits on the inner lining of arteries. Also called "bad" cholesterol.

Lp(a)   A lipoprotein that, when present in elevated levels, may cause blockages to increase in size and blood to thicken. Lp(a) is an inherited factor and cannot be controlled by lifestyle choices.

Lumpectomy   A procedure in which only the cancerous lump and a small amount of surrounding tissue are removed from the breast.

Lupus   A complex chronic inflammatory disorder in which the immune system forms antibodies that target healthy tissues and organs. Lupus can be a mild, moderate, or severe disease.

Luteinizing hormone (LH)   The hormone secreted by the pituitary gland that stimulates ovulation in the female.

Lyme disease   A type of inflammatory arthritis which is caused by a tiny, tick-borne bacterium. If Lyme disease is not treated, it can lead to cardiac problems, neurological disorders, or infectious arthritis (usually of the knees).

Lymphoma   A tumor, usually cancerous, that originates from lymph tissue that is part of the body's immune system.

M

Macromineral   One of the six major minerals—calcium, chloride, magnesium, phosphorus, potassium, and sodium.

Macular degeneration   Common eye disease associated with aging that gradually destroys sharp, central vision.

Malignant tumor   A tumor that is cancerous, capable of spreading to other tissues and invading adjacent areas.

Malnutrition   An imbalance between the body's nutritional needs and the intake or digestion of nutrients, which may result in disease or death. Malnutrition can be caused by an unbalanced diet, digestive problems, or absorption problems.

Mammography   A procedure in which a low-dose X ray of the breast is taken so as to detect tumors.

Managed care   A system of healthcare delivery that aims to manage utilization of services and cost of services, while measuring performance. The goal is a system that delivers value by giving people access to quality, cost-effective health care.

Mastectomy   Removal of the entire breast tissue and possibly underarm lymph nodes to treat cancer.

Mastitis   An infection in the breast, usually caused by bacterial infection. It results in localized pain, redness, and heat with symptoms of fever, nausea, and vomiting.

Masturbation   Excitation of one's own or another's genital organs, usually to orgasm, by manual contact or means other than sexual intercourse.

Maternal morbidity and mortality   Death or illness while pregnant or within a defined time period of the termination of pregnancy, irrespective of the duration and the site of the pregnancy, from any cause related to or aggravated by the pregnancy or its management but not from accidental or incidental causes.

Maternal serum alpha-fetoprotein screening   A prenatal screening test that measures a substance produced by the baby's kidneys found in the mother's blood between the thirteenth and twentieth weeks of pregnancy.

Medicaid   A joint federal/state health insurance program for low-income persons who receive public assistance or whose medical expenses "spend down" their income to qualify for the program. This program is administered by each state, and places fairly tight restrictions on payment for physician services and drugs. Also known as Title XIX.

Medicare   A health insurance program providing benefits to approximately 30 million elderly (aged 65 or older) and disabled Americans. It is funded by the federal government and administered by the Center for Medicare and Medicaid Services (CMS).

Melanocytes   Pigment-producing cells in the skin.

Melanoma   A cancer that originates within the melanocytes.

Melatonin   A hormone that is important in regulating the body's response to biological rhythms, such as the light-dark cycle.

Menarche   The initial onset of menstrual periods in a young woman.

Menopause   The cessation of regular menstrual periods by surgical or natural means. Also known as the climacterium or the "change of life."

Menstrual cycle   A recurring cycle (beginning at menarche and ending at menopause) in which the endometrial lining of the uterus prepares for pregnancy. If pregnancy does not occur, the lining is shed at menstruation. The average menstrual cycle is 28 days.

Metastasis   The spread of cancer from one part of the body to another. Cells in the metastatic tumor (the second tumor) are like those in the original tumor.

Mineral   A naturally occurring inorganic substance. These nutrients are essential in small amounts for regulating body functions.

Miscarriage   A pregnancy that terminates before the twentieth week of gestation because of fetal defects or pregnancy problems.

Mitral valve   The valve separating the left atrium and ventricle.

Modified radical mastectomy   Removal of the breast. Modified radical mastectomy is a less extensive procedure than radical mastectomy because the underlying chest wall muscles and some of the nearby lymph nodes are not removed. Also known as total mastectomy.

Monounsaturated fat   A type of fat that comes from both plant and animal sources and is liquid at room temperature and solid or semi-solid when refrigerated. Monounsaturated fats help to lower blood cholesterol.

Monozygotic twins   Two offspring developed from one fertilized egg that splits into equal halves. Monozygotic twins are of the same sex, share the same genes, and look nearly identical. Also called identical twins.

Mons veneris   A triangular mound over the pubic bone above the vulva.

Mood disorders (affective disorders)   Conditions characterized by extreme disturbances of mood.

Morbidity rate   The rate of illness in a given population over a period of time.

Mortality rate   The rate of death in a given population over a period of time.

Multiple sclerosis (MS)   An autoimmune disease that is characterized by the loss of the myelin covering of the nerve fibers of the brain and spinal cord.

Muscular endurance   The ability to withstand the stress of physical exertion.

Muscular strength   Physical power, such as the amount of weight one can lift, push, or press in a single effort.

Mycobacterium avium complex (MAC)   An infection contracted through contaminated food, soil, or water and affecting only those with weakened immune systems. MAC is an opportunistic infection of HIV/AIDS.

Myocardial infarction   Heart attack.

Myomectomy   Surgical removal of a uterine fibroid.

Myometrium   The smooth muscle layer of the uterine wall.

N

Narcotics   A class of drugs that includes the opiates—opium and its derivatives, morphine, codeine, and heroin—and some non-opiate synthetic drugs. All narcotics have sleep-inducing and pain-relieving properties.

Natural menopause   The failure of the ovaries to respond to the luteinizing and follicle-stimulating hormones that are produced in the anterior pituitary, which is under the control of the hypothalamus. As a result of this failure, ovulation becomes somewhat erratic. The mechanisms for these changes are not well understood. Menopause is considered complete once monthly periods have ceased altogether.

Neoplasm   A type of tumor that is a new growth of tissue serving no physiological function. The growth may be benign or malignant.

Neural tube defects   Defects of the spine and brain caused by failure of the neural tube to close during pregnancy.

Neuroblastoma   A cancer that originates from cells in the nervous system.

Nicotine   The addictive element in cigarettes. Nicotine has several effects on the body, including increasing blood pressure, increasing heart rate, and negating hunger.

Non-governmental organizations (NGOs)   According to the World Bank, "private organizations that pursue activities to relieve suffering, promote the interests of the poor, protect the environment, provide basic social services, or undertake community development." This term can be applied to any nonprofit organization that is independent from government, including a large charity, community-based self-help group, research institute, church, professional association, and lobby group.

Noninsulin-dependent diabetes Mellitus (NIDDM)   The most common type of diabetes. Approximately 90% to 95% of all people with diabetes have NIDDM. In this type of disease, the pancreas usually produces insulin but the insulin is not used effectively. Also referred to as type 2 diabetes or adult-onset diabetes.

Nonmelanoma   The most common cancers of the skin (usually basal cell and squamous cell cancers). Nonmelanoma cancers include all skin cancers except malignant melanoma.

Norplant   A hormonal method of birth control that prevents ovulation and is administered by implanting capsules of hormones under the skin of the inside part of the upper arm. The manufacturing of Norplant has been discontinued.

Nutrient   A substance essential to life that the body cannot produce on its own. Nutrients are provided by food and assist in the growth and development of the body.

Nutrition   The science studying the need for and the effects of food on an organism.

O

Obesity   The excessive accumulation of fat in the body; a condition of being 20% or more above ideal weight.

Obsessive-compulsive disorder (OCD)   An anxiety disorder that causes a person to have disturbing repetitive thoughts (obsessions), and to perform rituals or routines (compulsions) to get rid of the obsessions. The disorder is diagnosed only when the repetitive behaviors consume many hours each day and interfere with daily life.

Oligospermia   A condition in which few sperm are produced in the semen. Oligospermia is often the cause of male infertility.

Opportunistic infections   Infections that seldom cause disease in people with normal immune function but "take the opportunity" to cause disease in people with a present illness or a lowered immune system, such as caused by HIV/AIDS.

Opposed estrogen   Estrogen replacement therapy that is taken with the opposing effects of progestin.

Oral contraceptives   Birth control pills that cause the woman's own reproductive hormone cycle to be suppressed by the synthetic estrogen and progestin. Without the natural signals, either the ovary egg follicle cannot mature and ovulation does not occur or implantation of a fertilized egg becomes impossible.

Organic brain syndrome (OBS)   A general term refering to physical disorders that cause a decrease in mental function, usually not including psychiatric disorders. OBS is a common "diagnosis" of the elderly. It is not an inevitable part of aging, however. OBS is not a separate disease entity, but is a general term used to categorize physical conditions that can cause mental changes.

Orgasm   A series of muscular contractions of the pelvic floor muscles occurring at the peak of sexual arousal.

Orgasmic dysfunction   An inability to experience the orgasmic component of the sexual response cycle.

Orgasmic phase   Term used by Masters and Johnson to describe the third phase of the sexual response cycle in which the rhythmic muscular contractions of the pelvic floor occur.

Osteoarthritis   A disease in which the surface layer of cartilage erodes, causing bones under the cartilage to rub together. This friction results in joint pain, swelling, and loss of movement of the joints. Also called degenerative joint disease.

Osteopathic school   A school that focuses on natural medicine, which aims to restore function to the organism by treating the causes of pain and imbalance.

Osteopenia   Decreased calcification or density of bone. This descriptive term is applicable to all skeletal systems in which such a condition is noted.

Osteoporosis   An age-related, debilitating disorder characterized by a general decrease in bone mass and structural deterioration of bone tissue.

Ova   Female reproductive cells that are released in single units from the ovary. Also called eggs.

Ovaries Reproductive organ that produces ova, estrogen, and progesterone.

Overnutrition A form of malnutrition caused by overeating, insufficient exercise, and excessive intake of vitamins and minerals. Overnutrition can lead to overweight and obesity.

Overweight Having a body mass index (BMI) of 25 to 29.9.

Ovulation The release of a mature ovum from the graafian follicle of the ovary.

Ovum The female reproductive cell; an egg.

P

Panic disorder An anxiety disorder characterized by periods of intense fear known as panic attacks that are accompanied by physical symptoms (pounding heart, sweating, dizziness, chest pain, and so on) and emotional distress.

Pap smear A gynecological procedure in which a sample of cervical cells is examined for the presence of precancerous or cancerous cells.

Partial mastectomy Surgery to treat breast cancer that involves the removal of some breast tissue and some of the surrounding lymph nodes. Also called segmental mastectomy.

Patent ductus arteriosus A congenital condition common in premature babies in which the passageway between the pulmonary artery and aorta does not close.

Pelvic floor The muscles that provide the basis of support for a woman's uterus, bladder, and rectum.

Pelvic inflammatory disease (PID) A general term describing an infection of the internal female reproductive tract that can lead to infertility, chronic pain, or ectopic pregnancy. PID is usually caused by a sexually transmitted disease, such as chlamydia or gonorrhea, that spreads into the upper reproductive tract.

Perimenopause Refers to the years immediately preceding and following the last menstrual period.

Perineal Referring to the area of smooth skin between the vaginal opening and the anus, known as the perineum.

Perineum The area of smooth skin between the vaginal opening and the anus.

Peripheral artery disease A disease of the extremities (hands, arms, but mainly in the legs and feet) in which the blood supply is diminished, and sufficient oxygen and nutrients do not reach these areas properly. Because waste is not removed from these areas effectively, the affected person may experience symptoms that range from cramping and numbness to gangrene (tissue death), which may require amputation of the extremity.

Personality disorders Mental disorders that are characterized by distorted and inflexible thoughts and behaviors that make it impossible for a person to live a productive life or establish fulfilling relationships.

Phenylketonuria (PKU) A genetic disorder in which a crucial liver enzyme is absent. It may result in severe mental retardation if left untreated.

Phobia   An anxiety disorder characterized by a powerful and irrational fear of a particular object or situation.

Phytochemicals   Plant chemicals found in fruits and vegetables that protect the body from cancer by blocking the carcinogenic activities of certain substances in the human body.

Phytoestrogen   Chemicals found in plants that may act like the estrogen produced naturally in the body.

Placebo   A substance that is inactive, but given in the same dose and form as a real medication.

Placenta   An organ that develops after implantation to which the embryo attaches via the umbilical cord for nourishment and waste removal.

Placenta previa   A complication of pregnancy in which the birth canal becomes obstructed by the placenta.

Plaque   Fatty deposits on the lining of arteries.

Platelets   Disk-shaped structures in the blood needed for blood coagulation. Also called thrombocytes.

Pneumocystis carinii pneumonia (PCP)   A lung infection that affects those with damaged immune systems; the most common AIDS-related opportunistic infection in the United States.

Pneumonectomy   Removal of the lung.

Polycystic ovarian syndrome   A condition that is associated with the overproduction of male hormones, failure to ovulate, formation of cysts on the surface of the ovaries, inability to become pregnant, and abnormal hair growth on the body. Polycystic ovary syndrome occurs most often in women who are obese, and it generally can be reversed with weight loss. Also called polycystic ovarian disease (PCOD).

Polyps   Small benign growths that develop in the endocervical canal or colorectal region.

Polyunsaturated fats   A type of fat that is liquid at room temperature and when refrigerated. Such fats help lower both LDL and HDL cholesterol.

Postmenopause   Life after the final menstrual period.

Postpartum psychosis   The most severe of the psychiatric disorders that can develop in women after delivery. Symptoms of postpartum psychosis include depression, anxiety, irritation, tiredness, and sleep disturbances, as well as behavior that tends to change throughout the day from clear consciousness to total loss of reality.

Post-traumatic stress disorder (PTSD)   An anxiety disorder that usually begins within three months after a traumatic event. Its symptoms include flashback episodes, nightmares, and emotional numbness.

Preeclampsia   A complication of pregnancy characterized by high blood pressure, swelling caused by fluid retention, and high levels of protein in the urine. Also called toxemia.

Premature labor   Labor that begins before the completed ninth month of fetal gestation.

Premenopause   The entirety of a woman's reproductive life—from first menstruation to menopause.

Premenstrual dysphoric disorder (PMDD)   A condition associated with severe emotional and physical problems that are linked closely to the menstrual cycle; a more severe form of premenstrual syndrome (PMS).

Premenstrual syndrome (PMS)   A group of cyclic symptoms that occur in some women about a week before menstruation, including breast tenderness, abdominal bloating, fatigue, fluctuating emotions, and depression.

Premium   In terms of health insurance, a regular periodic payment.

Prevalence   The total number of people with a given condition at a point in time.

Primary prevention   Prevention of disease by reducing exposure to a risk factor that may lead to the disease. Primary preventive measures include healthy nutrition, regular physical activity, cessation of smoking, and safe sexual practices.

Private health insurance   Health insurance provided by third-party payers to individuals or employer groups either through indemnity or managed care systems.

Prodrome   Period of infectiousness before the first signs of infection are present.

Progestational phase   Second half of the endometrial cycle. Also known as the secretory phase.

Progesterone   The hormone produced by the corpus luteum of the ovary that causes the uterine lining to thicken.

Progestin   A natural or synthetic progestational substance that mimics some or all of the actions of progesterone. It is used in conjunction with estrogen in hormone replacement therapy.

Prolapsed cord   A complication of pregnancy in which the umbilical cord comes through the pelvis before the baby. It can result in a disrupted flow of oxygen to the baby due to a compressed cord.

Proliferation phase   The phase in the menstrual cycle in which the ovarian follicles mature.

Proportionality   A term relating to one of the themes of the USDA's new MyPyramid, which replaces the Food Guide Pyramid. Proportionality is displayed on the pyramid by the different widths of the food group bands. The widths suggest how much food a person should choose from each group. The widths are just a general guide, not exact proportions. For example, larger widths represent greater proportions of foods such as fruits, vegetables, and whole grains; smaller widths represent smaller proportions of foods that are high in saturated or trans fats, or have added sugars, cholesterol or salt.

Prostaglandins   A family of hormones present in many body tissues. The release of prostaglandins as uterine cells are shed is believed to be the cause of menstrual cramping.

Protein   A substance that is basically a compound of amino acids; one of the essential nutrients.

Protein-energy malnutrition (PEM)   A deficiency syndrome caused by the inadequate intake of protein and/or energy intake. PEM, the most destructive form of malnutrition, mainly affects infants and young children.

Psychedelic   A drug that produces a heightened sense of reality with visual hallucinations and, sometimes, psychotic-like behaviors.

Psychological dependence   An emotional or mental attachment to the use of a drug. Also called habituation.

Psychosis   A severe mental disorder characterized by a loss of contact with reality and severe personality changes.

Puberty   The stage of life between childhood and adulthood during which the reproductive organs mature and secondary sexual characteristics begin to develop. For girls, it is the time of the onset of menstruation, the development of breasts and body hair, and usually some level of growth spurt.

Public health insurance   Health insurance provided by government sources including Medicare, Medicaid, the Department of Defense (DOD), Veterans Administration (VA), and the Bureau of Indian Affairs.

Pulmonary arteries   Vessels that receive blood from the right ventricle to carry to the lungs for oxygenation.

Pulmonary stenosis   A condition in which the valve between the ventricle and pulmonary artery is defective and does not open properly.

Pulmonary veins   Vessels that return oxygenated blood from the lungs to the left atrium.

Purging   The use of vomiting, laxatives, or diuretics after a bingeing episode. Purging is characteristic of the eating disorder, bulimia nervosa.

Pus   Substance composed of dead bacteria, dead white blood cells, and fluid that is most commonly the result of an infection process.

R

Radiation therapy   Treatment with high-energy radiation from X rays or other sources.

Radical mastectomy   Removal of the entire breast, underlying chest muscles, and underarm lymph nodes following a diagnosis of breast cancer.

Rape   Any unwanted sexual acts, including forced vaginal or anal intercourse, oral sex, or penetration with an object.

Recommended Dietary Allowances (RDAs)   Daily nutrient allowances recommended for healthy adults by the National Research Council.

Recreational drugs   Drugs taken purely for fun.

Red blood cells   One of the formed elements in circulating blood. It contains hemoglobin and transports oxygen. Also called erythrocytes.

Reproductive tract infections (RTIs)   Infections caused by a variety of organisms that affect the upper reproductive tract, the lower reproductive tract, or both. Most infections are transmitted by sexual intimacy and, therefore, are referred to as sexually transmitted diseases (STDs).

Retrovirus   A virus that has the ability to take over certain cells and interrupt their normal genetic function.

Rheumatic heart disease   A heart condition resulting from a bacterial infection (*Strepto-coccus*) that has been inadequately treated. The infection can develop into rheumatic fever and damage the heart valves.

Rheumatoid arthritis   Chronic inflammatory disease of the joints that results from an autoimmune response.

Rh incompatibility   A condition that occurs when an Rh-negative mother and an Rh-positive father conceive a baby who inherits the father's Rh-positive blood type. This situation may present problems during pregnancy, labor, and delivery if the fetus's Rh-positive blood cells enter the mother's bloodstream.

Right atrium   One of the two upper chambers of the heart. It collects deoxygenated blood from the body.

Right ventricle   One of the two lower chambers of the heart. It pumps blood from the heart to the lungs to collect oxygen.

Rubella   An infectious disease often causing birth defects in pregnant women. Also called German measles.

S

Sarcoma   A cancer that originates in the connective tissue, such as cartilage, tendons, and bone.

Saturated fats   Fats that come primarily from animal sources.

Schizophrenia   A type of psychosis representing a complex group of diseases with symptoms that may appear gradually or suddenly and include hallucinations or delusions, disordered thinking, and an impaired ability to manage emotions and interact with others. Schizophrenia is the most chronic and disabling of the severe mental disorders.

Scleroderma   An autoimmune disease that is characterized by a thickening of the skin and internal organs, and by blood vessel disturbances.

Seasonal affective disorder (SAD)   A form of depression caused by seasonal shifts in daylight hours that affect a person's sleep-wake cycle.

Secondary prevention   Early detection and prompt treatment of disease. Example of secondary preventive measures include screening tools such as mammography and Pap smears, which may detect disease before it spreads, thereby preventing further complications from the disease.

Secondary sex characteristics   The physical characteristics other than genitals that indicate sexual maturity, such as breasts and body hair.

Secretory phase   The phase of the menstrual cycle in which the corpus luteum develops and secretes progesterone.

Sedative   A drug that depresses the central nervous system, resulting in sleep.

Segmental mastectomy   Surgery to treat breast cancer that involves the removal of some breast tissue and some of the surrounding lymph nodes. Also called partial mastectomy.

Segmentectomy   Surgery to removes a section of a lobe of a lung.

Selective estrogen receptor modulators (SERMs)   Compounds that bind with estrogen receptors and exhibit estrogen action in some tissues and anti-estrogen action in other tissues. Many menopausal women use SERMs as an alternative to estrogen replacement, and infertile women use them for ovulation induction.

Self-mutilation   Any self-directed, repetitive behavior that causes physical injury. Self-mutilation acts are not usually suicide attempts but rather behaviors meant to express or release emotional turmoil. Examples include skin cutting with razors or knives (the most common pattern); burning or biting oneself; picking one's skin or hair; and extreme injuries such as auto-enucleation (self-removal of the eye), castration, or amputation.

Septum   A dividing wall, such as that between the right and left sides of the heart.

Serotonin   A neurotransmitter (brain chemical) known to affect appetite.

Sex   An individual's biological status as male or female.

Sexual assault   Conduct of a sexual or indecent nature toward another person that is accompanied by actual or threatened physical force or that induces fear, shame, or mental suffering. The term is frequently used as an all-encompassing term for any type of unwanted sexual advance.

Sexual dysfunction   The inability of an individual to function adequately in terms of sexual arousal, orgasm, or in coital situations.

Sexual harassment   Behavior that may include unwanted sexual attention or advances and/or the use of threats or bribery to obtain sexual favors. The offensive conduct often interferes with a person's ability to perform regular duties at work and creates an intimidating or hostile working environment.

Sexual health   A state of physical, emotional, mental and social well-being related to sexuality.

Sexual orientation   One's erotic, romantic, and affectional attraction to people of the same sex, to the opposite sex, or to both sexes.

Sexually transmitted diseases (STDs)   Infections of the reproductive tract that are transmitted by sexual intimacy. STDS include chlamydia, gonorrhea, syphilis, herpes, genital warts, hepatitis, and human immunodeficiency virus (HIV) infections.

Sickle cell anemia   A debilitating genetic disorder of the blood characterized by sickle-shaped red blood cells, primarily affecting African Americans.

SIDS (Sudden Infant Death Syndrome)   The diagnosis given for the sudden death of an infant under one year of age that remains unexplained after a complete investigation, which includes an autopsy, examination of the death scene, and review of the symptoms or illnesses the infant had prior to dying and any other pertinent medical history. Because most cases of SIDS occur when a baby is sleeping in a crib, SIDS is also commonly known as crib death.

Sigmoidoscopy   A procedure that uses a thin, lighted tube to examine the rectum and lower colon.

Simple carbohydrate A sugar. It provides the body with glucose and a quick spurt of energy.

Simple mastectomy Complete removal of the breast but not the lymph nodes under the arm or chest muscles following a diagnosis of breast cancer.

Sitz bath A tub in which one bathes in a sitting position with hips and buttocks under water and legs out.

Sjögren's syndrome A chronic autoimmune disorder characterized by dry eyes and dry mouth and caused by decreased tear and salivary gland functioning.

Sodomy Oral and/or anal sex.

Spermicide A chemical that breaks down the cell walls of sperm. It is often used in conjunction with barrier contraception methods.

Sphygmomanometer A cuff device connected to a hose and measuring device to ascertain blood pressure.

Spina bifida A neural tube defect in which the spine does not close during fetal development and exposed nerves are thereby damaged, possibly causing paralysis and life-threatening infections.

Spontaneous abortion Unintentional ending of pregnancy before a fetus is viable; miscarriage.

Sputum A secretion that is produced in the lungs and the bronchi (tubes that carry the air to the lung). This mucus-like secretion may become infected, become bloodstained, or contain abnormal cells that may lead to a diagnosis. Sputum is what comes up with deep coughing.

Squamous cell carcinoma A nonmelanoma skin cancer that begins in the squamous cells of the outer layer of skin (epidermis). It usually first appears on areas of the skin exposed to the sun, such as the face, ear, neck, lip, and back of the hands, but it can also develop where skin has been injured, such as within scars, burns, or skin ulcers.

Staging The process of learning whether cancer has spread from its original site to another part of the body.

Stalking Behaviors directed toward a specific person that involve repeated visual or physical proximity; nonconsensual communication; verbal, written, or implied threats; or a combination of these behaviors that would cause fear in a reasonable person.

Statins A class of cholesterol-lowering drugs.

Stent An implantable steel screen that is placed at the site of arterial narrowing to keep an artery open.

Sterilization The permanent, often surgical, end to fertility by interrupting the mechanisms of normal reproductive action.

Sternum The breastbone.

Stillbirth Death occurring before or during birth of a fetus of sufficient size and age to be otherwise expected to survive.

Stimulants   Drugs that affect the central nervous system and increase the heart rate, blood pressure, strength of heart contractions, blood glucose level, and overall muscle tension.

Stress   The response, be it physical, mental, or emotional, that a person displays when subjected to any type of stressor. Stressors can range from daily hassles to life-altering events, and they are experienced and perceived by people in very different ways.

Stress urinary incontinence   The involuntary release or leaking of small amounts of urine; usually associated with sudden exertion.

Stroke (cerebrovascular accident)   A condition in which blood vessel damage occurs in the brain.

Substance abuse   The overuse, misuse, and/or addiction to any chemical substance such as alcohol, tobacco, or drugs, including over-the-counter medications, prescription medications, and illicit drugs.

Sudden infant death syndrome (SIDS)   The diagnosis given for the sudden death of an infant younger than one year of age that remains unexplained after a complete investigation, which includes an autopsy, examination of the death scene, and review of the symptoms or illnesses the infant had prior to dying and any other pertinent medical history. Because most cases of SIDS occur when a baby is sleeping in a crib, SIDS is also called crib death.

Suffragist   An advocate of the right to vote and the ability to exercise that right.

Superior vena cava   The venous trunk draining blood from the head, neck, upper limbs, and thorax to the heart.

Surrogacy   A procedure for treating infertility in which a woman is artificially inseminated with the sperm of an infertile woman's partner. She then carries the pregnancy to term for the infertile couple.

Synovium   The cells lining the inside of the joint capsule which surround and protect the joint. The synovium is responsible for creating synovial fluid, which provides protective lubrication to the joint.

Syphilis   A sexually transmitted bacterial infection that causes small, painless sores in the genital area, a rash and flu-like symptoms, and after many years, systemic damage.

Systolic   First reading of blood pressure which represents the amount of pressure the blood exerts against the wall of the artery when the heart contracts.

T

Tamoxifen   An antiestrogen drug that is used as a treatment for breast cancer; may also inhibit breast tumor growth.

Target heart rate   A rate 60 to 90 percent of the maximum heart rate at which the maximum benefit is derived from exercise.

Tay-Sachs disease   A genetic disorder characterized by the inability to process fat, ultimately resulting in death. It occurs almost exclusively among Jews of Eastern European ancestry.

T-cell   A cell that governs the immune system and assists the B-lymphocyte in producing antibodies; T-cells are reduced in a person with AIDS.

Tendonitis   Inflammation caused by friction from overuse of tendons (connective tissues that attach muscle to bone).

Teratogenic   The characteristic of producing a permanent abnormality in structure or function, causing growth retardation, or causing death when an embryo or fetus is exposed to a certain substance, organism or physical agent.

Tertiary prevention   Prevention measures that take place once a disease has advanced. They may involve alleviating pain, providing comfort, halting progression of an illness, and limiting disability that may result from disease.

Testosterone   A male sex hormone that plays a role in the development of functionally mature sperm and is responsible for the development and maintenance of male secondary sexual characteristics such as the deepening of the voice and the growth of facial hair; also secreted in small amounts by women.

Tetrahydrocannabinol (THC)   The primary psychoactive ingredient in marijuana and hashish.

Third-party payer system   A payment system whereby an insurer (or third party) pays for services rendered to an individual by a provider of care.

Thrombocytes   Disk-shaped structures in the blood needed for blood coagulation. Also called platelets.

Thrombus   A blood clot that blocks an artery.

Thrush   A yeast infection that infects the mouth.

Thyroid disease   Disease of the thyroid gland, often occurring from excess production of thyroid hormones (hyperthyroidism) or decreased production of thyroid hormones (hypothyroidism).

Thyroiditis   An inflammation of the thyroid gland. Chronic thyroiditis frequently results in lowered thyroid function (hypothyroidism).

Title IX   The portion of the Education Amendments of 1972 that prohibits sex discrimination in educational institutions that receive any federal funds. If educational institutions are found to violate Title IX, their federal funding can be withdrawn.

Tolerance   The body's ability to withstand the effects of a drug. Continued use of a drug may result in increased tolerance and decreased responsiveness.

Total hysterectomy and bilateral salpingo-oophorectomy   Surgical removal of the uterus performed in conjunction with the removal of both ovaries and the fallopian tubes.

Toxemia   A complication of pregnancy characterized by high blood pressure, swelling caused by fluid retention, and high levels of protein in the urine. Also called preeclampsia.

Toxic shock syndrome (TSS)   A rare but serious infection caused by strains of the bacteria *Staphylococcus aureus* (*S. aureus*). For reasons not fully understood, these bacteria release toxins (poisons) into the bloodstream after deep wounds, surgery, or tampon use (especially high absorbency tampon use).

Toxoplasmosis   A disease that is caused by the parasite *Toxoplasma gondii*, which is associated with contaminated cat litter or soil containing cat feces. Infection by this parasite can cause problems with the fetus during pregnancy. It also can affect a person with a compromised immune system and is considered an opportunistic infection of HIV/AIDS.

Trafficking   In regard to women, the use of force and deception to transfer women into situations of extreme exploitation; the recruitment, transportation, transfer, harboring, or receipt of persons, by the threat or use of force or the abuse of power for the purpose of exploitation.

Trans fats   Fats that are formed when vegetable oils are processed into margarine or shortening. Trans fats are found in snack foods such as potato chips, commercial baked goods with "partially hydrogenated vegetable oil" or "vegetable shortening," many types of fast food (e.g., french fries and onion rings), stick margarine, and some dairy products. These fats are solid or semi-solid at room temperature and raise levels of LDL cholesterol.

Transdermal therapy   Treatment applied to the skin; the medicine or substance is absorbed through the skin and enters the bloodstream.

Transgender   Anyone whose behaviors, thoughts, or traits differ from those traditionally ascribed to the person's sex.

Transient ischemic attack (TIA)   An event in which an artery closes momentarily in a spasm and may result in a brief memory lapse or garbled speech.

Transitioning   The process in which transsexuals work to change their appearance and societal identity so as to match their gender identity.

Transsexual   A person who wishes to be considered by society as a member of the opposite sex; a person who has undergone a sex change.

Transvaginal ultrasound   A method of imaging the genital tract in women. The ultrasound machine sends out high-frequency sound waves, which bounce off body structures and thereby create a picture. With the transvaginal technique, the ultrasound transducer (a hand-held probe) is inserted directly into the vagina.

Transvestitism   The practice of adopting the clothes, manner, or sexual role of the opposite sex.

Trichomoniasis   A vaginal infection caused by *Trichomonas vaginalis*, a single cell protozoan parasite with a whip-like tail that it uses to propel itself through vaginal and urethral mucus.

Tricuspid valve   A heart valve that has three points or cusps and is situated between the right atrium and the right ventricle.

Triglycerides   Fatty substances found in the body's fatty tissues. High levels of triglycerides are associated with an elevated risk of heart disease.

Tumor   An abnormal mass of tissue that results from excessive cell division. It may be either benign or malignant.

U

Ultrasound A procedure that uses high-frequency sound waves to project an image of structures inside the body, such as an organ or a fetus during pregnancy.

Undernutrition Poor health resulting from the depletion of nutrients due to inadequate nutrient intake over time.

Underweight An individual who is below the acceptable average weight for his or her height or body type.

Universal health insurance A system by which the government provides health insurance to all citizens, thereby controlling health insurance at the federal level.

Unopposed estrogen Estrogen replacement therapy that is taken without the opposing effects of progestin.

Unsaturated fats Fats that come from plants and include most vegetable oils.

Urethra The tube through which urine passes from the bladder to outside the body. In men, semen also passes through the urethra.

Urethritis Inflammation of the urethra, often caused by infection in the bladder or kidneys.

Urinary incontinence The inability to control the flow of urine from the bladder.

Uterus A hollow, muscular organ located in the pelvic cavity of females in which the fertilized egg becomes implanted and develops. Also called the womb.

V

Vacuum curettage The most widely used abortion technique in the United States. In this procedure, the cervix is first dilated. A vacuum curette—an instrument consisting of a tube with a scoop attached for scraping away tissue—is then inserted through the cervix into the uterus. The other end of the tube is attached to a suction-producing apparatus, which aspirates the contents of the uterus into a collection vessel.

Vagina A moist canal in females extending from the labia minora to the uterus.

Vaginal atrophy A condition often associated with menopause that refers to the thinning of the vaginal lining.

Vaginismus A relatively rare form of sexual difficulty in which a woman experiences involuntary spasmodic contractions of the muscles of the outer third of the vagina.

Varicocele A mesh of varicose veins in and around the testicle, which is associated with infertility and may have to be treated with surgery.

Vasectomy A male sterilization method whereby one or two small incisions are made just through the skin of the scrotum. The vas deferens is lifted through the incision, and the two ends are tied or cauterized to seal them.

Vasocongestion The engorgement of blood vessels in particular body parts in response to sexual arousal.

Vasoconstrictor　A compound that results in closing down—narrowing—of blood vessels.

Veins　Blood vessels that carry blood from the capillaries toward the heart.

Ventricle　The right or left lower blood-pumping chamber of the heart.

Ventricular fibrillation　A disturbance in heart rhythm.

Venules　Small veins.

Very–low-density lipoprotein (VLDL)　A type of lipoprotein made up mostly of triglycerides. As with LDL, high levels of VLDL increase the risk of atherosclerosis.

Vestibular bulbs　Part of the vast network of bulbs and vessels that engorge with blood during sexual arousal. Vestibular bulbs cause the vagina to increase in length and the vulvar area to become swollen.

Vestibule　The area of the vulva inside of the labia minora.

Vestibulitis　A recurring inflammation and burning sensation around the vaginal opening.

Villi　Short vascular projections attaching the fetus to the uterine wall.

Viruses　Small pathogens incapable of independent metabolism; can only reproduce inside living cells.

Vitamin　An organic substance needed by the body in a very small amount. The various vitamins have many different functions in metabolism and nutrition.

Vulva　The external genital organs of the female, including the labia majora, labia minora, clitoris, and vestibule of the vagina.

Vulvitis　Inflammation of the vulva.

W

Water-soluble vitamins　Vitamins used up or excreted in urine and sweat; must be replaced daily.

Western Blot Test　Laboratory test used to detect antibodies; Western blots are performed after two positive ELISA tests to test for HIV.

White blood cells　Elements in circulating blood that protect the body against pathogenic microorganisms. Also called leukocytes.

Y

Yeast infection　A vaginal infection caused most commonly by the fungal organism, Candida albicans. Symptoms of yeast infections include abnormal vaginal discharge; vaginal and labial itching and burning; redness and inflammation of the vulvar skin; pain with intercourse; and painful urination.

Yo-yo dieting　The practice of losing weight and then regaining it, only to lose it and regain it again. This practice makes it more difficult to succeed in future attempts to lose weight because thyroid hormone levels may drop very low in subsequent dieting, thereby significantly slowing basal metabolism.

Z

Zygote intrafallopian transfer (ZIFT)   A method of assisted reproductive technology in which a fertilized egg is placed in the fallopian tube, allowing the zygote to continue its cell division and become implanted in the uterus naturally.

Zygote   A fertilized egg.

INDEX

PHOTO CREDITS